## DATE DUE

| SE 9 '96 | | | |
|---|---|---|---|
| OC 21 '96 | | | |
| DE 6 '96 | | | |
| RENEW | | | |
| NV 10 97 | | | |
| MY 12 98 | | | |
| NO 18 98 | | | |
| AG 6 01 | | | |
| AP 21 03 | | | |
| | | | |
| | | | |
| | | | |
| | | | |
| | | | |
| | | | |

DEMCO 38-296

The Foot and Ankle in Sport

# THE FOOT AND ANKLE IN SPORT

**DONALD E. BAXTER, M.D.**
Clinical Professor
Department of Orthopedic Surgery
Baylor College of Medicine
and University of Texas
Health Science Center
Houston, Texas

*with 492 illustrations*

**M Mosby**

St. Louis  Baltimore  Berlin  Boston  Carlsbad  Chicago  London  Madrid
Naples  New York  Philadelphia  Sydney  Tokyo  Toronto

*Publisher:* Anne S. Patterson
*Editor:* Robert Hurley
*Developmental Editor:* Lauranne Billus
*Project Manager:* Linda Clarke
*Production Editor:* Allan S. Kleinberg
*Designer:* Nancy McDonald
*Manufacturing Supervisor:* Kathy Grone
*Cover Art:* Narda Lebo

FIRST EDITION

**Copyright © 1995 Mosby–Year Book, Inc.**

Printed in the United States of America
Composition by Graphic World, Inc.
Printing/binding by Walsworth

Mosby–Year Book, Inc.
11830 Westline Industrial Drive
St. Louis, MO 63146

**Library of Congress Cataloging in Publication Data**

Baxter, Donald E.
    The foot and ankle in sport/Donald E. Baxter. — 1st ed.
      p.   cm.
    Includes bibliographical references and index.
    ISBN 0-8016-6890-5
    1. Foot — Wounds and injuries.  2. Ankle — Wounds and injuries.  3. Sports injuries.  4. Foot — Abnormalities.  5. Ankle — Abnormalities.  I. Title.
  RD563.B39   1994
  617.5′85044 — dc20                94-34668
                                       CIP

95  96  97  98  99  /  9  8  7  6  5  4  3  2  1

# Contributors

**Champ L. Baker, Jr., M.D.**
President and Staff Physician
The Hughston Clinic, P.C.
Columbus, Georgia

**Donald E. Baxter, M.D.**
Clinical Professor, Department of Orthopaedic
    Surgery
Baylor College of Medicine and University of Texas
    Health Science Center
Houston, Texas

**Roy S. Benedetti, M.D.**
Chief, Foot and Ankle Service
Kaiser Permanente Medical Center
Anaheim, California

**James L. Beskin, M.D.**
Assistant Clinical Professor of Orthopaedics
Tulane University School of Medicine
New Orleans, Louisiana;
Peachtree Orthopaedic Clinic
Atlanta, Georgia

**R. Luke Bordelon, M.D.**
Opelousas, Louisiana

**Brian T. Chimenti, M.D.**
University of Colorado Health Science Center
Denver, Colorado

**Michael R. Clain, M.D.**
Clinical Instructor of Orthopaedics and
    Rehabilitation
Yale University
New Haven, Connecticut;
Greenwich Hospital
Greenwich, Connecticut

**Thomas O. Clanton, M.D.**
Clinical Associate Professor
University of Texas Medical School at Houston
Associate Team Physician
Rice University
Chief, Foot Service
Hermann Hospital
Houston, Texas

**Michael J. Coughlin, M.D.**
Associate Professor of Surgery, Division of
    Orthopaedics
Oregon Health Sciences University
Portland, Oregon;
Private Practice in Orthopaedic Surgery
Boise, Idaho

**Pamela F. Davis, M.D.**
Orthopaedic Surgeon
Trinity Medical Center
Moline, Illinois;
Illini Hospital
Silvis, Illinois

**J. Melvin Deese, Jr., M.D.**
Southeast Georgia Regional Medical Center
Brunswick, Georgia

**Jesse C. DeLee, M.D.**
Associate Professor
Department of Orthopaedics
University of Texas Health Science Center
San Antonio, Texas

**Carol Frey, M.D.**
Associate Clinical Professor of Orthopaedic Surgery
University of Southern California
Director
Orthopaedic Foot and Ankle Center
Los Angeles, California

**William G. Hamilton, M.D.**
Assistant Clinical Professor of Orthopaedic Surgery
Columbia University College of Physicians and
 Surgeons
Senior Attending Orthopaedic Surgeon
St. Luke's-Roosevelt Hospital Center
New York, New York

**Marion C. Harper, M.D.**
Clinical Professor
Vanderbilt University School of Medicine
Centennial Medical Center
Nashville, Tennessee

**Stan L. James, M.D.**
Courtesy Professor
Department of Exercise and Movement Science
University of Oregon
Orthopaedic Staff
Sacred Heart General Hospital
Eugene, Oregon

**Kenneth A. Johnson†**

**Donald C. Jones, M.D.**
Clinical Instructor
University of Oregon Health Science Center
Orthopaedic Consultant
University of Oregon Athletic Department
Sacred Heart Hospital
Eugene, Oregon

**James S. Lillich, M.D.**
Clinical Instructor, Foot and Ankle Service
Louisiana State University Medical
 Center-Shreveport
Willis Knighton Medical Center
Shreveport, Louisiana

**Lowell Dean Lutter, M.D.**
Clinical Associate Professor of Orthopaedic Surgery
University of Minnesota
Director, Health East-Minnesota Orthopaedic Foot
 and Ankle Center
Midway Hospital
St. Paul, Minnesota

**Roger A. Mann, M.D.**
Director, Foot Fellowship Program
San Leandro, California

**Angus M. McBryde, Jr., M.D.**
Professor and Chairman, Department of
 Orthopaedic Surgery
Director, Sports Medicine Service
University of South Alabama College of Medicine
Mobile, Alabama

**Laura A. Mitchell, M.D.**
New Mexico Orthopaedic Associates
Presbyterian Healthcare Systems
Albuquerque, New Mexico

**J. Bruce Moseley, Jr., M.D.**
Assistant Professor, Department of Orthopaedic
 Surgery
Baylor College of Medicine
Chief, Orthopaedic Service
Houston Veterans Affairs Medical Center
Team Physician, Houston Rockets
Methodist Hospital
St. Luke's Episcopal Hospital
Houston, Texas

**Glenn B. Pfeffer, M.D.**
Assistant Clinical Professor, Department of
 Orthopaedics
Chief, Orthopaedic Foot and Ankle Clinic
University of California School of Medicine
Chief, Orthopaedic Foot and Ankle Surgery
California Pacific Medical Center, Pacific Campus
San Francisco, California

**Ronald Quirk, F.R.C.S., F.R.A.C.S.**
Consultant
Australian Institute of Sport
Private Orthopaedic Practitioner
Melbourne, Australia

**G. James Sammarco, M.D., F.A.C.S.**
Volunteer Professor of Orthopaedics
University of Cincinnati Medical Center
The Christ Hospital
Cincinnati, Ohio

**Lew C. Schon, M.D.**
Attending Orthopaedic Surgeon, Department of
 Orthopaedics
Director, Dance Medicine Program
Foot and Ankle Center
Union Memorial Hospital
Baltimore, Maryland

**Saul G. Trevino, M.D.**
Associate Professor of Clinical Orthopaedic Surgery
Baylor College of Medicine
Chief of Foot and Ankle Service
Veterans Affairs Medical Center
The Methodist Hospital
Houston, Texas

†Deceased.

*To my wife, Frances, for her patience and understanding*

# Foreword

The study of sports medicine presents the clinician with a unique opportunity to test his diagnostic skills. This is because many of the problems observed in the athlete, particularly the elite athlete, are due to subtle biomechanical alterations that are often not a problem for the less athletic individual. The problem is even more magnified in the foot and ankle due to the increased stress and often repetitive nature of the stress on the lower extremities. A mild forefoot varus that is usually inconsequential in most people may be a problem for someone training 80 to 90 miles per week or a minor ankle impingement creating a disabling injury for a ballerina.

In *The Foot and Ankle in Sport* Dr. Donald E. Baxter has approached these problems in five sections. First, the reader is exposed to Athletic Evaluation through the eyes of Dr. Baxter, who has had years of experience in evaluating the subtle and not so subtle medical findings of elite athletes. In this chapter he shares with us many of the ways to detect minor changes that may be affecting the elite athlete. Next, the reader is presented with Sport Syndromes, which delves into the various neurologic, tendinous, and impingement syndromes. This section also discusses the various types of fractures and dislocations as well as the ever perplexing dermatological conditions of the foot. The third section of the book looks at Anatomic Disorders in which specific anatomic regions, such as the ankle, subtalar, and first metatarsophalangeal joint, are examined in detail in order to point out specific clinical entities in each area. Unique Problems associated with specific athletic endeavors, such as ballet, running, and the sports of elite athletes, are evaluated in the fourth section. This section correlates the previously presented material as it applies to a specific athletic event, giving the reader further insight into athletic needs. The book closes with a discussion of Shoe Wear and Orthotic Devices. This extremely important section discusses the detailed management of the athlete, particularly since shoe wear has become so event oriented. The concluding chapter discusses Physical Therapy and Rehabilitation, both of which play an important role in bringing the athlete and nonathlete back to full physical strength.

After reading through this book, I am sure everyone, whether family practitioner, orthopaedic resident, or practicing orthopaedist, will find their knowledge regarding the foot and ankle in sport greatly enhanced.

**Roger A. Mann, M.D.**

# Preface

The foot and ankle in sport includes a myriad of pathological processes and treatments. The foot and ankle undergoes hundreds of biomechanical forces with body weight, gravity, surfaces, and shoes being contending forces.

The foot and ankle must function perfectly in the athlete to allow optimal running, jumping, turning, and balance. The basketball player is a good example. The foot and ankle must allow quick starts, stops, acceleration, leaping, and proprioception in landing. The lateral ligaments of the ankle and subtalar joints as well as the Achilles tendon must withstand pressures far beyond sedentary activity.

Tennis, racquetball and squash players are at risk to rupture tendons; football players may get turf toe, ankle diastasis, Lisfranc's injury of the midfoot, or countless traumatic insults.

We could go on and on but you the reader will probably want to read the parts of this book that apply to your athletic patients and then use the book in your office, training room, or therapy clinic as a reference.

Many physicians, coaches, friends, and athletes have made this book possible. First, I must thank the contributing authors. These authors are leading experts in their fields; some are former foot and ankle fellows at the University of Texas Medical School in Houston or the Baylor College of Medicine in Houston, Texas. They are all friends and I appreciate their time and effort. I am deeply sad that Ken Johnson was tragically killed in a plane crash shortly after sending me his chapter on posterior tibial tendon problems. He wrote me a nice letter with the chapter in support of the book and my effort. I miss Ken as do all of us in the American Orthopaedic Foot and Ankle Society.

I am grateful to my former teachers, especially Roger Mann, for setting me off on the foot and ankle journey 20 years ago after I trained with him in Oakland, California. Also my gratitude to the teams, clubs, companies, coaches, athletes, and dancers who stimulated this book. These include Coach Jim McLatchie and the Houston Harriers Running Club, Coach Tom Tellez and the University of Houston Track Team, the Santa Monica Running Club, and Artistic Director Ben Stevens and the Houston Ballet.

I am grateful to my office staff who rounded up and helped to edit and type the various chapters. These include Nancy Metcalf, Michele Bryne, Carol Ann Tomlinson, and also Christopher Zinga, Foot and Ankle Fellow, Baylor College of Medicine.

Finally, a most important thanks goes to Tamara Miller for her beautiful art and medical illustrations. Her art has made the book easier to understand and more pleasant to read.

**Donald E. Baxter**
February 1994

# Contents

# Athletic Evaluation

# Chapter 1

# Athletic evaluation

**Donald E. Baxter**

Athletes commonly have problems with their feet and ankles. Usually the problems are only transient and respond to self-treatment, rest, or treatment by trainers.

If the problem persists, a careful history, functional physical examination, and appropriate diagnostic study must be performed.

## HISTORY

Forms may be used in taking a history to allow the athlete to make an outline of complaints while seated in the waiting room.

A chief complaint should be listed, and if there are secondary problems, these should also be listed. The most severe problems should be listed first with the duration and nature of the onset of the symptoms. Lesser problems should then be listed in order of their significance.

Other problems to discuss include the following:

1. Does the pain occur during activity or after the activity?
2. What previous treatment has the patient undergone?
3. What is the nature of the patient's training program? Is the patient a beginner, a recreational, noncompetitive athlete, or a competitive athlete? Has there been a recent increase in training? Has there been an increase in speed associated with the workouts?
4. Has there been a recent change in shoe wear? Are the shoes rotated between two or three types to avoid similar stresses? Does the patient note a specific abnormal-wear pattern?
5. Does the athlete use orthotic devices? Are the devices rigid or flexible? What symptoms were changed by their use?
6. Is the training surface hard or soft, circular or slanted?
7. Are there any related exercises used such as stretching or strengthening? Is there a systematic stretching or yoga program? Are weights used to build up strength in a balanced manner?
8. Are supplemental vitamins or minerals used? Does the athlete get adequate nutrition for his activities?

## PHYSICAL EXAMINATION

The physical examination must encompass the entire lower extremity and back. Not only should the examination be carried out with the patient sitting, but also in a prone or supine position and in a functional manner as well.

### Standing

With the patient standing, the back is observed for evidence of scoliosis, which results in malalignment of the spine. An increase in lumbar lordosis associated with weakened abdominal muscles should be observed. The level of the iliac wings gives a good idea as to leg length. The patient is asked to touch the floor with his hands to provide the examiner some idea as to the flexibility of the hamstrings and Achilles tendons. Overall alignment of the knees is important to determine abnormalities involving the patella as well as whether genu varum or valgum is present. Next the overall alignment of the foot is examined to determine if the feet have normal rotation. Is there an external rotational component to the lower leg? Is the heel in proper alignment, or does the athlete have excessive heel varus or valgus? Is there a pronated position to the foot, or is there a cavus deformity? The patient is asked to stand on the ball of the feet for observation of appropriate subtalar function and posterior tibial strength. Next the patient is asked to walk to determine if there is any evidence of femoral anteversion or femoral retroversion.

### Sitting

With the patient sitting, the leg lengths are again observed by having the runner place his back flat against the wall or chair back and extend the knees. By examining the patient in this manner, the possibility of pelvic obliquity is eliminated. While the leg lengths are noted, the tightness of the hamstrings and the sciatic nerve is tested. Next the patient's knee is examined and the patella is palpated while the knee is actively extended for observation of possible chondromalacia. The degree of malleolar torsion is noted as to symmetry. The ankle joint is examined for dorsiflexion and plantar flexion. The hindfoot is placed in a neutral position and the alignment of the forefoot is observed to determine if there is a neutral varus or valgus position. The pattern of callus formation on the plantar aspect of the foot is observed. The toes are carefully examined for any fixed or dynamic contractures.

### Supine

With the patient supine, the range of motion of the hips and knees is checked. The sciatic nerve can once again be evaluated while the athlete is supine.

### Prone

The examination of the patient in the prone position is important for evaluation of the Achilles tendon area. With the knee flexed to 90°, the heel-leg alignment is observed along with the configuration of the longitudinal arch. The Achilles tendon can also be palpated.

### Functional examination

If the exact cause of the problem is not clearly indicated or the problem is not clearly determined from the history and physical examination in the office, the athlete is observed while running or jumping at the track or gymnasium. This often gives some additional information which may expose a problem that occurs only after extreme exertion. For example, occasionally a track runner has symptoms in the foot only on the second or third lap of a mile race. Thus having the athlete run on a track will stimulate the problem and allow the examiner to observe the problem while it is symptomatic.

### DIAGNOSTIC STUDIES

To complete the patient's workup, one or more diagnostic studies may be indicated. The initial study

begins with routine radiographic films of the involved area. Disorders such as osteoarthritis, infection, osteochondritis, and tendon and ligament avulsions as well as the presence of extra ossicles can be diagnosed. A stress fracture, if over 3 to 4 weeks in duration, may be discovered by callus formation or by periosteal reaction. Weight-bearing views can provide information about foot alignment. In cases with suspected ligamentous instability of the ankle or Lisfranc's joint, stress views can be helpful. This is especially true when a Lisfranc-type injury is suspected and plain films reveal no abnormalities. Subtalar stress views are less predictable, and subtalar instability may need to be determined by excluding other diagnoses.

When symptoms are vague and the physical findings are difficult to interpret, a bone scan may be indicated. The bone scan is extremely helpful in the early diagnosis of stress fractures where plain x-rays are normal. A computed tomographic (CT) scan can assist in the evaluation of osteoarthritis in the ankle and subtalar joint as well as the smaller joints of the midfoot. Osteochondral lesions of the talus are well visualized with the CT scan, which can be instrumental in preoperative planning.

Magnetic resonance imaging (MRI) is becoming increasingly useful in the evaluation of foot and ankle disorders. MRI provides excellent contrast between bone marrow, tendons, cartilage, ligaments, muscles, and bone allowing clearer visualization of these structures. Tendon ruptures and areas of degenerative changes within tendons can be visualized. MRIs also allow assessment of articular cartilage and the presence of soft tissue masses. Ligament injuries of the foot and ankle can sometimes be confirmed by MRI.

### PRIMARY AND SECONDARY INJURIES

In assessing athletic injuries of the foot and ankle, it is important to determine which is the primary problem and what secondary problem the primary problem has caused. Often if one leg is injured, the opposite leg will develop an injury by overcompensating for the weaker leg. For instance, if a muscle is pulled in one leg, a stress fracture may occur in the opposite leg. If hyperpronation of the foot is present, patellar subluxation may occur secondarily.

There are numerous problems which develop in athletes. The physician should analyze the problems carefully and during the examination always ask whether the problem presented is primary or secondary.

Often the etiology of athletic injuries can be traced to a change or faults in the training schedule, the shoe type, or the running surface. Running diaries can be maintained to record how much training was done, the shoes that were worn, and the surface that was run on. Rapid weight changes also may result in musculoskeletal injury resulting from a nutritional deficiency. Not all biomechanical imbalances need to be corrected. Leg length inequalities that have never been treated and have not caused secondary problems may not need treatment. Mild pronational deformity that causes minimal problems may not require treatment.

## SURFACE INJURIES

Synthetic surfaces, which have replaced cinders and grass over the past 30 years, have increased the number of athletic records. However, these synthetic surfaces are also causing injuries as technically aided performances push the body toward and beyond the breaking point. Synthetic carpets are faster, longer lasting, and weatherproof, but it appears that muscles and bones are suffering from their use. Eliminating the skid phase of running seen with imperfect surfaces such as grass or cinders results in a more powerful push-off and more efficient running but more stressful forces in the joints as well. Synthetic surfaces cause shock vibrations to an extent not known on grass or cinders. This causes jarring, which can lead to damage to the ankle, foot, or lower leg. Shoe manufacturers are attempting to develop shoes that will cushion heel strike and lessen shear forces. This shoe design may eliminate some of the excessive torquing forces that occur when running on synthetic surfaces. When possible, athletes should train on a variety of surfaces, allowing the foot more padding and more skid.

## TORSIONAL JOINT INJURIES

Athletes should be encouraged not only to do linear stretching but also rotational stretching. If there is limited hip, pelvic, or back rotation, more torque is placed on the knee, leg, and ankle during running or jumping. For example, if there is an external rotation deformity of the hip, more torque is placed on the knee during running as the speed is increased and the lower extremity attempts to rotate inwardly. By doing internal rotational stretching of the hip, and having the runner or the athlete run with legs and feet slightly externally rotated, knee pain may be eliminated. Other rotational deformities can cause similar torquing problems. Congenital femoral retroversion and external tibial torsion often cause knee pain in running as the runner attempts to rotate the leg internally during the normal swing phase in foot plant. Rarely does femoral anteversion or internal tibial torsion cause problems, since these are more anatomic positions for running.

## SHORT-LEG SYNDROME

When a runner is evaluated, care should be taken to examine leg length. If there is a leg length inequality, there is often a history of repeat injuries to the short-leg. These may include stress fractures, medial knee strain from genu valgus, hyperpronation with resultant plantar fasciitis, or patellar subluxation. Iliotibial band tendinitis or lateral knee joint impingement may develop. A short-leg develops from a congenitally short tibia or femur or a fixed pelvic obliquity from scoliosis. Functional short-leg syndrome occurs by running on the same tilt of the road or in the same direction on a circular track. It can also occur from a flexion contracture in the knee or the ankle. If a short-leg is present, it is corrected by adding a lift to the interlining of the shoe. The insole of the running shoe is built-up gradually in one-eighth to one-fourth inch increments. The inside of the running shoe can be elevated approximately one-half inch if necessary. Should more elevation be needed, it must be made to the midsole of the shoe.

Occasionally problems develop in the long-leg. These problems include lateral hip pain, as the iliotibial band rubs over the greater trochanter of the longer leg. Iliotibial band problems also may develop on the lateral aspect of the knee in the longer leg. By placing a lift in the shoe of the shorter leg, the iliotibial band problem may be lessened.

## CONCLUSION

Once an overall evaluation is completed, a treatment plan is prescribed and a determination is made as to whether the athlete should discontinue the sport or may continue and simply alter the training regimen. Often the treatment plan, as well as the determination whether to play or not, is more complicated and difficult than actually determining the diagnosis.

# Sport Syndromes

# Chapter 2

# Functional nerve disorders

**Donald E. Baxter**

Some foot, ankle, and leg injuries in athletes are obvious, such as fractures, dislocations, and severe ligament injuries, while others are transient or occur only during athletic effort. These problems include impingements, synovitis, and nerve entrapments. Nerve problems of the foot, ankle, and leg include interdigital nerve compression, various entrapments of the posterior tibial nerve and its branches, entrapments of the superficial and deep peroneal nerves, as well as entrapments of the sural nerve.

Nerves are compressed by bony impingements, compartment syndromes, or as a secondary phenomenon to joint instability. Occasionally a double crush syndrome will confuse the examiner with the nerves of the lower extremity being compressed at two locations.

Many nerve problems are functional, which means that the nerve is compressed during functional activity of the athlete. For that reason, it is highly important to obtain a careful history as well as a static and functional physical examination. Standard tests do not always show the abnormality. Nerve conduction delays may occur only during a treadmill examination. Many of these problems will correct with changes in the activity, shoe changes, orthoses, or ankle braces.

## INTERDIGITAL NERVE

As the foot plantar flexes and the toes dorsiflex during push-off, the interdigital nerves between the second and third, and third and fourth metatarsals (Fig. 2-1/Plate 1) may be compressed by the intermetatarsal ligament. This causes neuritic radiation of pain into the affected web space and toes. Often the pain radiates proximally as well. With forefoot pain, it is important to make sure there is no proximal lesion,

such as a disk herniation causing radicular pains down the extremity into the foot. If such a lesion exists, there will be more proximal tenderness to the nerve, and nerves in all interspaces of the forefoot will be hypersensitive. It is also important to look for metabolic problems as a cause for diffuse neuralgias. On physical examination, the palpation should be carried out between the metatarsal heads as well as the metatarsals themselves. Stress fractures present as tender metatarsals. Capsulitis is another painful malady as well as subluxation of the metatarsophalangeal joint.

For ballet dancers and basketball players with interdigital syndromes, the dancer or the athlete should first use a wider shoe. A metatarsal pad changes the relative position of the metatarsals, as does an arch support. By preventing excessive pronation, pressure is alleviated from the third, fourth, and fifth metatarsal heads. A three-sixteenth to one-quarter-inch metatarsal pad placed proximal to the heads lifts the second, third, and fourth metatarsal heads, thus changing the mechanics of the foot.

Cortisone injections should be avoided in athletes who have interdigital neuromas. This causes fat atrophy and degeneration of the volar plate or collateral ligaments. With degeneration of the collateral ligament or volar plate, toes may develop angular deformities at the metatarsophalangeal joint.

If pain persists despite conservative treatment, the nerve is excised. If possible, with an athlete, the intermetatarsal ligament is left intact, allowing more rapid recovery and preventing instability of the metatarsals. If the neuroma, however, extends under the metatarsal ligament, it may be necessary to cut the metatarsal ligament to avoid recurrence of pain and a stump neuroma. When the nerve is excised, the nerve

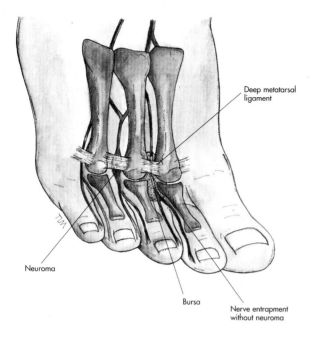

Neuroma

Deep metatarsal ligament

Bursa

Nerve entrapment without neuroma

**Fig. 2-1.** Interdigital neuroma.

is first cut proximally and then distally. This prevents retraction of the nerve after the initial incision of the nerve.

If a typical neuroma is present in an athlete and surgery is considered, the following procedure may be used:

1. An incision is made on the dorsum of the foot.
2. The nerve is identified in the affected interspace just distal to the intermetatarsal ligament. This is done with blunt dissection.
3. A portion of the intermetatarsal ligament is released.
4. The nerve is grasped with a hemostat and pulled distally.
5. The affected nerve is cut proximally underneath the intermetatarsal ligament back, well proximal to the enlarged portion of the nerve.
6. The nerve is then cut distally and the nerve is removed.
7. The wound is closed in an anatomic fashion and a compressive dressing is applied.

Occasionally two nerves are involved. Even though this is extremely rare, it does occur (see Case Study 1). By avoiding the dorsal cutaneous nerves to the middle toe when two nerves are removed, the middle toe loses sensation only to the plantar aspect and thus maintains protective sensation to the dorsum of the toes.

**Case Study 1.** This international middle-distance runner had a bunion, which caused an incompetent first metatarsal and thus shifted the weight to the lateral metatarsals. Over the ensuing 3 years, pain developed in the second and third

interspaces of the forefoot. Using one incision between the third and fourth metatarsal heads, a large neuroma was identified and excised. By carefully retracting the skin, the second and third interspace could be exposed through the same incision. Care was taken to avoid damaging the dorsal cutaneous nerves. Inspection of the second and third interspace revealed a large neuroma as well. This nerve was also removed proximal to the metatarsal ligament.

After surgery, when the athlete returns to athletic activity, the forefoot should be strapped with circumferential adhesive tape, which adds comfort during athletic activity. Taping should be maintained for 4 weeks or as needed. An arch support and metatarsal pad should be continued until all symptoms have subsided.

## DISORDERS OF THE TIBIAL NERVE AND ITS BRANCHES
### Tarsal tunnel syndrome

The tarsal tunnel is a fiberosseous tunnel formed by the flexor retinaculum or laciniate ligament, the medial wall of the calcaneus, the posterior portion of the talus, the distal tibia, and the medial malleolus. The structures within the canal include the posterior tibial nerve and its branches, the tendons of the posterior tibialis, the flexor digitorum longus, the flexor hallucis, and the posterior tibial artery and vein. Although there is considerable variability, the posterior tibial nerve usually divides from 0 to 2 cm proximal to an imaginary line drawn from the tip of the medial malleolus to the calcaneal tuberosity. Approximately 1 to 2 cm distal to this line, the lateral plantar nerve and the medial plantar nerve enter two tunnels within the abductor hallucis muscle. These canals are divided by a fibroseptum and are approximately 2 cm long.[8] The calcaneal nerve is the most posterior branch of the posterior tibial nerve and may pierce the laciniate ligament or may exit between it and the fascia of the abductor hallucis muscle.

The posterior tibial nerve may be compressed at several locations (Fig. 2-2/Plate 2). A high tarsal tunnel syndrome exists when compression of the posterior tibial nerve occurs at the lower edge of the gastrocnemius muscle in the middle aspect of the posteromedial tibia. The traditional tarsal tunnel occurs behind the medial malleolus under the retinacular ligament. Other more distal tarsal tunnel syndromes can occur affecting the various branches of the posterior tibial nerve.

## PROXIMAL POSTERIOR TIBIAL NERVE
### High tarsal tunnel syndrome

In evaluating tarsal tunnel syndromes or pain along the distribution of the posterior tibial nerve, nerve studies are important. Electromyelograms and nerve

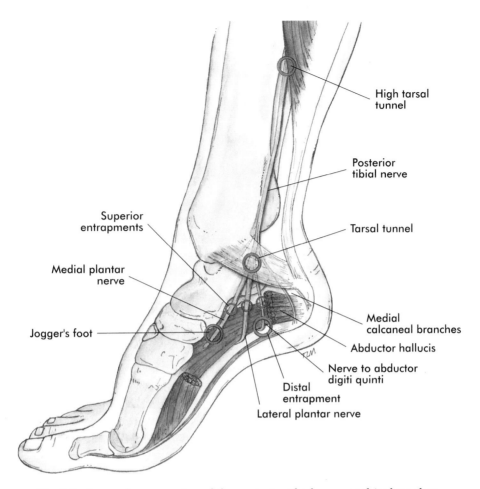

**Fig. 2-2.** Areas of compression of the posterior tibial nerve and its branches.

conduction studies are indicated. These studies are not always positive, especially if the nerve compression is present only during the activity. If the study is positive, however, a more confident diagnosis is made.

For athletes with a high tarsal tunnel syndrome and compressive neuropathy, which occurs in the lower leg, attempts should be made to rest the extremity so that the nerve irritation subsides. This can be done by immobilizing the foot and leg in a cast-brace or a splint, by doing physical therapy to the leg to decrease inflammation, and possibly by using a longitudinal arch support to invert the foot. Flexibility exercises also should be used to stretch structures about the ankle and leg.

If surgery is performed, it is often the inclination of the surgeon to release the entire nerve along the distal course of the posterior tibial nerve. Since the athlete often has pain distal to the site of compression, there is pain from the site of compression distally into the ankle and into the hindfoot and forefoot. The surgeon should release the nerve at its most proximal site of compression, avoiding unnecessary nerve dissection

distally. By avoiding excessive release, morbidity is lessened and recovery is more rapid.

If surgery is performed for a high tarsal tunnel syndrome, it is important to determine the exact location of the compression in the lower leg by careful physical examination along with electrodiagnostic studies. If surgery is performed, the following procedure is used:

1. Make a small incision over the area of compression.
2. Go down to the tight fascial structures in the area of compression and release just the area of tight compression over the neurovascular structure. This often necessitates releasing the fascia about the lower gastroc at its attachment to the posterior tibia.
3. Once this area of compression has been released, it is not necessary to identify the neurovascular structures nor is it necessary to release the nerve more distally unless compression is thought to exist in a more distal area.
4. Once the surgery is completed, the wound is

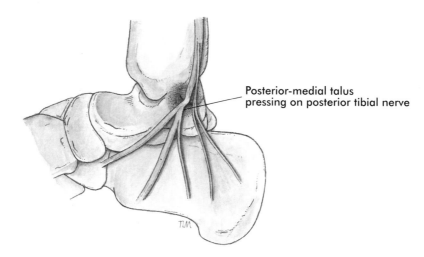

Posterior-medial talus
pressing on posterior tibial nerve

**Fig. 2-3.** Compression by the talus on the posterior tibial nerve.

irrigated and the skin and subcutaneous tissues are closed with an interrupted vertical mattress suture.

Postoperatively the athlete is maintained on crutches for several days and then gradually resumes weight bearing. If the dissection has not been extensive, the patient can resume athletic activities as early as 3 weeks postoperatively. If the dissection has been extensive, non–weight bearing and conservative treatment will be more prolonged.

## POSTERIOR TIBIAL NERVE
### Tarsal tunnel syndrome

The traditional tarsal tunnel syndrome occurs behind the medial malleolus under the retinacular ligament (Fig. 2-2/Plate 2). The compression may occur from a posterior bony prominence of the talus (Fig. 2-3/Plate 3). With a hypermobile subtalar joint, the posterior tibial nerve is stretched by a prominence of the posteromedial talus. If an os trigonum is present, it may rotate medially and press on the flexor hallucis longus tendon and posterior tibial nerve. Tarsal tunnel syndromes also result from ganglionic cysts.

For an athlete with tarsal tunnel syndrome, conservative treatment consists of using a longitudinal arch support or a medial sole and heel wedge within the athletic shoe. Stretching exercises of the posterior tibial muscle should be done, as well as the gastrocsoleus muscle. Edema should be eliminated with antiinflammatory medications, elevation, or support stockings. If necessary, a short-leg walking cast can be applied until symptoms subside.

In performing tarsal tunnel surgery, care is taken to only release the retinaculum. The fat is not stripped away from the nerve, thus avoiding excessive scarring. The area of compression is located, and the incision planned before surgery so that minimal dissection is needed. It is important to decide preoperatively the length of the incision and the location of the release. The incision's location is changed only with an unexpected finding. Often the nerve is not seen but only the yellowish perineural fat. Since veins and arteries follow the course of the nerves, they can be used as landmarks as well.

When surgery is performed for a tarsal tunnel syndrome, the following procedure is used:

1. An incision is made in the area of compression, usually behind the medial malleolus.
2. The incision is carried down, exposing the retinacular ligament, and if the area of compression occurs in the area of the retinacular ligament, this retinacular ligament is incised. Care is taken to avoid exposing the nerve, and once the fatty tissue around the nerve is identified, dissection is stopped.
3. It is important to make sure the superior edge of the abductor hallucis muscle is released. This tight fascial structure around the abductor hallucis muscle often is the source of compression in tarsal tunnel syndrome.
4. Once the posterior tibial nerve has been released, as well as the branches extending underneath the abductor hallucis muscle, dissection is stopped.
5. The wound is irrigated and closed with interrupted sutures in the skin and subcutaneous tissues.

Other causes of nerve stretching or nerve compression are edema or an unstable joint. If the nerve is chronically compressed medially because of an unstable lateral ankle joint, the lateral ligaments should be repaired in addition to releasing the affected medial nerve. If edema is present, the leg should be elevated

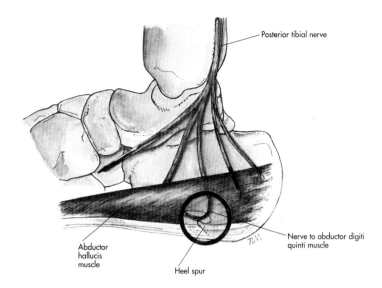

Posterior tibial nerve

Nerve to abductor digiti quinti muscle

Abductor hallucis muscle

Heel spur

**Fig. 2-4.** Compression of the first branch of the lateral plantar nerve.

appropriately and compressive wrap should be used to see if the problem can be corrected without surgery.

Postoperatively the athlete is maintained on crutches until all of the initial trauma of surgery subsides. If the dissection has been minimal, the athlete can begin resuming weight bearing as early as 1 week. If the dissection has been extensive, non–weight bearing is extended until it is safe to allow weight bearing, thus avoiding separation of the incisional site. Appropriate compressive dressings are applied until all edema subsides. If the athlete is extremely active, it may be necessary to consider cast immobilization during the initial 2 weeks of recovery.

## BRANCHES OF THE POSTERIOR TIBIAL NERVE
### Distal tarsal tunnel syndrome

Distal tarsal tunnel syndromes occur in several areas (Fig. 2-2/Plate 2). The first branch of the lateral plantar nerve can be compressed at the superior abductor hallucis longus muscle or at the location of the inferior abductor hallucis longus muscle where it joins the plantar fascia (Fig. 2-4/Plate 4).

According to several recent anatomic and clinical studies, entrapment of the first branch of the lateral plantar nerve occurs between the deep fascia of the abductor hallucis longus and the medial caudal margin of the quadratus plantae muscle.[19] Athletes with hypermobile pronated feet may be particularly susceptible to chronic stretching of the nerve. Hypertrophy of the abductor hallucis muscle or the quadratus plantae muscle may also explain the occurrence of this condition.[2,3,5]

Athletes who suffer from entrapment of the first branch of the lateral plantar nerve complain of chronic heel pain. Often the pain is increased by

running and can even occur when the athlete runs on the ball of the foot. Pain radiates to the medial inferior aspect of the heel and proximally into the medial ankle region of the foot. The pain may even radiate across the plantar aspect of the heel to the lateral aspect of the foot. Often the pain is worse in the morning when there is engorgement of the venous plexus veins adding to the compression. Unless there is more proximal entrapment of the nerve, patients usually do not complain of numbness in the heel or the foot. The average duration of symptoms was 22 months in the Baxter and Pheffer series.[3] Athletes frequently give a history of having tried stretching programs, heel cups, nonsteroidal antiinflammatory medications, and injections.

The physical examination must be performed with thorough knowledge of the anatomy of this region. More proximal and distal nerve entrapments must be excluded by palpation along the entire course of the posterior tibial nerve and its branches. The pathognomonic findings in these patients include tenderness over the first branch of the lateral plantar nerve deep to the abductor hallucis muscle. Pressure on the point of compression reproduces the symptoms and radiation of pain proximally and distally.

Extended conservative care should be offered to the athlete with entrapment of the first branch of the lateral plantar nerve. Often, with conservative care and rest, the nerve compression subsides. Other conservative treatments include heel pads or longitudinal arch supports, ice treatment, or local friction massage.

If all conservative treatment fails and surgery is considered, the following procedure is performed (Figs. 2-5 and 2-6/Plates 5 and 6):

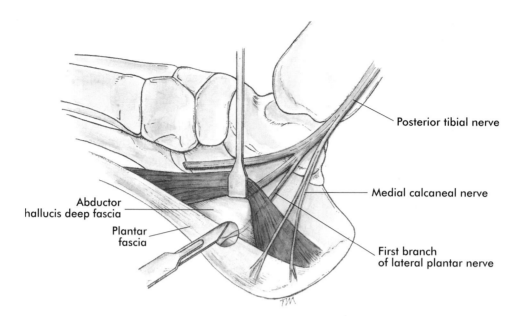

**Fig. 2-5.** Hourglass affect of nerve as it goes over quadratus plantae muscle. Deep fascia of the abductor muscle being windowed.

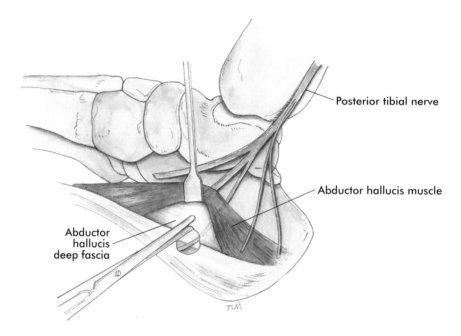

**Fig. 2-6.** Deep fascia of abductor hallucis being divided from inferior to superior.

1. An oblique incision is made on the medial aspect of the heel. This incision is obliquely placed just distal to the calcaneal sensory nerve and directly over the first branch of the lateral plantar nerve.
2. The incision is carried down through the skin and subcutaneous tissues, exposing the origin of the abductor hallucis muscle.
3. The superficial fascia of the abductor muscle is incised and the abductor muscle is retracted superiorly.

4. This exposes the deep fascia of the abductor hallucis muscle and the plantar fascia.
5. A rectangular wedge is removed, removing the medial one third of the plantar fascia and the lower one third of the plantar fascia and the lower one fourth of the deep abductor fascia.
6. Then by releasing the deep fascia more proximally, the first branch of the plantar nerve can be decompressed. This compression usually occurs between the abductor hallucis muscle and the quadratus plantae muscle.

After surgery is performed, the athlete is maintained on crutches for 4 days. He is then allowed to start touching his foot down and gradually places more weight on the heel of his foot. Compressive dressings are applied for 2 weeks until all swelling subsides, and then the athlete may resume the use of a soft athletic shoe with a padded heel insert. At 4 weeks following surgery, the athlete can resume training as tolerated, even though symptoms often last for 2 to 4 months.

## MEDIAL PLANTAR NERVE
### Jogger's foot

After the medial plantar nerve travels underneath the flexor retinaculum, it courses deep to the abductor hallucis muscle. The nerve runs along the plantar surface of the flexor digitorum longus tendon and passes through the master knot of Henry (Fig. 2-7/ Plate 7). The nerve continues along the medial border of the foot, ramifying into branches that lie on the medial and lateral aspects of the flexor hallucis longus tendon.

Medial plantar nerve entrapment classically affects joggers (jogger's foot). Although it has been reported most commonly in men, in my experience, there is no gender predilection.

Medial plantar nerve entrapment occurs in the region of the master knot of Henry. Most patients with this syndrome run with excessive forefoot abduction, heel valgus, or with hyperpronation of the foot. There is often a history of a previous ankle injury with a chronically unstable lateral ankle or forefoot. If excessive adduction or abduction of the forefoot is seen at the talonavicular joint, the medial plantar nerve may be compressed underneath the master knot of Henry. Arch supports, especially those that are built-up, may compress the nerve. Kopell and Thompson[10] describe the entity associated with hallux rigidus. They postulated that overactivity of the tibialis anterior caused by the patient attempting to lift the arch of the foot to avoid pain contributed to the syndrome. Kopell and Thompson also thought that medial plantar nerve denervation resulted in increased stress in the first metatarsophalangeal joint, which ultimately led to arthrosis.[10]

In patients with medial plantar nerve compression, the pain often radiates distally into the medial toes and may radiate proximally into the ankle. The pain is worse with running on level ground, especially curves, but may be induced by workouts on stairs. Not uncommonly, the patient reports the onset of the syndrome associated with the use of a new orthosis.

Most characteristically tenderness occurs on the medial plantar aspect of the arch in the region of the navicular tuberosity. The pain may be reproduced by everting the heel or by having the patient stand on the

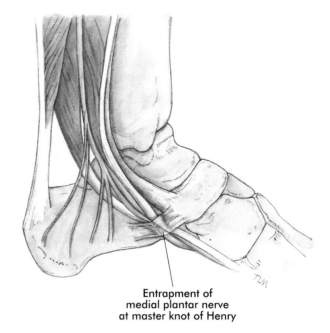

Entrapment of
medial plantar nerve
at master knot of Henry

**Fig. 2-7.** Jogger's foot.

ball of the foot. Tinel's sign may be found. Decreased sensation usually is present only after the patient has been running.

For treatment of jogger's foot, the physician should first try a heel lift or a medial longitudinal arch support. These are used to limit pronation of the foot and thus limit irritation of the medial plantar nerve in the area of the talonavicular joint.

Should conservative treatment fail, an operation is performed in the following manner:

1. An incision is made just beneath the talonavicular joint.
2. The incision is extended to the naviculocalcaneal ligament, releasing a portion of the tight fascial structures surrounding the medial plantar nerve.
3. Once the tight structures are released and the perineural fat is identified, the wound is irrigated and closed with interrupted sutures.
4. A compressive dressing is applied.

Crutches are used for 4 to 7 days postoperatively, depending on the extent of dissection. Compressive dressings are maintained for 2 weeks until the sutures are removed. Athletic gravity training is not resumed until approximately 6 weeks postoperatively.

## LATERAL PLANTAR NERVE COMPRESSION

With previous plantar fascia releases, the athlete may subsequently develop entrapment of the lateral plantar nerve. When the plantar fascia is released, the plantar fascia and its surrounding structures displace distally. This puts an abnormal pull on the abductor hallucis muscle and the foramen of the lateral plantar nerve. Because of the anatomic location of the lateral plantar nerve, there may be a secondary tethering following the release of the plantar fascia. For that reason, if possible, only a portion of the plantar fascia should be released, thus preventing distal traction.

## MEDIAL HALLUCAL NERVE

Rarely the medial hallucal nerve will be entrapped as it exits the distal abductor hallucis muscle. With this syndrome pain occurs under the medial aspect of the first metatarsophalangeal joint in the area of the tibial sesamoid. This condition is often mistaken for tibial sesamoiditis. If the radiograph does not show osteonecrosis of the tibial sesamoid, the medial hallucal nerve should be carefully examined. This condition may occur when the great toe deviates into hallux valgus, when there is extremely prominent tibial sesamoid pressing on the nerve, or if there is excessive hypertrophy of the abductor hallucis muscle compressing the medial hallucal nerve as it exits the fascia of the abductor hallucis muscle. The neuritic Tinel sign is usually positive first proximally to the tibial sesamoid bone.

## DEEP PERONEAL NERVE
### Anterior tarsal tunnel syndrome

The deep peroneal nerve lies between the extensor digitorum longus and the tibialis anterior muscles in the proximal one third of the leg. It travels between the extensor digitorum longus and the extensor hallucis longus in the region approximately 3 to 5 cm above the ankle joint. This is just below the inferior edge of the extensor retinaculum. Approximately 1 cm above the ankle joint, the nerve divides, giving off a lateral branch that innervates the extensor digitorum brevis muscle. This occurs in the region underneath the oblique superomedial band of the inferior extensor retinaculum. The medial branch of the deep peroneal nerve continues alongside the dorsalis pedis artery underneath the oblique inferomedial band of the inferior extensor retinaculum. The nerve may be compressed in this region between the retinaculum and the ridges of the talonavicular joint. The nerve continues distally between the extensor hallucis brevis and the tendon of the extensor hallucis longus. The nerve supplies sensation to the first web space in the adjacent borders of the first and second digits.[20]

The deep peroneal nerve may become entrapped in several locations (Fig. 2-8/Plate 8). The most commonly described entrapment is the *anterior tarsal tunnel syndrome,* which refers to the entrapment of the deep peroneal nerve under the inferior extensor retinaculum. Entrapment may also occur as the nerve

passes under the tendon of the extensor hallucis brevis.[10] Additionally entrapment has been described under the superior edge of the inferior retinaculum where the extensor hallucis longus tendon crosses over the nerve.[4,10,15] Compression by underlying dorsal osteophytes of the talonavicular joint or an os intermetatarseum (between the bases of the first and second metatarsals) has previously been described in runners.[17]

Trauma often plays a role in this syndrome. Many of these patients have a history of recurring ankle sprains. As the foot plantar flexes and supinates, the nerve is placed under maximal stretch, especially at the anterior ankle joint and over the talonavicular joint. Thus with repetitive ankle sprains, nerve entrapment may occur. Tight-fitting shoes or ski boots have been implicated as inciting factors.[6,11,12,15] Occasionally a jogger will tie a key in the lacing of his shoe. The external compression of this key may cause localized pressure to the deep peroneal nerve. External compression may also occur in athletes who do sit-ups with their feet hooked under a rigid bar. Fracture residuals or osteophytes in the region of the distal tibia, talus, navicular, cuneiforms, or metatarsal bases put undue pressures on the nerve as well. The presence of edema or ganglia can result in deep peroneal compressive neuropathy.

Patients with compression of the deep peroneal nerve complain of pain in the dorsum of the foot with occasional radiation into the first web space. The pain usually occurs during athletic activities and subsides with rest and removal of the shoe. The pain is described as spasmodic, dull, aching, or sharp. Patients frequently give a history of recurrent sprains or previous trauma.

As with other syndromes examination should begin with the spine. Palpation of the common peroneal nerve around the neck of the fibula is critical because entrapment of the nerve in this location may give rise to recurrent sprained ankles from peroneal weakness. Palpation should continue along the entire course of the deep peroneal nerve, the anterior compartment of the leg, and the dorsum of the foot. Tenderness in the anterior compartment, especially after a workout, may indicate exertional compartment syndrome. Depending on the area of entrapment, the pain may be brought on by either dorsiflexion or plantar flexion of the foot. Decreased sensation in the first web space may be noted. If the compression occurs before the bifurcation of the nerve, there may be atrophy or weakness of the extensor digitorum brevis.

For anterior tarsal tunnel syndrome, all attempts should be made to ascertain that no compression occurs on the nerve by external structures such as

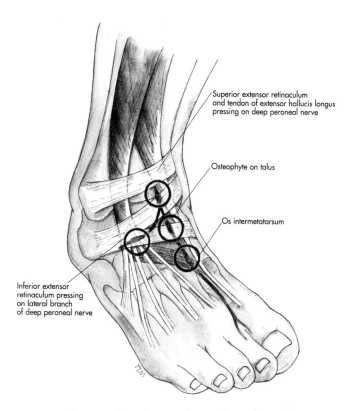

Superior extensor retinaculum
and tendon of extensor hallucis longus
pressing on deep peroneal nerve

Osteophyte on talus

Os intermetatarsum

Inferior extensor
retinaculum pressing
on lateral branch
of deep peroneal nerve

**Fig. 2-8.** Anterior tarsal tunnel syndrome.

tight shoelaces or poorly fitting shoes. If the ankle is unstable, appropriate bracing or taping should be used for the ankle to eliminate instability of the ankle, which may cause secondary compression of the deep peroneal nerve. Occasionally a short-leg walking cast or a cast-brace is used to rest the affected ankle or foot and allow the irritated nerve to recover.

Should all conservative treatment fail and surgery is performed, the following technique is used:

1. The exact location of entrapment is identified whether at the anterior ankle or the talonavicular joint or distally at the first metatarsal tarsal joint, and a small incision is made.
2. The incision is carried down, care being taken to avoid excessive dissection or stripping of tissues around the nerve.
3. The tight structures surrounding the deep peroneal nerve are identified and carefully released. If possible, the surrounding fatty tissues are left intact protecting the nerve and, if possible, only a small area of the nerve is released.
4. If any offending bony structures are pressing the nerve, these bony exostoses or prominences are removed.
5. The wound is irrigated and carefully closed, closing only the skin and subcutaneous tissues. The nerve is protected from raw bony surfaces

by placing soft tissues between the bone and the nerve.

Postoperatively a bandage or cast is applied, care being taken not to cause any abnormal pressure about the nerves or bones of the dorsal foot. Non–weight bearing is maintained for 4 to 7 days. Swimming and biking is resumed as tolerated after the sutures are removed. Running and jumping may be initiated after all swelling and pain subside.

## SUPERFICIAL PERONEAL NERVE
### Anterolateral compartment syndrome

The superficial peroneal nerve is a branch of the common peroneal nerve. It courses through the anterolateral compartment, innervating the peroneus brevis and longus. Traveling between the anterior intermuscular septum and the fascia of the lateral compartment, it pierces the deep fascia approximately 10.5 to 12.5 cm above the tip of the lateral malleolus. The nerve then becomes subcutaneous. At approximately 6.5 cm above the lateral malleolus, it divides into two branches (the intermediate and the medial dorsal cutaneous nerves). The intermediate dorsal cutaneous nerve usually provides sensation to the dorsal aspect of the lateral dorsal aspect of the ankle, as well as the fourth toe and portions of the third and fifth toes. The medial dorsal cutaneous nerve provides

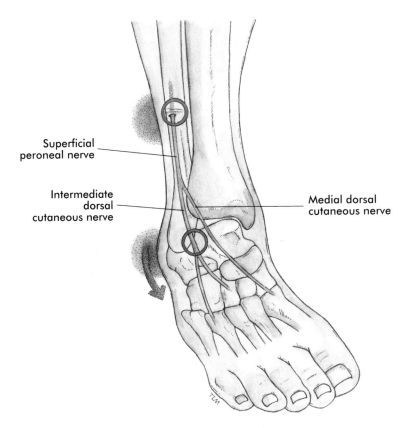

Superficial
peroneal nerve

Intermediate
dorsal
cutaneous nerve

Medial dorsal
cutaneous nerve

**Fig. 2-9.** Anterolateral compartment syndrome. Superficial peroneal nerve entrapment.

sensation of the dorsomedial aspect of the ankle as it extends forward to the medial aspect of the hallux, as well as the second and third toes.[20]

The point of entrapment of the nerve occurs at its exit point from the deep fascia, according to clinical and anatomic studies. In most cases the fascia ledge impinges on the exiting nerve. Fascial defects with muscle herniation exacerbate the impingement. Styf[22] described a short fibrous tunnel between the anterior intermuscular septum and the fascia of the lateral compartment. In almost half of these cases, he described a fibrotic, low compliant tunnel that may predispose to local compartment syndrome.[22] Chronic ankle sprains, a major underlying factor, subjects the nerve to recurrent stretching (Fig. 2-9/Plate 9). A previous anterior compartment fasciotomy may cause shifting of the fascia with resultant stretching and impingement of the nerve. Occasionally two nerves exist or the nerve can be in the anterior compartment, as a variation of normal anatomy.

Patients complain of a history of pain over the outer border of the distal calf and the dorsum of the foot and ankle. Pain can be present for several years intermittently. Roughly one third of patients have numbness and paresthesias along the distribution. Occasionally patients only complain of pain at the junction of the middle and distal thirds of the leg with or without the presence of local swelling. The pain is typically worse with physical activity ranging from walking, jogging, and running to squatting. Nocturnal pain is rare. Relief by conservative measures is uncommon.* Approximately 25% of patients with the syndrome have a history of prior trauma to the extremity, most commonly, an ankle sprain.

The physical examination should include an evaluation of the lower back. The region where the common peroneal nerves sweeps around the neck of the fibula must also be examined. Point tenderness is usually elicited where the nerve emerges from the deep fascia approximately 10.5 to 12.5 cm above the tip of the distal fibula. Styf[22] described three provocative tests to suggest a diagnosis. The patient actively dorsiflexes and everts the foot against resistance while the physician palpates the nerve impingement site. In the second and third tests, the physician passively plantar flexes and inverts the foot, first without pressure over the nerve, and then with percussion along the course of the nerve.[22]

Conservative treatment for the entrapment of the superficial peroneal nerve should be directed at avoiding pressure on this structure and preventing ankle and subtalar instability. By preventing ankle

*References 1, 9, 13, 14, 16, 21, 22.

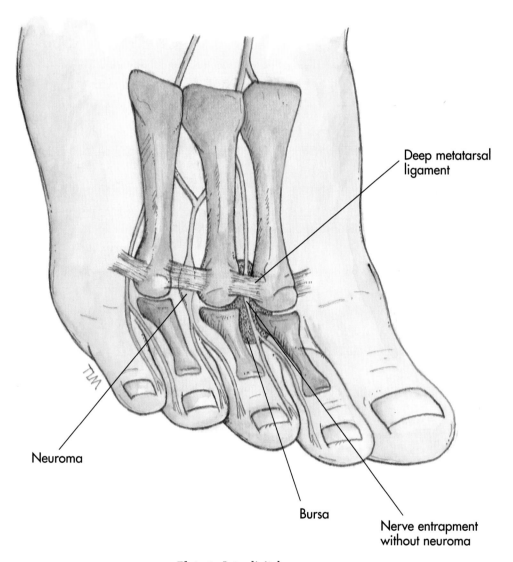

Deep metatarsal ligament

Neuroma

Bursa

Nerve entrapment without neuroma

**Plate 1.** Interdigital neuroma.

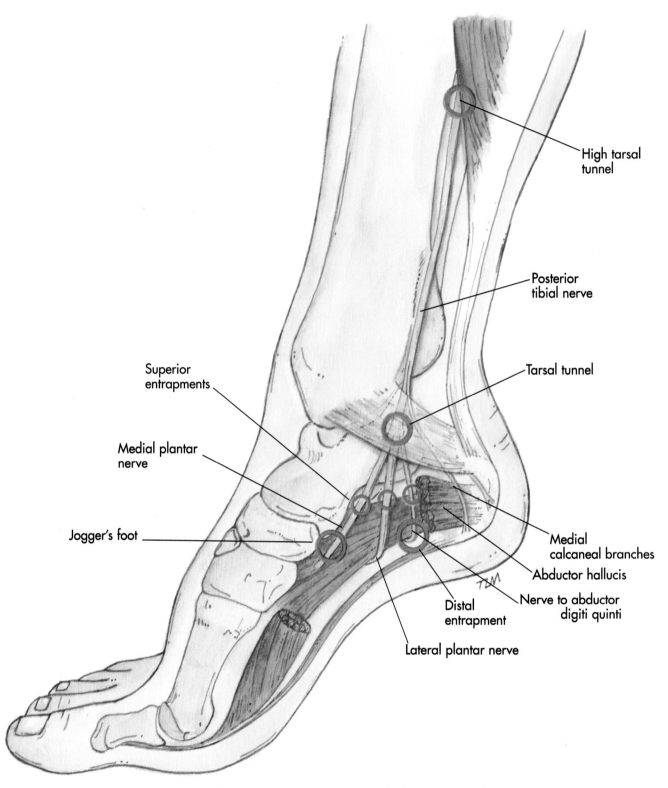

High tarsal
tunnel

Posterior
tibial nerve

Tarsal tunnel

Superior
entrapments

Medial plantar
nerve

Jogger's foot

Medial
calcaneal branches

Abductor hallucis

Nerve to abductor
digiti quinti

Distal
entrapment

Lateral plantar nerve

**Plate 2.** Areas of compression of the posterior tibial nerve and its branches.

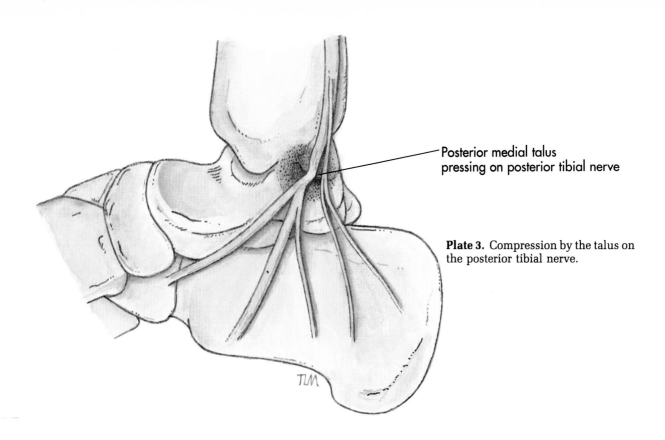

Posterior medial talus
pressing on posterior tibial nerve

**Plate 3.** Compression by the talus on
the posterior tibial nerve.

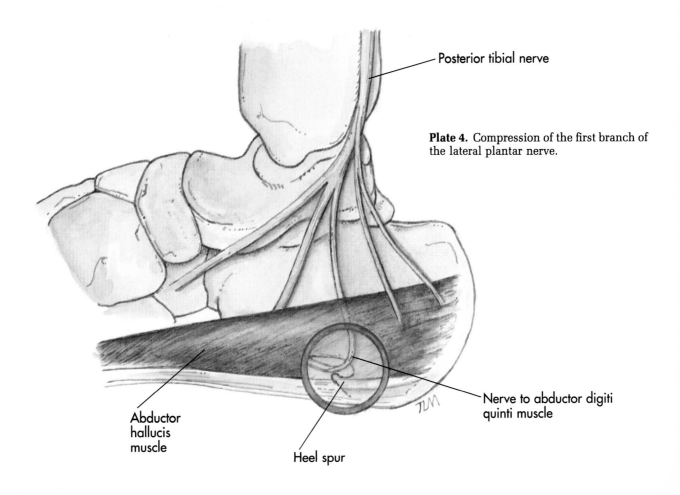

Posterior tibial nerve

**Plate 4.** Compression of the first branch of
the lateral plantar nerve.

Nerve to abductor digiti
quinti muscle

Abductor
hallucis
muscle

Heel spur

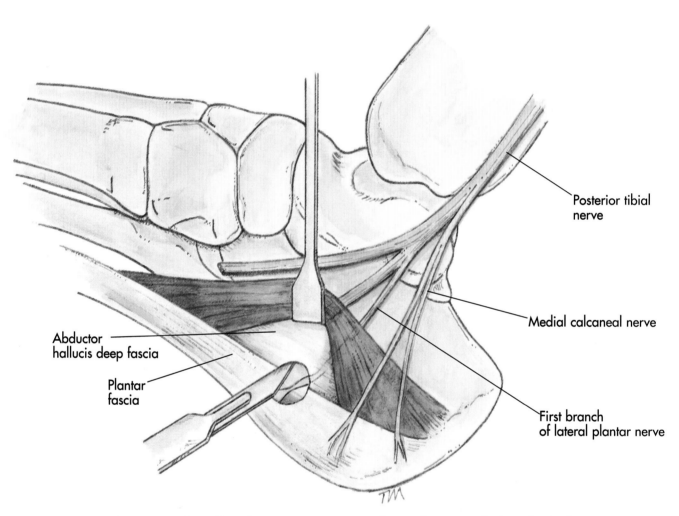

Posterior tibial nerve

Medial calcaneal nerve

First branch of lateral plantar nerve

Abductor hallucis deep fascia

Plantar fascia

**Plate 5.** Hourglass effect of nerve as it goes over quadratus plantae muscle. Deep fascia of the abductor muscle being windowed.

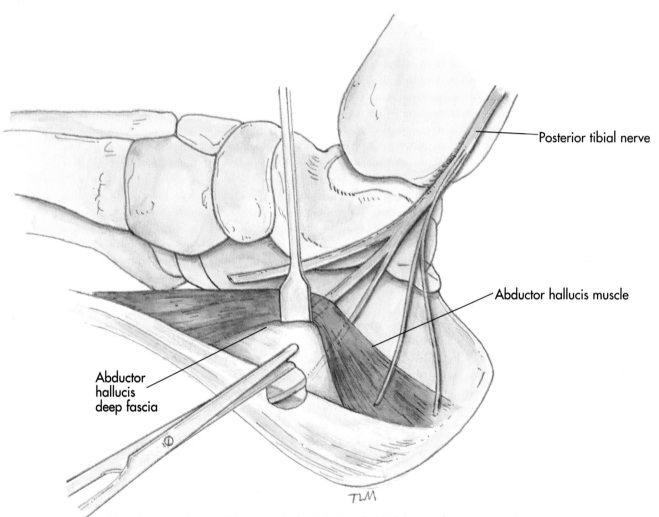

Posterior tibial nerve

Abductor hallucis muscle

Abductor
hallucis
deep fascia

TLM

**Plate 6.** Deep fascia of abductor hallucis being divided from inferior to superior.

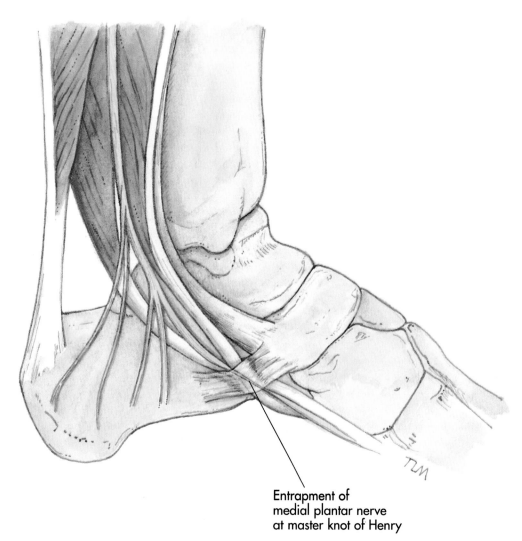

Entrapment of
medial plantar nerve
at master knot of Henry

**Plate 7.** Jogger's foot.

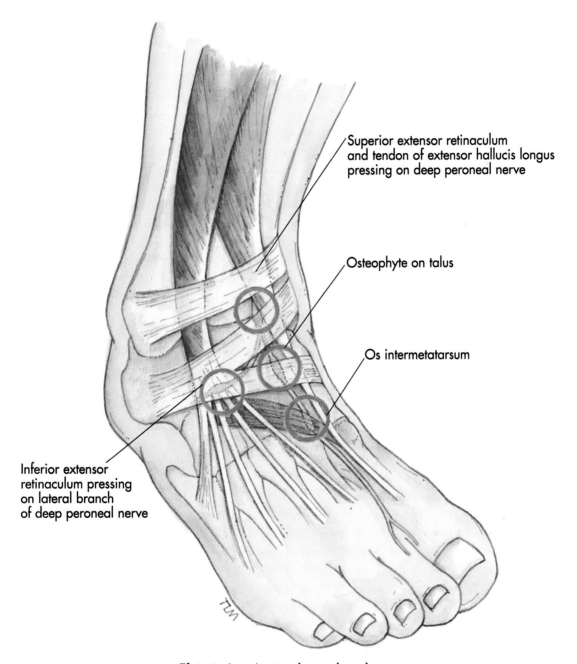

Superior extensor retinaculum
and tendon of extensor hallucis longus
pressing on deep peroneal nerve

Osteophyte on talus

Os intermetatarsum

Inferior extensor
retinaculum pressing
on lateral branch
of deep peroneal nerve

**Plate 8.** Anterior tarsal tunnel syndrome.

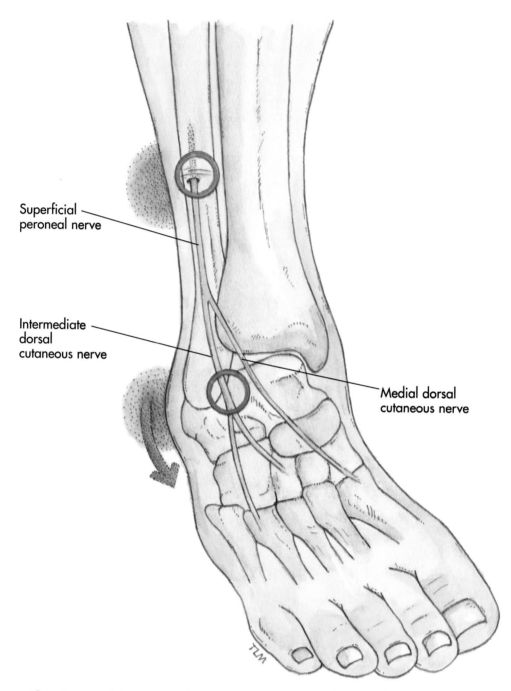

Superficial peroneal nerve

Intermediate dorsal cutaneous nerve

Medial dorsal cutaneous nerve

**Plate 9.** Anterolateral compartment syndrome. Superficial peroneal nerve entrapment.

and subtalar instability, the nerve is not placed on stretch.

If the syndrome has been present for an extended time and is caused by a lateral compartment syndrome or muscle herniation, surgery is usually the only method to correct the problem. Surgery is carried out in the following way:

1. A two- to three-inch incision is made in the skin and subcutaneous tissues over the exit of the superficial peroneal nerve from the lateral compartment of the leg.
2. Soft tissue dissection is carried out, care being taken to protect the nerve and identify the exit of the superficial peroneal nerve.
3. The fascia is released from the superficial peroneal nerve, extending the opening in the fascia where the nerve exits the lateral compartment and becomes superficial.
4. Care is taken to ascertain that the entire compression of the nerve is released.
5. Following this, irrigation is performed and the skin and subcutaneous tissues are closed with interrupted sutures.

Should the ankle be unstable, the surgeon may need to stabilize the ankle instability in addition to releasing the superficial peroneal nerve. Postoperatively a compression dressing is used until the swelling subsides and then progressive ambulation and activities are allowed, depending on the symptoms present. Activities usually can be resumed within 3 weeks if dissection has not been excessive or traumatic.

## SURAL NERVE ENTRAPMENT

The medial sural nerve runs between the heads of the gastrocnemius muscle and penetrates it deep aponeurosis approximately halfway up the leg. Subsequently it anastomoses with the peroneal communicating nerve and travels along the border of the Achilles tendon next to the short saphenous veins. Two centimeters above the ankle, it gives off branches: one supplies sensation to the lateral heel, and the other frequently anastomoses with the lateral branch of the superficial peroneal nerve. The nerve then runs inferior to the peroneal sheaths in a subcutaneous position. As it reaches the tuberosity of the fifth metatarsal, the nerve ramifies, providing sensation to the lateral aspect of the fifth toe and the fourth web space.[20]

**Case Study 2.** This athlete had pain in the plantar foot and heel. The pain and numbness occurred intermittently and followed the distribution of the posterior tibial nerve. Initially a classic tarsal tunnel syndrome was thought to

exist with compression behind the medial malleolus under the retinacular ligament.

On nerve conduction studies, the nerve did not show traditional slowing at the retinacular ligament, but slowing of the nerve conduction at a higher level in the area of the distal gastrocnemius muscle. A deep posterior compartment syndrome caused this high tarsal tunnel syndrome. This syndrome was corrected by releasing the deep posterior compartment. Four weeks later, all pain had subsided.

At the time of surgery, the patient was given a regional anesthetic doing a field block of the area to be released. A 3-inch-long incision was made in the area of the distal gastroc muscle. The deep posterior compartment was released over a 4-inch area, thus eliminating the pressure on the posterior tibial nerve. No tourniquet was used for this operation.

**Case Study 3.** A 26-year-old male professional major league baseball player had intermittent problems in his right heel for 2 years. He had increasing difficulty during workouts with exacerbation of the pain when he ran. This especially occurred on hard surfaces. He had used heel pads, taping, and medications with incomplete and inconsistent relief of his symptoms. The athletic trainer tried different therapeutic modalities including ultrasound, ice, heat, and various massage treatments. On the physical examination of the baseball player, there was localized tenderness along the proximal and medial aspect of the plantar fascia. Tenderness was also noted at the edge of the abductor hallucis next to the plantar fascia along the course of the first branch of the lateral plantar nerve. There were no neurological deficits. The posterior tibial nerve proximally was not tender. A roentgenogram showed some localized spurring in the right os calcis, with the calcification occurring just dorsal to the plantar fascia in the substance of the flexor brevis muscle. Since the patient had failed conservative treatment and did not feel he could complete spring training, he elected to have surgery.

With the patient given an ankle block anesthetic, he underwent release of the first branch of the lateral plantar nerve. One fourth of the medial plantar fascia was released as well as the deep fascia of the abductor hallucis muscle (Figs. 2-5 and 2-6). The spur was excised even though it was thought that nerve compression was causing his pain. One week after surgery the patient was able to put some pressure on his heel without discomfort. After 12 postoperative days, the sutures were removed. Moist heat and ice treatments with gentle stretching of the Achilles tendons was instituted. Eight weeks after the procedure, he was able to resume full sports activity. He has competed over the past 4 years without any loss of speed or affect to his batting average.

**Case Study 4.** One patient, an avid walker, had a long history of rigidus. She subsequently developed medial plantar neuralgia. It was theorized that this was on the basis of abductor hallucis and flexor brevis muscle spasm, which was her unconscious attempt to splint the first metatarsophalangeal joint against dorsiflexion.

**Case Study 5.** A 23-year-old marathon runner stated that while training he would note his foot to "give way" on the third lap of the mile. Occasionally he had a burning, numbing sensation that radiated into the great toe and to the second toe. This had been present for 3 years and had prevented him from entering international competition. Significantly he had had repeated lateral ankle sprains on the ankle of the affected foot. He also had hypermobility in the forefoot in relation to the hindfoot and excessive migration of the navicular bone on the head of the talus. It appeared that he had forefoot abduction when he was running around the track, during which time his symptoms were most prominent. The only time his symptoms developed was after his training sessions. For that reason, he was asked to run on the track and after 1 mile, an examination was carried out.

The examination revealed some localized tenderness at the knot of Henry. The structures of the foot were identified in the area of symptoms. The patient was taken to surgery and given a regional anesthetic to the foot and ankle; the nerve was released by releasing part of the knot of Henry. It was found to be compressed with the fatty tissue around the nerve being compressed in a chronic manner. After release of the nerve in this local area, the patient was allowed to resume training 4 weeks after the operation. By 3 months he was competing. Over the past 5 years, he has had no recurrence of the previous symptoms and has been able to return to international competition.

**Case Study 6.** A major league baseball pitcher had severe pain of his medial hallucal nerve under the tibial sesamoid. On x-ray, he was found to have a bifurcate tibial sesamoid with some separation. Because of chronic pain, it was elected to take out the avascular necrotic portion of the tibial sesamoid. At the time of surgery, the medial hallucal nerve was found to be thickened and compressed against the prominent tibial sesamoid. In addition to taking out the fragmented pole of the tibial sesamoid, the medial hallucal nerve was carefully displaced more dorsally, and the nerve was released from its proximal exit from the abductor hallucis muscle. Awareness of this nerve syndrome will prevent the surgeon from unnecessarily removing a sesamoid bone or damaging the nerve during sesamoid excision.

**Case Study 7.** A 19-year-old college 800-m runner complained of aching pain in the dorsum of the foot exacerbated by running the first turn of the second lap of the 800 m. The pain was relieved by rest and removal of the shoe. The pain increased until he was compelled to return from European competition. Attempts at diminishing the pain by rest, nonsteroidal antiinflammatory medications, massage, and physical therapy were only temporarily successful. As soon as any serious training was resumed, the syndrome recurred.

On physical examination the patient had point tenderness over the talonavicular joint with radiation of dull pain into the first web space. The pain increased with plantar flexion and supination of the foot. Roentgenograms revealed an osteophyte on the dorsum of the talus as it articulated with the naviculum. At surgery the osteophyte was found to be in the vicinity of the deep peroneal nerve. The capsule was opened. The inferior retinaculum was partially released and the osteophyte was excised. By 3 months the runner

was once again competing. He has had no more problems in this area over the past 8 years.

**Case Study 8.** A 20-year-old female collegiate champion was referred for a fusion of the first metatarsal tarsal joint because of continuous pain. This problem had been evaluated by several doctors, with many diagnostic studies. On physical examination there was a local area of pain at the base of the first and second metatarsals. On x-ray, the faint outline of a bony exostosis could be seen extending dorsally from the first metatarsal. This was seen on the lateral x-ray. A decision was made to explore the region and release the deep peroneal nerve. At the time of surgery, a small accessory bone was found between the bases of the first and second metatarsals, compressing the deep peroneal nerve as it migrated over the first metatarsal tarsal joint. By carefully releasing the nerve, retracting it and removing the bone, the runner was able to return to national competition. She was able to return to running within 4 weeks.

**Case Study 9.** A 28-year-old male ballet dancer developed chronic instability of his ankle. The chronic instability worsened to the point that he was unable to dance. He was taken to surgery and the lateral ligaments were repaired. He returned to dancing but had a continued problem with extreme dorsiflexion. With dorsiflexion a sharp pain developed in the anterior ankle.

Using a regional anesthetic to the anterior ankle, a 1.5-inch longitudinal incision was carried out. The superior transverse retinacular ligament was partially released at the anterior ankle joint. The deep peroneal nerve was released. Postoperatively the pain subsided. The dancer returned to his ballet with good stability in the ankle and elimination of the anterior ankle pain.

Sural nerve entrapment may occur anywhere along its course. Several cases have been described in runners who sustained fractures of the base of the fifth metatarsal following severe plantar flexion in inversion injuries.[7,18] Recurrent ankle sprains may lead to fibrosis and subsequent nerve entrapment.[18] Ganglia of the peroneal sheaths or calcaneocuboid joint have been reported.[18] In one case a patient had Achilles peritendinitis that was irritating the sural nerve posterior to the Achilles peritendon sheath (see Case Study 10). This chronic pain syndrome responded to a release of the casing around the sural nerve. Fractures of the os calcis (see Case Study 11) may entrap the sural nerve also.

**Case Study 10.** A twenty-six-year-old male middle-distance runner described a 2-year history of pain along the Achilles tendon bilaterally. Initially the pain was controlled with antiinflammatory medications, heel lifts, and stretching exercises. The patient was a competitive 400- and 800-m runner but had difficulty training because of the pain. On physical examination he had tenderness along the course of the Achilles tendon, but there was a point of severe pain at one isolated location. This tenderness was noted approximately 6 cm proximal to the calcaneus along the lateral aspect of the tendon. Under a field block, an incision was made along the lateral aspect of the Achilles tendon. The sural nerve was identified and found to be tightly adherent to the aponeurotic band posterior to the Achilles tendon, right in the location of maximal pain. After releasing the aponeurosis, the nerve was displaced laterally and a portion of the peritenon was debrided. The Achilles tendon itself was intact with no evidence of degeneration. Pathologic reports confirmed edematous, fibroconnective tissues with areas of local hemorrhage. Postoperatively the patient was placed in a short-leg cast. The following week, he was put in an off-the-shelf removable ankle-foot orthosis (AFO) brace. After 1 month he was instructed to increase his activities and wean himself from the brace gradually. By 8 weeks the patient was doing well with the exception of some minor stiffness. Over the course of the next 2 months, he was able to resume his running with no further reported pain for 3 years.

**Case Study 11.** A 43-year-old avid golfer was evaluated for lateral ankle pain 4 years after sustaining a closed calcaneal fracture. The initial injury had been treated in a cast, and the fracture healed in acceptable position. However the patient continued to have pain in his foot in the area distal to the tip of the fibula. This was thought to be due to subtalar arthritis. Three years before being evaluated, he was seen by another physician. It was thought that his symptoms were coming from an osteophytic spur, which was removed. However he continued to have sharp pains that radiated down the fifth metatarsal and proximally into the ankle.

On questioning the patient, it was evident that progressive activities did not exacerbate the pain nor did swelling occur. The pain was more constant in nature and radiated into the foot and up into the leg. Interestingly the patient had a history of a disk excision from his back 7 years before evaluation. On physical examination the patient had point tenderness distal to the fibula. Compression over this region produced a sharp pain in the lateral aspect of the heel that radiated proximally into the leg and distally into the foot, reproducing his symptoms.

With the patient given a regional anesthetic without the use of a tourniquet an incision was made over the lateral aspect of the heel. The sural nerve was identified and decompressed from the area of the peroneal tendons. It was found to be rubbing along the lateral subtalar joint. The nerve was moved anteriorly into the subcutaneous fatty tissues away from the scar of the previous surgery and away from the bony exostosis of the subtalar joint. Postoperatively the patient had relief from the constant pain. By 2 months the patient had returned to full activities, resuming golf with complete resolution of his symptoms.

Patients frequently give a history of an acute twisting injury or recurrent ankle sprain. There are neurologic symptoms with shooting pain and paresthesias. On physical examination the sural nerve is examined from the popliteal fossa to the toes. Local tenderness and a positive Tinel sign are characteristic. Occasionally numbness is noted.

## SUMMARY

Although neuropathies in the athlete's foot, ankle, and leg are uncommon, they are often underdiagnosed. This is primarily due to the complex interplay of factors required for their presentation. The physician should be aware of their possible occurrence, as well as the anatomy and course of the nerves. Often the problem occurs only during functional activity and is not present during the routine static examination.

Other problems should also be considered when a nerve syndrome is entertained. Metabolic processes such as diabetes or abuse of alcohol can cause neuropathies. A double crush syndrome or pain from a higher source should also be considered.

Finally, if surgery is performed for chronic problems, only the area of constriction is released, without interfering with the nerve itself. Release the fascia but leave the peroneal fat intact. Stabilize the joint if instability is a factor. To treat athletes effectively, physicians must be able to perform an accurate history, examination, and a functional physical examination and be aware of nerve syndromes of the foot, ankle, and leg.

## REFERENCES

1. Banerjee T, Koons DD: Superficial peroneal nerve entrapment: report of two cases, *J Neurosurg* 55:991, 1981.
2. Baxter DE, Thigpen CM: Heel pain: operative results, *Foot Ankle* 5:16, 1984.
3. Baxter DE, Pfeffer GB: Treatment of chronic heel pain by surgical release of the first branch of the lateral plantar nerve, *Clin Orthop* 279:229, 1992.
4. Borges LF et al: The anterior tarsal tunnel syndrome: report of two cases, *J Neurosurg* 54:89, 1981.
5. Cozen L: Bursitis of the heel, *Am J Orthop* 3:372, 1961.
6. Gessini L, Jandolo B, Peitrangel A: The anterior tarsal tunnel syndrome: report of four cases, *J Bone Joint Surg* 66A:786, 1984.
7. Gould N, Trevino S: Sural nerve entrapment by avulsion fracture at the base of the fifth metatarsal bone, *Foot Ankle* 2:153, 1981.
8. Heimkes B et al: The proximal and distal tarsal tunnel syndromes: an anatomic study, *Int Orthop* 11:193, 1987.
9. Kernohan J, Levack B, Wilson JN: Entrapment of the superficial peroneal nerve: three case reports, *J Bone Joint Surg* 67B:60, 1985.
10. Kopell HP, Thompson WAL: *Peripheral entrapment neuropathies*, Malabar, FL, 1976, RE Krieger Publishing.
11. Krause KH, Witt T, Ross A: The anterior tarsal tunnel syndrome, *J Neurol* 217:67, 1977.
12. Lindenbaum BL: Ski boot compression syndrome, *Clin Orthop* 140:19, 1979.
13. Lowdon IMR: Superficial peroneal nerve entrapment: a case report, *J Bone Joint Surg* 67B:58, 1985.
14. Mackey D, Colbert DS, Chater EH: Musculocutaneous nerve entrapment, *Ir J Med Sci* 146:100, 1977.
15. Marinacci AA: Neurological syndrome of the tarsal tunnels, *Bull LA Neurol Soc* 33:98, 1968.
16. McAuliffe TB, Fiddian NJ, Browett JP: Entrapment neuropathy

of the superficial peroneal nerve: a bilateral case, *J Bone Joint Surg* 67B:62, 1985.

17. Murphy PC, Baxter DE: Nerve entrapment of the foot and ankle in runners, *Clin Sports Med* 4:753, 1985.

18. Pringle RM, Protheroe K, Mukherjee SK: Entrapment neuropathy of the sural nerve, *J Bone Joint Surg* 56B:465, 1974.

19. Rondhuis JJ, Huson A: The first branch of the lateral plantar nerve and heel pain, *Acta Morphol Neerl Scand* 24:269, 1986.

20. Sarrafian SK: *Anatomy of the foot and ankle: descriptive, topographic, functional,* Philadelphia, 1983, Lippincott.

21. Sridhara CR, Izzo KL: Terminal sensory branches of the superficial peroneal nerve: an entrapment syndrome, *Arch Phys Med Rehabil* 66:789, 1985.

22. Styf J: Entrapment of the superficial peroneal nerve: diagnosis and results of decompression, *J Bone Joint Surg* 71B:131, 1989.

# Chapter 3

# Impingement syndromes

## William G. Hamilton

"Impingement" is derived from the Latin verb *impingere* meaning "to force against." The periosteum is composed of two layers: the superficial (fibrous) layer and the deep (cambium) layer. The cambium layer has osteogenic potential. This can be seen following conditions that strip the periosteum from the underlying bone (i.e., tumors and fractures). In impingement one bone repetitively striking the other can stimulate the cambium layer to form osteophytes. Once the osteophytic prominence forms, impingement occurs more easily so that the impingement spur, once formed, frequently increases in size and eventually may break off, forming a loose body. Conservative treatment should be aimed at breaking this repetitive cycle so that the impingement spurs do not grow and produce irritation. In ballet we tell the dancer not to "hit bottom" in their plié (knee-bend) when they land from a jump and the ankle is forced into maximum dorsiflexion. These restrictions are often difficult to follow or are too restrictive—so if the symptoms warrant, and conservative treatment is not working, surgery is usually indicated.

## GENERAL TECHNIQUE TIPS FOR OSTEOPHYTE REMOVAL

1. Get adequate exposure and visualization. If you are using the arthroscope and struggling, open it up and do the job right.
2. Make your skin incisions carefully to avoid incisional neuromas. Nothing is more discouraging than a good clean-out that is spoiled by a hypersensitive scar.
3. Be sure you get all the osteophytes out; there can be hidden spurs or more than one. If there is any doubt, it is best to take an x-ray in the operating

room at the end of the case to make sure nothing has been missed.
4. If the patient is not allergic to bees (bone wax is derived from beeswax), I use bone wax to cover the raw areas of bone to prevent bleeding and hopefully to prevent regrowth of the osteophyte.

## SPECIFIC ANATOMIC AREAS
### The interphalangeal joint of the hallux

Dorsal impingement with spur formation similar to that seen in the first metatarsophalangeal (MP) joint can occur in this joint. It can be a sign of degenerative joint disease (DJD) but usually is secondary to stiffness and lack of motion in the adjacent MP joint. When hallux rigidus forms in the first MP joint, the interphalangeal (IP) joint will be forced into excessive dorsiflexion in an attempt to compensate for the lack of motion in the proximal joint. This at times can be dramatic. I once saw a female dancer who was born with congenital ankylosis of both first MP joints. They were almost totally rigid. She had Grecian (Morton's) feet with short first rays and had developed 90 degrees of dorsiflexion in her IP joints so that she had a full demipointe relevé. Rigidity in this joint can be treated similarly to the condition found in the first MP joint. One should remember, however, that this joint is very forgiving and surgery is rarely necessary.

### The metatarsophalangeal joint of the hallux

*Hallux rigidus* is one of the most common foot problems seen in athletes, especially older athletes. It comes in three stages or degrees: (1) dorsal impingement spurs are present but joint itself is normal (ideal case for cheilectomy); (2) dorsal spurs and some mild DJD within the joint (mixed results with a "radical cheilectomy"); and (3) dorsal spurs secondary to obvious DJD (poor results with cheilectomy—the patient needs fusion or an arthroplasty).

*Nonsurgical treatment* involves shoe modifications to accommodate the deformity and the peripheral osteophytes that accompany it. This consists of stretching the area of the shoe around the first MP joint with a cobbler's swan to avoid pressure on the osteophytes, and putting rocker bars and a stiff sole in the athletic shoes and footwear.

*Operative treatment* consists of four choices: (1) cheilectomy, (2) radical cheilectomy, (3) resection or capsular arthroplasty, and (4) first MP fusion.

The type of cheilectomy that I prefer is the type popularized by Mann and Coughlin.[18] They emphasize that you need to remove more than you think—usually the upper one quarter to one third of the articular portion of the metatarsal (MT) head. You also need to mobilize the sesamoids by blunt dissection, for they often are anchored by adhesions and limit dorsiflexion, even after removal of the osteophytes. I try to obtain 90 degrees of dorsiflexion at the time of the surgery and hope to get 50% to 60% of this later. I use bone wax to cover the raw surfaces and emphasize early motion as soon as the incision is healed. I perform this as an outpatient operation with an ankle block, but caution the patient that it can take much longer than they anticipate before they have their "end result." This is one of the few occasions in which I do not have patients wear a postoperative shoe. Instead, I try to get them walking in a soft sneaker as soon as possible for joint mobilization. If motion does not return as fast as it should, I send patients to a physical therapist for more vigorous mobilization. Mann and Coughlin report around 90% excellent/good results with their cheilectomies.[18] My results have not been that good. I may be operating on some joints that are too far gone for this procedure. The salvage procedure for a failed cheilectomy is either an arthroplasty or preferably a first MP fusion.

The *radical cheilectomy* is similar to the cheilectomy just described, but more bone is removed and a resection of the dorsal portion of the base of the proximal phalanx, matching the resection performed on the MT head is also performed (Fig. 3-1).

If the patient has first and second MTs that are relatively the same length, has a destroyed joint, and wants to preserve some MP motion, I perform a *capsular arthroplasty*. The patient needs to be warned that this may not work, and, if it does, it may not hold up over time. If it fails, an MP fusion can be performed for salvage. The operation is basically a resection arthroplasty, but the thick dorsal capsule of the joint including the distal insertion of the extensor hallucis brevis (EHB) is pulled down between the MT head and

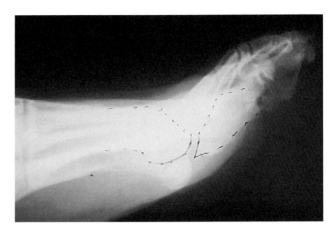

**Fig. 3-1.** Radical cheilectomy. Note removal of the dorsal portion of both the metatarsal head and the proximal phalanx.

the base of the resected proximal phalanx and sutured to the stumps of the flexor brevi, distal to the sesamoids. One must be careful not to remove too much of the proximal phalanx, 25% to 30% at most. If the extensor hallucis longus (EHL) tendon is tight, it should be lengthened to prevent the hallux from riding upward. I perform a tenotomy of the EHB proximally so that the whole dorsal sleeve of the MP joint, including EHB insertion can be pulled down into the gap between the bones. I have had mixed results with this procedure, sometimes surprisingly good and sometimes disappointing. If the first ray is foreshortened, this procedure does not work as well, because the patient almost certainly will develop a transfer lesion under the second MT head. Better results will be obtained in patients who have first and second MTs that are nearly the same length.

The *first MP fusion* is a more reliable long-term solution for arthritic joints in most athletes (other than dancers, who *must* have MP joint motion). There are many different methods of performing this operation. The reader should consult one of the standard textbooks on foot surgery for the various types of first MP fusions currently in use.[13,14,18] My own preference is a cup-and-dome fusion using reamers, an intramedullary toe wire, and a "box" stitch around the joint with heavy monofilament nylon suture. The position of fusion should be in very slight dorsiflexion and 10 to 15 degrees of valgus. If the hallux is longer than the other toes, some shortening should be performed as part of the fusion to make it proportional to the other digits.

*Silastic implants* and total joint replacements of the first MP joint have been abandoned by all reputable foot surgeons, because the long-term results have been so poor. They simply cannot hold up under the

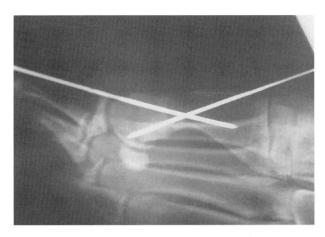

**Fig. 3-2.** Hallux elevatus secondary to dorsal displacement of the metatarsal following a metatarsal osteotomy.

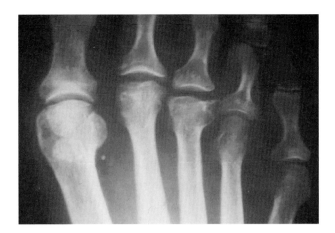

**Fig. 3-3.** A rare case of multiple Freiberg's disease.

demands of active athletes. The paradox of silicone is that "the people who need it, you can't use it in; the people you can use it in, don't need it."

There is a special type of hallux rigidus that is secondary to *hallux elevatus.* It usually occurs when a first MT osteotomy for correction of a bunion deformity allows the first ray to dorsiflex at the osteotomy site. The proximal phalanx subluxes plantarward as the MT head moves upward and the joint becomes rigid, initially without DJD or osteophytes. It can also occur in neurological conditions that produce weakness in the peroneus longus. (In normal foot mechanics the first ray is held plantarward by the pull of the peroneus longus insertion into the plantar aspect of the base of the first MT.) On physical examination dorsiflexion is markedly reduced or absent. If the proximal phalanx is reduced onto the MT head by translating it upward (similar to the MP Lachman test), dorsiflexion returns to the joint.

*Conservative management* involves making an orthosis with an elevation beneath the base of the great toe to place it in alignment with the head of the first MT. This sometimes works, but usually surgery is required to bring the first MT down into proper alignment with the proximal phalanx.

The *operation* I prefer in this situation is a horizontal crescentic plantar flexion osteotomy transfixed with crossed Kirschner wires (K-wires) at the site of the deformity. It is usually done in conjunction with a cheilectomy (Fig. 3-2).

### The lesser metatarsophalangeal joints

Dorsal impingement in these joints is usually associated with *Freiberg's disease.*[31]

This condition is no more common in athletes and dancers than it is in the general population. One should remember, however, that it can be symptomatic for as long as 6 months before it appears on x-ray

and should be considered in unexplained metatarsalgia in young patients. A bone scan will usually confirm the diagnosis before radiographic changes. Freiberg's infraction comes in the following four variations:[31]

**Type I.** The head of the MT dies and then heals by "creeping substitution" (Phemister[24]). In this form it may heal completely, with little or no collapse, leaving the articular surface intact and almost as good as it was before the event occurred, surgery often is not necessary.

**Type II.** The head collapses during revascularization, the articular surface settles and remains intact, but peripheral osteophytes form along the dorsal margin of the joint, limiting dorsiflexion. This type is amenable to a dorsal clean-out (cheilectomy), which should leave the joint intact and restore dorsiflexion. (The surgeon should remember to remove more bone than he/she thinks is necessary when this operation is performed.)

**Type III.** The head collapses and the articular surface loosens and falls into the joint, leaving the joint totally destroyed. Obviously simply removing the osteophytes will not suffice in this case—an arthroplasty is required. All the necrotic bone must be excised from the MT head and all the dorsal osteophytes must be removed. Usually the plantar portion of the head is left when this has been done. The surgeon should be generous in the excision to have full dorsiflexion later, but the entire MT head should not be removed. Either a dorsiflexion osteotomy of the MT head or a capsular arthroplasty, similar to the one described for use in the first MP joint, can be useful in this situation.

**Type IV.** Multiple heads are involved in the process (Fig. 3-3). This type is rare and may actually be a form of epiphyseal dysplasia. Each MT head must be evaluated and treated individually.

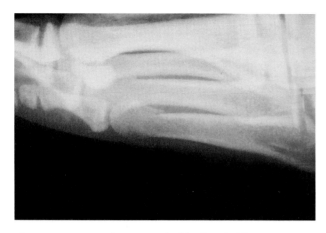

**Fig. 3-4.** Boxer's fracture of the distal fifth metatarsal *(arrow)*.

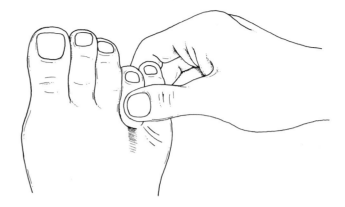

**Fig. 3-5.** Lachman test of the MP joint.

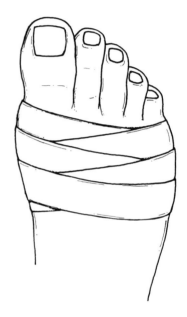

**Fig. 3-6.** Taping to control MP instability.

A Freiberg-like syndrome can occur in the fifth MT head following an undisplaced, or minimally displaced, fracture of the distal MT shaft, similar to the "boxer's fracture" of the fifth metacarpal (Fig. 3-4).

**Lesser MP joint instability**

Metatarsalgia is not common in the young, healthy athletic population. When it is encountered, one should suspect either early Freiberg's disease or MP instability.[31] This subtle problem often goes unrecognized because the x-rays and bone scan are normal. The patient presents with isolated metatarsalgia. There is plantar tenderness under the MT head and dorsal tenderness where the phalanx subluxes on top of the head when the patient relevés or goes up on the ball of the foot. The subluxed phalanx pushes the head of the metatarsal downward, producing the metatarsalgia, the so-called "dropped metatarsal." It is easily recognized on physical examination if one remembers to observe for it. The Lachman test of the MP joint will be positive.[31] The base of the proximal phalanx is grasped in the fingers and an anteroposterior force is applied. The instability is easily recognized when the phalanx dislocates on top of the MT head (Fig. 3-5).

*Conservative treatment* consists of padding to unweight the painful MT head and taping or wearing a toe retainer to try to control the instability (Fig. 3-6). It often is a frustrating situation for the dancer/athlete because they do not want to undergo surgery, but once the ligaments and plantar plate are stretched, they can be tightened again only by surgery. The *surgical options* for this problem in a dancer are tricky. The usual operations for this condition (stabilizing procedures such as the Girdlestone-Taylor operation[18]) are appropriate for athletes because they stabilize the joint but they also limit dorsiflexion—an unacceptable solution for dancers, gymnasts, and so on. I have

had success in a limited number of dancers and athletes with a resection arthroplasty, especially in the fourth MP joint—a joint that seems especially prone to this problem. As previously noted, one should not remove too much of the proximal phalanx (¼ to ⅓ at most), remove the plantar condyles of the MT head, use a toe wire, and remove it early (2 weeks).

**Idiopathic synovitis**

Idiopathic synovitis[30] is characterized by MP swelling, the so-called "sausage toe." Its cause is controversial. (It is not usually caused by systemic inflammatory diseases, but of course these need to be ruled out.) It is usually associated with laxity of the joint and MP instability. Whether the looseness irritates the joint and leads to chronic synovitis or whether the synovitis loosens the joint is not known. Conservative therapy involves stabilizing the joint by taping or toe retainers (Fig. 3-6), reduced activities, and antiinflammatory medication and, if necessary, one or two (at most!) intraarticular injections of steroids. If this fails, exploration and appropriate surgery is indicated. Often at surgery one sees articular damage that explains why the joint did not respond to conservative therapy. Surgical choices include (1) extensor tendon lengthening with resection of the plantar condyles of the MT head, (2) Girdlestone-Taylor[18] procedure, (3) DuVries-type arthroplasty,[18] and (4) resection arthroplasty with partial webbing to the adjacent phalanx.

### Medial midfoot impingements

True impingements in the midfoot are rare. Occasionally accessory ossicles can be seen between the bases of the MTs or the cuneiforms; symptoms may warrant their removal. These bones, more often than not, will be asymptomatic.

An isolated osteophyte on the dorsum of the midfoot can occasionally cause entrapment of the deep peroneal nerve or irritation of the EHL tendon as they pass over it. In these cases removal may be necessary.

The painful accessory navicular is not due to impingement and is discussed elsewhere.

### Lateral midfoot impingements

In the lateral midfoot three related conditions are a combination of impingement and subluxation: (1) derangement of the cuboid base of the fourth and fifth MT, (2) cuboid subluxation, and (3) sinus tarsi syndrome.

*Subluxation of the cuboid*[19] and derangement of the cuboid base of the fourth and fifth MTs are frequently seen together. The subluxing cuboid is a common but poorly recognized condition. It presents as lateral midfoot pain and an inability to "work through" the foot. Pressing on the plantar surface of the cuboid in a dorsal direction is painful. The normal dorsal/plantar joint play is reduced or absent when compared with the uninjured side. (Because of this immobility, the condition has sometimes been referred to as a *locked cuboid.*) Frequently there is a shallow depression on the dorsal surface and a palpable fullness on the plantar aspect of the cuboid and subtle forefoot valgus. Documentation by x-ray, CT scan, or MRI, is difficult due to the normal variations found in the relationship between the cuboid and its surrounding structures. The diagnosis must be made on the basis of the history and physical findings. Treatment involves recognition of the pathology and manual reduction by a therapist or physician familiar with the condition, and follow-up to be certain that it remains in place. Therapists and orthopedists involved in the care of athletes and dancers should be aware of the subluxed cuboid and be able to recognize it when it

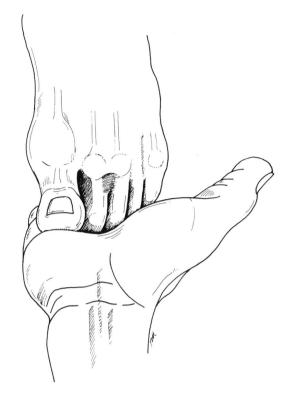

**Fig. 3-7.** A "dropped" fourth metatarsal head due to elevation of its base. (From Marshall PM, Hamilton WG: Cuboid subluxation in ballet dancers, *Am J Sports Med* 20:170, 1992.)

occurs. When the cuboid subluxes plantarward, the base of the fourth and/or fifth MTs are frequently elevated, causing the head of the fourth MT to be depressed (Fig. 3-7, Table 3-1).

There are usually two types of cuboid subluxations: acute and chronic/recurrent. Treatment consists of recognition and manual reduction by a therapist familiar with the condition. The cuboid must then be held in place by taping and padding for several weeks to prevent recurrence. If the subluxation has gone unrecognized, and the joint has been subluxed for any length of time, reduction can be difficult. The forefoot valgus must be corrected and the lateral column lengthened manually before the reduction can be performed. In the chronic condition, it may not be possible to keep the cuboid reduced if it goes in and out at random. In these cases athletes can often be taught to reduce the subluxation themselves (Fig. 3-8).

*Sinus tarsi syndrome*[30] is a controversial condition that produces pain deep in the sinus tarsi that increases with activity and is exacerbated by impact (jumping and running) and pronation. It frequently, but not always, is a sequel to a sprained ankle. On physical examination there is discrete tenderness, or a "trigger point" deep in the sinus tarsi, and forceful abduction-pronation of the heel and midfoot may be

**Table 3-1.** Cuboid subluxation

| Symptoms | Signs |
|---|---|
| Lateral midfoot pain | Tender plantar mass |
| Weakness in push-off | Decreased joint play |
| Inability to "work through" the foot | Shallow depression over the cuboid |
| Function limited by pain | Subtle forefoot abduction |

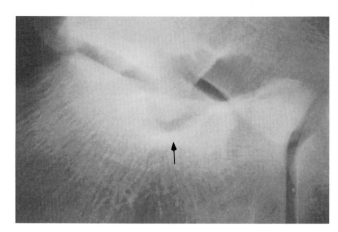

**Fig. 3-9.** Sinus tarsi syndrome; note osteophytes *(arrow)*.

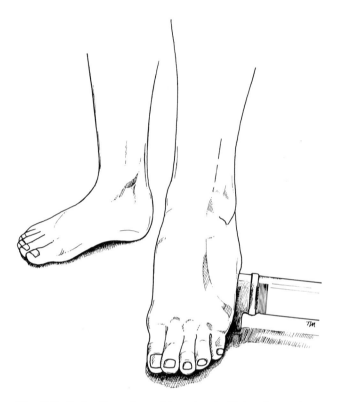

**Fig. 3-8.** Reduction of a subluxed cuboid by the patient.

painful. The condition can usually be confirmed with an injection of ½ cc of lidocaine into the trigger point. If the pain is relieved by the local anesthetic, a second injection of ¼ to ½ cc of corticosteroids can often be highly effective. The condition is thought to have several etiologies: (1) soft tissue entrapment, (2) osteophyte impingement (Fig. 3-9), and (3) neural entrapment (motor nerve to the extensor digitorum brevis [EDB]).[15] It can be difficult to differentiate this syndrome from subtalar dysfunction, and osteophytes can be found in the sinus tarsi that are not causing symptoms. The two areas are anatomically close together. One of the best ways to differentiate one from the other is to pay close attention to subtalar motion. Mann and Coughlin have shown[18] how important subtalar motion is to normal foot mechanics. Subtle loss of this motion, such as arthrofibrosis of the subtalar joint from bleeding into the joint in conjunc-

tion with an ankle sprain, can cause residual symptoms after the sprain has healed.

*Conservative treatment* consists of antiinflammatory medication, physical therapy, a medial heel wedge or arch support to open up the sinus tarsi, and, if necessary, the previously mentioned cortisone injection. If symptoms persist, and the diagnosis has been confirmed with lidocaine, surgical exploration and clean-out is indicated. This is one area where an injection—if it can be placed in the right spot—is often dramatically effective and will avoid surgery in many cases. Finally, the sinus tarsi syndrome is often found in conjunction with lateral ankle ligament laxity and, in these cases, sinus tarsi exploration and debridement should be considered if ankle ligament reconstruction is planned.

**The ankle**

When considering ankle impingement, one should remember the basic anatomy of the ankle. The talus sits sidesaddle upon the os calcis so that the axis of the talus is roughly in line with the first web space of the foot and the axis of the os calcis is lined up with the fourth web space (Fig. 3-10). In *dorsiflexion*, bony impingement occurs anteromedially between the neck of the talus and the anterior lip of the tibia. In plantar flexion bony impingement occurs *posterolaterally* between the os calcis and the posterior lip of the tibia. Therefore anteromedial and posterolateral problems are usually associated with bony impingement, whereas anterolateral and posteromedial problems are usually soft tissue in origin rather than bony (there is no bony impingement in these areas).

*Anterior ankle* is an extremely common location for impingement, but impingements can be found in all quadrants around the ankle: anterior, lateral, posterior, and medial.

**Anterior (medial, central, lateral).** *Anteromedial* ankle pain often comes from impingement of the

Superior view

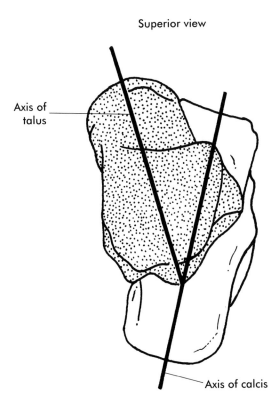

Axis of
talus

Axis of calcis

**Fig. 3-10.** Axis of talus versus axis of os calcis.

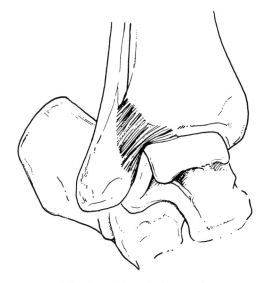

**Fig. 3-11.** Basset's ligament.

anterior portion of the medial malleolus against an impingement spur on the medial shoulder of the talus. This spur is hard to see on an x-ray because it cannot be visualized on standard lateral radiographs. It can often be palpated on physical examination and should be looked for in any anterior ankle clean-out. It is easy to miss!

*Anterocentral* is the location of the classic anterior ankle impingement. It comes in the following four types:

1. *Spurs are primarily on the lip of the tibia* — This type is ideal for arthroscopic debridement. Under direct vision the lip of the tibia can be removed fairly easily with a thin osteotome. Care should be taken not to damage the dome of the talus either by holding the ankle in maximum dorsiflexion or by using an osteotome with blunt edges, as described by Scranton and McDermott.[28]

2. *Spurs are primarily on the neck of the talus* — This type is more difficult to perform with the arthroscope, because the osteophytes are often within the capsular insertion on the neck of the talus, and it is necessary to strip off the capsule distally to visualize the pathology. It is easy to miss some of the osteophytes, so an x-ray may be needed at the end of the case to assure adequate removal.

3. *Spurs are present on both the lip of the tibia and the neck of the talus,* sometimes with loose bodies that have broken off the osteophytes. This type is common and is the most difficult to deal with. In the early 1980s I thought professional dancers would return to dancing sooner if their anterior clean-outs could be done with the arthroscope. I found that, in all but the most uncomplicated cases, it took 3 months for them to return whether the operation was performed with the arthroscope or with a small anterior arthrotomy. Use of the arthroscope was often taking over an hour and required an x-ray to be certain that I had not missed anything, whereas the arthrotomy took 30 to 40 minutes. I thought that I was doing a better job faster with the open technique. I have therefore gone back to a small anterior arthrotomy on these complex cases.

4. *Multiple anterior osteophytes can be present secondary to frank osteoarthritis of the ankle* — Anterior clean-out in these cases is of questionable effectiveness and probably should not be performed for this condition.

*Anterolateral* ankle pain is not usually due to bony impingement, because the tibia and talus do not come together in this location. Difficulties in this area are usually due to one of two recently described conditions: Basset's ligament and Ferkel's phenomenon.

*Basset's ligament*[1] is an abnormal distal slip of the anterior tibiofibular ligament running down so far on the lateral malleolus that the lateral shoulder of the talus impinges against it when the ankle is plantar flexed (Fig. 3-11). It is difficult to diagnose but, when present, can be resected with the arthroscope.

*Ferkel's phenomenon*[2] is a build-up of scar tissue and synovitis in the anterolateral gutter of the ankle, usually following trauma. It causes symptoms similar to Basset's ligament and is also amenable to arthroscopic debridement.

*Anterior syndesmosis pathology* is usually not the result of impingement, but can cause anterolateral ankle pain that is exacerbated by dorsiflexion of the ankle as the wide portion of the talus spreads the malleoli and places tension on the anterior tibiofibular ligament:

1. A sprain of the syndesmosis, the "high ankle sprain" can sometimes take an extraordinarily long time to heal.
2. The "Tillot" fragment is an avulsion fracture of the insertion of the ligament into the tibia. On rare occasions the avulsion can occur on the fibular side.
3. Synovial hernias into rents in the tibiofibular ligament have been described.[20]

*Lateral ankle* can be a complex site of pain and discomfort, and an accurate diagnosis in this area can be difficult. Symptoms in this area often have their onset following ankle sprains. The original trauma can often be mild—for example, a first-degree sprain with no resultant lateral instability. *Cuboid subluxation* and the *sinus tarsi syndrome* were discussed earlier. Other conditions to consider are:

1. The *"meniscoid" of the ankle*[33] is thought to be soft tissue trapped between the lateral shoulder of the talus and the lateral malleolus. It can usually be seen and corrected by arthroscopy.
2. *An avulsion fracture of the anterior process of the os calcis*[11] is not an impingement. It is an avulsion fracture at the origin of the EDB. It can usually be diagnosed on physical examination by the specific tenderness at the anatomical site or pain with pronation-supination of the forefoot. Persistent symptoms may warrant excision of the fragment (Fig. 3-12).
3. *Lateral process fracture of the talus*[10] can also cause impingement beneath the lateral malleolus.
4. *Accessory ossicle, the os subfibulare,* which had been asymptomatic, can be loosened by injury and become symptomatic.
5. *Avulsion fracture at the tip of the fibula* can become trapped in or under the lateral ankle joint and become symptomatic. The bony fragment is often in the insertion of the calcaneofibular ligament. If it is small, it should be excised and the stump of the ligament sutured into the tip of the lateral malleolus. If it is large, it can often be reattached with a screw or K-wire.

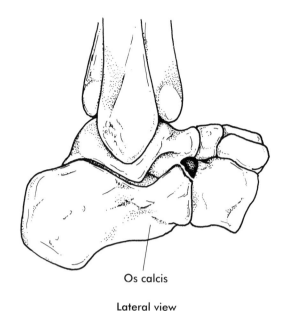

Os calcis

Lateral view

**Fig. 3-12.** Fracture of the anterior process of the os calcis.

Infrequently the same situation can be found at the anterior edge of the lateral malleolus at the insertion of the anterior talofibular (ATF) ligament (Fig. 3-13).

In ankle sprains usually the ATF ligament either is avulsed from the bone or tears in its midsubstance. On rare occasions it can avulse its insertion in the bone and become symptomatic.

6. *Impingement under the tip of the fibula following os calcis fractures* is a common complication of this injury. Often it is difficult to differentiate the impingement pain from subtalar joint pain. A small injection of a local anesthetic beneath the tip of the lateral malleolus, but not into the subtalar joint, can indicate how much of the pain is coming from the impingement versus an arthritic subtalar joint. If the pain relief with the local anesthetic is dramatic, it might be worthwhile to excise this portion of the os calcis before recommending a subtalar fusion (Fig. 3-14).
7. *Peroneal dysfunction,* while not an impingement, can also produce pain in this area and should be considered in the differential diagnosis. This includes peroneal subluxation, longitudinal splits in the tendons,[26] and even fracture of the os peroneum with retraction of the peroneus longus[32] (Fig. 3-15).

*Posterior ankle pain* is common in athletes such as dancers, gymnasts, and ice skaters who must work in the equinus position. A review of posterior ankle anatomy will help explain the two common pain syndromes found in this area (Tables 3-2, 3-3). The

Posterior view

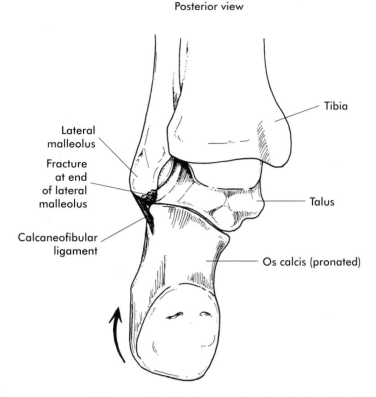

**Fig. 3-13.** Fracture of the tip of the fibula trapped under the lateral malleolus.

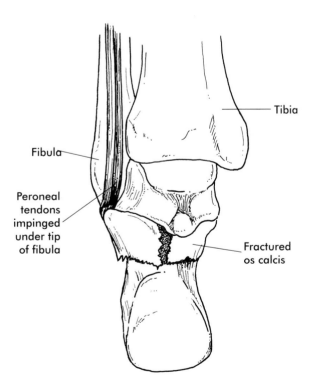

**Fig. 3-14.** Impingement under the tip of the fibula, following a fracture of the os calcis.

posterior aspect of the talus has two tubercles: the medial and the lateral (Fig. 3-16). The lateral tubercle is the origin of the posterior talofibular ligament. It can be small or large. When it is large it is referred to as the *posterior process* of the talus or a Stieda process. In 7% to 11% of people this posterior process is separate from the talus and connected by a fibrous synostosis; it is then called the *os trigonum (OT)*.[3] The OT is the second most common accessory bone in the foot, the accessory navicular being the most common.[27] Bony impingement can occur posterolaterally when the trigonal process or OT is compressed between the posterior lip of the tibia and the superior portion of the os calcis in extreme plantar flexion (Fig. 3-17).

The flexor hallucis longus (FHL) tendon passes through the fibroosseus tunnel between the two posterior tubercles as it runs from its origin on the proximal fibula (laterally) to its insertion in the distal phalanx of the hallux (medially) (Fig. 3-18). Chronic tendinitis and dysfunction within this tunnel can produce posterior medial pain, "dancer's tendinitis."[4-7] Thus there are usually two sources of posterior ankle pain: lateral (trigonal impingement) and medial (flexor hallucis longus [FHL] tendinitis).

**Posterolateral ankle pain.** The *posterior impingement syndrome of the ankle,* or *talar compression syndrome,*[6,12,25] is the natural consequence of full

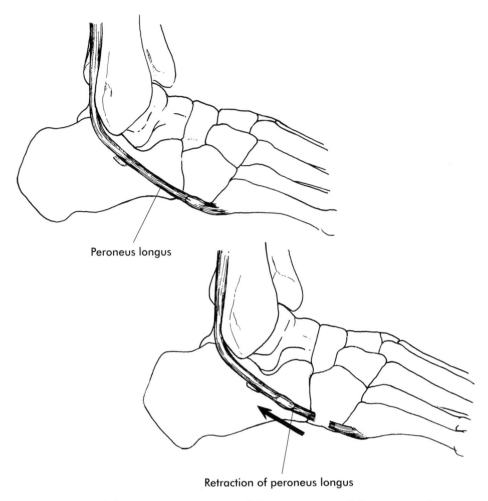

Peroneus longus

Retraction of peroneus longus

**Fig. 3-15.** Retraction of the os peroneum *(arrow)*, following rupture of the peroneus longus tendon.

weight-bearing in maximal plantar flexion of the ankle in the demipointe or full pointe position, especially if an OT or trigonal process is present. It presents as posterolateral pain in the back of the ankle when the posterior lip of the tibia closes against the superior border of the os calcis. It can be confirmed on physical examination by (1) tenderness behind the peroneal tendons in back of the lateral malleolus (it is often mistaken for peroneal tendinitis) and (2) pain with forced passive plantar flexion of the ankle, the *"plantar flexion sign."*

This syndrome is often, but not always, associated with an OT or trigonal process in the back of the ankle. As previously noted, the posterior aspect of the talus normally has two tubercles: the medial and lateral. Between the two tubercles lies the fibroosseus tunnel and the FHL tendon (Fig. 3-19). Most people who have an OT are not aware of its presence, and the posterior impingement syndrome is rare in most athletes. In dancers it may or may not be symptomatic, and the degree of symptoms is not always related to its size.

Large OTs can be minimally symptomatic and small ones can sometimes be disabling. Usually the symptoms are mild and, on the whole, the OT is more often asymptomatic than symptomatic. Many world-famous ballerinas have asymptomatic OTs, and they work with them without any trouble. It is important to stress this fact to the dancer when discussing the problem, because the condition is frequently overdiagnosed by paramedical practitioners who may recommend surgery unnecessarily, perhaps due to the dramatic appearance of the bone on the x-ray. It is best seen on a lateral view of the ankle en pointe or in full plantar flexion (Fig. 3-17). The diagnosis can be confirmed, if necessary, by injecting 0.5 cc of a local anesthetic into the posterior soft tissues behind the peroneal tendons. If the pain that was present is relieved by this small injection, the diagnosis is almost certain.

Treatment of the posterior impingement syndrome should be graded. The first step, similar to tendinitis, is modification of activities ("Don't do what hurts!"), NSAIDS (if the dancer is over age 16), and physical

Posterior view of talus                    Superior view of talus

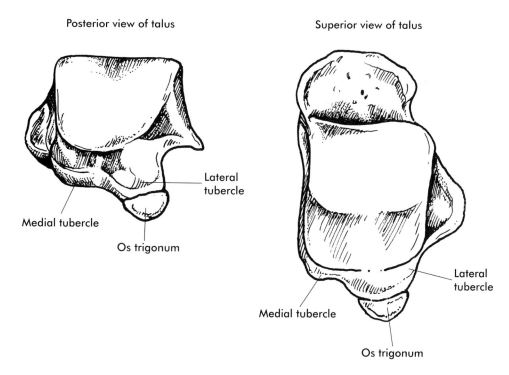

Fig. 3-16. Anatomy of the posterior talus.

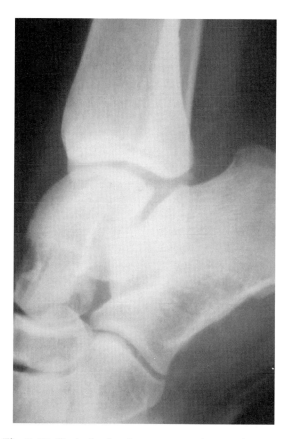

Fig. 3-17. Posterior impingement on the os trigonum.

therapy. In cases where this approach has failed, or the symptoms recur, an injection of ¼ to ½ cc of a mixture of a long- and a short-acting corticosteroid can often give dramatic and permanent relief of symptoms. Before injecting the steroid preparation, the diagnosis should be confirmed with a local anesthetic. If the local anesthetic does not relieve the symptoms, there is no point in injecting the steroids. It should be stressed that the OT is not usually a surgical problem; most dancers with an OT do not need to have it removed surgically.

Occasionally OT does cause enough disability to warrant surgical excision, but, as with most elective surgery, it is indicated only after the failure of conservative treatment in a serious dancer at least 16 years of age or older. If the problem is an isolated OT with no medial symptoms, it can be approached posterolaterally between the FHL and the peroneals (with the sural nerve protected). Not infrequently there is a combined problem of FHL tendinitis and posterior impingement. In these patients the postero-medial approach is used so that the neurovascular (NV) bundle can be isolated and protected. A tenolysis of the FHL and removal of the adjacent OT can then be performed safely.

Other causes of posterolateral ankle pain include:

1. A previously asymptomatic OT may become persistently symptomatic following an ankle sprain due to disruption of its ligamentous connections and a subtle shift in position.

Medial view

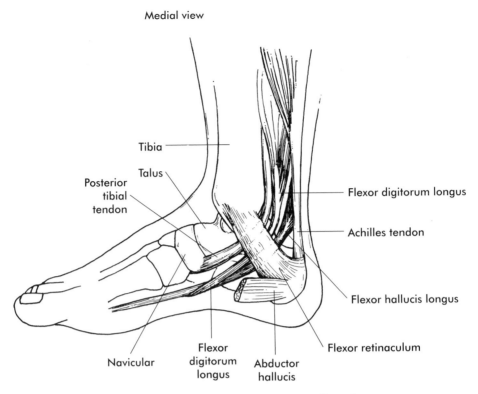

**Fig. 3-18.** Medial anatomy of the flexor hallucis longus.

2. Posterior impingement can follow an ankle sprain that stretches out the lateral ligaments that hold the talus under the tibia in the relevé.[7] As the talus slips forward, the posterior lip of the tibia comes to rest upon the os calcis. The treatment for this type of posterior impingement is to tighten the lateral ankle ligaments (preferably by the Brostrom-Gould procedure).[9] If the drawer sign can be corrected, the posterior impingement usually disappears.

3. A *posterior pseudomenisus* or plica in the posterior ankle,[7] with or without an OT, can cause the posterior impingement syndrome in the absence of an OT or loose ligaments. We have seen bucket-handle tears in this structure causing locking and other mechanical symptoms more often seen in the knee than the ankle.

### Excision of the os trigonum using the lateral approach

Under anesthesia the patient is placed in the lateral decubitus position with a pneumatic tourniquet in the leg or thigh over cast padding. (Because dancers have increased external rotation of the hip, it is extremely difficult to perform this operation with the patient supine.) A curvilinear incision is made at the level of the posterior ankle mortise in line with the posterior border of the peroneal sheath. The sural nerve is identified or carefully avoided in the subcutaneous tissues. The dissection is carried down in the interval between the peroneal tendons laterally and the muscle belly of the FHL medially. A posterior capsular incision is then made with the ankle in neutral or slight dorsiflexion. The OT or trigonal process (a Stieda process) can be found on the superior surface of the posterior talus just on the lateral side of the FHL tendon between the ankle and subtalar joints. It has attachments on all its sides (1) *superior*—the posterior capsule of the talocrural joint; (2) *inferior*—the posterior talocalcaneal ligament, at times thick and fibrous; (3) *medial*—the FHL tunnel with its sheath; and (4) *lateral*—the origin of the posterior talofibular ligament.

The bone can be removed by circumferential dissection. Be careful not to stray too far medially—the posterior tibial (PT) nerve rests upon the FHL tunnel. The proximal entrance of this FHL tunnel can be opened if there are muscle fibers attaching distally on the FHL tendon that crowd into the tunnel when the hallux is brought into dorsiflexion (see Tomasen's sign[32]). One should not dissect medial to the FHL tendon without adequate visualization; there are branches of the PT artery that can bleed. Check for loose bodies; I have found them even in the FHL tunnel. The foot should be brought into maximum plantar flexion to look for any residual impingement.

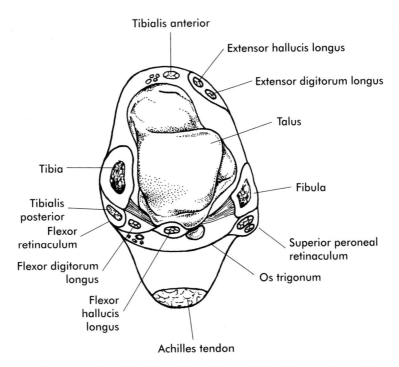

**Fig. 3-19.** Superior view of relationship of flexor hallucis longus to os trigonum.

At times it is necessary to remove more of the posterior lateral tubercle. Frequently there is a facet on the cephalad portion of the os calcis that articulated with the OT, and this can be large enough to impinge against the posterior lip of the tibia after the OT has been removed. Bone wax should be used to cover raw bony surfaces. Careful hemostasis will prevent a post-operative hematoma that can delay recovery and make early motion difficult for the patient. A layered closure is then performed with catgut stitches. I usually close the wound with a running absorbable suture and Steri-strips. The patient is placed in a bulky dressing and weight bearing with crutches is begun as tolerated. The dancer is encouraged to swim and progress to barre exercises as discomfort subsides. Average return to full dancing is 2 to 3 months.

**Posteromedial ankle pain.** *Tendinitis of the flexor hallucis longus tendon* (FHL) behind the medial malleolus of the ankle is so common in dancers that it is known as *dancer's tendinitis*.[4-8] It is less common in athletes and, when present, is often misdiagnosed as PT or Achilles tendinitis. The FHL is the "Achilles tendon of the foot" for the dancer. It passes through a fibroosseus tunnel behind the talus like a rope through a pulley. As it passes through this pulley, it is easily strained. When strained, rather than moving smoothly in the pulley, it begins to bind. This binding causes irritation and swelling, which, in turn, causes further binding, irritation, and swelling—setting up the familiar cycle: because it is swollen and irritated,

it binds; and because it binds, it is swollen and irritated. If a nodule or partial tear is present, triggering of the big toe may occur—*hallux saltans* (Fig. 3-20) or the tendon may become completely frozen in the sheath causing *pseudohallux rigidus*. This tendinitis typically responds to the usual conservative measures. Rest is an important component of the therapy so that the chronic cycle previously described can be broken. NSAIDs can help, but they should be used only as part of an overall treatment program and not as medicine to kill the pain so that the patient can continue dancing and ignore the symptoms. As with other tendon problems, steroid injections should be avoided. On some occasions, in professional or high-level amateur dancers and athletes, FHL tendinitis may be recurrent and disabling. In these cases operative tenolysis may be indicated (but only after the failure of conservative therapy). The situation is similar to De Quervain's stenosing tenosynovitis in the wrist.

FHL tendinitis usually occurs behind the medial malleolus, but it can occasionally be found at the knot of Henry under the base of the first MT where the FDL crosses over the FHL, and under the head of the first MT where it passes between the sesamoids. A fibrous subtalar coalition may be present in the posteromedial ankle mimicking FHL tendinitis or tarsal tunnel syndrome. This condition should be suspected when there is less than normal subtalar motion on physical examination.

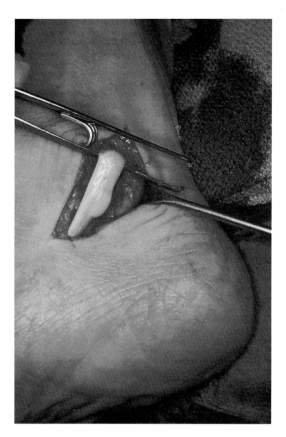

**Fig. 3-20.** A nodule in the FHL tendon causing triggering of the great toe; "hallux saltans."

The differential diagnosis of posterior ankle pain includes the following:

1. Posterior process (Shepherd's)[28] fracture; hairline, or stress
2. FHL tendinitis (dancer's tendinitis)
3. Peroneal tendinitis
4. Posteromedial localized talocalcaneal coalition
5. Osteoid osteoma

Operative treatment is indicated when conservative therapy has failed. The posterior clean-out can be performed from either the medial or lateral side of the Achilles tendon. The lateral approach should be used if the patient has an isolated posterior impingement without a history of FHL tendinitis or medial difficulties. A medial incision is indicated if they have a combined problem of FHL tendinitis and posterior impingement or if they primarily have FHL tendinitis with an incidental OT that you wish to remove along with a FHL tenolysis. The medial incision is safer and more utilitarian because you can work safely on the lateral side from the medial, but it is dangerous to work medially from the lateral approach, because you cannot isolate and protect the NV bundle from that side.

**Table 3-2.** FHL tendonitis vs. posterior impingement of the ankle

| FHL tendonitis | Posterior impingement |
| --- | --- |
| Posteromedial | Posterolateral |
| Tenderness over FHL tendon | Tenderness behind fibula |
| Pain or triggering with motion of the hallux | Pain with plantar flexion of the ankle |
| ± Tomasen's sign[33] | Plantar flexion sign |
| Mistaken for PT tendinitis | Mistaken for peroneal tendinitis |

### Tenolysis of the flexor hallucis longus and excision of the os trigonum from the medial side

This procedure can be performed with the patient supine because dancers usually have increased external rotation of the hip and knee that allows easy visualization of the posterior ankle from the medial side. A bloodless field is desirable, so I use a tourniquet on the distal thigh over cast padding. For this reason, the procedure cannot be performed with the patient under local anesthesia or an ankle block. A curvilinear incision is made over the NV bundle behind the medial malleolus beginning just above the superior border of the os calcis and continuing to a line just posterior to the tip of the medial malleolus (Fig. 3-21, *A*). This incision should be made carefully. The deep fascia and lacinate ligament in this area are often thin. If the incision is made too enthusiastically, the surgeon may find himself in the midst of the NV bundle before he had planned to be there. The deep fascia is then divided carefully to avoid damage to the artery and nerve beneath it.

At this point you must decide whether to go in front of the bundle or behind it. The posterior approach can take you into the variable neural branches to the os calcis. It is safer to go anterior to the bundle. All branches of the tibial nerve at this level go posteriorly, so the safe plane is between the posterior aspect of the medial malleolus and the NV bundle. The bundle can be taken down off the back of the malleolus by blunt dissection (Fig. 3-21, *B*). Often there are several small vessels here that need to be ligated, but once the bundle is mobilized it can be held with a blunt retractor such as a loop or Army-Navy retractor (never with a rake) (Fig. 3-21, *C*). The PT nerve is much larger than one expects; it is usually about the size of a pencil (Fig. 3-21, *D*). The surgeon should examine the NV bundle carefully. There are frequent anatomical variations within the tarsal tunnel. Both the nerve and the artery divide into medial and lateral plantar

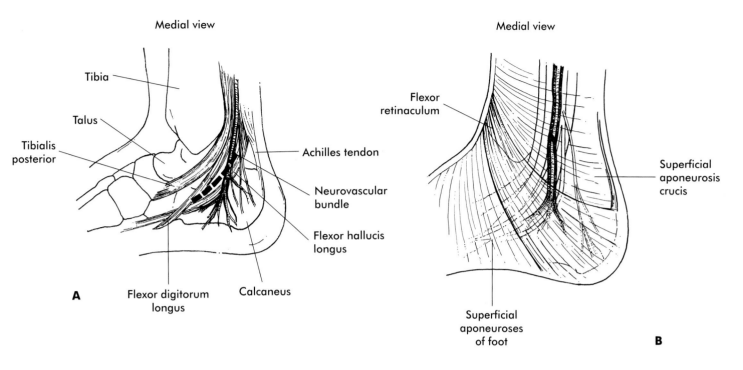

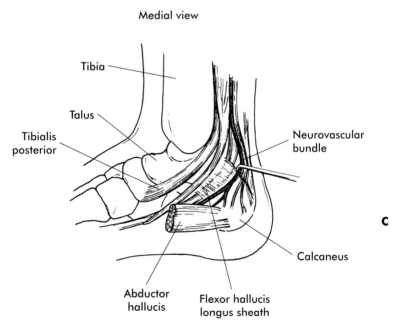

**Fig. 3-21. A,** Posteromedial incision. **B,** Neurovascular bundle beneath a thin layer of fascia. **C,** Neurovascular bundle taken down from the posterior medial malleolus.

*Continued.*

branches as they leave the tarsal canal. It is not unusual for one or both to divide above this area, leading to reduplication within the tunnel. There may also be reduplication of the tendons—the flexor hallucis accessorius. With the NV bundle retracted posteriorly, the FHL is easily identified by moving the

hallux (Fig. 3-21, *E*). The thin fascia overlying the muscle fibers of the FHL is opened proximally, and a tenolysis is performed by opening the sheath from proximal to distal (Fig. 3-21, *F*). Usually it is stenotic and tough, and the FHL can often be seen entering it at an acute angle. Care should be taken distally

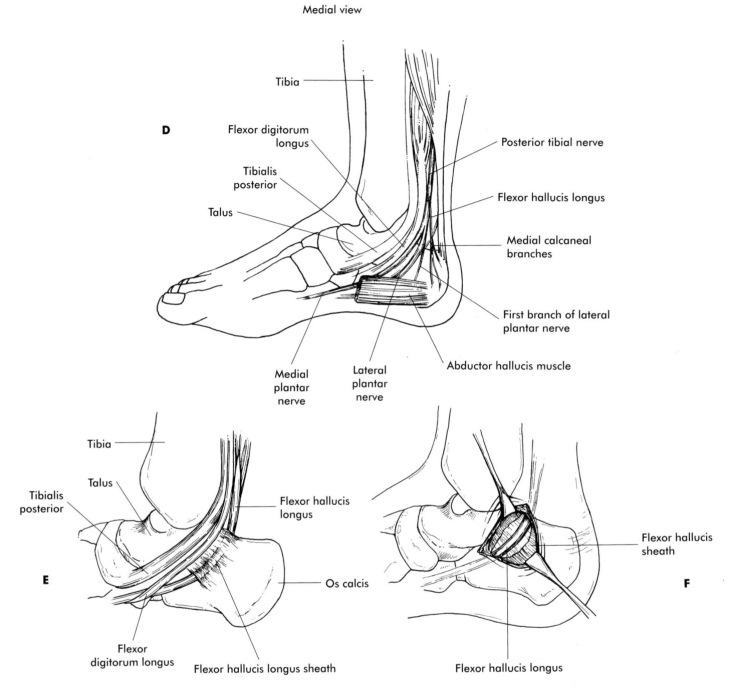

Medial view

Tibia

**D**

Flexor digitorum longus

Tibialis posterior

Talus

Posterior tibial nerve

Flexor hallucis longus

Medial calcaneal branches

First branch of lateral plantar nerve

Abductor hallucis muscle

Medial plantar nerve

Lateral plantar nerve

Tibia

Talus

Tibialis posterior

Flexor hallucis longus

**E**

Os calcis

Flexor digitorum longus

Flexor hallucis longus sheath

Flexor hallucis sheath

**F**

Flexor hallucis longus

**Fig. 3-21, cont'd. D,** Posterior tibial nerve. **E,** FHL sheath. **F,** FHL sheath opened.

because the FHL tunnel and the nerve are close together here. As the tenolysis approaches the area of the sustentaculum tali, the sheath thins so that there no longer seems to be anything to divide. The tendon should by retracted with a blunt retractor and inspected for nodules or longitudinal tears. If present, these should be debrided carefully or repaired. At this point the FHL can be retracted posteriorly with the NV bundle. The OT or trigonal process will be found just

on the lateral side of the FHL tunnel. If the posterior aspect of the talus cannot be visualized, a capsulotomy should be performed. If there is difficulty in visualizing the OT, it helps to identify the superior border of the os calcis, and the subtalar joint (by moving the os calcis into adduction and abduction). The subtalar joint is then dissected from medial to lateral, and this will take you underneath the OT. Once identified, it can be removed by circumferential

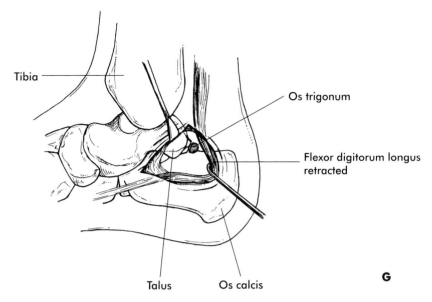

**Fig. 3-21, cont'd. G,** Removal of the os trigonum.

**Table 3-3.** Medial versus lateral posterior ankle pain in athletes and dancers

| Posteromedial | Posterolateral |
| --- | --- |
| FHL tendinitis | Posterior impingement (OT syndrome) |
| Soleus syndrome | Fx. trigonal process (Shepherd's fracture) |
| PT | Peroneal tendinitis |
| Posteromedial fibrous tarsal coalition | Pseudomeniscus syndrome |

dissection (Fig. 3-21, *G*). Care should be taken to stay on the bone when performing this part of the procedure. This can sometimes be somewhat difficult, especially if the OT is large. Once it is removed, the posterior ankle joint should be inspected for remnants, bone fragments or loose bodies, soft tissue entrapment, or a large articular facet on the upper surface of the os calcis that articulated with the OT. If this is present, it may need to be removed with a thin osteotome. (The FHL sheath is *not* closed.) The wound is then irrigated, checked for any residual impingement by putting the foot in maximum plantar flexion and closed in layers with plain catgut. I begin weight bearing as tolerated with crutches as soon as possible and proceed with swimming and physical therapy when the wound is healed. If the tenolysis is performed without excision of the OT, the recovery period is about 6 weeks. If the OT is removed along with the tenolysis, the recovery time is 8 to 12 weeks. It is important to get patients moving early to prevent stiffness. In dancers with a rather large OT it is

necessary to warn them that, once it is removed, the ankle doesn't just drop down into maximum plantar flexion. They must realize that the bone has been there since they were born and removing it does not lead to immediate motion. The increased plantar flexion is obtained slowly and can be accompanied by many strange symptoms, both anteriorly and posteriorly, as the soft tissues adjust to the new range of motion.

**THE MEDIAL ANKLE**

PT tendinitis, so common in athletes, is rare in dancers—an example of altered kinesiology producing altered patterns of injury. Working primarily in the equinus position produces less stress on the PT tendon but more on the FHL tendon as it passes through its pulley behind the medial malleolus. In addition, dancers are selected for, and usually have, cavus feet and these are less prone to PT tendonitis. Indeed, more often than not, a dancer diagnosed with PT tendinitis, on careful examination, will be found to have FHL tendinitis instead (dancer's tendonitis).

Medial sprains of the ankle are rare because the medial structures are strong and rigid compared with the lateral ones. Persistent symptoms on the medial side may be due to an unrecognized fracture of the sustentaculum tali that can be picked up on a bone scan, or a localized fibrous tarsal coalition. Sprains of the medial ankle do occur, usually from landing off balance with sudden pronation, but again, this is more likely to produce a sprain of a portion of the deltoid ligament than a strain of the PT tendon, although this can occur. The sprain usually affects the portion of the ligament under tension when the force was applied: the anterior deltoid if the foot was in equinus, the

**Table 3-4.** Differential diagnosis of medial ankle pain in athletes and dancers

| Occurrence | Anatomic location |
| --- | --- |
| Most common | PT tendinitis (athletes) |
| | FHL tendinitis (dancers) |
| Common | Deltoid ligament strain |
| Rare | FDL tendinitis |
| | Soleus syndrome |

middle deltoid if it was plantargrade, and the posterior portion if the foot was in dorsiflexion (rare). An accessory bone, the os subtibiale, may be present in the deep layer of the deltoid; this bone can be involved in the sprain, becoming symptomatic when it had not been before. The treatment of these medial sprains and strains in the acute phase consists of the usual RICE regimen, an Aircast, crutches if necessary, and physical therapy. An x-ray should be taken to rule out bone or epiphyseal injury. Recovery is usually uneventful. Occasionally a trigger point can form in the deltoid, usually around a chip fracture or accessory ossicle. These may require a corticosteroid injection if they do not respond to conservative therapy. Occasionally surgical excision will be necessary. Nodules may form on the EDL or PT tendons following medial strains, but these usually are asymptomatic.

In dancers the most common cause of pain around the medial malleolus comes from "rolling in" (pronating) to obtain proper turnout (Table 3-4). This produces a chronic strain on the deltoid ligament and is one of many overuse syndromes seen in dancers.

Contusion of the medial prominence of the tarsal navicular can occur. This usually happens when one foot is brought forward past the other and, as it passes the navicular, strikes the medial malleolus of the other ankle. These contusions usually heal with symptomatic treatment. On rare occasions a fracture of the medial tubercle can occur or disruption of an accessory navicular. When this occurs, the injury should usually be treated in a short-leg walking cast or cam-walker for 4 to 6 weeks to prevent the injury from becoming chronic.

Strains of the spring ligament and plantar fascia can be mistaken for medial ankle pain, but a careful physical examination should make the diagnosis apparent.

A rare cause of medial ankle pain is an unrecognized fracture of the "colliculus" located on the medial portion of the posterior tibia. This occult injury can be difficult to diagnose. It usually can be documented by a bone scan and CT scan.

Another cause of medial pain just above the medial malleolus is the soleus syndrome.[21] This presents as chronic pain resembling a shinsplint, but is too far distal on the posteromedial tibial metaphysis to be a true shinsplint. It is caused by an abnormal slip in the origin of the soleus muscle. The condition, similar to the compartment syndrome, is much more common in athletes than dancers. It usually responds to conservative therapy. On rare occasions subcutaneous release of the tight band may be necessary.

**REFERENCES**

1. Bassett FH et al: Talar impingement by the anterior-inferior tibiofibular ligament, *J Bone Joint Surg* 72-A:55, 1990.
2. Ferkel RD et al: Arthroscopic treatment of anteriorlateral impingement of the ankle, *Am J Sports Med* 19:440, 1991.
3. Grant JCB: *A method of anatomy*, Baltimore, 1958, Williams & Wilkins.
4. Hamilton WG: *"Dancer's tendonitis" of the FHL tendon*, Durango, CO, 1976, American Orthopedics Society for Sports Medicine.
5. Hamilton WG: Tendonitis about the ankle joint in classical ballet dancers; "Dancer's tendonitis," *J Sports Med* 5:84, 1977.
6. Hamilton WG: Stenosing tenosynovitis of the flexor hallucis longus tendon and posterior impingement upon the os trigonum in ballet dancers, *Foot Ankle* 3:74, 1982.
7. Hamilton WG: *Foot and ankle injuries in dancers*. In Yokum L, editor: *Sports clinics of North America*, Philadelphia, 1988, Williams & Wilkins.
8. Hamilton WG: *Ballet*. In Reider B, editor: *The school-age athlete*, Philadelphia, 1991, WB Saunders.
9. Hamilton WG, Thompson FM, Snow SW: The modified brostrom procedure for lateral ankle instability, *Foot Ankle* 14:1, 1993.
10. Hawkins LG: Fractures of the lateral process of the talus, *J Bone Joint Surg* 52A:991, 1970.
11. Harburn T, Ross H: Avulsion fracture of the anterior calcaneal process, *Phys Sports Med* 15: 1987.
12. Howse AJG: Posterior block of the ankle joint in dancers, *Foot Ankle* 3:81, 1982.
13. Jahss MJ: *Disorders of the foot*, ed 2, Philadelphia, 1988, WB Saunders.
14. Johnson KA: *Surgery of the foot and ankle*, New York, 1989, Raven Press.
15. Kenzora JE, Copeland CE: Nerve entrapment in the sinus tarsi syndrome, *Orthop Consult* 13:1, 1992.
16. Kleiger B: Mechanisms of ankle injury, *Orthop Clin North Am* 5:127, 1974.
17. Kleiger B: Anterior tibiotalar impingement syndromes in dancers, *Foot Ankle* 3:69, 1982.
18. Mann RA, Coughlin MJ: *Surgery of the foot and ankle*, ed 6, St Louis, 1993, Mosby–Year Book.
19. Marshall PM, Hamilton WG: Cuboid subluxation in ballet dancers, *Am J Sports Med* 20:169, 1992.
20. McLaughlin HL: *Trauma*, Philadelphia, 1960, WB Saunders.
21. Michael RH, Holder LE: The soleus syndrome, *Am J Sports Med* 13:87, 1985.
22. Newell S, Woodie A: Cuboid syndrome, *Phys Sports Med* 9:71, 1981.
23. Parkes JC et al: The anterior impingement syndrome of the ankle, *J Trauma* 20:895, 1980.
24. Phemister DB: Necrotic bone and the subsequent changes which it undergoes, *JAMA* 64:211, 1915.

25. Quirk R: The talar compression syndrome in dancers, *Foot Ankle* 3:65, 1982.
26. Sammarco JG, DiRaimondo CV: Chronic peroneus brevis tendon lesions, *Foot Ankle* 9:163, 1989.
27. Sarrafian SK: *Anatomy of the foot and ankle*, Philadelphia, 1983, JB Lippincott.
28. Scranton PE, McDermott JE: Anterior tibiotalar spurs: a comparison of open versus closed debridement, *Foot Ankle* 13: 125, 1992.
29. Shepherd FJ: A hitherto undescribed fracture of the astragalus, *J Anat Physiol* 17:79, 1882.
30. Taillard W et al: The sinus tarsi syndrome, *Int Orthop* 5:117, 1981.
31. Thompson FM, Hamilton WG: Problems of the second metatarso-phalangeal joint, *Orthopedics* 10:83, 1987.
32. Thompson FM, Patterson AH: Rupture of the peroneus longus tendon, report of three cases, *J Bone Joint Surg* 71-A:293, 1989.
33. Tomasen E: *Diseases and injuries of ballet dancers*, Denmark, 1982, Universitetsforlaget I. Arhus.
34. Wolin I et al: Internal derrangement of the talofibular component of the ankle, *Surg Gyn Obs* 91:193, 1950.

# Chapter 4

# Posterior tibial tendon

**Kenneth A. Johnson**

The recognition of pain and disability related to difficulties with the tibialis posterior tendon (TPT) has evolved through the efforts of multiple workers. An important contribution by Kettelcamp and Alexander[10] described this problem of tendon loss; approximately 20 years ago Goldner et al[5] suggested a method of tendon transfer for complete disruption of that tendon. But it has been primarily over the past 10 years that difficulties of the TPT were emphasized, stages clarified, and results of treatment determined.[4,7,8,11-13] This chapter describes the stages of presentation of TPT problems and reviews the evolving concepts of presentation as well as formulates a plan of treatment.

## DIAGNOSIS

The stages of TPT dysfunction[9] are important in understanding the problem as well as leading to a treatment rationale (Table 4-1). In essence stage I represents peritendinitis and/or tendon degeneration but with a normal length of tendon. Stage II represents a still mobile hindfoot but with the tendon elongated and insufficient. Mild deformity may be present. Stage III is an extension of the difficulties, with not only the tendon elongated but the hindfoot deformed in a highly significant valgus deformity, which may be fixed (see Case Study 1 below). Each of these stages is discussed with regard to pain symptoms, physical findings, and changes seen on radiographs.

**Case Study 1.** A 56-year-old patient was seen for pain involving her left ankle. Two years previously she began having pain with her walking activities. There was no specific traumatic incident. After several months she saw an orthopedic surgeon who diagnosed a tibialis posterior tendinitis. Steroids were injected in this area; 5 weeks later the patient noticed a snap in the medial aspect of her ankle

with weight bearing and subsequent flattening of the arch of her foot and a feeling of instability. The mild-to-moderate pain across her midfoot area increased with activity. She tried antiinflammatory agents without significant relief.

On physical examination she was unable to rise up on the ball of that foot and was not able to invert the hindfoot on the single heel rise test. She tried inlays and arch supports, but these too had not relieved her pain symptoms. She has been laid off from her employment as a department store clerk because of an inability to stand for prolonged periods.

She was treated surgically by a transfer of her FDL to the undersurface of the navicula and 6 weeks of postoperative immobilization. She subsequently has had good relief of her pain symptoms, although she still has some hindfoot deformity and has not been able to return to her previous occupation.

## Stage I: tendon length normal

In the nonathletic population many TPT problems may remain unrecognized because the pain is only mild to moderate. Patients may have an ache along the medial aspect of the hindfoot that is exacerbated by physical activity; these people probably have modified their activities to be less vigorous. For athletes, of course, such a problem can be significant and eliminate the possibility of participating in strenuous physical activity that includes running. Initially it is difficult for patients to localize discomfort; however, they almost always point to the medial aspect of the hindfoot and with close questioning along the course of the TPT about the tip of the medial malleolus down to the major attachment of that tendon to the undersurface of the navicular. The onset of pain has been gradual, and it is uncommon that an inciting episode will be related. Young athletes may remember a twisting episode with subsequent pain that was exacerbated by further physical activities. Older

**Table 4-1.** Changes associated with various stages of TPT dysfunction

|  | Stage 1 | Stage 2 | Stage 3 |
|---|---|---|---|
| TPT condition | Peritendinitis and/or tendon degeneration | Elongation | Elongation |
| Hindfoot | Mobile, normal alignment | Mobile, minimal valgus position | Fixed, moderate-to-severe valgus position |
| Pain | Medial: focal, mild to moderate | Medial: along TPT, moderate | Medial: possible lateral, moderate |
| Single heel rise test | Mild weakness | Moderate weakness | Marked weakness |
| "Too-many-toes" sign with forefoot abduction | Normal | Positive (mild) | Positive (marked) |
| Pathology | Synovial proliferation, degeneration | Synovitis, tendon frayed | Marked degeneration |
| Treatment | Conservative: 3 months; surgical: 3 months with synovectomy, tendon debridement, rest | Transfer FDL* for TPT | Subtalar arthrodesis |

From Johnson KA, Strom DE: Tibialis posterior tendon dysfunction, *Clin Orthop* 239:196, 1989.
*Flexor digitorum longus.

middle-aged athletes are more likely to experience a gradual onset of pain in the medial aspect of the ankle with moderate exercise.

The point of maximal tenderness for a stage I problem corresponds with the area of pain—that is, from along the tendon just before it passes around the medial malleolus down to its navicular insertion. This site of tenderness corresponds well with the areas of TPT pathologic abnormalities noted at surgery. Swelling is best appreciated by viewing the hindfoot with the patient standing and from a posterior vantage. Looking specifically at the area just inferior to the medial malleolus, it becomes evident that swelling is present. In stage I, however, the alignment of the hindfoot/forefoot will still be normal since the tendon is of a normal length.

Testing for strength of the TPT is accomplished with the single heel rise test (Fig. 4-1). Again while viewing the patient from the posterior aspect, the patient is asked to rise up on the ball of the affected foot while the other foot is held off the ground. The patient may use a door or a wall for balance. When the pain is coming from the TPT in a stage I abnormality, the patient usually is unable to rise up on the forefoot but complains of pain. At this early stage I there is little in the way of secondary deformity, and the standing roentgenogram changes will be minimal. If the diagnosis is in question, a magnetic resonance imaging (MRI) study will demonstrate an increased signal about the tendon, indicating fluid in the tendon sheath and peritendinitis.

### Stage II: tendon elongated, hindfoot mobile with mild deformity

The changes from stage I to stage II evolve over

months to years. It is, of course, important during the early stages to diagnose and treat the patient appropriately to avoid the progression. In stage II the pain increases in severity and may even be present after cessation of weight bearing. The pain will still be located along the TPT, but now the tendon has been disrupted and secondary changes are developing. Swelling and tenderness again are present inferior to the medial malleolus when viewed posteriorly.

In stage II the single heel rise test becomes even more abnormal because the tendon has been elongated and weakened. The tibialis posterior muscle tendon unit is a prime stabilizer of the hindfoot by virtue of its position posterior to the access of the ankle joint and medial to the subtalar joint. It provides plantar flexion of the ankle and more importantly inversion of the hindfoot. This tendon's excursion is short and the muscle is powerful.[15] Thus even a relatively mild elongation of the tendon decreases its function significantly. Again, this muscle-tendon unit is tested by the single heel rise test. The normal sequence for a single heel rise test is as follows. First, the TPT is activated, which inverts and locks the hindfoot, thus providing a rigid hindfoot structure. Next, the gastroc-soleus group pulls up the posterior calcaneus and the heel rise is completed. With elongation of the TPT, the initial heel inversion is weak and the patient either rises up incompletely without locking the heel or does not rise up on the ball of the foot at all. Looking specifically for the absence of the initial heel inversion is important in diagnosing stage II tendon elongation.

Another helpful diagnostic sign is that of "too many toes" (Fig. 4-2); when the hindfoot is viewed from the posterior aspect, more toes are seen lateral to the ankle

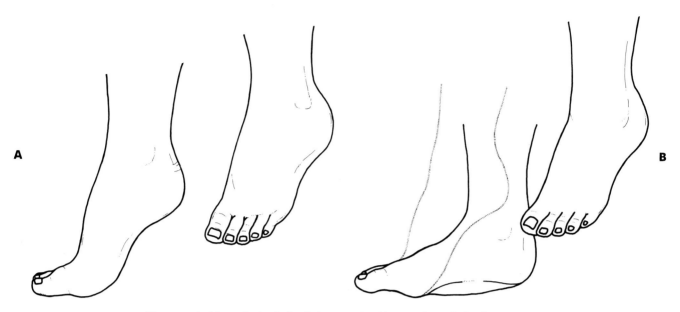

Fig. 4-1. **A,** Normal single heel rise test. **B,** Abnormal single heel rise test.

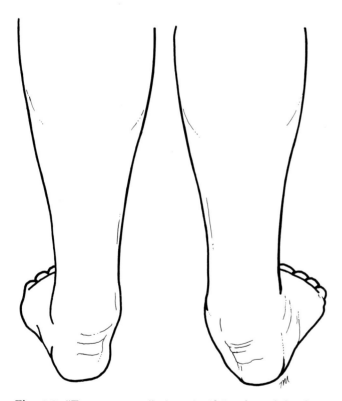

Fig. 4-2. "Too-many-toes" sign signifying lateral forefoot rotation. Two and one-half toes seen on the left foot, four toes on the abnormal right foot.

than are seen on the opposite normal side. As the heel goes into increased resting eversion and the forefoot goes into abduction, too many toes are seen on the affected side. The number of extra toes seen is a recordable measurement of the degree of deformity.

Changes on routine standing roentgenograms now become evident. If one thinks of the foot as consisting of only two pieces (Fig. 4-3), the changes of TPT abnormalities are understandable. One part of the foot is the talus, which can only flex and extend in the ankle mortise. The second part of the foot is the calcaneus, navicular, and everything distal from those bones. The second part of the foot then can move in the varus/valgus position with the forefoot deviating out into abduction as the calcaneus rotates from beneath the talus. With rotation of the sustentaculum of the calcaneus from beneath the talus, the talus then goes into slight plantar flexion. This explains the changes on the anteroposterior view of an increased angle between the talus and the calcaneus (Fig. 4-4), an uncovering of the lateral aspect of the talar head by the navicular, and an abducted position of the forefoot. From the lateral view the angle between the calcaneus increases. As the talus goes into a plantar-flexed position, a sag at the talonavicular joint is evident. The normal alignment of the longitudinal axis of the talus through the navicular and down through the cuneiform and in a straight line with the first metatarsal is disrupted. The break in this longitudinal axis is at the talus to navicular area because of the plantar flexion of the talus.

If the diagnosis is uncertain, MRI will show a tendon discontinuity.[1] Usually, however, the physical examination provides the appropriate diagnosis.

### Stage III: tendon elongated, hindfoot moderately to severely deformed

With stage III changes in the hindfoot due to disruption of the TPT, pain may transfer to the lateral aspect of the hindfoot and be present over the sinus

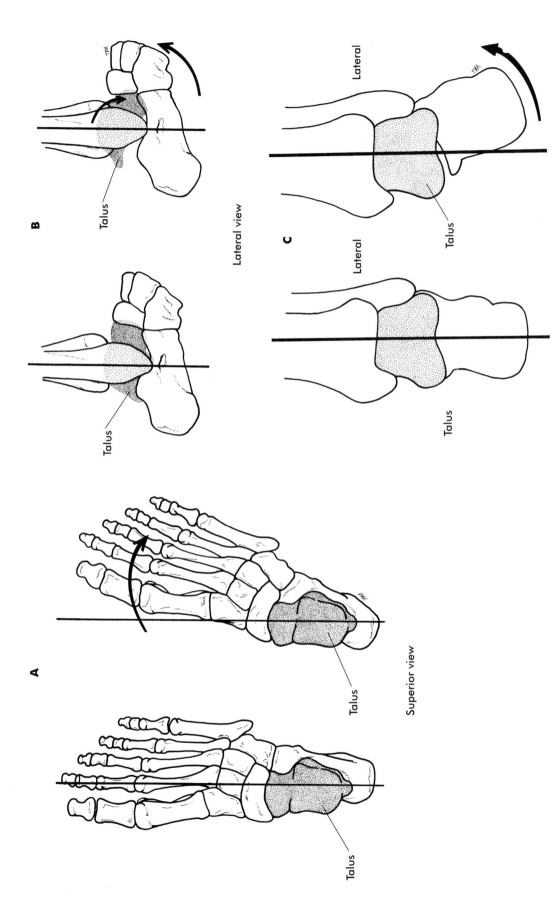

**Fig. 4-3. A,** Anteroposterior foot view shows the two-piece deformity. The calcaneus-navicular-cuboid and distal foot bones rotate lateralward from beneath the talus. **B,** As the sustentaculum of the calcaneus moves lateralward, the talus rotates plantarward. **C,** Anteroposterior ankle view diagrams the increased hindfoot valgus as the calcaneus is allowed to displace lateralward.

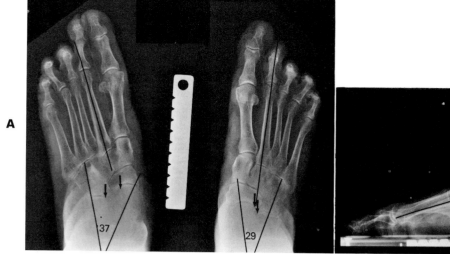

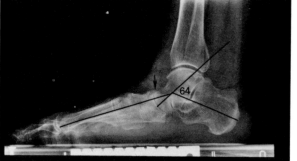

**Fig. 4-4. A,** This radiograph shows the increased angle of 37 degrees on the left between the long axis of the talus and calcaneus. Also the long axis of the second metatarsal does not bisect the hindfoot talus and calcaneus long-axis angle. Also, the medial cortex margin of the talar head will separate *(arrows).* **B,** This lateral view shows the increased angle between the calcaneus and talus with a sag *(arrow)* at the talonavicular joint.

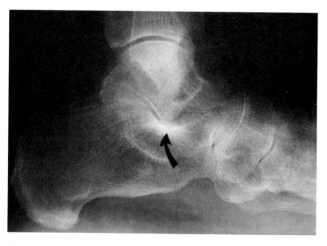

**Fig. 4-5.** Impingement of the anterior portion of the posterior talar facet on the superior aspect of the calcaneus produces a reactive sclerosis called the "white sign" *(arrow).*

tarsi. This occurs because the bony projection at the anterior margin of the posterior facet impinges on the superior aspect of the calcaneus in the sinus tarsi region (Fig. 4-5). Pressing on the sinus tarsi produces the pain symptoms as well as forcefully presses the foot into the deformed position. Stage III pain may be suggestive of degenerative arthritis, since it may be present long after the inciting activity ceases.

In stage III deformity is the most significant change. When viewed posteriorly, the hindfoot eversion and forefoot abduction are moderate to severe. The single heel rise test again demonstrates the absence of locking of the hindfoot in inversion, along with an

almost complete inability to rise up on the ball of the foot; the too-many-toes sign will be more apparent, and the patient is readily aware that the foot has become flat (Fig. 4-6).

On roentgenogram the changes described under stage II are present but more marked. If this deformity has been present for some time, joint narrowing in the subtalar region and osteophyte formation may appear.

If a technetium scan is performed, the delayed views will show uptake of the isotope at the site of sinus tarsi impingement by the anterior margin of the posterior talar facet.

## TREATMENT

By understanding the diagnostic signs and symptoms of TPT difficulties, along with the roentgenographic abnormalities, the pathologic changes can be anticipated and a treatment program suggested.

### Stage I: tendon length normal

At this stage the length of the tendon appears normal. There will usually be a combination of inflammation about the tendon evidenced by fluid in the tendon sheath and synovial proliferation. Sometimes the amount of fluid is predominant with minimal synovial changes; in other instances synovial changes are marked with only minimal fluid. Changes in the tendon also vary from just an off-white color to longitudinal split tears within the tendon substance. The tendon may be mildly enlarged with a bulbous configuration (Fig. 4-7). In patients with significant

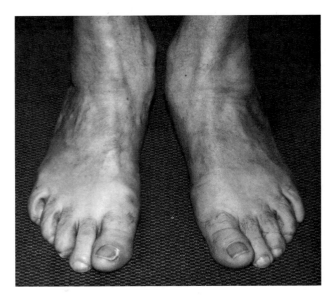

**Fig. 4-6.** This patient has an elongation of the left tibialis posterior tendon with a pes planus deformity.

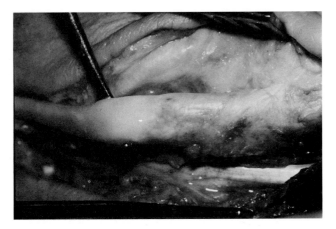

**Fig. 4-7.** Bulbous configuration of tibialis posterior tendon degeneration.

peritendinitis and synovial inflammation, the underlying diagnosis may be rheumatoid arthritis or one of the rheumatoid variants.

Treatment of the stage I TPT difficulties should initially be nonoperative. A systemic antiinflammatory agent such as aspirin in an antiinflammatory dose should be used for several weeks. Sometimes a simple orthosis in the shoe or even just avoiding aggravating footwear is indicated. Decreasing or eliminating the sports activities that exacerbate the pain would be suggested. Cross-training into an activity such as swimming or strength development and avoiding running-type motions with that inflamed tendon is appropriate. Steroid use about this tendon is controversial.[3] Steroid injection should not be done around the tendons of the lower extremities for inflammatory problems because of the risk of tendon weakness and subsequent rupture.

Surgical treatment of stage I TPT difficulties is undertaken if conservative measures are not successful. In the presence of continued inflammation after about 3 months of conservative treatment, surgical treatment would be appropriate. Particularly in stage I, surgical treatment should halt the progression of the disease and mitigate against the much more extensive surgical treatment for stage II and stage III abnormalities.

Surgical treatment for stage I TPT problems involves opening the sheath of the TPT from the musculotendinous junction all the way to its insertion. A 1-cm pulley posterior to the malleolus is maintained usually about an area where the tendon is not involved. This release is followed by a synovectomy and debridement of the flaps of tendon if present. If the

tendon is enlarged to more than one and one half times its normal size, a midsubstance wedge is removed to debulk the tendon; the resultant wedge defect is then sutured closed. The longitudinal split tears can be sutured with a burying of the knot technique. The roof of the tendon sheath is removed particularly distal to the medial malleolus so that it will not reconstitute itself. Initially after wound closure a bulky compressive dressing is applied with the hindfoot in a neutral position. Approximately 3 days later, a short-leg walking cast is applied for 3 weeks.

This treatment method is often successful in stopping the inflammation and tendon degeneration that would otherwise proceed to stage II changes.

### Stage II: tendon elongated, hindfoot mobile, mildly deformed

In stage II the tendon can show significant degeneration over a length of several centimeters (Fig. 4-8). If the tendon has been elongated for some months, the TPT proximal to the medial malleolus which is not primarily involved will have a peculiar whitefish flesh appearance. Pulling in the tendon will give a stiff feeling as the muscles attaching to the tendon have become stiffened. Adhesions form around the tendon in its sheath, and the tendon will have a change to firmness in its consistency.

Conservative measures for stage II changes may be suggested in older persons with mild pain and perhaps some systemic condition that mitigates against surgical care. Conservative measures include antiinflammatory agents, low-heeled high-top shoes, and perhaps a more extensive shoe insert such as a UCBL orthosis.

Surgical treatment for stage II elongated TPT and mildly deformed hindfoot has been accomplished by substitution transfer of adjacent tendons. Probably the most common transfer is that of the flexor digitorum

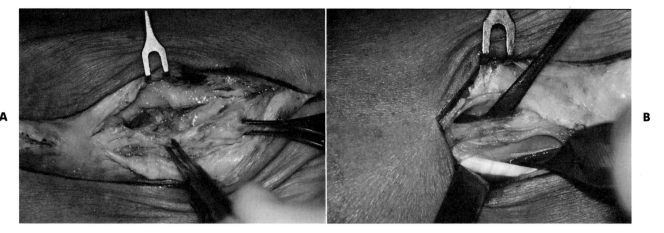

**Fig. 4-8. A,** Marked degeneration of the tibialis posterior tendon for several centimeters before its insertion on the navicular. **B,** Marked degeneration proximal to the medial malleolus in the same patient. This is probably a secondary change due to the absence of stress on the tendon from distal elongation and degeneration.

longus (FDL) to substitute for the TPT (Fig. 4-9). This transfer entails transecting the FDL distally and reinserting it into the undersurface of the navicular through a drill hole. It is not necessary that the distal portion of the FDL be tenodesed to the adjacent flexor hallucis longus. The intrinsic toe flexors are so strong in the foot that leaving this distal stump of the FDL alone will not cause functional loss to the toes. Without this transfer of the FDL to the flexor hallucis longus, a longer extent of FDL can be harvested to transfer to the undersurface of the navicular.

The FDL to be transferred is left in its own sheath and then brought up just inferior to the stump of the tibialis posterior and inserted into the navicular bone. The tendon is pulled tight as the hindfoot is placed in an inversion and forefoot adduction. If the TPT muscle is not stiff to tendon tension, the proximal portion of the TPT can be attached to the transferred FDL tendon to provide increased strength. If the muscle, however, is nonyielding and fibrotic, this proximal attachment is not done. Because the FDL seems to be so expendable, liberal use of this transfer seems reasonable. The results of transfer of the FDL for an elongated TPT have been quite good. Unfortunately patients do not always achieve relief of their deformity but usually do obtain relief of the pain symptoms.[2] Helal[6] has suggested that a transfer of the medial half of the tibialis anterior tendon into the navicular bone is an appropriate substitute for loss of the TPT. This certainly seems appropriate; however the experience with this transfer has not been extensive. To not only achieve pain relief, but also increased function, it may be that a combination of a transfer of the FDL into the undersurface of the navicular as well as the lateral half of the tibialis anterior into the superior aspect of the

navicular will be necessary to improve the hindfoot alignment as well as achieve pain relief.

It is evident from experience, however, that when the deformity is moderate to severe or the hindfoot has become increasingly stiff, the treatment for a stage III condition should be used.

### Stage III: tendon elongated, hindfoot significantly deformed and stiff

The tendon changes in a stage III abnormality mimic those of stage II but with more severe involvement. The increased deformity has occurred because the static supports of the foot have been elongated and the foot has gone into a more fixed pes planus deformity. When this amount of deformity is present, a tendon transfer against such a significant deformity has not been effective. Instead, realignment of the hindfoot followed by an arthrodesis procedure is used. There is controversy as to the site of the appropriate arthrodesis. It has been suggested that an arthrodesis should be done at the subtalar joint, the talonavicular joint, the talonavicular and calcaneocuboid; or perhaps a triple arthrodesis should be done for a stage III abnormality. In fact, all of these arthrodeses probably are of benefit since blocking any one of the hindfoot joints will to a certain degree effectively block the entire hindfoot—that is, motion at the subtalar, talonavicular, and calcaneocuboid joints are coupled motions; when one is blocked all three are impaired. Probably the most direct approach to the deformity, however, would be at the subtalar joint where the calcaneus has rotated out from beneath the talus and has allowed the talus to go into a plantar-flexed position. At the time of surgery, placing the calcaneus back under-

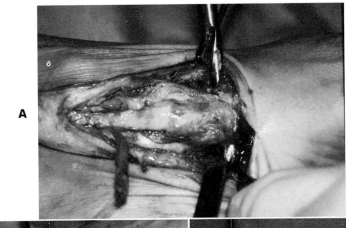

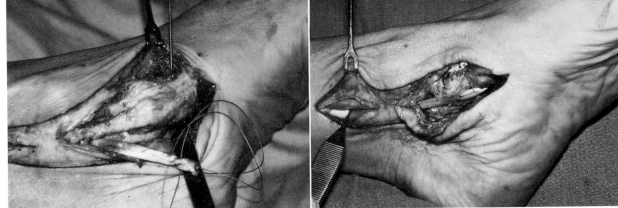

**Fig. 4-9. A,** For a stage II degeneration of the tibialis posterior tendon, transfer of the flexor digitorum longus is done. The drill is inserted through the tuberosity of the navicular. **B,** Here a suture is shown passing through the navicular drill hole in preparation to pulling the tendon of the flexor digitorum longus through from a plantar to dorsal direction. **C,** The tendon of the flexor digitorum longus was left in its own sheath and brought through the navicular tuberosity and sutured. Because of tendon scarring and muscle stiffness of the tibialis posterior, the proximal tenodesis of the flexor digitorum longus (thumb forcep) to the tibialis posterior was not done.

neath the talus so that the hindfoot valgus is normal and then completing the arthrodesis by inserted bone graft into the subtalar area is appropriate. For such a subtalar arthrodesis, morcellated bone graft from the anterior iliac crest inserted into the subtalar joint with temporary fixation by a Steinmann pin across the neck of the talus into the calcaneus has been effective.[14] Cast immobilization is necessary for 10 weeks after the arthrodesis: the first 6 weeks without weight bearing, the last 4 weeks with weight bearing. Such an arthrodesis is an effective procedure since it does correct the static hindfoot deformity and gives good relief of pain. However hindfoot motion in the subtalar joint is then absent, and the ability to adapt to uneven surfaces is lost. In the middle-aged to older recreational athlete, loss of such motion is readily accepted to eliminate the previous pain and hindfoot deformity.

## SUMMARY

It is necessary that the diagnosis be made early so that nonoperative measures may be used. If these nonoperative measures are not successful, surgical treatment while the tendon is still of a normal length is appropriate and should break the cycle of peritendinous inflammation and tendon degeneration. If the patient does have elongation of the tendon, and mild deformity is present, transfer of the FDL and/or the medial half of the anterior tibial tendon to the navicula may be appropriate. For this tendon transfer, however, pain relief is usually satisfactory but correction of the deformity has not been consistent. If the tendon has elongated, the deformity is moderate to severe, and the hindfoot has become less mobile, an arthrodesis of the hindfoot is suggested. Various options are present, but a personal preference is an arthrodesis of the subtalar joint with bone grafting from the iliac crest so as not to disturb the hindfoot articulations in the mid and distal portions of the foot.

Problems of the TPT can be disabling particularly for the middle-aged athlete. Early diagnosis and treatment is necessary.

## REFERENCES

1. Alexander IJ et al: Magnetic resonance imaging in the diagnosis of disruption of the posterior tibial tendon, *Foot Ankle* 8:144, 1987.
2. Bourne MH, Johnson KA, Campbell DA: Treatment of tibialis posterior tendon dysfunction by transfer of the flexor digitorum longus tendon, unpublished data presented at American Orthopaedic Foot and Ankle Society Meeting, 1989.
3. Ford LT, DeBender J: Tendon rupture after local steroid injection, *South Med J* 72:827, 1979.
4. Funk DA, Cass JR, Johnson KA: Acquired adult flat foot secondary to posterior tibial tendon pathology, *J Bone Joint Surg* 68A:95, 1986.
5. Goldner JL et al: Progressive talipes equinovalgus due to trauma or degeneration of the posterior tibial tendon and medial plantar ligaments, *Orthop Clin North Am* 5:39, 1974.
6. Helal B: Cobb repair for tibialis posterior tendon rupture, *J Foot Surg* 29:349, 1990.
7. Jahss JH: Spontaneous rupture of the tibialis posterior tendon: clinical findings, tenographic studies, and a new technique of repair, *Foot Ankle* 3:158, 1982.
8. Johnson KA: Tibialis posterior tendon rupture, *Clin Orthop* 177:140, 1983.
9. Johnson KA, Strom DE: Tibialis posterior tendon dysfunction, *Clin Orthop* 239:196, 1989.
10. Kettelkamp DB, Alexander HH: Spontaneous rupture of the posterior tibial tendon, *J Bone Joint Surg* 51A:759, 1969.
11. Leach RE, DeIorio E, Harney RA: Pathologic hindfoot conditions in the athlete, *Clin Orthop* 177:116, 1983.
12. Mann RA, Thompson FM: Rupture of the posterior tibial tendon causing flat foot, *J Bone Joint Surg* 67A:556, 1985.
13. Mueller TJ: Ruptures and lacerations of the tibialis posterior tendon, *J Am Podiatr Med Assoc* 74:109, 1984.
14. Russotti G, Cass JR, Johnson KA: Isolated talocalcaneal arthrodesis, *J Bone Joint Surg* 70A:1372, 1988.
15. Sutherland DH: An electromyographic study of the plantar flexors of the ankle in normal walking on the level, *J Bone Joint Surg* 48A:66, 1966.

# Chapter 5

# Injuries to the tibialis anterior, peroneal tendons, and long flexors and extensors of the toes

**G. James Sammarco**

Several types of problems occur in the tendons of the extrinsic foot muscles at the ankle, which affect function in sports. Contact sports, running sports, and sports requiring static posturing for short periods put great demand on these muscles, which may exceed their physiologic capacity. In younger athletes tears may occur within the substance of the tendon. In older athletes complete rupture of the tendon may occur at its insertion. Tendinitis is common, since high-impact sports create loads on the foot that are several times body weight, while the foot may not be in a position to give proper support.

Endurance sports, which require aerobic conditioning in a repeated cycle of phasic activity for many thousand times, produce overuse syndromes, leading to attritional wear within the tendon substance. This chapter outlines important conditions of several tendons in the ankle and foot that are frequently injured. Because of their size, function, and anatomic placement, these injuries are sometimes difficult to diagnose and treat.

## TIBIALIS ANTERIOR

The tibialis anterior muscle takes origin from the anterior tibia, interosseus membrane, and crural fascia. Its tendon runs beneath both the superior and inferior extensor retinacula in its own tunnel to insert on the medial cuneiform and the medial border of the

proximal first metatarsal. Because it crosses the ankle from the anterior compartment and passes medially, it is at risk to direct trauma from a kick or from striking a blunt object. The function of the tibialis anterior is to dorsiflex the ankle and supinate the foot. It stabilizes the foot in the latter part of stance phase of gait and extends the foot at the beginning and middle portions of the swing phase of gait.

### Tendinitis

Tibialis anterior tendinitis may manifest in acute and chronic forms. Symptoms of acute tendinitis are pain anteriorly at the ankle with tenderness over the anterior ankle, specifically on palpation along the course of the tendon as the foot is actively dorsiflexed against resistance. Occasionally crepitus is palpable, but since the tendon lies deep beneath the superior perineal retinaculum, swelling usually is not evident. The patient complains of pain on activity, which is usually relieved with rest. This occurs following a period of rest and is a sign of poor conditioning. It must be differentiated from an anterior compartment syndrome, which is associated with symptoms of increased pain proximally in the anterior compartment of the calf, or from a medial tibial syndrome, in which symptoms occur behind the medial malleolus as well as from stress fractures of the distal tibia. Chronic tendinitis presents with similar symptoms.

These occur often above the superior extensor retinaculum in the musculotendinous junction of the muscle. Fullness over the tendon anterior to the ankle joint, or as the tendon splays out distally toward its insertion, may be visible. Symptoms of chronic tendinitis are usually present for more than 6 weeks and often are ignored by athletes who may be in training. Weekend athletes are also subject to this condition due to the cyclical nature of their rest/use program with a more extended period of rest.

Treatment for tibialis anterior tendinitis is symptomatic. For acute symptoms, rest, elevation, ice over the affected area, and an elastic compression bandage are indicated. Limited weight bearing with crutches and a posterior splint are indicated if symptoms are severe enough to alter the gait pattern. Nonsteroidal antiinflammatory drugs (NSAIDs) are prescribed if the patient is able to tolerate salicylates. A physical therapy program with gentle stretching and active range of motion, both non–weight bearing and weight bearing, is also prescribed. Occasionally surgical intervention, including tenosynovectomy with repair of longitudinal rents in the tendon, is indicated. This is followed by 3 weeks of immobilization with a gatched walker cast boot (Bledsoe®) set at zero degrees of motion. Ten degrees of dorsiflexion and ten degrees of plantar flexion are permitted in the boot after 3 weeks, progressing to 20 degrees of dorsiflexion and 20 degrees of plantar flexion after 5 weeks. A power-building and flexibility program is then instituted. Recurrence is uncommon if the patient is taught a good conditioning program and adheres to it.

### Laceration

Lacerations of the anterior tibial tendon occur through direct trauma, such as striking the ankle against a piece of equipment. An acute laceration results in a sudden weakness in dorsiflexion of the ankle. There is retraction of the proximal tendon segment since the tibialis anterior muscle contracts as much as 6 cm from the distal segment of the tendon. Symptoms include increased use of the accessory dorsiflexors of the ankle and foot, specifically the extensor hallucis longus and extensor digitorum longus. The toes hyperextend with dorsiflexion of the ankle. Tenting of the skin on the anterior foot and ankle, which normally occurs over the intact tibialis anterior, is lost. Compared with the opposite side, the tendon is not palpable at the dorsomedial aspect of the foot distal to the ankle.

Swelling of the retracted proximal tendon stump may mimic that of a ganglion cyst or tumor anterior to the ankle. Although radiographs fail to reveal symptoms other than soft tissue swelling locally, magnetic resonance imaging (MRI) will clearly distinguish the disruption of the tibialis anterior tendon as well as its attendant edema.

In the young or middle-aged athlete, recommended treatment is direct surgical repair of the tendon, with 0-0 braided Dacron suture on a tapered needle. Postoperatively, the foot is held in dorsiflexion of 5 degrees in a cast for 3 weeks, and then in a neutral position for an additional 3 weeks. Forces in the muscle are high, and early mobilization of this tendon allows the repair to pull apart. Chronic lacerations of the tendon can occur as a result of significant trauma but may go unrecognized if the skin is not violated (Fig. 5-1). In such a circumstance, the tendon is crushed and simply pulls apart in its substance. Although the symptoms of pain and weakness are the same as acute tears initially, the pain subsides within 2 to 3 weeks, leaving an abnormal gait. The ankle must now be flexed with the weaker accessory dorsiflexors consisting of the extensor hallucis longus and extensor digitorum longus. Moreover, coordination and strength are decreased considerably. If the tendon is not fixed in contraction, a direct repair should be made. There may be a gap between the two ends of the tendon secondary to contracture of the muscle proximally and the bulbous proximal end of the tendon. The bulbous stump is debrided and trimmed to its original shape, and a plantaris tendon graft is used to bridge the gap between tendon ends. An alternative is to use one of the long-toe extensors, harvested through the same incision for a tendon graft. If this graft is chosen, the proximal and distal ends of the host tendon are tenodesed with a 2-0 braided Dacron suture on a tapered needle to the extensor tendon of an adjacent toe so as to retain the extension function to that toe. The extensor tendon graft may be doubled on itself to provide extra strength. The tendon graft is sutured end to end proximally and distally into the respective ends of the tibialis anterior tendon with an 0-0 braided Dacron suture. The extensor retinaculum is not closed because the resultant bow stringing of the tendon does not cause significant loss of function. Postoperative treatment is the same as for acute injuries for the first 6 weeks. Gentle active range of motion is permitted in a gatched walker boot set at 10 degrees of dorsiflexion and 10 degrees of plantar flexion following this. Return to sport is permitted when strength is increased to 90% of the other leg. A chronic tear of the tibialis anterior in older athletes, although it does decrease function, may not reduce it significantly enough to restrict casual play and therefore may need only observation without surgery. My experience is that it does affect return to a high level of performance and the patient should be so informed.

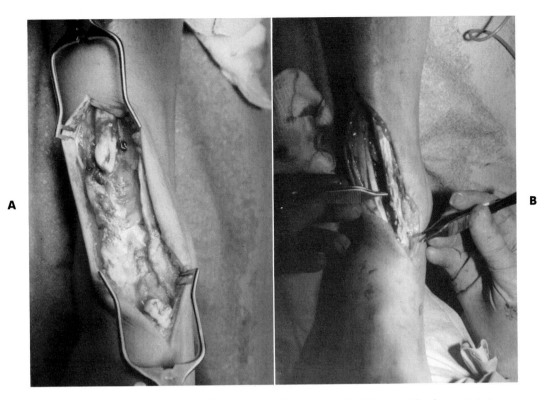

**Fig. 5-1. A,** Operative photograph of 20-year-old soccer goalie. He struck his leg sustaining a laceration, which was sutured. Unrecognized at the time was a lacerated anterior tibial tendon. At surgery 6 weeks later, the tendon ends have retracted and cannot be approximated. (Forefoot is at *bottom* of field.) **B,** An extensor digitorum tendon graft was used to bridge the gap. Immobilization for 6 weeks followed by protected ambulation and a supervised physical therapy program resulted in excellent recovery with normal function within 1 year. Two years post-injury, his function remains normal.

## Avulsion of the tibialis anterior tendon

Avulsion of the tibialis anterior tendon (see box on p. 56) from its insertion on the medial aspect of the foot occurs in younger athletes who are poorly conditioned and in "weekend" athletes.[30] Active seniors who walk for sport and exercise also suffer this injury.[7] An associated risk factor is diabetes mellitus. The mechanism is attributed on occasion to high-impact trauma on the dorsum of the foot, or to striking the foot against a solid object while in the process of dorsiflexing the ankle. The patient feels an immediate pain in the midfoot and has difficulty dorsiflexing the ankle and in weight bearing. Swelling and ecchymosis often occur. In the occasional senior athlete, even though play is discontinued, home remedies including NSAIDs and elevation are tried. An antalgic gait ensues, but the pain subsides over 1 to 3 weeks. Dorsiflexion is provided by the secondary extensors of the foot. The proximal end of the tendon retracts beneath the superior retinaculum and presents as a tumor mass anterior to the ankle. Pain subsides and the patient often seeks treatment because of the sudden development of a mass on the

anterior ankle. Radiographs are of little value except to exclude bony involvement. If function is satisfactory, and the patient is able to tolerate the moderate limitation, which includes weak dorsiflexion of the ankle during gait and fatigue, surgical intervention may not be necessary.

In high-performance athletes, however, surgical intervention is recommended through advancement and reattachment of the tendon, augmented by the use of a plantaris tendon graft or one of the long extensor tendons to a lesser toe (see the foregoing). If physical examination fails to convince the examiner that an avulsion has occurred, MRI will demonstrate the mass beneath the peroneal retinaculum anterior to the ankle representing the retracted tendon. This bulbous mass is two to three times the width of the tendon. Surgical repair differs from a midsubstance tear of the tendon in that the distal end of the tendon graft must be secured to the dorsomedial side of the proximal first metatarsal. Since the tendon retracts and remains fixed beneath the superior extensor retinaculum, the tendon must be mobilized and advanced as well as debrided so

---

**Avulsion of anterior tibial tendon**

- Older athlete
- Mass anterior to ankle
- Absence of anterior tibial tendon tenting skin on dorsum of foot
- Extension of hallux and lesser toes with dorsiflexion of ankle

---

that the tendon graft will function after healing. The graft is doubled on itself through a drilled hole in the proximal first metatarsal or secured using bone anchors. Postoperatively a cast is applied with the ankle in 5 degrees of dorsiflexion and slight supination. After 3 weeks the foot is brought into a neutral position to prevent development of contracture of the foot and ankle in dorsiflexion. After 6 weeks of immobilization, physical therapy including active and passive range of motion, whirlpool, balance board (Baps board), and isokinetic testing is initiated. Competitive athletes are permitted to return to play when 90% of the function of the opposite foot is achieved. The author found recurrence of this injury rare (see Case Study 1).

**Case Study 1.** A 65-year-old male walks 3 miles a day, trips on the sidewalk, and feels a sharp pain on the medial aspect of his foot. Swelling develops and he has difficulty dorsiflexing his foot for the first week. After the swelling subsides, he notices that a mass has developed anterior to his ankle. Physical examination reveals a mass on the anterior ankle, which is slightly tender and rubbery hard (Fig. 5-2). Dorsiflexion of the foot reveals no palpable tibialis anterior tendon proximal to its insertion on the anteromedial aspect of the midfoot. The patient uses his toe extensors to dorsiflex the ankle. A diagnosis of avulsion of the tibialis anterior tendon is made and surgery is counseled. At operation an avulsed and retracted tibialis anterior tendon is found beneath the superior extensor retinaculum anterior to the ankle. The tendon is advanced and reattached to the medial aspect of the proximal first metatarsal. Cast immobilization with the foot and ankle in neutral position is prescribed for 6 weeks postoperatively, after which a supervised therapy program is instituted. Six months following surgery, the patient has a functional ankle with satisfactory dorsiflexion and returns to his preinjury activity level.

### Intratendinous lesions

The two most common tumors of the tibialis anterior are ganglion and giant cell tumor of tendon sheath. The intratendinous ganglion can be differentiated from a retracted stump of a torn tendon since the function of the tendon remains intact and the secondary extensors of the ankle do not overfunction in dorsiflexion. The ganglion is often loculated and

can extend for distances of 4 to 6 cm within the tendon. A mass is present beneath the inferior peroneal extensor retinaculum. If the mass becomes large or tender, the treatment of choice is a simple excision conducted through a linear incision over the tendon, with care taken to ensure preservation of the cutaneous nerves. Repair of the tendon is indicated if the ganglion has invaded the tendon and created rents within its substance. Immobilization for 2 weeks postoperatively, after which an active program with power-building and flexibility exercises under supervision, is then prescribed. Giant cell tumor of tendon sheath is the most common solid tumor of the foot associated with the tibialis anterior. Excision is recommended through the same approach as for a ganglion. All tumor tissue should be removed since remaining portions of this benign tumor tend to reoccur locally. The tumor characteristically is encased in a membrane and migrates along the tendon sheath. It is easily distinguishable by its yellow-orange color and reticulated pattern on gross examination. It becomes loculated as it passes along the tendon sheath. Postoperatively, active range of motion with a rehabilitation program is begun as soon as the wound heals, since the tendon is not destroyed by the tumor and is thus intact.

### PERONEUS BREVIS TENDON

The peroneus brevis muscle takes origin in the lateral compartment of the leg, from the lower two thirds of the fibulae body and two intermuscular septa adjacent to the bone. There is a long, musculotendinous junction with muscle fibers inserting on the tendon from midcalf down to, and often beyond, the lateral malleolus for a distance of 2 to 3 cm. At the lateral malleolus the tendon lies closest to the bone in the groove on the posterior fibula, pressed against it by the peroneus longus tendon. As it passes behind the lateral malleolus, it makes an oblique turn anteriorly over the calcaneofibular ligament into its own tendon sheath above the trochlea lateralis of the calcaneus. The tendon then crosses the cuboid to insert on the fifth metatarsal styloid. The special function of the peroneus brevis is that it is the strongest abductor of the foot. It also functions as a secondary flexor of the ankle and foot evertor. This serves to stabilize the foot during gait, particularly in the final portion of stance. Because of this, the tendon is at risk of injury during the combined motions of a supinated foot and dorsiflexed ankle. Such positioning occurs with high loads during sports activities.

### Tendinitis

Tendinitis usually occurs when resuming play after an unconditioned period. Such periods are

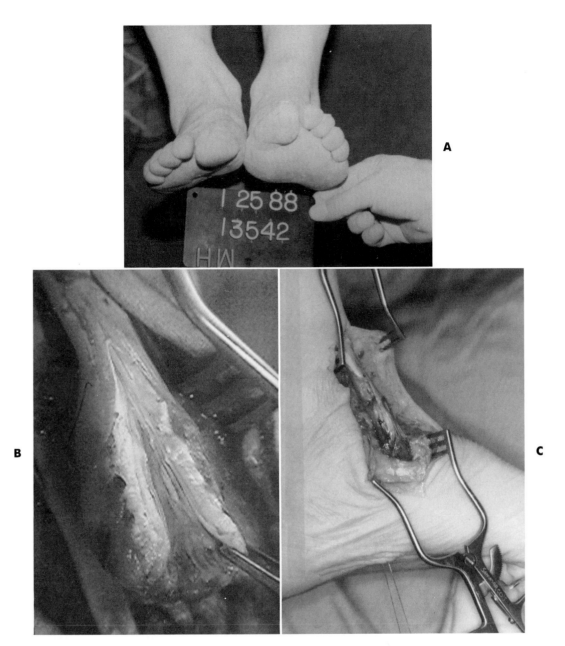

**Fig. 5-2. A,** A 65-year-old aerobic walker with avulsion of the left anterior tibial tendon. Note the mass anterior to the ankle where the bulbous tendon end has retracted. Note also the absence of the anterior tibial tendon tenting the skin on the left but present on the right. Note the use of the accessory dorsiflexors of the ankle, the extensor hallucis longus, and the extensor digitorum longus contracting to achieve ankle dorsiflexion. This is noticeably absent on the normal right side. **B,** Operative photograph of the retracted end of the avulsed tibialis tendon. The tendon has been split lengthwise, revealing retracted torn tendon elements in organizing hematoma. **C,** The tendon has been advanced and reattached onto the first metatarsal with 0-0 Dacron braided sutures. (Forefoot is to *right* of field.) Four years later, the patient is asymptomatic with normal gait and function.

followed by intensive practice schedules or dance class to prepare for competition or performance. Symptoms of pain develop behind and distal to the lateral malleolus. Swelling and tenderness occur along the tendon sheath and may be visible since the tendon lies subcutaneously.[24] Radiographs are useful to exclude bony abnormalities, arthritis, or fracture. Treatment consists of ice packs, taping the ankle, and NSAIDs. If symptoms subside within 48 hours, active gentle range of motion and a gradual increase in activity is resumed. The athlete is permitted to perform for short periods if symptoms remain mild and do not increase. Ballet dancers are particularly susceptible to this condition since they spend long periods of time standing in half-pointe — that is, on the ball of the foot (demipointe) — during dance class and rehearsal. Therefore they should be counseled to perform a regular schedule of warming-up. Chronic tendinitis often develops over several weeks or months and is a true overuse syndrome. Minimal swelling and tenderness occur.

Tendon inflammation may be a precursor to longitudinal rents within the tendon.[44] When such swelling and tenderness occur in the absence of increased athletic activity, it is usually associated with rheumatoid arthritis or other seronegative arthritides. In difficult to diagnose cases, or in those that must be differentiated from lateral ankle ligament injuries, MRI may be indicated.[15,19,21,32] Fluid accumulation around the tendon is visible on T2-weighted studies. Treatment includes a program of warm-ups with slow stretching, NSAIDs, taping of the ankle, and use of an ankle brace during contact sports. In recalcitrant cases surgical debridement through a lateral incision over the tendon is indicated. Care is taken to avoid the sural nerve and its branches in the area, since a neuroma of this nerve can be painful and disabling. A tenosynovectomy is recommended. The tendon sheath is not closed distal to the lateral malleolus. A splint is applied for 10 days, followed by a supervised ankle rehabilitation program. Prognosis of this condition is good. I do not recommend injection of corticosteroids in or about the peroneal tendons. In addition to weakening the tendon by intratendinous injection, extravasation of steroids outside the tendon sheath may cause subcutaneous tissue atrophy as well as skin atrophy, depigmentation of the skin, and increased tenderness over the tendon, making it difficult to wear a shoe.

### Styloid (avulsion) fracture of the peroneus brevis tendon insertion

Sudden inversion of the foot against the contracting peroneus brevis muscle can produce an avulsion of the fifth metatarsal styloid. Such a fracture usually includes a portion of the articular surface. Tenderness, swelling, and pain on ambulation occur immediately. In addition to the tendon, the capsular attachments of the fifth metatarsocuboid joint may be injured. This fracture occurs commonly in athletes with poor conditioning. Tenderness at the styloid is an important diagnostic finding. Radiographs confirm the presence of a fracture, usually extending into the fifth metatarsocuboid joint. This injury can be treated with an elastic bandage and crutches or, if symptoms warrant, a cast or cast boot (Bledsoe) immobilization for up to 4 weeks. If a cast or cast boot is used, weightbearing is permitted. The fracture should not be confused with the os vesalianum, an accessory sesamoid present in 0.1% of cadaver specimens, or with an open fifth metatarsal styloid apophysis in immature athletes.[8a] In difficult to diagnose cases in which no bony involvement is visible on plain films, MRI will confirm the clinical suspicion of an avulsed tendon. Peroneal tendon avulsion without a bony fragment is, however, uncommon. Although delayed unions are not uncommon, nonunions are. In the event that a nonunion occurs, it may not be symptomatic and does not require treatment. A symptomatic nonunion, however, may be treated in two ways. If the fragment is small and involves less than 50% of the articular surface, excision of the fragment with reattachment of the remaining portion of the tendon to the fifth metatarsal is recommended. This is done through drill holes in the proximal metatarsal, using a 2-0 braided Dacron interrupted suture. If the avulsed proximal fragment comprises 50% or more of the articular surface of the fifth metatarsal, open reduction with internal fixation using a lag screw and washer is recommended. This should be inserted through a lateral incision over the styloid, and the screw head can be passed through the insertion of the peroneus brevis tendon into the proximal fragment so that the head of the lag screw lies deep to the peroneus brevis tendon insertion. Rehabilitation following acute fracture is started after 4 weeks. Radiographs are taken at regular intervals to ensure healing is progressing. Shoe modification with a stiff insole and a semirigid orthosis protects the midfoot from increased flexion. A conditioning program stressing peroneal strengthening exercises is an important rehabilitation adjunct. Recurrence of this fracture is uncommon.

### Peroneus brevis tendon tear

The position of the peroneus brevis tendon in the fibular groove posterior to the lateral malleolus predisposes it to increased stress as it is sandwiched between the peroneus longus tendon and bone. Moreover, differential shear stresses within the tendon itself can contribute to the formation of longitu-

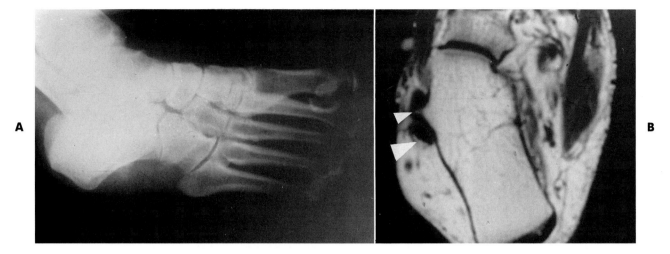

**Fig. 5-5. A,** An oblique x-ray of the foot of a 25-year-old male baseball player with acute onset of lateral foot pain. Note that the os peroneum has migrated proximally from its normal position beneath the cuboid to the calcaneal trochlea lateralis. **B,** An MRI reveals the tendon and os peroneum *(lower arrow)* retracted proximally and held at the trochlea lateralis *(upper arrow).* Excision of the sesamoid, advancement of the tendon with tendon graft, were the treatment. One year later the man was playing baseball with good function but still had mild aching in the foot.

tendons. They present with symptoms of pain along the lateral foot and have been reported in the middle-aged athlete as well as in patients with generalized diseases such as diabetes. Tenderness occurs over the os peroneum at the cuboid with fullness over the lateral calcaneus.[26,42,43] A mass representing a portion of the os peroneum may be present but is small and may be overlooked. If the tendon is intact, longitudinal rents—which may extend from the os peroneum to lateral malleolus— may be confused with tears of the peroneus brevis tendon. Radiographs show a fragmented os peroneum. MRI reveals longitudinal degenerative tears in the tendon and fluid in the tendon sheath. If the tendon is ruptured, it will migrate proximately to bind at the trochlea lateralis of the calcaneus.

Without complete rupture of the tendon, immobilization for 2 weeks in a gatched walker boot is indicated, followed by a rehabilitation program stressing flexibility and power-building exercises. Improvement in conditioning techniques and adequate stretching before running again is prescribed. NSAIDs are recommended. An Aircast® may be indicated until symptoms subside, since it helps control ankle and subtalar motion on inversion. An ankle brace is recommended on return to sports. An orthotic in the shoe, made of semirigid material, may relieve the stress on the tendon.

If symptoms persist, surgical debridement and tenosynovectomy are suggested. This is accomplished with a direct repair of the tendon, using a running 4-0 braided Ethibond suture and burying the knots on either end of the repair. Excision of the degenerated tissue within the tendon is also performed. When complete disruption has occurred, the proximal tendon stump is mobilized. If the tendon can be advanced, this is an indication that the muscle is still functional and has not contracted. If not, reattachment of the tendon to the distal stump can be performed by tendon graft using half of the peroneus brevis tendon harvested through the same operative field. The peroneus brevis tendon lies dorsal to the peroneus longus tendon (see Acute Rupture section). If the torn peroneus longus tendon is retracted and the muscle contracted and fixed, its function will be significantly reduced. The tendon should be attached to the lateral calcaneus so that it may still function as an accessory ankle flexor and lateral stabilizer of the foot. The patient should be counseled, however, concerning the possibility of progressive elevation of the first metatarsal head, if this "dorsal bunion" has not already occurred. In children pes cavovarus has been reported.[9] Rarely both tendons of the peroneus longus and peroneus brevis are ruptured. This is usually associated with severe chronic lateral ankle ligament instability. If both tendons are retracted and fixed, attachment to the lateral calcaneus is recommended.

Rehabilitation is begun after 4 weeks of immobilization, and the patient should continue use of an ankle brace until asymptomatic. A semirigid orthotic of metatarsal length is prescribed. Prognosis for return to play is good; however the period for return is often over 3 months (see Case Study 3).

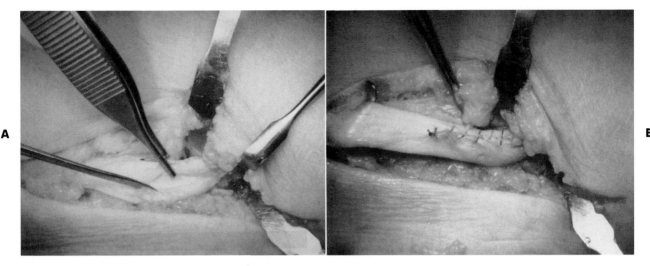

**Fig. 5-6. A,** Operative photograph of a 40-year-old male with a 4-cm tear of the peroneus longus tendon. (Forefoot is to the *right* of the field.) Note how the tear extends distally beneath the cuboid (the os peroneum is not visible in the field). **B,** The tear was repaired with 4-0 braided Dacron running suture. The patient was immobilized for 3 weeks and thereafter began a supervised physical therapy program. Significant symptoms of pain remained for 1 year postoperatively. The patient returned to playing tennis 4 months after surgery but 2 years following surgery still has discomfort during play.

**Case Study 3.** A 40-year-old experienced tennis player stretched for a backhand volley and felt a sharp pain over the lateral aspect of his midfoot. He was unable to continue play. Examination revealed tenderness over the lateral aspect of the midfoot (Fig. 5-6). Radiographs were normal. Over the next 3 weeks the pain increased and swelling developed on the lateral aspect of his heel. Examination revealed tenderness over the course of the peroneus longus tendon beneath the lateral ankle in the region distal to the trochlea lateralis of the calcaneus. Surgical intervention was counseled. At operation, a 4-cm-long tear of the peroneus longus tendon was noted, extending proximally from the os peroneum. It was bound within the tendon sheath at the trochlea lateralis. This was repaired. Postoperatively the patient was immobilized in a cast for 3 weeks, after which an Aircast was applied and gentle active range of motion begun with a supervised physical therapy program. Three months following surgery the patient was playing tennis again, using an ankle brace. He stated that he felt more comfortable in a prescribed orthosis. One year following the injury, the patient had minimal symptoms of aching on the lateral side of his foot but was unrestricted in his activities.

## FLEXOR HALLUCIS LONGUS

The flexor hallucis longus muscle rises in the deep posterior compartment of the calf. From its attachment on the interosseus membrane, lower two thirds of the fibula and intermuscular septa, it passes from the deep compartment into its own tunnel at the posterior aspect of the talus. It then passes beneath the sustentaculum tali of the calcaneus to the master knot of Henry, where it crosses deep to the flexor digitorum

longus tendon. Here it gives off a slip of tendon that then inserts on the medial fibers of the flexor digitorum longus tendon. It then passes beneath the first metatarsal between the sesamoids to insert on the distal phalanx of the hallux. The anatomic position puts this tendon at risk for injuries in various places. Like all polyarthrodial muscles, the extrinsic muscles of the foot—both in the anterior and posterior compartments of the leg—have a complex function. The muscle functions as a flexor of the distal and proximal phalanges of the hallux, thus aiding in flexion of the midtarsal joints and supination of the foot as well as plantar flexion of the ankle.

### Tendinitis

Acute tendinitis occurs most commonly at the posterior ankle where the tendon passes behind the ankle beneath the sustentaculum tali.[4] This injury is common in dancers and has been termed "dancer's tendinitis." Although less common than Achilles tendinitis, it often occurs in inexperienced dancers and in athletes who are suboptimally conditioned and return to high-intensity sports activity. Tendinitis also develops when athletes change sports without properly conditioning themselves for the new activity. Symptoms begin within several days following a change of technique or at the beginning of a new season. When the dancer rises on the ball of the foot, pain occurs in the posterior aspect of the ankle. This is usually vague and occurs with flexion of the ankle and foot. Passive dorsiflexion of the ankle with great toe extension, and in particular interphalangeal extension, can predispose to tripping and weakened resistance to flexion of the hallux in the playing shoe. Direct repair with or without tendon graft is indicated (see the section, Tibialis Anterior). Although untreated disruption of the tendon can lead to flexion of the hallux interphalangeal joint, performance may not be significantly affected. If this is the case, repair is not necessary. Interphalangeal joint flexion can, however, cause pain due to weight bearing on a flexed distal phalanx. In addition, the player may have difficulty slipping the foot into a shoe. In this case correcting the flexed phalanx is performed by arthrodesis or proximal phalangeal condylectomy. Both procedures will stiffen the joint and prevent flexion. Injections of corticosteroids on the dorsum of the foot should be performed with caution. It is my opinion that the minimal subcutaneous tissue predisposes the patient to tissue atrophy as well as skin depigmentation. Moreover sterile abscess has been reported.

## REFERENCES

1. Arrowsmith SR, Fleming LL, Allman FL: Traumatic dislocations of the peroneal tendons, *Am J Sports Med* 11:142, 1983.
2. Bianchi S, Abdelwahab IF, Tegaldo G: Fracture and posterior dislocation of the os peroneum associated with rupture of the peroneus longus tendon, *Can Assoc Radiol J* 42:340, 1991.
3. Brand JC Jr, Smith RW: Rupture of the flexor hallucis longus after hallux valgus surgery: case report and comments on technique for abductor release, Comment in *Foot Ankle* 12:132, 1991; *Foot Ankle* 11:407, 1991.
4. Burman M: Stenosing tenosynovitis of the foot and ankle, *Arch Surg* 67:686, 1953.
5. Buschmann WR, Cheung Y, Jahss MH: Magnetic resonance imaging of anomalous leg muscles: accessory soleus, peroneus quartus and the flexor digitorum longus accessorius, *Foot Ankle* 12:109, 1991.
6. Cowell HR, Elener V, Lawhon SM: Bilateral tendonitis of the flexor hallucis longus in a ballet dancer, *J Pediatr Orthop* 2:582, 1982.
7. Crosby LA, Fitzgibbons TC: Unrecognized laceration of tibialis anterior tendon: a case report, *Foot Ankle* 9:143, 1988.
8. Cross MJ et al: Peroneus brevis rupture in the absence of the peroneus longus muscle and tendon in a classical ballet dancer. A case report, *Am J Sports Med* 16:677, 1988.
8a. Dameron TB Jr: Fractures and anatomical variations of the proximal portion of the fifth metatarsal, *J Bone Joint Surg* 57A:788, 1975.
9. DeLuca PA, Banta JV: Pes cavovarus as a late consequence of peroneus longus tendon laceration, *J Pediatr Orthop* 5:582, 1985.
10. Elmslie RC: Recurrent subluxation of the ankle joint, *Ann Surg* 100:364, 1935.
11. Garth WP: Flexor hallucis tendinitis in a ballet dancer, *J Bone Joint Surg* 63A:1489, 1981.
12. Gilula LA et al: Ankle tenography: a key to unexplained symptomatology. Part II: diagnosis of chronic tendon disabilities, *Radiology* 151:581, 1984.
13. Harrington KD: Degenerative arthritis of the ankle secondary to longstanding lateral ligament instability, *J Bone Joint Surg* 61A:354, 1979.
14. Hecker P: Etude sur le peroneir due tarse: veriations des peroniers lateraux, *Arch Anat Histol Embryol* 3:327, 1924.
15. Kerr R, Forrester DM, Kingston S: Magnetic resonance imaging of foot and ankle trauma, *Orthop Clin North Am* 21:591, 1990.
16. Korovessis P et al: Simultaneous rupture of the tibialis posterior and flexor digitorum longus tendons in a closed tibial fracture, *J Orthop Trauma* 5:89, 1991.
17. Krakow KA: Acute traumatic rupture of a flexor hallucis longus tendon: a case report, *Clin Orthop* 261, 1980.
18. LeDouble AF: *Traits des variations du systems musculaire de l'homme et de leur signification au point de vue de I. Anthropoligie et zoologique*, Vol 2, Paris, 1897, Schleicher Freres.
19. Liou J, Totty WG: Magnetic resonance imaging of ankle injuries, *Top Magn Reson Imaging* 3:1, 1991.
20. Menz P, Nettle WJ: Closed rupture of the musculotendinous junction of extensor hallucis longus, *Injury* 20:378, 1989.
21. Mink JH, Duetsch AL, Kerr R: Tendon injuries of the lower extremity: magnetic resonance assessment, *Top Magn Reson Imaging* 3:23, 1991.
22. McCarroll JR, Ritter MS, Becker TE: Triggering of the great toe: a case report, *Clin Orthop* 184, 1983.
23. Munk RL, Davis PH: Longitudinal rupture of the peroneus brevis tendon, *J Trauma* 16:803, 1976.
24. Parvin RW, Fort LT: Stenosing tenosynovitis of the common peroneal tendon sheath, *J Bone Joint Surg* 38A:1352, 1956.
25. Peacock KC, Resnick EJ, Thoder JJ: Rupture of the peroneus longus tendon. Report of three cases, *J Bone Joint Surg(A)* 72:306, 1990.
26. Peacock KC, Resnick EJ, Thoder JJ: Fracture of the os peroneus with rupture of the peroneus longus tendon. A case report and review of the literature, *Clin Orthop* 223, 1986.
27. Pozo JL, Jackson AM: A rerouting operation for dislocation of peroneal tendons: operative technique and case report, *Foot Ankle* 5:42, 1984.
28. Rasmussen RB, Thyssen EP: Rupture of the flexor hallucis longus tendon: a case report, *Foot Ankle* 10:288, 1990.
29. Regan TP, Hughston JL: Chronic ankle "sprain" secondary to anomalous peroneal tendon: a case report, *Clin Orthop* 123:52, 1977.
30. Rimoldi RL et al: Acute rupture of the tibialis anterior tendon: a case report, *Foot Ankle* 12:176, 1991.
31. Romash MM: Fracture of the calcaneus: an unusual fracture pattern with subtalar joint interposition of the flexor hallux longus. A report of two cases, *Foot Ankle* 12:32, 1992.
32. Rosenberg ZS, Cheung Y, Jahss MH: Computer tomography scan and magnetic resonance imaging of ankle tendons: an overview, *Foot Ankle* 8:297, 1988.
33. Rosenberg ZS et al: Peroneal tendon injury associated with calcaneal fractures: CT findings, *AJR* 149:125, 1987.
34. St Pierre R, et al: A review of lateral ankle ligamentous reconstructions, *Foot Ankle* 3:114, 1982.
35. Sammarco GJ, Miller EH: Partial rupture of the flexor hallucis longus tendon in classical ballet dancers, *J Bone Joint Surg* 61A:149, 1979.
36. Sammarco GJ, DiRaimondo CV: Chronic peroneus brevis tendon lesions, *Foot Ankle* 9:163, 1989.
37. Sammarco GJ, DiRaimondo CV: Surgical treatment of lateral ankle instability, *Am J Sports Med* 16:501, 1988.
38. Sammarco GJ, Brainard BJ: Asymptomatic anomalous peroneus brevis in a high jumper, *J Bone Joint Surg* 73A:131, 1991.
39. Shoda E et al: Longitudinal ruptures of the peroneal tendons. A report of a rugby player, *Acta Orthop Scand* 62:491, 1991.
40. Snyder RB, Lipscomb AB, Johnson RK: The relationship of tarsal coalitions to ankle sprains in athletes, *Am J Sports Med* 9:313, 1981.

41. Stark HH et al: Bridge flexor tendon grafts, *Clin Orthop* 242:51, 1989.

42. Tehranzadeh J, Stoll DA, Gabriele OM: Case report 271. Posterior migration of the os peroneum of the left foot, indicating a tear of the peroneal tendon, *Skeletal Radiol* 12:44, 1984.

43. Thompson FM, Patterson AH: Rupture of the peroneus longus tendon: report of three cases, *J Bone Joint Surg (A)* 72:306, 1990; *J Bone Joint Surg (A)* 71:293, 1989.

44. Webster FS: Peroneal tenosynovitis with pseudo-tumor, *J Bone Joint Surg* 50A:153, 1968.

45. Winfield P: Treatment of undue mobility of the ankle joint following severe sprains with avulsion of the anterior and middle bands of the external ligaments, *Acta Chir Scand* 105:299, 1953.

# Chapter 6

# The achilles tendon

## Michael R. Clain

### ANATOMY AND BIOMECHANICS

The gastrocnemius and soleus muscles coalesce distally and insert into the Achilles tendon. The gastrocnemius spans two joints: the knee and the ankle. Placing it under an extreme and rapid eccentric contracture (knee extension and ankle dorsiflexion) has been implicated etiologically in acute complete Achilles tendon ruptures.[46] In the area of noninsertional tendinitis, 2 to 6 cm proximal to the calcaneus, the tendon internally rotates just before inserting into the bone (i.e., the posterior fibers become lateral). This may result in localized torque stresses, causing tendinitis. The tendon itself is surrounded by a paratendon, not a synovial sheath. This enveloping structure may be involved in the disease process of noninsertional tendinitis. In fact, Kvist et al[38,39] have found marked metabolic changes in peritendinitis with a proliferation of pathologic myofibroblast cells.

The tendon itself inserts distal to the posterosuperior calcaneal tuberosity on the inferior portion of the calcaneus. The retrocalcaneal bursa is a normal lubricating structure between the tendon and the bone just proximal to its insertion. Both the tuberosity and the retrocalcaneal bursa are involved in early insertional tendinitis. A second subcutaneous bursa between the tendon and skin is variably present. The posterosuperior tuberosity of the calcaneus can be highly prominent. If excessively prominent, it is called a *Haglund deformity*.[22] The exact definition of a Haglund deformity is controversial. It was probably best defined by Pavlov et al, in 1982[55] (Fig. 6-1). They established the concept of parallel pitch lines. An initial line is from the plantar aspect of the anterior tubercle and the plantar aspect of the medial tubercle. A line is drawn parallel to that from the posterior lip

of the talar articular facet. A Haglund deformity would be defined as one in which bone is seen to extend excessively above the upper pitch line. The bony prominence associated with chronic inflammation of the retrocalcaneal bursa mechanically abrades and chemically erodes the Achilles tendon at its insertion.

Lagergren and Lindholm[41] performed a classic cadaveric angiographic study of the blood supply to the Achilles tendon, reported in 1958/1959. They found that the most tenuously supplied region was that 2 to 6 cm proximal to the calcaneus insertion. This correlates with the area of involvement in noninsertional tendinitis and indeed most complete subcutaneous ruptures. This vascular explanation has more recently been implicated as a cause for tendinitis and ruptures in other anatomic locations. Posterior tibialis tendinitis and supraspinatus tendinitis of the rotator cuff are but two examples.[19,58]

Biomechanically the Achilles is subjected to large stresses. The plantar flexor muscles are the dominant group during stance phase. The stress that the Achilles experiences varies between 2000 and 7000 N.[7,61] This is equivalent to 10 times body weight repetitively exerted on the Achilles tendon. The more rigorous the activity, the greater the stress. Further, since the Achilles inserts into the calcaneus, talar calcaneal motion will place an uneven rotational force on the tendon fibers. Clement et al[12] and James et al[31] have implicated "functional overpronation" as an etiologic factor in noninsertional tendinitis.

The pronated foot normally imparts an internal rotation force on the tibia, whereas knee extension imparts an external rotation force through the tibia. The hypothesis is that during midstance the foot remains pronated for a relatively long period of the

71

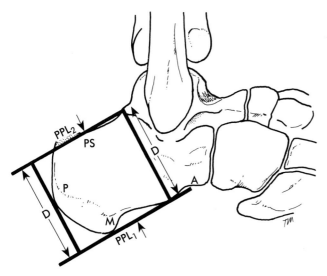

**Fig. 6-1.** The parallel pitch lines (PPLs) determine the prominence of the posterior superior tuberosity of the calcaneus (PS). The lower PPL (PPL$_1$) is the baseline, constructed from the inferior line of the Fowler and Philip angle. A perpendicular (D) is constructed between the posterior lip of the talar articular facet (T) and the baseline. The upper PPL (PPL$_2$) is drawn parallel to the baseline at distance D. A posterior superior tuberosity touching or below PPL$_2$ is normal, whereas one extending above it is considered excessively prominent.

gait cycle. While the foot remains pronated excessively, normal knee extension occurs and the Achilles experiences unusually high forces secondary to these contradictory rotational forces. In an Achilles rupture, a concentric or eccentric sudden and rapid contracture overcomes the tendon, causing it to rupture.[4]

Thus the mechanical and vascular anatomy, combined with biomechanical overload, may predispose an individual to developing tendinitis or even a complete rupture.

## ACHILLES TENDINITIS

Achilles tendinitis is a common problem. It is an overuse syndrome that can be caused by many factors. Specific anatomic characteristics combined with biomechanical variation may predispose an individual to developing a problem with the Achilles tendon. Excessive mileage, improper training techniques, and inadequate shoe wear have been implicated in causing Achilles tendinitis. The incidence of Achilles tendinitis among runners is reported to vary from 6.5% to 18%.[11,36]

It is helpful to organize Achilles tendinitis into "insertional" and "noninsertional" Achilles tendinitis.[9a] Noninsertional tendinitis occurs just proximal to the tendon insertion on the calcaneus in or around the tendon substance. Insertional tendinitis involves the tendon/bone interface and may be associated with

a bony protuberance of the os calcis. Appropriate categorization ensures that treatment is problem specific.

### Incidence

Achilles tendinitis is quite common. In a study by Bovens et al from The Netherlands in 1989,[4] 115 volunteers were closely supervised in a marathon preparation training program. The subjects were untrained volunteers who were followed for all injuries, with the stated goal of marathon participation within 18 months. The subjects were individually supervised by experienced coaches with particular attention to physiologic training and injury prevention. During the study period, 11% of injuries involved the Achilles tendon. There was a direct correlation of injuries with the intensity level of the training program. Interestingly the incidence of injuries on the left side significantly exceeded those on the right side, which was thought to be related to road-running techniques.

A recent study by Leppilahti et al[44] revealed that 7% of their patients at a sports medicine clinic had overuse injuries of the Achilles tendon. Krissoff and Ferris,[36] writing in 1979, reviewed runners injuries. They found an 18% incidence of Achilles tendinitis. Clement et al[11] reported on a retrospective review of 1650 patients in 1981 who presented at a sports medicine clinic with a specific complaint. Six percent of the injuries were Achilles peritendinitis (7.9% of injuries in men and 3.2% in women). Men consistently have a disproportionately higher number of Achilles injuries than women.[12,37,44]

Most of the reviews of the incidence of injuries have been done in runners.[4,10,11,36] Presumably this is because they are the easiest group to standardize (e.g., mileage per week). Clinical experience indicates that others are also at high risk. Specifically these include middle-aged weekend athletes, dancers, tennis players, racquetball players, soccer players, and basketball players. The common thread seems to be repetitive impact loading associated with jumping.

### Noninsertional tendinitis

Most reports of diseases of the Achilles tendon limit their study to those of noninsertional Achilles tendinitis.* In 1976 Puddu et al[57] proposed a classification system for noninsertional diseases of the Achilles tendon. They described three entities: peritendinitis, peritendinitis with tendinosis, and tendinosis. In peritendinitis, inflammation is limited to the peritendon. Many cases resolve with nonoperative treatment. If the disease is persistent, resection of the

*References 4, 10, 12, 21, 36, 39, 40, 51, 57, 63.

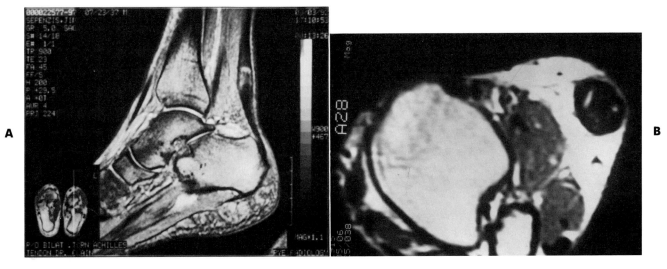

**Fig. 6-2. A,** MRI of noninsertional tendinitis. **B,** Axial cut noninsertional tendinitis.

peritendon alone usually resolves the problem. Additionally, surgical exploration would verify that, in fact, the tendon itself was not involved.

Peritendinitis with tendinosis describes a second stage of inflammation in which a portion of the Achilles tendon itself is involved in the disease process. The tendon may feel thicker and perhaps nodular. At exploration it will have lost some of its normal glistening appearance, and there may be areas of focal degeneration and even a partial tear. These patients are at risk for complete rupture. If they come to surgery for persistent tendinosis, a repair of the tendon with a possible augmentation procedure needs to be considered.

The third entity as described by Puddu et al is pure tendinosis. This is usually a presumptive diagnosis made at the time of an acute rupture of the Achilles tendon. These patients are typically middle-aged, weekend athletes. Most deny any symptoms related to the Achilles tendon before rupture, but on pathologic examination, evidence of chronic macroscopic and microscopic degeneration is found.

Clinically the symptoms include pain, usually 2 to 6 cm proximal to the insertion (the zone of decreased vascularity and fiber rotation). The pain is often worse in the morning and after exercise. With progression of the disease, pain can become constant on walking or running. Many individuals with an acute rupture, however, have no prodrome of pain at all.

On physical examination in the early stages of noninsertional tendinitis, several signs are present. Often localized tenderness and crepitus may be evident. The tendon may be thickened. Dorsiflexion may be limited by comparison to the other side. Radiographic examination may reveal calcification in or about the tendon. Magnetic resonance imaging

(MRI) can be helpful in assessing whether tendinosis is present (Fig. 6-2).

Treatment of noninsertional tendinitis at the early stages is nonoperative. Antiinflammatory measures such as medication, rest of the tendon, local ice massage, electrostimulation, and contrast baths may be instituted. Most patients improve relatively rapidly. In the rehabilitation phase, an Achilles tendon stretching program should be instituted.[59] An incline board backstage at major ballet companies has been reported to have dramatically decreased the incidence of Achilles tendinitis among the dancers[23] (Fig. 6-3). The use of orthotic devices may be considered. A heel lift, or if the patient seems to overpronate, a medial arch support may symptomatically be helpful. Kvist et al[37] recommend assessing overpronation by asking the patient to do a knee bend and observing the medial arch for evidence of collapse. The use of cortisone is discouraged in noninsertional tendinitis because of the risk of rupture.[37] In fact, cortisone was shown to be ineffective in a blinded study of 28 patients in England.[13]

If symptoms persist, operative intervention may be indicated. Some surgeons operate as early as 3 months after the initiation of treatment; others prefer to wait for a year or more.*

Kvist and Kvist[40] from Finland reported in 1980 on the operative treatment of chronic calcaneal paratendinitis. Between 1961 and 1978 they performed 201 operations. Their procedure was performed early, after 2 to 3 months of failed nonoperative therapy. The procedure basically involved release of the crural fascia on both sides of the tendon, release of adhesions, and trimming of the paratendon if hypertro-

*References 10, 40, 51, 57, 60, 63.

phied. They reported excellent/good results in 194 of 201 cases. The disease process by extrapolation seems to have been predominantly Puddu group I.

The other large series in the literature is from Belgium. Nelen et al[51] reported in 1989 on 170 cases. Their patients were symptomatic for an average of 18 months before surgery. For Puddu group I the procedures described by Kvist were performed. For Puddu group II—in addition to resection of the fascia—debridement and repair of the tendon itself was performed in 26 cases. A turndown flap was necessary in 24 cases because of extensive debridement. Eighty-six percent of patients had only a fascial release and good/excellent results. Seventy-three percent with resection of diseased tissue had good/excellent results. Schepsis and Leach[60] reported in 1987 on their results. They performed a similar procedure to that described, including resection of the fascia and debridement as indicated of the Achilles tendon itself. Their patients were symptomatic on average for 3 years. Of 24 patients with pure noninsertional tendinitis, 22 had good/excellent results. Earlier studies with smaller numbers by Clancy et al,[10] Gould and Korson,[21] Snook[63] and basically agreed with the focus of these larger series.

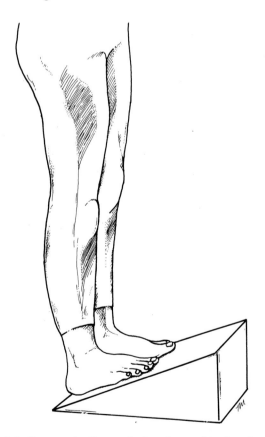

**Fig. 6-3.** Feet gradually worked to base of incline board. Stretch should be felt in calf (gastroc) muscle, not in Achilles tendon.

The literature thus supports operative intervention after a course of nonoperative therapy. The decision should be made after an assessment of multiple factors such as duration and intensity of discomfort, thoroughness of rehabilitation, and athletic demands of the patient. We believe peritendinitis should be treated by resection of the peritendon. Peritendinitis with tendinosis requires resection of the peritendon and debridement of the tendon itself, with a possible augmentation flap. A small group of patients may benefit from an additional tendon transfer procedure. These include patients in whom the remaining tendon substance is insufficient. The simplest transfer procedure was the plantaris tendon in the repair.[47] Other transfer options are discussed later.

### Insertional tendinitis

Insertional Achilles tendinitis is considered to be a separate entity. Unfortunately little in modern sports literature addresses this problem.[9a,60,62] Most of what has been written primarily addresses the "pump bump."[14,16,22,34] Radiographically there may be some overlap with a Haglund deformity. But in the case of the pump bump, the problem is largely one of a bony posterolateral prominence, often with overlying bursitis associated mainly with women's shoe wear. The Achilles is minimally involved with a pump bump. Shoe modification with local padding and antiinflammatory measures may be helpful. Occasionally resection of the prominent tuberosity is necessary.[14]

Schepsis and Leach,[60] writing in 1987, included 14 of 45 cases involving insertional Achilles tendinitis alone. The inflammation of the tendon may be associated with retrocalcaneal bursitis as well as a Haglund deformity. The combination of chronic overuse associated with retrocalcaneal bursitis and bony impingement probably creates a chronic inflammatory response with chemical attrition and mechanical abrasion of the Achilles tendon. Often this results in calcification of the tendon substance.

Clinically the symptoms include pain at the bone/tendon junction. Often the pain is worse after exercise and may become constant. On physical examination the tendon is tender in a specific location, often posterolaterally. With chronicity it becomes thickened. Occasionally a defect in the tendon may be palpated, particularly if a localized steroid injection has been used. Often the gastroc-soleus complex is relatively tight. That is, there is less dorsiflexion on the affected side than the normal side. If the problem is bilateral, dorsiflexion is barely to the neutral position with the knee extended. Radiographically a Haglund deformity is usually present. In chronic cases the bone/tendon junction becomes calcified with a spur extending into the tendon itself (Fig. 6-4).

Nonoperative therapy includes measures similar to those used in noninsertional tendinitis. Antiinflammatory medications, ice massage, and contrast baths can be used. Immobilization in acutely inflamed cases, followed by Achilles rehabilitation with stretching, is often indicated. Orthotic devices may be useful. A simple heel lift in working shoes might be effective. In a runner—if the tenderness is localized—for example, to the posteromedial Achilles, a one-eighth-inch heel-to-toe medial wedge in the sole of the running shoe may be indicated (Fig. 6-5). The wedge is extended into the forefoot, since most of the stance phase of the running gait cycle is spent on the forefoot. A lateral wedge can be used for posterolateral tendinitis.

Operative treatment may be recommended only after failure of conservative measures.[60,62] In general we recommend a two-incision technique, medial and lateral to the Achilles. The first incision is made on the symptomatic side. The Haglund deformity is aggressively resected, as is the chronically inflamed retrocalcaneal bursa (Figs. 6-6 and 6-7). The Achilles tendon is inspected from anterior to posterior. Often there is a defect in the substance. The inflamed or degenerated tissue is resected, and any calcified tissue is removed sharply. The second incision adds little morbidity and will ensure complete decompression. Immobilization is dependent on the degree of tendon compromise. Usually 1 month in a cast followed by a course of rehabilitation is preferred. In failed cases, as well as in patients with severe tendon compromise, a tendon transfer procedure may be indicated.

Achilles tendinitis includes two basic groups: insertional and noninsertional. Treatment is predicated on the appropriate categorization. Most patients respond to a multifaceted, nonoperative approach. Some will require surgery. A few will be operative failures or have tendon compromise so extensive that a transfer procedure is indicated. Like other orthopedic disorders, a systematic approach to Achilles tendinitis enables the physician to deliver the most effective treatment to the individual patient.

## ACHILLES TENDON RUPTURE

The history obtained in patients with a ruptured tendo Achillis is remarkably consistent. Typically the individual is a middle-aged, weekend, male athlete. He reports that he thought his partner had just swung a racquet with full force at his heel. A pop is often heard. Upon turning he realized no one was behind

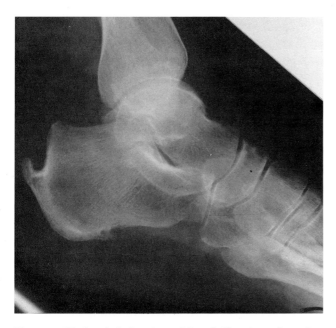

**Fig. 6-4.** Haglund deformity with calcification of tendon insertion.

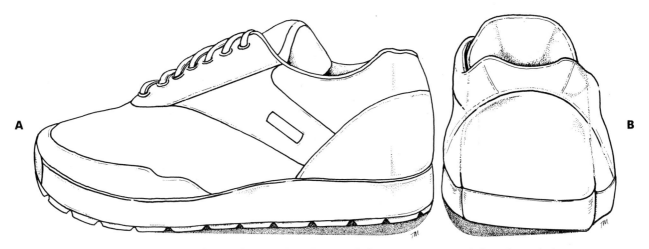

**Fig. 6-5. A,** One-eighth-inch medial wedge (medial view). **B,** One-eighth-inch medial wedge (back view).

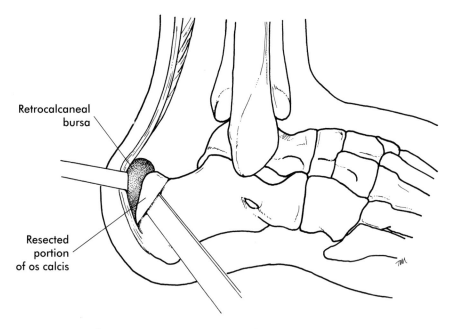

**Fig. 6-6.** Aggressive resection of Haglund deformity.

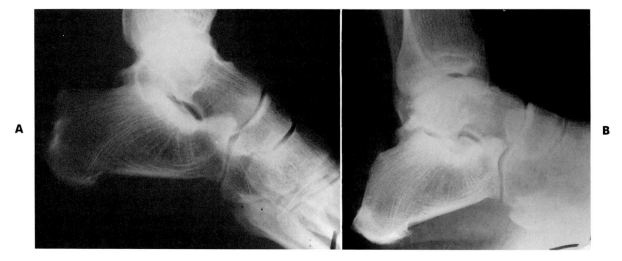

**Fig. 6-7. A,** Preoperative insertional Achilles tendinitis. **B,** Postoperative insertional Achilles tendinitis.

him. Most individuals are disabled enough to seek medical attention immediately, but some are not. Only when the latter group fails to recover from this presumed "sprain" do they then present. There may have been a history of symptomatic Achilles tendinitis before the event, but that is not usually the case.[1,17,36] Histologically virtually all patients with an acute rupture of the Achilles tendon have preexisting tendinitis.[33,57]

**Diagnosis**

Physical examination of a suspected ruptured tendo Achillis should involve the following five components:

1. The Thompson-Doherty squeeze test[65]
2. Palpation of the medial head of the gastrocnemius
3. Palpation of a gap in the tendon
4. O'Brien's needle test
5. Assessment of heel resistance strength

The Thompson-Doherty squeeze test involves placing the patient prone with the knee at 90 degrees of flexion. A squeeze of the calf musculature normally results in passive plantar flexion. A positive Thompson-Doherty test is an absence of passive plantar flexion. This also incorporates the second test, which is necessary to rule out a tear of the medial head of the gastrocnemius muscle. Tenderness in that area (or calf pain with the Thompson-Doherty test) indicates a probable medial gastrocnemius tear. A palpable gap is usually present in an Achilles rupture, particularly in an acute situation. This is best felt with the patient prone, the foot over the edge of the examining table, and the patient actively dorsiflexing the ankle.[62] O'Brien's[53] needle test involves placing a needle 10 cm proximal to the superior border of the calcaneus into the tendon substance. If, on passive motion of the foot, the needle is seen to swivel, the Achilles is intact. An absence of motion indicates a positive O'Brien test. The final assessment is that of heel resistance strength. The examiner grasps the foot in neutral and instructs the patient to plantar flex. With an intact Achilles, the grasp is easily broken. If the Achilles is torn, the posterior tibial, peroneal, and flexor tendons will fail to break the grasp.[15] In an acute case usually palpation of a gap and a positive Thompson-Doherty test will suffice. But with a delayed presentation, the other three techniques may be indicated.

Radiography may indirectly be useful in establishing the diagnosis but generally is not of great importance. MRI and ultrasonography may have a role in the unusual or perplexing case.[54] But in general the diagnosis is clinical, based on history and physical examination[25,52] (Fig. 6-8).

### Etiology

Three factors are thought to be involved in predisposing an individual to an acute rupture of the Achilles tendon. The first is mechanical. Rapid push-off with the knee extended, or sudden, unexpected dorsiflexion with a misstep has been postulated as a mechanism.[1] The second factor is vascular. The tendon that ruptures usually will do so in the zone of relatively diminished blood supply about 2 to 6 cm proximal to the calcaneus.[40] The third component involves the quality of the tissue substance. Many studies[33,37,57] have revealed that the ruptured Achilles tendon will have preexisting degenerative pathologic changes. Specifically these include hypoxic, mucoid, lipomatous, and calcific changes. Thus, overall, it is a pathologic and usually asymptomatic Achilles tendon subjected to an unusually rapid and extreme force that will fail and rupture.

### Treatment

There is no clear consensus on the appropriate treatment for a rupture of the Achilles tendon. When treatment is delayed, most workers feel that operative treatment is indicated, since the tendon will have begun to heal inappropriately lengthened.[8] In an acute situation, however, there are two schools of

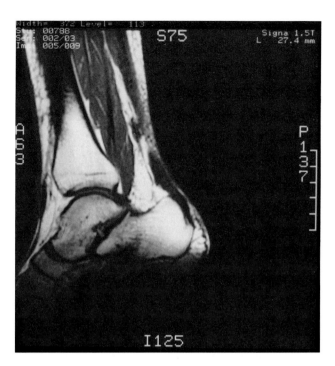

**Fig. 6-8.** MRI of Achilles tendon rupture.

thought. The first involves nonoperative treatment, which has been most strongly advocated by Lea and Smith.[42,43] Their treatment involves short-leg casting for 8 weeks followed by a 2.5 cm heel lift for another 4 weeks. The principal complication is rerupture, which is reported to vary between 10% and 35%.*

The second option is open repair, which includes a multitude of techniques, has a lower rerupture rate (<6%), but adds the risk of surgical and anesthetic complications including infection, skin slough, sural nerve injury, and an adherent scar. The advocates of open treatment believe that the lower risk of rerupture associated with better long-term strength and endurance outweigh the surgical risks in most active individuals.[2,27-29] This debate is unresolved.

I favor a case-by-case approach. In young, generally athletic individuals, I favor operative intervention. In older persons, particularly those with systemic disease such as diabetes mellitus, I prefer nonoperative treatment.

### Nonoperative

The protocol as described by Lea and Smith[42,43] is appropriate for closed treatment. It involves application of a walking cast initially in the gravity equinus position (i.e., not forced equinus). Over 8 weeks the foot is brought closer to neutral. At 2 months I prefer a heel lift in a removable cast boot with a rocker sole for a further month. Physical therapy is initiated to

*References 20, 27, 28, 42, 43, 52.

mobilize the foot and strengthen it at 12 weeks. The temptation to shorten the period of protection must be resisted to minimize the possibility of rerupture.[25,52]

### Operative

A review of *Campbell's Operative Orthopaedics*[56] details the history of operative Achilles tendon repair. These methods include simple suture, use of the plantaris,[47] peroneus brevis,[64] turndown flaps,[3] and fascial strips[6] to augment the repair. Synthetic substances such as carbon fiber[68] and the use of other techniques such as a percutaneous approach[5,48] and local anesthesia[9] have been advocated. The fundamental concern is to provide a strong repair and to minimize the two potential major complications: skin slough and rerupture.

In an acute rupture we prefer a spinal anesthetic. The patient is placed prone. Radiographs are checked to ensure that a bony avulsion has not occurred. An important step is to preoperatively assess the tension of the Achilles tendon on the uninjured side with the knee flexed. This should be the goal in terms of the appropriate tensioning to be achieved on the operative site. We prefer not to use a tourniquet. The incision is made medial to the tendon, safely away from the sural nerve and should be generous to minimize skin tension. Skin flaps and unnecessary retraction are avoided. The paratendon is incised and the tendon inspected; the ends are minimally debrided. An incision is made in the anterior paratendon to aid in closure posteriorly. The repair is performed using a modified Kessler stitch using two individual #5 nonabsorbable sutures with the knot in the repair. Tensioning is critical and is based on the preoperative assessment of the other side. The repair is strengthened with an absorbable suture about the edges, which adds to the strength of the repair.[67] We prefer not to "overstuff" the tendon space by the use of extensive augmentation techniques in a straightforward acute rupture. The paratendon is closed, and then skin is closed using nylon sutures. A short-leg cast is applied with the foot in equinus. We protect the repair for 7 to 8 weeks in a cast, after which the patient begins therapy and uses a removable cast boot. Most patients are unprotected at 10 to 12 weeks. A full return to vigorous sports can take 5 to 6 months.

In late ruptures of several weeks, the standard technique is used. In delayed treatment we prefer to perform a transfer procedure to augment the repair with the peroneus brevis, the flexor digitorum longus (FDL), or the flexor hallucis longus (FHL).

The history and physical examination in an acute Achilles rupture are usually diagnostically conclusive. Further testing is of little added value. Treatment is controversial. We prefer a closely supervised nonoperative approach in older, more debilitated patients. In younger, athletic individuals, we prefer an open procedure with meticulous attention to detail. Both methods require lengthy immobilization and rehabilitation. An Achilles rupture can be a devastating injury from which an athlete should completely recover, provided the treatment protocol is well executed and not injudiciously accelerated.

### TRANSFER PROCEDURES

Basically there are three substantial musculotendinous units that could be used in a transfer procedure: the peroneus brevis, the FDL, and the FHL. Teuffer in 1974[64] and Turco and Spinella in 1987[66] described use of the peroneus brevis in acute Achilles tendon ruptures as an augmentation procedure. Mann et al in 1991[49] described the use of the FDL in chronic Achilles ruptures. Hanson[24] has recommended use of the FHL as a transfer. We have had experience with all three procedures. The peroneus brevis does not give as much length as the FDL and FHL. It is, however, a substantial tendon that can be harvested from the lateral side. Thus if there is an existing lateral incision, one may use the peroneus brevis.

The FDL and the FHL require a medial approach as well as dissection at the knot of Henry. Length is more than sufficient, especially if the FHL is cut at the interphalangeal joint of the great toe. The line of pull of the FDL might impinge on the neurovascular bundle if it is not dissected proximally, since it normally lies anterior to the bundle. This is not a concern with the FHL since its position is more posterior. There is no information in the literature as to whether the FDL or FHL is a superior transfer. In the transfer procedure for posterior tibial tendon rupture, most workers prefer to use the FDL.[30,32,50] This preserves the role of the FHL in push-off and stabilization of the medial longitudinal arch. However a study of the late sequelae of unrepaired lacerations of the FHL in young athletes failed to reveal disability.[18]

Thus the decision as to which medial transfer procedure to perform should be based upon prior incisions, the amount of tendon needed, and the presence or absence of flexible claw toes. Generally the FDL will turn out to be the most appropriate donor. Technically we adequately mobilize the tendon proximally. The FDL is then released at the crossover site with the FHL (knot of Henry). The peroneus brevis would be released at the base of the fifth metatarsal. The tendon may then be woven through the Achilles. It is then secured through a drill hole in the calcaneus extending from the superior tuberosity out either the medial (FHL and FDL) or lateral (peroneus brevis) side. The tendon transfer is then sutured back onto the Achilles with the ankle in about 5 to 10 degrees of plantar flexion. Postoperative immobilization is 6 to 10 weeks in a progression of casts and cast-braces. Return to full activity is at 3 to 5 months.

**Case Study 1.** A 63-year-old executive complained of left heel pain at the insertion of the Achilles tendon, which had been problematic for over a year. At the time of our initial evaluation, he had received 8 months of physical therapy that gave him little relief. In fact, the pain had gotten worse over time. He was highly active, playing tennis several times a week and was playing basketball until recently.

He had had an extensive rheumatologic workup, including a Lyme titer, all of which were negative.

The patient was noted to have tight tendo Achillis bilaterally. He was markedly tender at the insertion of the Achilles tendon, particularly on the medial side. Review of x-rays showed a large Haglund deformity with some calcific involvement in the insertion of the Achilles tendon.

The patient had clearly failed nonoperative therapy. It was recommended to him that he undergo operative resection of the Haglund deformity with debridement of the Achilles and resection of the calcific bodies within the insertion of the Achilles. Surgery proceeded through two incisions, a large portion of bone decompressing posteriorly. He was kept weight bearing in a cast for 5 weeks and then began physical therapy. At 3½ months he was able to return to a full level of activity, including playing tennis without pain, although some swelling still occurred in the foot.

**Case Study 2.** A 33-year-old male physician sustained an Achilles tendon rupture while playing tennis. He reviewed the literature and elected nonoperative treatment and was treated initially elsewhere in a long-leg cast for 4 weeks. He then came under our care.

We switched him to a short-leg gravity equinus cast that was switched to a walking boot with a heel lift for the final 4 weeks of the 3 month treatment. He was then begun on a course of physical therapy to regain flexibility and strengthen. Biodex testing at about 7 months from the date of injury revealed symmetric strength but slightly less endurance on the affected side. The patient is now 1 year from the injury and is functioning normally, jogging and playing tennis without difficulty.

**Case Study 3.** A 32-year-old male ruptured his Achilles tendon while playing squash. He was taken to surgery where an open repair was performed and was kept immobilized initially in a cast and then in a cast boot for 9 weeks. He began physical therapy at 8 weeks.

Strength has progressed, with the patient finally able to return to normal sporting activities at about 5½ months from the date of injury.

## REFERENCES

1. Arner O, Lindholm A: Subcutaneous rupture of the Achilles tendon: a study of 92 cases, *Acta Chir Scand* 239(suppl):1, 1959.
2. Beskin JL et al: Surgical repair of Achilles tendon ruptures, *Am J Sports Med* 15:1, 1987.
3. Bosworth DM: Repair of defects in the tendon Achilles, *J Bone Joint Surg* 38A:111, 1956.
4. Bovens AMP et al: Occurrence of running injuries in adults following a supervised training program, *Int J Sports Med* 10:S186, 1989.
5. Bradley JP, Tibone JE: Percutaneous and open surgical repairs of Achilles tendon ruptures, *Am J Sports Med* 18:188, 1990.
6. Bugg EI, Boyd EM: Repair of neglected rupture or laceration of the Achilles tendon, *Clin Orthop Rel Res* 56:73, 1968.
7. Burdett RG: Forces predicted at the ankle during running, *Med Sci Sports* 14:308, 1982.
8. Carden DG et al: Rupture of the calcaneus tendon, *J Bone Joint Surg* 69B:416, 1987.
9. Cetti R, Christensen SE: Surgical treatment under local anesthesia of Achilles tendon rupture, *Clin Orthop* 173:204, 1983.
9a. Clain MR, Baxter DE: Achilles tendonitis, *Foot Ankle* 13:482, 1992.
10. Clancy WG, Neidhart D, Brand RL: Achilles tendinitis in runners: a report of five cases, *Am J Sports Med* 4:46, 1976.
11. Clement DB et al: A survey of overuse running injuries, *Phys SportsMed* 9:47, 1981.
12. Clement DB, Taunton JE, Smart GW: Achilles tendinitis and peritendinitis: etiology and treatment, *Am J Sports Med* 12:179, 1984.
13. DaCruz DJ et al: Achilles paratendinitis: an evaluation of steroid injection, *Br J Sports Med* 22:64, 1988.
14. Dickinson PH et al: Tendo Achilles bursitis, *J Bone Joint Surg* 48A:77, 1966.
15. Elstorm, Pankovich A: Muscle and tendon surgery of the leg. In Evarts CM: *Surgery of the musculoskeletal system,* ed 2, 1990, Churchill Livingstone.
16. Fowler A, Philip JF: Abnormality of the calcaneus as a cause of painful heel, *Br J Surg* 32:494, 1945.
17. Fox JM et al: Degeneration and rupture of the Achilles tendon, *Clin Orthop* 107:221, 1975.
18. Frenette JP, Jackson DW: Lacerations of the flexor hallucis longus in the young athlete, *J Bone Joint Surg* 59A:673, 1977.
19. Frey C, Shereff M, Greenridge N: Vascularity of the posterior tibial tendon, *J Bone Joint Surg* 72A:884, 1990.
20. Gilles H, Chalmers J: The management of fresh ruptures of the tendo Achilles, *J Bone Joint Surg* 52A:337, 1970.
21. Gould N, Korson R: Stenosing tenosynovitis of the pseudosheath of the tendo Achilles, *Foot Ankle* 1:179, 1945.
22. Haglund P: Beitrag Zur Uliwik der Achillesse Have, *Z Orthop Chir* 49:49, 1928.
23. Hamilton WG: Personal communication, 1991.
24. Hansen S: Personal communication, 1991.
25. Hattrup SJ, Johnson KA: A review of ruptures of the Achilles tendon, *Foot Ankle* 6:34, 1985.
26. Hooker CH: Rupture of the tendo calcaneus, *J Bone Joint Surg* 45B:360, 1963.
27. Inglis AE et al: Ruptures of the tendo Achilles, *J Bone Joint Surg* 58A:990, 1976.
28. Inglis AE, Sculco TP: Surgical repair of ruptures of the tendo Achilles, *Clin Orthop* 156:160, 1981.
29. Jacobs D et al: Comparison of conservative and operative treatment of Achilles tendon rupture, *Am J Sports Med* 6:107, 1978.
30. Jahss MH: Spontaneous rupture of the tibialis posterior tendon: clinical finds, tenographic studies, and a new technique of repair, *Foot Ankle* 3:158, 1982.
31. James SL, Bates BT, Osternig LR: Injuries to runners, *Am J Sports Med* 6:40, 1978.
32. Johnson K: Tibialis posterior tendon rupture, *Clin Orthop Rel Res* 177:140, 1983.
33. Kannus P, Jozsa L: Histopathologic changes preceding spontaneous rupture of a tendon, *J Bone Joint Surg* 73A:1507, 1992.

34. Keck SW, Kelly PJ: Bursitis of the posterior part of the heel, *J Bone Joint Surg* 47A:267, 1965.

35. Kleinman M, Gross AE: Achilles tendon rupture following steroid injection, *J Bone Joint Surg* 65A:1345, 1983.

36. Krissoff WB, Ferris WD: Runners' injuries, *Phys SportsMed* 7:55, 1979.

37. Rust M: Achilles tendon injuries in athletes, *Ann Chir Gynaecol* 80:188, 1991.

38. Kvist M et al: Chronic Achilles paratenonitis in athletes: a histological and histochemical study, *Pathology* 19:1, 1987.

39. Kvist M et al: Fine structural alterations in chronic Achilles paratenonitis in athletes, *Path Res Pract* 180:416, 1985.

40. Kvist H, Kvist M: The operative treatment of chronic calcaneal paratendinitis, *J Bone Joint Surg* 62B:353, 1980.

41. Lagergren C, Lindholm A: Vascular distribution in the Achilles tendon, *Acta Chir Scand* 116:491, 1958/59.

42. Lea RB, Smith L: Non-surgical treatment of tendo Achilles rupture, *J Bone Joint Surg* 54A:1398, 1972.

43. Lea RB, Smith L: Rupture of the Achilles tendon nonsurgical treatment, *Clin Orthop Rel Res* 60:115, 1968.

44. Leppilahti J et al: Overuse injuries of the Achilles tendon, *Ann Chir Gynaecol* 80:202, 1991.

45. Levy M et al: A method of repair for Achilles tendon ruptures without cast immobilization, *Clin Orthop Rel Res* 187:199, 1984.

46. Ljungqvist R: Subcutaneous partial rupture of the Achilles tendon, *Acta Orthop Scand* 113(suppl):1, 1968.

47. Lynn TA: Repair of the torn Achilles tendon, using the plantaris tendon as a reinforcing membrane, *J Bone Joint Surg* 48A:268, 1966.

48. Ma GWC, Griffith TG: Percutaneous repair of acute closed ruptured Achilles tendon, *Clin Orthop Rel Res* 128:247, 1977.

49. Mann RA et al: Chronic rupture of the Achilles tendon: a new technique of repair, *J Bone Joint Surg* 73A:214, 1991.

50. Mann RA, Thompson FM: Rupture of the posterior tibial tendon causing flat foot, *J Bone Joint Surg* 67A:556, 1985.

51. Nelen G, Martens M, Burssens A: Surgical treatment of chronic Achilles tendinitis, *Am J Sports Med* 17:754, 1989.

52. Nistor L: Surgical and non-surgical treatment of Achilles tendon rupture, *J Bone Joint Surg* 63A:394, 1981.

53. O'Brien T: The needle test for complete rupture of the Achilles tendon, *J Bone Joint Surg* 66A:1099, 1984.

54. O'Keefe D, Mamtora H: Ultrasound in clinical orthopaedics, *J Bone Joint Surg* 74B:488, 1992.

55. Pavlov H et al: The Haglund syndromes: initial and differential diagnosis, *Radiology* 144:83, 1982.

56. Philips BB: *Traumatic disorders.* In Crenshaw AH, editor: *Campbell's operative orthopaedics,* ed 9, St. Louis, 1992, Mosby–Year Book, p 1903.

57. Puddu G, Ippolitto E, Postacchini F: A classification of Achilles tendon disease, *Am J Sports Med* 4:145, 1976.

58. Rathbun JB, MacNab I: The microvascular pattern of the rotator cuff, *J Bone Joint Surg* 52B: 540, 1970.

59. Reese RC, Burruss TP: *Athletic training techniques and protective equipment.* In Nicholas J, Hershman E, editors: *The Lower extremity and spine in sports medicine,* St Louis, 1986, Mosby.

60. Schepsis AA, Leach RE: Surgical management of Achilles tendinitis, *Am J Sports Med* 15:308, 1987.

61. Scott SH, Winter DA: Internal forces at chronic running injury sites, *Med Sci Sports Exercise* 22:357, 1990.

62. Singer KM, Jones DC: *Soft tissue conditions of the ankle and foot.* In Nicholas J, Hershman E, editors: *The lower extremity and spine in sports medicine,* St Louis, 1986, Mosby.

63. Snook GA: Achilles tendon tenosynovitis in long-distance runners, *Med Sci Sports* 4:155, 1972.

64. Teuffer AP: Traumatic rupture of the Achilles tendon. Reconstruction by transplant and graft using the lateral peroneus brevis, *Orthop Clin North Am* 5:89, 1974.

65. Thompson TC, Doherty JH: Spontaneous rupture of tendon of Achilles: a new clinical diagnostic test, *J Trauma* 2:126, 1962.

66. Turco VJ, Spinella AJ: Achilles tendon ruptures, *Foot Ankle* 7:253, 1987.

67. Urbaniak JR et al: *Tendon suturing methods: analysis of tensile strengths.* In *AAOS Symposium on tendon surgery in the hand,* St Louis, 1975, CV Mosby.

68. Weiss AB et al: *The use of carbon fiber composites.* In Jahss M, editor: *Disorders of the Foot and Ankle,* ed 2, Philadelphia, 1991, Saunders.

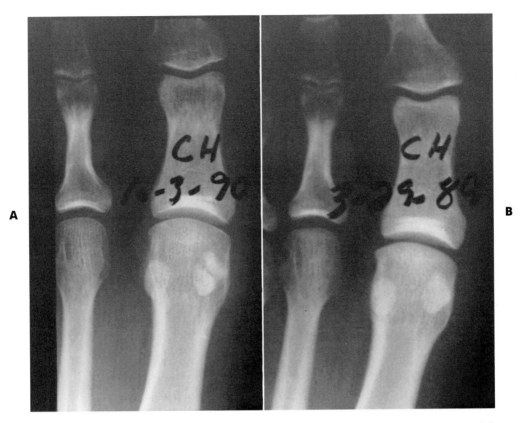

**Fig. 7-2.** Rarely are there premorbid films showing intact sesamoids. Here a 23-year-old runner with subacute symptoms 2 years before bone grafting. **A,** Two to four months after the onset of symptoms. **B,** Unquestioned medial sesamoid stress fracture with resorption, irregularity, and nonunion.

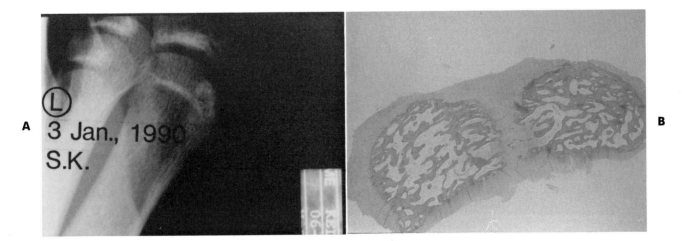

**Fig. 7-3.** A 20-year-old college basketball player with a sesamoid stress fracture ununited after 8 weeks of immobilization in a short-leg cast. Bone grafting failed and medial sesamoidectomy was necessary. **A,** Nonunion following bone grafting. Note the dense distal fragment suggesting avascular necrosis. **B,** Sesamoid nonunion at excision.

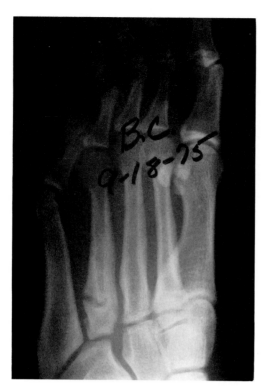

**Fig. 7-4.** Proximal metatarsal stress fractures are less common but occur in runners, here in the fourth metatarsal.

Less critical or not-at-risk fractures require "keeping the level of activity below that which causes pain." This principle implies not only decreasing the activity but in many cases substitution or total abstinence. For running-based sports, swimming, biking, walking, race walking, cross-country skiing, NordicTrack and other circuit training, general and muscle-specific exercises will help. Eccentric muscle strengthening has an important role to play in ongoing postinjury rehabilitation.

Treatment for stress fractures should be implemented on the basis of history, symptoms, physical examination, and a positive bone scan—whether conventional x-ray findings are diagnostic or nondiagnostic.[14,24,25]

Orthoses within shoes—whether running shoes, soccer shoes, basketball shoes, tennis shoes or other athletic shoes—can reroute stress proximally, distally, medially, or laterally. External electrical bone stimulation units can be and are appropriately used for selected ununited stress fractures of the foot but have no routine therapeutic role. I have not used implanted bone stimulators in the foot and ankle. The tarsalnavicular with recalcitrant symptoms and delayed union may require bone stimulation to prevent its high morbidity complications (see the section on Specific Stress Fractures).

Rehabilitation, substitution, activities with reduc-

tion in the inciting activity, promptness of resuming pain-free sports-specific activity status are variables in timing the training pattern for return to competition. There is necessary emphasis on anatomy of the stress fracture radiographically. But its specific treatment, rehabilitation, and length of time before return to recreation or competition depends on the length of time significant ongoing stress was applied to the part after the stress fracture was clinically present and before treatment was begun.

## SPECIFIC STRESS FRACTURES
### Great toe sesamoids

Stress fracture of the hallux sesamoids is one of the injuries involved in the great toe metatarsophalangeal (MtP) joint.[28] During running, more than half the weight-bearing load travels through the great toe complex. Three times body weight can be the osseous load that crosses the sesamoid—particularly the medial sesamoid. The medial sesamoid stress fracture is 10 times more common than the lateral (Fig. 7-1). Runners (Fig. 7-2), basketball players (Fig. 7-3), volleyball players, and any leg-based athlete can incur sesamoid injuries. So-called "turf toe" and in fact all medial forefoot trauma (both repetitive stress and acute stress) often directly or indirectly involve the sesamoid. The sesamoid,[32] for example, can be completely sequestered with acute injury and lie free. Repetitive stress following acute dorsiflexion injury of the great toe MTP joint with secondary sesamoid problems constitutes one common basic pathology of turf toe.

Six weeks in a fully extended short-leg cast is necessary for initial treatment. Radiographic lack of union by linear tomography with continued symptoms after 6 months warrants consideration of surgery. Excision, partial excision, or preferably bone grafting is performed, depending on the varying presence and size of multiple fragments, presence of osteochondritis, type of foot (cavovarus), overlying bursa,[36] and so on. Hallux sesamoids are a common site of delayed or nonunions.[9]

### Metatarsals one through four

The first metatarsal stress fracture is harder to see radiographically at 3 to 4 weeks than metatarsals two through five. X-rays generally show overlap or undershooting of the great toe since it is larger, denser, and has cortical and cancellous components. An additional and often confusing residual proximal physeal plate/line, creating a minimal sclerotic appearance, can be present in the first metatarsal. Second, third, and fourth metatarsal stress fractures are common. They rarely displace or comminute and rarely contribute to load shift, plantar callosity, and so on (Fig.

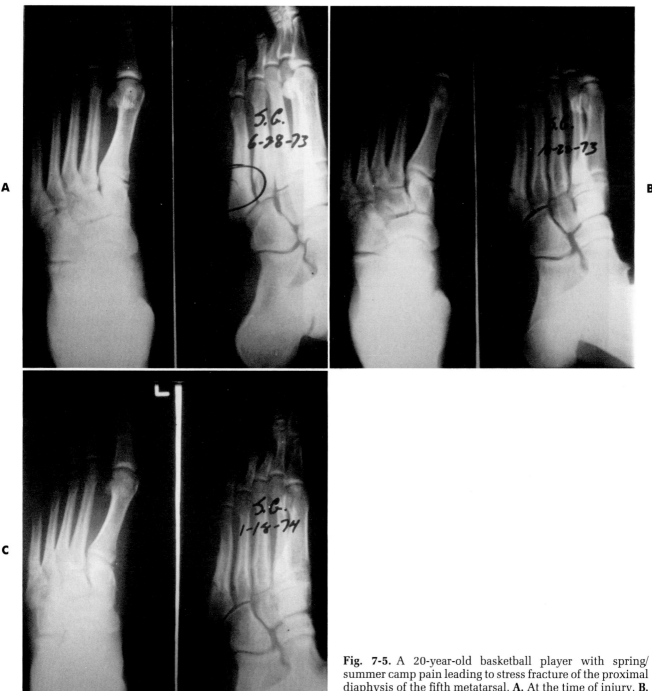

**Fig. 7-5.** A 20-year-old basketball player with spring/summer camp pain leading to stress fracture of the proximal diaphysis of the fifth metatarsal. **A,** At the time of injury. **B,** Completion of the fracture radiographically 4 months after presentation, including 6 weeks of casting. **C,** Early obscuring of the fracture site 6½ months after presentation.

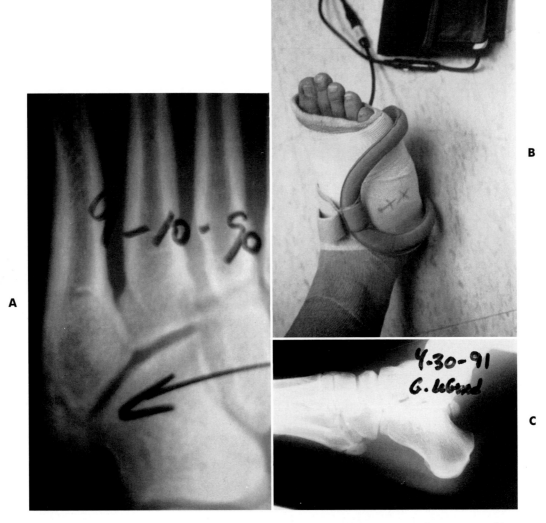

**Fig. 7-6.** Proximal fifth metatarsal avulsion fracture may fail to unite. This 19-year-old collegiate soccer player needed 10 months, including 10 weeks of casting and, at 6 months, bone stimulation for 10 hours daily. **A,** Healing fracture. **B,** A bone stimulation unit plus casting allowed eventual union. **C,** Eventual union at 10 months following injury.

7-4). The base of the second metatarsal is a more common site of injury in adult dancers. This is the most common stress fracture that can become intraarticular at the tarsal metatarsal interval. Special care should be taken to avoid delayed union or return to competition.[26]

### Base fifth metatarsal

Though the midshaft and neck of the fifth metatarsal can be involved, the proximal diaphysis (Fig. 7-5) and the proximal avulsion fracture are both common, disabling, and often undertreated.

Known but not publicized[3,49] and thoroughly differentiated by Dameron in 1975,[30] the proximal diaphyseal fracture (1.5-cm segment distal to the tuberosity), which may be acute or subacute, tends toward delayed or nonunion, stress refracture and significant morbidity. Intramedullary fixation with or without bone grafting can be necessary. The treatment is individualized. Certain high-level athletes may need early surgical treatment. Medullary sclerosis at an ununited fracture site encourages bone grafting and intramedullary screw. Criteria for stress fracture[6] are appropriately described, thus enabling classification.[20] Certainly stress fracture is a distinctly different entity from the acute fracture of this bone secondary to a single traumatic episode, even though both may progress to delayed union or nonunion.[41]

Proximal fifth metatarsal avulsion-type fractures have traditionally been treated by "Ace bandage,

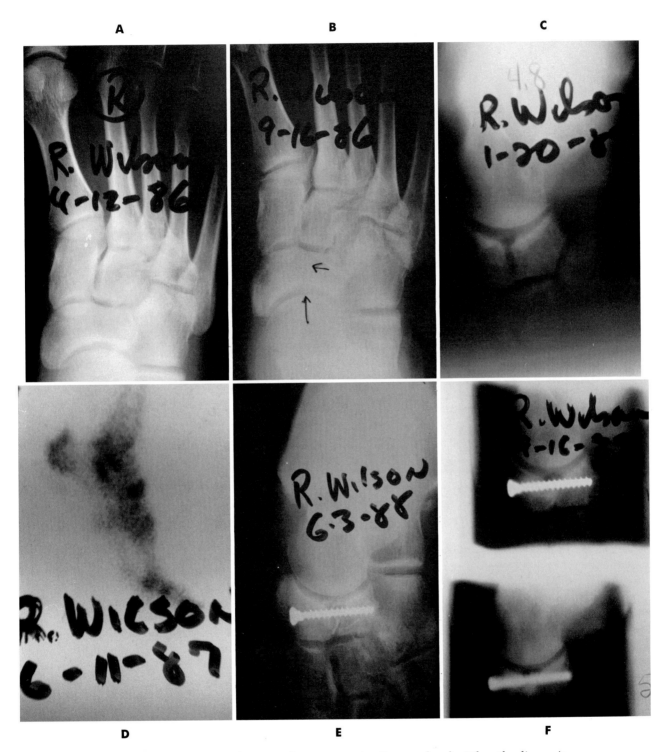

**Fig. 7-7.** The tarsonavicular stress fracture must be diagnosed early. When the diagnosis is delayed, treatment, as in this case, can be prolonged and involved. **A,** Initial AP foot. **B,** Typically positioned stress fracture at the time of initial diagnosis. **C,** Widened fracture site and nonunion. **D,** Bone scan still positive. **E,** Screw fixation but with articular involvement. **F,** Union but with apparent articular defect and probable long-term talonavicular osteoarthritis.

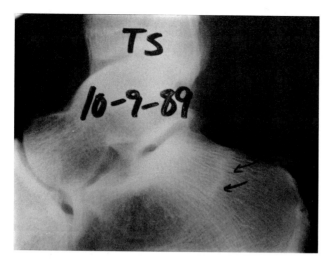

**Fig. 7-8.** This runner had typical stress fractures of the os calcis. Arrows indicate typical condensation of bone parallel to the subtalar joint.

crutches, and early ambulation" as tolerated. A subset of this avulsion-type fracture (type III)[23] may fail to unite. Surgery may be necessary[39] but bone stimulation offers a noninvasive option (Fig. 7-6).

### Tarsonavicular

The well-described tarsonavicular stress fracture[11,15,51,52] often needs more sophisticated workup both for diagnosis confirmation, extent of bony involvement, and possible articular cartilage involvement. Diagnosis delays are frequent and are due to a low index of suspicion and false-negative x-rays[11] (Fig. 7-7). In addition to baseline plain film imaging, baseline tomography, CT, technetium bone scan or MRI is necessary. Anatomic plain films or tomographic views 15 degrees off the normal anteroposterior view must be used.[37]

Significant disability can result with delayed diagnosis, premature resumption of athletics, lack of recognition of delayed union etc. The protocol for treatment at the present time should include 6 weeks of casting, verification of union by CT, and resumption of leg-based athletics at 12 to 18 weeks after initiation of treatment. No specific anatomic or individual correlating factors have been found.[50] If displacement of the fragments, delayed union beyond 12 weeks posttreatment, or frank nonunion is present, bonegrafting with optional internal fixation is indicated (Fig. 7-7). Accommodative semirigid custom orthoses should be used with return to training, athletics, and recreation.

### Cuneiform

The cuneiform bones function less variably (or more predictably) within the midfoot in their pro-

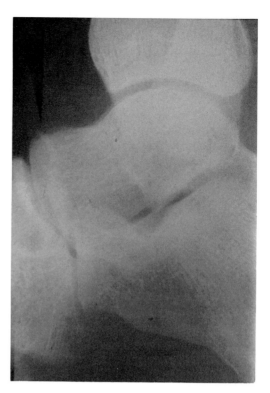

**Fig. 7-9.** Talar stress fractures are rare and parallel to the talonavicular joint.

tected and unexposed stress absorptive roles. They rarely incur stress fracture.[34]

### Talus and os calcis

Talus stress fractures are rare. Os calcis stress fractures are relatively common. Both occur roughly parallel to their joint in proximity, are condensations within cancellous bone, and do not involve articular interruption (Figs. 7-8 and 7-9). Both require 6 weeks of rest with activity below the level that causes pain. This implies casting, with or without weight bearing, depending on pain level—but simple substitution may suffice. Diagnosis is by lateral foot films. Os calcis fractures can occasionally become symptomatically recalcitrant. Neither completes to frank fracture. Minimally symptomatic os calcis stress fractures may be difficult to image and can mimic retrocalcaneal bursitis, posterior ankle impingement problems, and plantar fasciitis.

### Lateral malleolus (distal fibula)

Stress fracture of the fibula is the long-described, simple, uncomplicated prototype stress fracture.[29] This not-at-risk fracture is seen in distance runners. Often thought to be an ankle sprain or peroneal tenosynovitis, its treatment after recognition is straightforward. Reduction of stress below the level at which symptoms occur permits early monitored

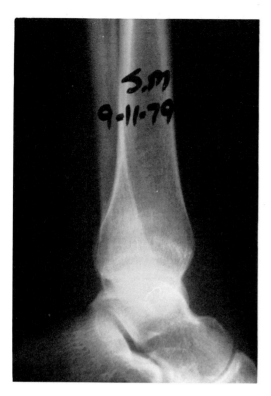

Fig. 7-10. Distal tibial stress fractures occur in cancellous bone. This distal tibial stress fracture in a 25-year-old patient, just proximal to the distal epiphyses, was never fully treated. Symptoms persisted 23 months. A separate condensation column is seen on the lateral view. The fracture healed promptly with recognition.

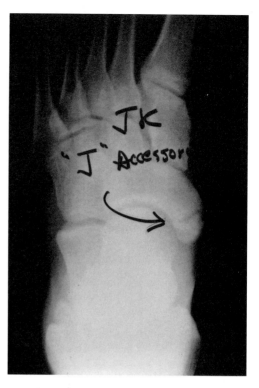

Fig. 7-11. This accessory navicula had "stress loosening" with high-impact aerobics and eventually required excision.

return to running-based sports. Substitution is only temporarily necessary. Three to four weeks is necessary for full recovery.

### Distal tibial metaphysis

Activities that add some angular or torque stress, as well as linear stress, to repetitive loading often are in the causative history. Unlike cortical bone with its periosteal blush, this predominantly cancellous fracture radiographically appears as a transverse condensation of bone (Fig. 7-10), often missed on plain films until at least 3 weeks after the onset of symptoms. Others are misdiagnosed as a "sprained ankle." Many remain unrecognized with clinical reliance only on initially negative films.

### Medial malleolus

Medial malleolar stress fractures can potentially displace. I have not seen that happen. Cancellous in nature, transverse condensation of bone is usually seen at joint level. Union occurs quickly, much as with the lateral malleolus and distal tibia at the ankle. This infrequent frank fracture on radiographs in high-performance athletes may require percutaneous fixation.[44]

An assortment of stress fracture-like problems occur in the ankle and foot. Avascular necrosis that can involve the talus (osteochondritis dissecans), navicular (Köhler's bone disease), and metatarsal head (Freiberg's disease) can all have repetitive stress as part of the etiology for the problem. The accessory navicular and os trigonum can mimic stress fracture with stress loosening at the synchondrosis on a repetitive stress basis. Nonoperative measures usually suffice. The accessory navicular (Fig. 7-11) or the posterior ankle-impinging elements occasionally need excision. Ossification into the plantar fascia and heelcord insertions may fracture and become symptomatic. Even exostoses involving the talus and navicula may undergo impingement or traction repetitive stress with avulsion.

### SUMMARY

Stress fractures of the foot and ankle culminate a complex set of circumstances. The magnitude of the repetitive inciting activity initiates the bone's effort to accommodate to this significant stress. Multiple global factors overlap the local factors that determine the bone's ability to accommodate to that stress. Global factors include sex, race, conditioning, prior similar stress, shoes, and surfaces. Local factors include the bone, the part of the bone involved, and the specific type of stress involved (i.e., shear, compressive, tensile). Given the significant repetitive stress circumstance, the single most important factor in clinically determining whether stress fracture develops is the duration of that stress (i.e., same level running in a runner). When clinical symptoms affect use/performance due to this prolonged stress, positive imaging is necessary to further confirm the diagnosis of and characteristics of the stress fracture. Basic treatment includes cessation of and substitution for the sports activity. With at-risk stress fractures such as the tarsonavicular, necessary aggressive approach avoids morbidity. Rehabilitation implies reforming strength of the extrinsic and intrinsic muscles of the legs and changing any identified anatomic, environmental, or training causes. This can modulate and better return the athlete to sports-specific activity.

## REFERENCES

1. Burr DB et al: Bone remodeling in response to in vivo fatigue microdamage, *J Biomech* 18:189, 1985.
2. Butler JE, Brown SL, McConnell BG: Subtrochanteric stress fractures in runners, *Am J Sports Med* 10:228, 1985.
3. Carp L: Fracture of the fifth metatarsal bone, with reference to delayed union, *Ann Surg* 86:308, 1927.
4. Chisin R et al: Clinical significance of nonfocal scintigraphic findings in suspected tibial stress fractures, *Clin Orthop Rel Res* 220:200, 1987.
5. Dameron TB Jr: Fractures and anatomical variations of the proximal portion of the fifth metatarsal, *J Bone Joint Surg* 57A:788, 1975.
6. DeLee JC, Evans JP, Julian J: Stress fracture of the fifth metatarsal, *Am J Sports Med* 35:697, 1992.
7. Floyd WN et al: Roentgenologic diagnosis of stress fractures and stress reactions, *South Med J* 80:433, 1987.
8. Frieberg O: Leg length asymmetry in stress fractures: a clinical and radiological study, *J Sports Med* 22:485, 1982.
9. Garcia JE, Grabhorn LL, Franklin KJ: Factors associated with stress fractures in military recruits, *Mil Med* 152:45, 1987.
10. Gardner LI et al: Prevention of lower extremity stress fractures: a controlled trial of a shock absorbent insole, *Am J Public Health* 78:1563, 1988.
11. Goergen TG et al: Tarsal navicular stress fractures in runners, *AJR* 136:201, 1981.
12. Groshar D et al: Stress fractures and bone pain: are they closely associated? *Injury* 16:526, 1985.
13. Guo XE et al: Finite element modeling of fatigue damage accumulation in trabecular bone, 38th Orthopaedic Research Society, 1992, p. 164.
14. Ha KI et al: A clinical study of stress fractures in sports activities, *Orthopaedics* 14:1089.
15. Hunter L: Stress fracture of the tarsal navicular, *Am J Sports Med* 9:217, 1981.
16. Johnson LC et al: Histogenesis of stress fractures, *J Bone Joint Surg* 45A:1542, 1963.
17. Johnson LC et al: Histogenesis of stress fractures, *J Bone Joint Surg* 45A:1542, 1963.
18. Johnson LK: The kinetics of skeletal remodeling symposia, structural organization of the skeleton, Bergsma, and Milch. Birth defects, Original Article Series, National Foundation, II:66, 1966.
19. Keller TS et al: Fatigue of immature baboon cortical bone, *J Biomech* 18:297, 1985.
20. Lehman RC et al: Fractures of the base of the fifth metatarsal distal to the tuberosity: a review, *Foot Ankle* 7:245, 1987.
21. Leveton L: March (fatigue) fracture of the long bones of the lower extremity and pelvis, *Am J Surg* 71:222, 1946.
22. Li G et al: Radiographic and histologic analysis of stress fracture in rabbit tibias, *Am J Sports Med* 13:285, 1985.
23. Mann RA: *Surgery of the foot.* In *Fractures and dislocations of the foot,* p 737.
24. Markey KL: Stress fractures, *Clin Sports Med* 6:405, 1987.
25. Matheson GO et al: Scintigraphic update of $^{99m}$Tc at nonpainful sites in athletes with stress fractures, *Sports Med* 4:65, 1987.
26. Matheson GE et al: Stress fractures in athletes: a study of 320 cases, *Am J Sports Med* 15:46, 1987.
27. Mauch M, Currey JD, Sedman AJ: Creep fracture in bones with different stiffness, *J Biomech* 25:11, 1992.
28. McBryde AM: Great toe metatarsophalangeal joint problems. In Reider B, editor: *Sports Medicine: The School Age Athlete,* Philadelphia, 1991, WB Saunders, p. 406.
29. McBryde AM, Bassett FH III: Stress fracture of the fibula, *GP* 38:120, 1968.
30. McBryde AM: Disorders of the ankle and foot, *Clin Sports Med:* 466.
31. McBryde AM: Stress fractures in athletes, *J Sports Med* 3:212, 1975.
32. McBryde AM: Stress fractures in athletes, *Am J Sports Med* 1:190, 1981.
33. McBryde A Jr: Stress fracture in runners, *Clin Sports Med* 4:1985.
34. Meurman OA, Elfving S: Case reports. Stress fracture of the cuneiform bones, *Br J Radiol* 53:157, 1980.
35. Michel et al, Translators: 37th Orthopaedic Research Society, 156, 1991.
36. Micheli LJ, Sohn RS, Solomon R: Stress fractures of the second metatarsal involving Lisfranc's joint in ballet dancers, *J Bone Joint Surg* 67-A:1372, 1985.
37. Pavlov H, Torg JS, Freiberger RH: Tarsal navicular stress fractures: radiographic evaluation, *Radiology* 148:641, 1983.
38. Pester S, Smith PC: Stress fractures in the lower extremities of soldiers in basic training, *Ortho Rev* 21:297, 1992.
39. Rettig AC, Shelbourne D, Wilckens J: The surgical treatment of symptomatic nonunions of the proximal (metaphyseal) fifth metatarsal in athletes, *Am J Sports Med* 20:50, 1992.
40. Rupani HD et al: Three-phase radionuclide bone imaging in sports medicine, *Radiology* 156:187, 1985.
41. Sammarco GJ: Be alert for jones fractures, *Phys SportsMed* 20:101, 1992.
42. Santi M, Sartoris DJ: Diagnostic imaging approach to stress fractures of the foot, *J Foot Surg* 30:85, 1991.
43. Schwellnus MP, Jordaan G, Noakes TD: Prevention of common overuse injuries by the use of shock absorbing insoles, *Am J Sports Med* 18:636, 1990.
44. Shelbourne KD et al: Stress fractures of the medial malleolus, *Am J Sports Med* 16:60, 1988.
45. Siddiqui AR: Bone scans for early detection of stress fractures, *N Engl J Med* 198:1033, 1978.
46. Smith JW, Arnoczky SP, Hersh A: The intraosseous blood supply of the fifth metatarsal: implications for proximal fracture healing, *Foot Ankle* 13:143, 1992.
47. Stafford SA et al: MRI in stress fracture, *AJR* 147:553, 1986.
48. Stanitski CL, McMaster JH, Scranton PE: On the nature of stress fractures, *Am J Sports Med* 6:391, 1978.
49. Stewart IM: Jones' fracture: fracture of the base of the fifth metatarsal, *Clin Orthop* 16:190, 1960.
50. Ting A et al: Stress fractures of the tarsal navicular in long-distance runners, *Clin Sports Med* 7:89, 1988.

51. Torg JS et al: Stress fractures of the tarsal navicular, *J Bone Joint Surg* 5:700, 1982.
52. Towne L, Blazina M, Cozen L: Fatigue of the tarsal navicular, *J Bone Joint Surg* 52A:376, 1970.
53. Uhthoff HK, Jaworski ZF: Periosteal stress-induced reactions resembling stress fractures, *Clin Orthop Rel Res* 199:284, 1985.
54. Yokoe K, Mannoji T: Stress fracture of the proximal phalanx of the great toe, *Am J Sports Med* 14:240, 1986.
55. Zwas ST, Elkanovitch R, Frank G: Interpretation and classification of bone scintigraphic findings in stress fractures, *J Nucl Med* 28:452, 1987.

# Chapter 8

# Traumatic fractures and dislocations

Jesse C. DeLee

Fractures and dislocations of the foot are among the most common injuries in the musculoskeletal system. With the recent explosion in interest in athletic endeavors, the foot and ankle have been exposed to a variety of new stresses.[24] In a recent report on the incidence of injuries in football, foot and ankle injuries ranked second in frequency of injury and composed 20% of all injuries reported.[32] The disability and time away from sports resulting from these injuries and their frequency warrant close attention in their diagnosis and management.[71] The following general comments on fractures and dislocations of the foot are meant to establish the basic principles of diagnosis and management.

## CLINICAL DIAGNOSIS

In evaluating patients with trauma to the foot, it is essential to obtain a thorough history. A detailed history of the mechanism by which the injury occurred will direct the examiner in the physical and radiographic examination.[50] In addition, it will provide a clue to the degree of soft tissue injury associated with the fracture.

Once the history is taken, the physical examination must be carried out systematically. Klenerman[80] emphasizes that although forefoot injuries are easily diagnosed, midfoot injuries often go undetected. Because of the high incidence of multiple fractures or fracture-subluxations in the injured foot,[50] careful palpation for points of tenderness is performed to detect any area of occult injury.[24,105] Evaluation of the range of motion of the tibiotalar, subtalar, midtarsal, and metatarsophalangeal joints is carried out within the limits of pain as part of a routine examination. A careful motor examination of intrinsic and extrinsic muscles and a sensory examination are recorded both before and after treatment. Vascular examination to assess the quality of palpable pulses or Doppler flow should also be recorded, as well as possible venous obstruction or engorgement.

## RADIOGRAPHIC DIAGNOSIS

Radiographs are considered only after a careful history and physical examination. The standard views used in evaluating the foot are the anteroposterior, lateral, and oblique views. The lateral view of the foot is indicated in evaluating fractures of the calcaneus, neck and body of the talus, and the midtarsal bones. Metatarsal overlap limits the usefulness of the lateral view in evaluation of the metatarsals and phalanges. The oblique view is particularly useful in evaluating the calcaneocuboid joint and in overcoming metatarsal overlap noted on the lateral view. Additional radiographs, such as the anteroposterior view of the ankle, are useful in evaluating the articular surface of the talus and the lateral aspect of the calcaneus. Axial views of the heel, special views of the subtalar joint, polytomography, and arthrography are also indicated in certain instances. Use of computed tomography and magnetic resonance imaging (MRI) will be extended in evaluating fractures and dislocations in the foot as experience with their use increases.

## TREATMENT

The prime objectives in the treatment of fractures and dislocations of the foot are (1) avoiding stiffness and loss of mobility; (2) preventing bony prominences, which may result in pressure phenomena from the use of a shoe; and (3) restoring the articular surfaces. The goal of treatment of fractures and dislocations is a flexible plantigrade foot with good bony alignment.

Once the diagnosis is certain, dislocations and fractures of the foot should be reduced as soon as possible. The reduction is easier to obtain before swelling occurs and before the hematoma between the fracture fragments organizes. Additionally, gross displacement of dislocations and fractures can result in localized pressure on the skin with vascular compromise and skin loss. Immediate reduction of the displacement can limit these complications. A perfect anatomic result does not necessarily ensure that mobility will be maintained. In fact, McKeever[94] emphasizes that all too often a perfect radiograph is seen, but the foot is so stiff that the patient cannot walk without pain. However Klenerman[80] emphasizes the importance of restoring the foot to its normal shape, even in cases in which joint mobility cannot be achieved. Chapman[20] emphasizes the importance in anatomical restoration of joint surfaces within the foot and advocates open reduction and internal fixation where applicable to restore joint continuity. In addition, Klenerman[80] stresses that mobility of joints of the foot, so essential in normal function, is not likely to be regained if joint surfaces remain notably incongruous. He also emphasizes that although a period of immobilization may be beneficial to soft tissue healing, it can lead to stiffness of joints—even those not involved in the injury—because of hemorrhage and extravasation about the adjacent joints.

Giannestras and Sammarco[53] emphasize that, since the foot is a weight-bearing structure, the preservation of soft tissue is as important as the reduction of the fracture. They note that patients experience a great deal of difficulty attempting to walk on scarred soft tissue, even if the bones of the foot are anatomically reduced.[53] Heck[63] also stresses the concept that fractures and dislocations of the foot are not solved simply by restoration of the continuity of a bone or joint complex, but rather by the simultaneous treatment and rehabilitation of the soft tissues. He emphasizes that the response to treatment of injuries to soft parts of the foot adjacent to a fracture is dependent on their early recognition and proper management. If for any reason one does not obtain supple soft tissues about the fracture, the final result will be impaired function of the foot and toes.

Lapidus and Guidotti[81] strongly emphasize the need for early mobilization in injuries of the foot. They note that the only two indications for immobilization of a fracture or dislocation are (1) maintaining the reduction of the fragments and (2) eliminating motion between fragments to prevent nonunion. They note that immobilization of a badly injured foot 6 weeks or longer (the time usually required for bony union) almost invariably produces fibrous ankylosis of the small joints of the foot, with resultant muscular atrophy and limitation of joint motion. Chapman[20] stresses that if a stable reduction can be accomplished by internal fixation, earlier institution of joint motion is possible and should be encouraged. However, if cast immobilization is required, leaving the toes free so that motion at the metatarsophalangeal joints can be encouraged will help decrease edema and stimulate muscle function in the calf and foot.

Early weight bearing decreases the period of disability following injury. Chapman[20] emphasizes that immobilization of the foot in a non–weight-bearing mode is accompanied by muscular atrophy, myostatic contracture, decreased joint motion, proliferation of connective tissue and capsular structures, internal synovial adhesions, and cartilaginous degeneration. He believes early weight bearing prevents the development of osteoporosis, decreases swelling by early muscle contraction, and permits slight motion in the small joints of the foot (even in a cast), which helps to prevent stiffness. In situations in which postoperative immobilization is indicated without weight bearing, consideration can be given to bivalving the short-leg cast and instituting early motion without weight bearing. Once motion is restored, immobilization can be continued until union occurs. The stability of the fracture or dislocation must be considered before this method is recommended. If full weight bearing needs to be delayed, Omer and Pomerantz[105] suggest using a patellar tendon-bearing plaster cast or brace to relieve weight stress while allowing mobilization. Lapidus and Guidotti[81] recommend early mobilization combined with swimming pool walking exercises for treatment of fractures of the ankle or tarsal bones. These swimming pool walking exercises are performed on a daily basis. Walking is started in the deepest part of the pool so that the buoyancy of the patient's body in the water results in a weightless state. The patient is instructed to walk as though walking on normal ground. Although Lapidus and Guidotti[81] recommend the initial treatment of some fractures of the foot in this manner, if immobilization of an unstable fracture is required, I have found this treatment method highly useful when motion is allowed. Although a whirlpool used for soaking before instituting range-of-motion exercises is helpful in improving range of motion, it does not allow actual weight bearing with support of the water as does swimming pool walking. Evaluation of stability, determined at the time of reduction, will help decide if

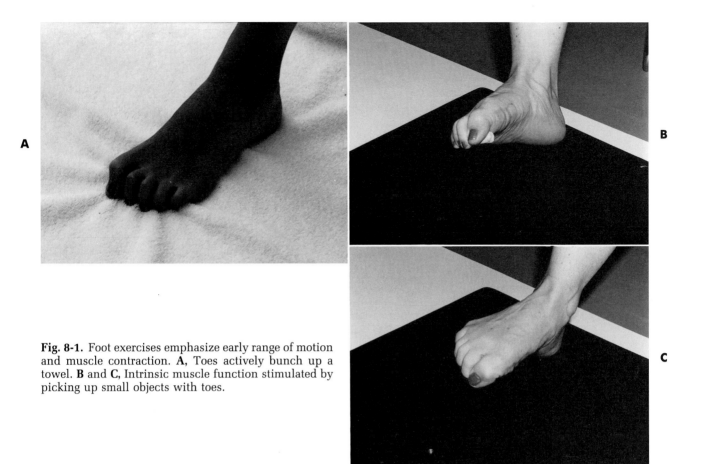

**Fig. 8-1.** Foot exercises emphasize early range of motion and muscle contraction. **A,** Toes actively bunch up a towel. **B** and **C,** Intrinsic muscle function stimulated by picking up small objects with toes.

early weight bearing, with its known benefits, can be instituted.

Following the period of fracture immobilization, an intensive rehabilitation program, specialized for the foot, should be instituted to ensure restoration of joint function and muscle strength. McKeever[94] points out that injuries to the foot result in crushing, stretching, or tearing of the soft tissues in addition to fractures. This produces hemorrhage, which extravasates through the soft tissue and infiltrates the tissue interstices. The result is dense intraarticular and extraarticular adhesions and fibrosis, all of which severely limit the normal flexibility of the foot. In addition, this can be accompanied by demineralization of bone and can result in a reflex sympathetic dystrophy of the limb. McKeever's opinion[94] is that prolonged immobilization of a foot distended with blood is a common precursor to this disabling syndrome.

I use an Aircast over support hose to support the foot and allow progressive motion of the foot and ankle joints. Exercises with the foot, including bunching a towel with the toes (Fig. 8-1, *A*) and picking up small objects with the toes (Fig. 8-1, *B* and *C*) help to institute muscle contraction and range of motion to the foot and ankle.

I have found the use of an elastic bandage for gentle resisted dorsiflexion–plantar flexion, inversion-eversion, and abduction-adduction helpful early in restoring both joint motion and muscle power (Fig. 8-2). Later, strengthening exercises, including resisted ankle plantar flexion–dorsiflexion and inversion-eversion are added as pain permits. Proprioceptive exercises are instituted when strength allows painless ambulation. A simple means of proprioceptive training is the use of a board placed on a cylinder (Baps board), which helps in two-dimensional retraining (Fig. 8-3). Eventually placing the board on half of a round ball will introduce three-dimensional tilt for proprioception education.

Stretching exercises for the Achilles tendon and gentle stretching of the subtalar, midtarsal, and metatarsophalangeal joints is also indicated. The metatarsophalangeal joints can be actively assisted in their range of motion, again, using an elastic bandage (Fig. 8-2, *B*). If swelling occurs during this period of rehabilitation, consideration is given to a compression dressing such as a Jobst compression stocking. Con-

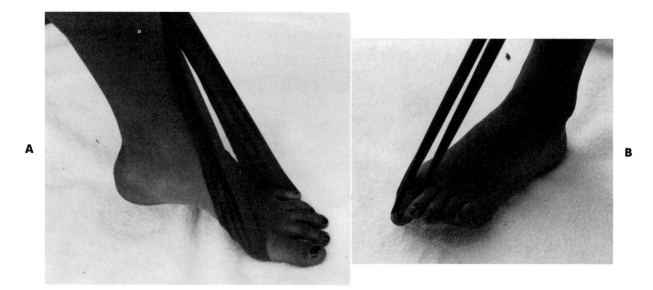

**Fig. 8-2.** Elastic bands of differing resistance supply gentle resistance for strengthening and range of motion. **A,** Ankle dorsal plantar flexion. **B,** Metatarsophalangeal joint motion.

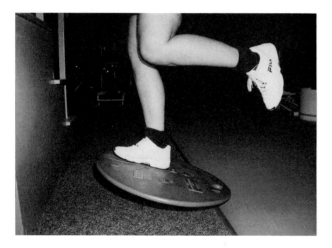

**Fig. 8-3.** Use of a Baps board to retrain proprioception.

trast baths alternating heat and cold are used later if recurrent swelling becomes a permanent problem.

After rehabilitation is complete, the use of a longitudinal arch support, particularly for midtarsal injuries, and a protective liner in the shoe made of a material such as Plastizote to relieve the plantar aspect of the foot are indicated to restore weight-bearing function.

## FRACTURES OF THE BASE OF THE FIFTH METATARSAL

Fractures of the base of the fifth metatarsal are the most common metatarsal fracture, and there is confusion in the literature regarding their treatment.[53] Fractures of the base of the fifth metatarsal have been

**Table 8-1.** Stewart's classification of fractures of the base of the fifth metatarsal[121]

| Type | Description |
|------|-------------|
| IA | Fracture of the junction of the shaft and base (Fig. 8-5, *A*) |
| IB | Comminuted |
| IIA | Fracture of the styloid process without articular involvement (Fig. 8-5, *B*) |
| IIB | Fracture with joint involvement (Fig. 8-5, *C*) |

classically termed the *Jones fracture* after Sir Robert Jones described the injury in his own foot in 1902.[73] Jones actually described a transverse diaphyseal fracture of the fifth metatarsal, three fourths of an inch from the base. This fracture is a less common injury than avulsion of the fifth metatarsal tuberosity with which the Jones fracture has been confused.[73,109] The transverse proximal diaphyseal fracture described by Jones often develops delayed union or nonunion.[5,26,75] Recently Zelko et al,[136] Kavanaugh et al,[75] and DeLee et al[33] have reported difficulty treating fractures of the proximal fifth metatarsal in which the diagnoses were initially missed or were actually fifth metatarsal stress fractures.

In an effort to clarify fractures of the base of the fifth metatarsal, Stewart[121] introduced a classification of these fractures (Table 8-1). Type I fractures are fractures at the junction of the metatarsal shaft and the base. This type is subdivided into two groups: non-comminuted fractures (IA) and comminuted fractures

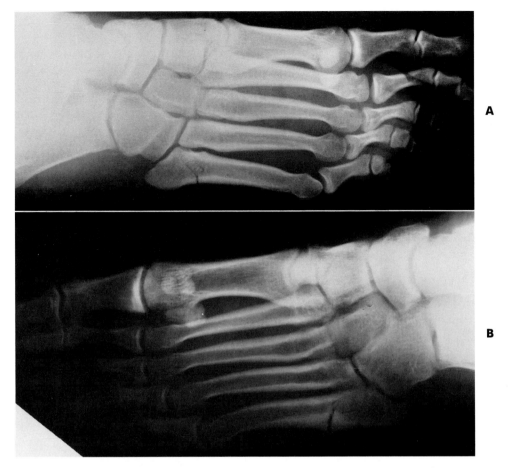

**Fig. 8-4.** Classification of Zelko et al[136] for fractures of the base of the fifth metatarsal. **A,** Group I: Acute fracture of the proximal diaphysis. **B,** Group II: Acute fracture of the diaphysis through an area of preexisting periosteal reaction.

*Continued.*

(IB). Type II fractures involve only the styloid process. This type is also subdivided into two groups: those with joint involvement (IIB) and those without joint involvement (IIA). See Figure 8-5 on page 101. Stewart formulated treatment recommendations based upon this classification system.

Zelko et al[136] and Torg et al[125] divided fractures of the fifth metatarsal occurring at the metaphyseal diaphyseal junction into four subgroups based upon their clinical history and initial roentgenographic findings.[136] Group I patients have an acute traumatic injury and no prior symptoms (Fig. 8-4, *A*). Roentgenographs demonstrate an acute fracture line with no chronic changes. Group II patients have sustained an acute injury but previously had mild symptoms on the lateral border of the foot (Fig. 8-4, *B*). Roentgenographs demonstrate a lucent fracture line with some periosteal reaction. Group III patients present with traumatic reinjury after one or more previous injuries. Radiographs in these patients demonstrate a lucent fracture line with periosteal reaction and often in-

tramedullary sclerosis (Fig. 8-4, *C*). Finally, group IV patients present with a history of chronic pain or multiple injury episodes. X-rays demonstrate a lucent fracture line with sclerotic margins (Fig. 8-4, *D*).

To simplify the discussion of these injuries, I use a classification system incorporating the systems of both Stewart[121] and Zelko et al[136] (Table 8-2).

I view these fractures as being of three distinct types: I, II, and III. Type IA, nondisplaced acute fractures at the junction of the shaft and base; type IB, acute comminuted fractures at the junction of the metatarsal shaft and base; type II, fractures at the junction of the metatarsal shaft and base with clinical and roentgenographic evidence of previous injury. To be classified a type II fracture, patients must have a history of prodromal symptoms along the lateral aspect of the foot before their acute fracture and/or an x-ray suggesting chronic reaction to stress — that is, a radiolucent fracture line, periosteal reaction, heaped-up callus on the lateral cortical margin, and intramedullary sclerosis that obviously preceded the acute epi-

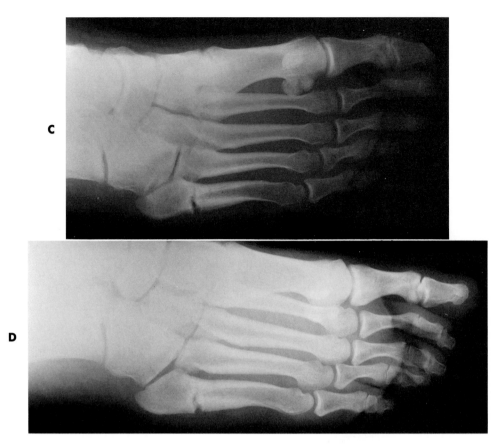

**Fig. 8-4. cont'd.   C,** Group III: Fracture of the proximal diaphysis of the fifth metatarsal. Note lucent fracture line and periosteal reaction. **D,** Group IV: Fracture of the proximal diaphysis of the fifth metatarsal. Note lucent line, periosteal reaction, and intramedullary sclerosis.

sode of pain[33] (Fig. 8-4, *D*). Type IIIA are fractures of the styloid process without joint involvement; type IIB are fractures of the styloid process with involvement of the fifth metatarsocuboid joint.

Stress fractures involving the proximal shaft of the fifth metatarsal (distal to the tuberosity) are different in their behavior from other metatarsal stress fractures. Zelko et al[136] found them slow to heal, predisposed to reinjury, and often causing prolonged disability, particularly in young athletes.[136] Kavanaugh et al[75] also stressed that this injury frequently occurs in young athletes and may be the source of prolonged disability. Its occurrence in basketball players has been emphasized by several authors.[33,75] Kavanaugh et al[75] found that 41% of patients with fractures of the fifth metatarsal related a history of discomfort over the lateral aspect of the foot at least 2 weeks prior to the roentgenographic evidence of the fracture (type II). Zelko et al[136] found roentgenographic evidence of a lucent fracture line with periosteal reaction in 14 of 21 patients at the time of initial fracture.

**Table 8-2.** Author's classification of fractures of the base of the fifth metatarsal (From Mann/Coughlin: *Surgery of the foot and ankle,* 6th ed, Mosby, 1993, Philadelphia.)

| Type | | Description |
|---|---|---|
| I | | Acute fractures at the metaphyseal-diaphyseal junction |
| | A | Nondisplaced |
| | B | Displaced and/or comminuted |
| II | | Fractures at the metaphyseal-diaphyseal junction with clinical and/or radiographic evidence of previous injury (i.e., pain, sclerosis, etc.) |
| III | | Fractures of the styloid process of the fifth metatarsal |
| | A | Without involvement of the fifth metatarsocuboid joint |
| | B | With involvement of the fifth metatarsocuboid joint |

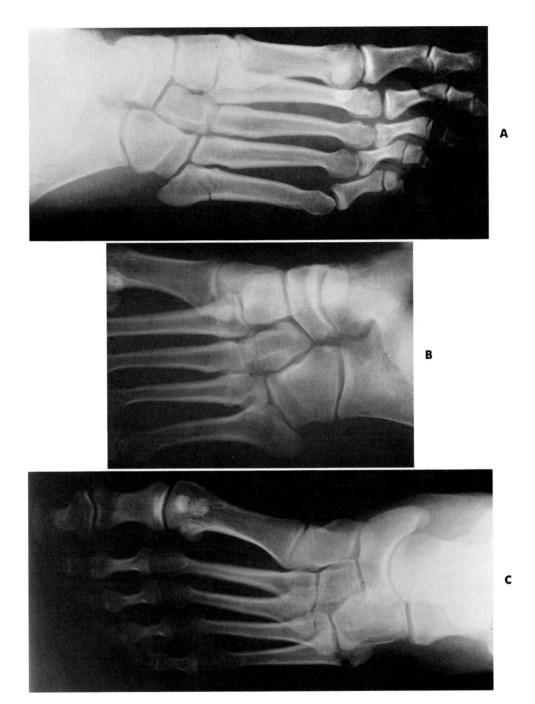

**Fig. 8-5. A,** Acute fracture of the junction of the shaft and base of the fifth metatarsal. **B,** Fracture of the styloid process not involving the joint. **C,** Fracture of styloid process with joint involvement.

## Anatomy

Due to the articulation between the base of the fifth metatarsal and the cuboid, and that between the bases of the fifth and fourth metatarsals, fractures of the base of the fifth metatarsal can be intraarticular in either of these two joints.[121]

Jones[73] stressed that the base of the fifth metatarsal is closely bound to the cuboid and to the fourth metatarsal by strong ligaments on every side. He believed these ligaments are so strong, dislocation of the base at the time of fracture is "the rarest of accidents." He did not mention the function of the insertion of the peroneus brevis tendon in this fracture. Kavanaugh et al,[75] based upon the anatomical dissection of five fresh specimens, confirmed Jones's observations on the thickness and strength of these ligaments. They stressed that the diaphyseal fracture reported by Jones occurs 0.5 cm distal to the splayed insertion of the peroneus brevis and almost invariably just distal to the joint between the fourth and fifth metatarsals. It was their opinion that the firm capsular attachments of the metatarsocuboid joint helped to stabilize the joint, thereby concentrating fracture forces at the metaphyseal-diaphyseal junction. The strong tendon of the peroneus brevis inserts on the dorsolateral aspect of the base of the fifth metatarsal over a relatively large area. This insertion has given rise to the theory that avulsion fractures occur due to contracture of this muscle.[53,108]

The base or proximal end of the fifth metatarsal presents a flair, the tuberosity, which protrudes down and laterally beyond the surfaces of the shaft of the metatarsal and the adjacent cuboid.[28] Dameron[28] emphasized the individual variations in the size and shape of this tubercle. Stewart noted that the amount the styloid process overhangs the metatarsocuboid joint appears to vary and invites isolated fractures when it is relatively long.[121]

In discussing delayed union of fractures of the fifth metatarsal, Carp[17] presented the thesis that poor blood supply to the shaft of the fifth metatarsal was responsible for the tendency to delayed union.

## Mechanism of injury

Direct and indirect mechanisms of injury have been given responsibility for this fracture.[53] Jones's[73,74] original description clearly delineated the mechanism of his own injury: "While dancing, I trod on the outer side of my foot, my heel at the moment being off the ground. Something gave midway down my foot, and I at once suspected a rupture of the peroneus longus tendon." The marked prominence of the tuberosity of the fifth metatarsal beyond the lateral line of the shaft of the metatarsal on the lateral border of the anterior

two thirds of the foot makes it particularly at risk to direct trauma.[53,96]

Fractures of the tuberosity of the fifth metatarsal by indirect violence are more common due to the number of structures that attach to the prominence.[22] These include the peroneus brevis tendon, a portion of the adductor digiti quinti muscle, the outer portion of plantar fascia, occasionally the abductor ossei metatarsi quinti muscle, and finally the flexor brevis minimi digiti muscle.[22,87] Lichtblau[87] stressed the importance of an active role by the peroneus brevis tendon in pulling the base of the metatarsal away from the shaft. According to Lichtblau, because the peroneus brevis muscle contracts during the stance phase, it is already contracted when an inversion stress is applied to the weight-loaded and plantar-flexed foot. Due to its insertion into the base of the fifth metatarsal, the tendon of the peroneus brevis holds firmly as the shaft is pulled away from it. Avulsion of the base from the rest of the fifth metatarsal is the result. Giannestras and Sammarco[53] also note that a plantar flexion, inversion stress placed on the forefoot, accompanied by contraction of the peroneus brevis muscle, avulses the styloid at the base of the fifth metatarsal where the tendon inserts.

Kavanaugh et al[75] used cinematography and force platform analysis in an effort to mimic the position of the foot at the time of the original injury. They concluded that either a vertical or a mediolateral force, or a combination of the two, acts on the base of the fifth metatarsal in conjunction with a posterior ground (braking) force, bringing the patient up on the metatarsal heads and concentrating the vertical and mediolateral forces on the lateral metatarsal. They postulated that inability or failure of the foot to go into inversion at that moment produces the large vertical and mediolateral ground forces responsible for the injury.[75]

Increased stress on the foot, secondary to increased activity, and prolonged running may produce stress fractures of the proximal diaphysis of the fifth metatarsal.[33,75,136] Although these stress fractures have been reported in most sports (i.e., football, soccer, tennis, and track), basketball players are most frequently affected and are the group most difficult to treat.[33,75,136]

## Clinical diagnosis

**History.** Careful evaluation of the patient's history is essential to distinguish fractures of acute onset from stress-type fractures.[33,75,136] According to Kavanaugh et al[75] there may be no history of a specific injury; an aching sensation on the lateral aspect of the foot may be the initial symptom of a roentgenographically

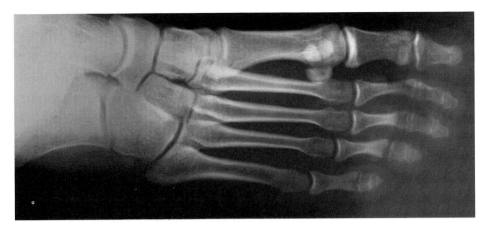

**Fig. 8-6.** Os peroneum.

diagnosable fracture. Zelko et al[136] and Torg et al[125] also emphasized prodromal symptoms of pain at the fracture site several weeks before any acute injury occurs. Alternatively, patients with an acute fracture give a history of a twisting injury to the ankle or a sudden inversion of the foot.

### Physical examination

Localized tenderness over the base of the fifth metatarsal and/or proximal metatarsal shaft helps to clinically distinguish this fracture from an injury to the lateral ligaments of the ankle.[53,128,132,135] Accentuation of the pain by inversion of the foot helps confirm the diagnosis.[22,53,132] Initially, swelling may be minimal, but it increases, particularly if the foot is held dependent for any length of time.[53,128,135] Edema and ecchymosis in the area of the fracture will be present if the patient's diagnosis and treatment is delayed beyond the first 24 hours.[53] Jones[73] noted there was generally no crepitus, no deformity, and no mobility on manipulation. However, Stewart[121] emphasized the importance of searching for abnormal mobility at the fracture site.

### Roentgenographic diagnosis

Anteroposterior and oblique roentgenographs are the most valuable in demonstrating the fracture.[53,121] On the lateral roentgenograph, displacement and intraarticular involvement may not be as clearly demonstrated. The oblique roentgenograph, clearly demonstrating the joint space between the bases of the fourth and the fifth metatarsal and the cuboid, is essential to detect both intraarticular involvement and displacement.

In evaluating fractures in the area of the base of the fifth metatarsal, congenital anomalies of ossification must be kept in mind.[132] Dameron[28] investigated the secondary center of ossification (apophysis) in the proximal end of the fifth metatarsal. He was unable to

demonstrate this accessory ossification center in children under 8 years of age, and found that the apophysis was united to the shaft of the bone before the age of 12 years in girls and before the age of 15 years in boys. He reported that 22% of the children he examined demonstrated such a secondary center of ossification.

Distinction between this accessory center of ossification and a fracture is essential in this age group. The roentgenographic characteristics of a normal apophysis that differentiates it from a fracture include (1) the apophyseal line traverses the tubercle in a direction parallel to the long axis of the shaft and (2) the apophysis does not extend proximally into the metatarsal joint or medially into the joint between the fourth and fifth metatarsals.[28] Fractures, on the other hand, are usually oriented at right angles to the shaft of the fifth metatarsal, and the fracture usually involves one or both articulations between the fifth metatarsal and the cuboid or between the fourth and fifth metatarsals.

Additionally, two accessory bones may be present near the base of the fifth metatarsal and must be distinguished from a fracture. The os peroneum, a sesamoid bone located within the tendon of the peroneus longus as it curves under the cuboid, and the os vesalianum, a secondary ossicle in the peroneus brevis, were both mentioned by Dameron (Fig. 8-6).[28] The os peroneum was noted in 15% of roentgenographs. The os vesalianum was present in only 1 of a 1000 feet in the study, and the location was proximal to the insertion of the peroneus brevis on the proximal tip of the fifth metatarsal. A smooth sclerotic opposing surface of this bone and most of the proximal portion of the fifth metatarsal should differentiate it from a fracture.[28] Additionally, O'Rahilly stresses that the os vesalianum is usually found bilaterally.[106]

When a fracture is diagnosed, evaluation of the roentgenograph is essential to determine whether the fracture is acute, or whether a preexisting stress reaction is present. A radiolucent fracture line, periosteal reaction, and callus on the lateral cortical margin with intramedullary sclerosis present at the time of the initial complaint suggest a stress reaction to bone.[33] Zelko et al[136] discovered a lucent fracture line with periosteal elevation in 14 of their 21 patients on initial roentgenographic evaluation.

## Treatment

Treatment of fractures of the base of the fifth metatarsal depends on the type of fracture present. Type I fractures (fractures at the junction of the shaft and base of the fifth metatarsal) can produce significant problems in treatment. Stewart[121] believes when comminution of these fractures is present, allowing abnormal mobility between the shaft and the base of the fifth metatarsal, consideration should be given to open reduction and internal fixation to decrease motion and accelerate union.

Giannestras and Sammarco[53] believe transverse fractures of the base of the fifth metatarsal should be treated with rest. They prefer short-leg walking cast immobilization for 5 to 6 weeks and state that such transverse fractures usually heal without complications. Dameron,[28] however, reported that patients with this fracture are generally younger than patients with fractures of the tuberosity. While he found that patients with fractures of the tuberosity (type II) uniformly responded to conservative treatment, 5 of 20 fractures involving the proximal shaft (type I fractures) required bone grafts for nonunion, and the time elapsed before roentgenographic and clinical union was often prolonged. He was unable to determine, however, if initial treatment of these fractures influenced the result. He therefore recommended treatment be individualized according to the demands of the patient and that early bone grafting be considered in high-performance athletes. Arangio[5] also emphasized the problem with healing in these fractures and recommended cross pinning the fracture in an effort to accelerate union. After an extensive review of the literature, he found that 38% of patients with acute fractures in this area developed delayed union and that 14% developed definite nonunions.

In evaluating type IA fractures—that is, acute nondisplaced fractures at the junction of the metaphysis and diaphysis, one must distinguish between acute fractures and fractures with a delayed diagnosis or with evidence of long-standing stress reaction of bone.[33] I classify fractures at the metatarsal diaphyseal junction with x-ray evidence of preexisting stress reaction in bone as type II fractures. Kavanaugh et al[75] reported 22 patients with fractures of the diaphysis of the fifth metatarsal of which 9 complained of discom-

fort over the lateral aspect of the foot at least 2 weeks before injury. In 41% of their patients, the clinical picture was consistent with the stress fracture evident on the initial roentgenographs. They found no such fracture united when treated conservatively in a varsity basketball player, and two thirds of patients treated conservatively in their series developed delayed union or nonunion. Even patients who developed union in a non–weight-bearing short-leg cast required 10 to 12 weeks of treatment. The authors advocated the use of intramedullary screw fixation of this fracture in professional athletes due to the time required for union. Following this treatment athletic competition was allowed in 6 weeks. Zelko et al[136] also stressed the importance of refractures in these patients. Carp[17] cited delayed union in 5 of 20 patients with fractures of the fifth metatarsal and ascribed this to poor blood supply. Zelko et al[136] classified fractures of the base of the fifth metatarsal into four groups for treatment purposes. Group I patients (Fig. 8-4, A)—those classified as having an acute traumatic injury and no prior symptoms—do well following plaster immobilization. These patients correspond to my type I category. Patients with preexisting clinical or x-ray evidence of stress reaction made up groups II, III, and IV. Group II patients—those with acute traumatic injury but with minor prior symptoms—also do well when treated by plaster immobilization (Fig. 8-4, B). However, this group of fractures requires more aggressive treatment in athletes, particularly basketball players. In group III patients—those who suffered a reinjury and in whom there was a lucent fracture line with periosteal reaction—consideration is given to bone grafting (Fig. 8-4, C). In group IV patients—those with chronic symptoms, multiple reinjuries, lucent lines at the fracture, dense sclerotic margins, and periosteal callus—direct primary bone grafting is the recommended means of treatment (Fig. 8-4, D). Zelko et al found that although many of these fractures will heal in athletes if they are willing to restrict activities for a prolonged period, the incidence of refracture is relatively high. In their group IV patients, bone grafting was performed using a tibial cortical cancellous inlay graft after thorough curettage of the sclerotic bone, which had obliterated the medullary canal. Following this treatment, the patient returned to activity within 3 months. Dameron[28] also recommended early bone grafting of these fractures in professional athletes, whereas symptomatic treatment was usually effective in sedentary patients.

DeLee et al[33] reported 10 cases of stress fractures of the base of the fifth metatarsal in athletes.[33] All 10 patients had prodromal symptoms and x-ray evidence of preexisting stress reaction of bone. These patients were treated by axillary screw fixation (Fig. 8-7). In all

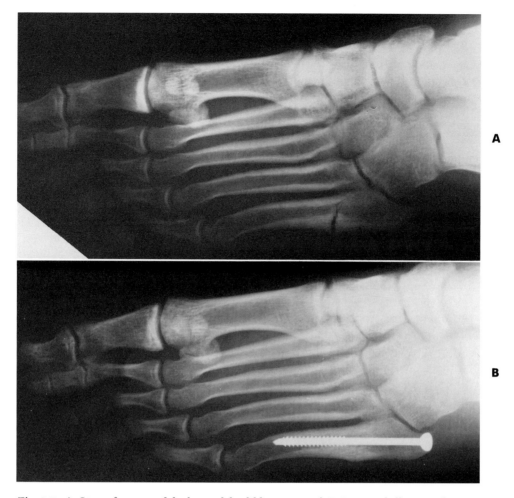

**Fig. 8-7. A,** Stress fracture of the base of the fifth metatarsal. **B,** Intramedullary axial screw fixation of stress fracture.

10 the fractures united within 6 weeks, and the patients returned to activity. DeLee et al recommend this form of treatment due to shorter disability time and lack of refracture. Minor discomfort over the screw head in the tuberosity of the metatarsal was decreased by countersinking the screw head. Slight discomfort underneath the fifth metatarsal head was eliminated by the use of shoe inserts.

Lehman et al[83] concluded that although fractures with delayed union may eventually heal if treated conservatively, an active athlete with delayed union or established nonunion will benefit from operative intervention. Although these authors admit that intermedullary screw fixation has the advantages of not opening the fracture site, is a shorter procedure, and has decreased healing time, they believe the complications are significant. These include screw fracture, the screw missing the medullary canal, and complaints of pain over the protruding screw heads. They emphasize that complications were not reported by Torg et al[125] following bone grafting. The authors

conclude that fractures with no intermedullary sclerosis should be treated with non–weight-bearing casts for 6 to 8 weeks. Fractures with intramedullary sclerosis, particularly in serious athletes, benefit from treatment. Also, those patients with nonunion of a fracture with dense sclerotic bone adjacent to the fracture line require surgical treatment. These authors believe the treatments of choice are medullary curettage and bone grafting or closed intermedullary screw fixation, but prefer medullary curettage and bone grafting because of the decreased risk of complications.

Recently Zogby and Baker[137] reported 10 patients with Jones fractures. These patients were treated conservatively in a short-leg non–weight-bearing cast. The cast was removed when the patients were able to bear weight on the affected foot without pain. All competitive athletes returned to their preinjury level of competition within 12 weeks. The authors conclude that nonoperative treatment of chronic or subacute fractures without intermedullary sclerosis compares favorably with surgical treatment in returning athletes to play.

Acker and Drez[1] reported three patients with fractures of the fifth metatarsal diaphysis, which fit the criterion of stress fractures. All roentgenograms demonstrated a lucent fracture line with periosteal reaction on the initial films. These patients were treated in short-leg walking casts until pain subsided. Patients were allowed to return to athletic activity when roentgenograms demonstrated healing, which occurred within 6 weeks in all patients. The authors conclude surgical treatment should be performed only in those patients in whom conservative treatment fails and recurrent pain develops.

In type III fractures—that is, fractures involving only the tuberosity of the base of the fifth metatarsal—two groups are present. The fracture may be extra-articular (type IIIA) or intraarticular (type IIIB). In undisplaced fractures of the styloid process seen within the first 48 hours of injury, Giannestras and Sammarco[53] recommend the use of a snug Elastoplast dressing or Gibney-type adhesive strapping. Patients are initially given crutches for partial weight bearing. The authors believe that a walking cast for such undisplaced fractures is unnecessary. In displaced extraarticular fractures of the styloid process, a below-the-knee walking cast is used for 4 to 6 weeks. Even though union may not be present roentgenographically, as long as a fracture is asymptomatic the cast is removed at 4 to 6 weeks.

Stewart[121] also believes the treatment of these fractures should be largely symptomatic and include the supporting footwear or strapping with or without padding around the tender prominence. He believes that unless the fracture is intraarticular, there is no indication for open reduction. Stone[122] himself suffered this fracture and recommends treatment by simple support of the foot. Stone found that after a Gibney basketweave strapping of the fracture, the foot became extremely painful with prolonged weight bearing. Even a walking cast did not stop the pain with prolonged weight bearing. He therefore recommends the use of a padded metal foot splint incorporated into short-leg cast. After about a week the cast is removed and the padded metal foot splint is applied to the foot with a snug Ace bandage. The patient then walks in a canvas boot. After 2 weeks of this treatment, the fracture is usually pain-free. Stone's basic concept is to treat the fracture with the goal of relieving pain. He stresses that reduction in the period of disability can be obtained by avoiding the use of a short-leg cast for periods as prolonged as 6 weeks. He also stresses that even though the fracture heals with a fibrous union roentgenographically, such a fibrous union is usually not symptomatic.

Pearson[108] found that treatment of these fractures by infiltration of the fracture site with procaine followed by strapping of the foot produced better results (with less time off work) than treatment by strapping alone or with plaster. Christopher[22] also recommends simplified treatment and suggests immobilization in a plaster cast for 2 to 3 weeks followed by massage.

According to Coker and Arnold,[24] fractures of the tuberosity heal quickly both clinically and roentgenographically. They report that symptomatic treatment alone suffices and that plaster immobilization is not required. Giannestras and Sammarco[53] distinguished between displaced and nondisplaced avulsion fractures of the styloid process, recommending 4 to 6 weeks of short-leg cast immobilization only in displaced fractures.

In type IIIB fractures—that is, fractures of the tuberosity of the fifth metatarsal which are intraarticular—Stewart[121] suggests open reduction and internal fixation in an effort to reconstruct the fifth metatarsocuboid joint, especially when these avulsion fractures consist of a large fracture fragment. However, he emphasizes tenderness in the healed skin incision overlying the bony prominence on the foot after open reductions. Pritsch et al[111] presented a case in which there was marked lateral and rotational displacement of the tuberosity fragment. He stressed the need for accurate open reduction and internal fixation to restore the articular surface of the fifth metatarsocuboid joint. He mentioned that with this degree of displacement, an alternative would be removal of the fragment and reinsertion of the peroneus brevis tendon into the metatarsal shaft.

Pearson[108] stresses that the presence of bony union is not considered important and that the final roentgenograph demonstrates a 19% nonunion rate in this fracture. However, all of his nonunions were painless. Although the literature implies that avulsion fracture of the fifth metatarsal heal with little difficulty or residua (whether by fibrous or bony union), Lichtblau[87] reported a case of a painful nonunion of the fracture of the base of the fifth metatarsal. He believes the activity of the peroneus brevis muscle is important not only in causation of the fracture, but also may assist in the production of nonunion. For this reason, he recommends restriction of weight bearing for the initial 3 weeks to avoid nonunion. Gould and Trevenio[57] reported three cases of sural nerve entrapment following avulsion fracture of the base of the fifth metatarsal. They emphasize the sural nerve is stretched over the displaced fragment, producing pain at the fracture site and distally along the course of the sural nerve. Clinically patients note bulging of the skin, local pain that increases with shoe wear, a positive Tinel sign, and dysesthesias distal to the fracture in the distribution of the sural nerve. They report prompt recovery following removal of the ununited fragment and neurolysis of the sural nerve.

**Author's preferred method of treatment**

Careful evaluation of anteroposterior, lateral, and oblique roentgenographs of the foot is critical to detect the presence of stress changes in the bone that antedate any acute fracture. In those patients in whom no evidence of stress is present, treatment is undertaken as follows.

In acute type IA fractures involving the metaphyseal diaphyseal junction, I prefer short-leg cast immobilization with early weight bearing. The fracture is immobilized for 4 to 6 weeks or until union is present. Often 8 to 12 weeks is required before there is roentgenographic and clinical evidence of union. In type IB fractures in athletes—where there is comminution and increased mobility at the fracture site—I prefer cross pinning to stabilize the fracture and promote union.

The treatment of type II fractures (fractures at the metaphyseal diaphyseal junction with evidence of preexisting stress reaction of bone) is based upon the patient's level of activity. In high-performance athletes with no evidence of intermedullary sclerosis, I consider an attempt at conservative treatment using a non–weight-bearing cast until pain subsides. Cast immobilization is maintained until there is evidence of bony union. Patients are then fitted with a molded arch support with a snug-fitting shoe. They are allowed to return to sports if radiographs reveal healing of the fracture. If patients have recurrent pain following resumption of activities, operative treatment is recommended. The risk in this form of treatment is loss of time from athletic activities should conservative treatment fail.

In high-performance athletes in whom there is a preexisting stress reaction of bone including intermedullary sclerosis, or in whom a loss of time from athletic participation due to failed conservative treatment is not acceptable, I proceed directly to intermedullary screw fixation.

Following axial screw fixation, patients are treated in a short-leg non–walking cast for 2 weeks. The cast is then removed and the foot is placed in a hard-soled shoe. Either a wooden shoe of the postbunionectomy type or a standard tennis shoe with a semiflexible steel sole insert is used to protect the foot. Progressive weight bearing is then begun. Patients are usually allowed to return to competitive sports when pain over the fifth metatarsal and the incision is gone. A soft-sole insert with protective padding over the lateral border of the foot at the base of the fifth

metatarsal will prevent pressure over the screw head or under the fifth metatarsal head when patients return to activity.

In patients with minimal activity levels, I use a period of immobilization in a short-leg walking cast. Following casting the decision for intramedullary screw fixation is then based upon progression toward union. I have not used bone grafting of the fracture site in treatment of type II fractures.

In type IIIA fractures (the fracture is extraarticular and involves the tuberosity of the base of the fifth metatarsal), I prefer symptomatic treatment. Strapping the foot with or without a sturdy arch support is used until patients become asymptomatic. In patients with marked displacement of the fracture, a short-leg walking cast is used until pain allows treatment by strapping. In all cases plaster immobilization is used only for patients in whom strapping or arch supports do not alleviate pain. Weight bearing is begun as soon as pain allows.

In patients with type IIIB fractures (fractures of the tuberosity involving the fifth metatarsocuboid joint), open reduction is recommended to restore articular congruity in highly competitive athletes (Fig. 8-8). However, in the majority of patients, I have found little disability from allowing these fractures to heal in the displaced position. Should such a malunion produce symptoms, excision of the displacement fragment and advancement of the peroneus brevis tendon is undertaken.

**TARSOMETATARSAL DISLOCATIONS**

The tarsometatarsal joint—consisting of the bases of the five metatarsals and their articulation with the three cuneiforms and the cuboid—is named after Lisfranc, a French surgeon in the army of Napoleon who originally described an amputation through that joint.[19,46,62,103] Dislocations and fracture-dislocations of the tarsometatarsal joint are rare injuries and are reported to occur at the rate of 1 injury per 55,000 people per year.* English[42] reports only 0.2% of all fractures involve this joint. Lenczner et al,[84] Bassett,[10] and O'Regan[107] report the injury was more common when the horse was the major means of transportation. Today, motorcycle accidents produce a similar mechanism of injury.[35] An increase in the incidence of motor vehicle accidents is believed by Lenczner et al[84] to be responsible for an increasing incidence of injuries to the tarsometatarsal joint. According to Myerson,[102] 81% of patients had sufficient additional major injuries to be considered as polytrauma patients.

Faciszewski et al[43] recently reported 15 patients

*References 3, 31, 42, 62, 110, 133.

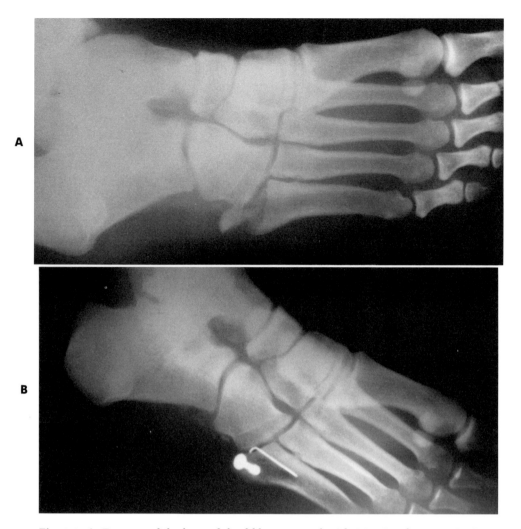

**Fig. 8-8. A,** Fracture of the base of the fifth metatarsal with joint involvement. **B,** Open reduction and internal fixation to restore articular congruity.

with "subtle" injuries to the Lisfranc joint, defined as a diastasis between the bases of the first two metatarsals of 2 to 5 mm. One third of their patients' injuries were sports related. In my experience these subtle injuries to the Lisfranc joint are more frequent in sports than true Lisfranc's dislocations and are often overlooked. Additionally, Coker and Arnold[24] and O'Donoghue[104] report injuries to the tarsometatarsal joints are occurring with increasing frequency in athletic events.

Due to the fact that the metatarsals may be displaced with or without an associated fracture and may be displaced in a dorsal, ventral, medial, lateral (or any combination) direction in relation to the hindfoot, a working classification is essential in understanding the diagnosis and treatment of these injuries.[110] One must distinguish between a total dislocation in which all the metatarsals are dislocated and partial dislocations in which some, but not all, of the metatarsals are dislocated from the tarsometatar-

sal joint.[103,131] Finally, especially in sporting activities, it is essential to recognize the group of patients with subtle injuries to the Lisfranc joint and to distinguish them from true dislocations. These injuries are far more frequent than Lisfranc's dislocations and are often overlooked. In this injury pattern, the base of the second metatarsal is subluxated laterally and dorsally, resulting in a diastasis between the bases of the first and second metatarsals.

Although these dislocations present with a great deal of individual variation, they generally have similar patterns of displacement.[20] Various classifications of tarsometatarsal dislocations have been presented.* Quenu and Kuss[112] proposed a simple and useful classification, which divides all these injuries into three types of dislocations:

1. Homolateral dislocations in which all five metatarsals are displaced in the coronal plane.

*References 20, 21, 62, 107, 110, 112.

2. Isolated dislocations in which one or two metatarsals are displaced in the coronal plane.
3. Divergent dislocations in which there is separation between the first and second metatarsals, and the displacement occurs in the sagittal as well as the coronal plane.

The simplicity of this classification system has made it attractive to many authors reporting tarsometatarsal injuries.[4,53,82]

Alternatively O'Regan[107] uses a simple classification system based upon displacement. Uniform dislocations are those in which all the metatarsals are displaced in the same direction, whereas divergent dislocations are those in which the first metatarsal moves medially away from the remaining four metatarsals. O'Regan[107] and Granberry and Lipscomb[59] emphasized that fractures involving the tarsometatarsal joint are usually present with these dislocations.

Hardcastle et al[62] used the classification of Quenu and Kuss as a basis for the classification they developed and upon which they believe treatment can be based (Fig. 8-9).

**Type A (Total):** In these injuries there is incongruity of the entire tarsometatarsal joint. Displacement is in one plane, which may be sagittal, coronal, or combined.

**Type B (Partial):** In these injuries there is incongruity of a part of the tarsometatarsal joint. The displaced segment is in one plane, which may be sagittal, coronal, or combined.

There are two types of partial dislocations whose treatment and prognosis differ:

1. *Medial dislocations*—displacement affects the first metatarsal either in isolation or combined with displacement of one or more of the second, third, or fourth metatarsals.
2. *Lateral dislocations*—displacement affects one or more of the lateral four metatarsals. The first metatarsal is not affected.

**Type C (Divergent):** In these injuries there may be partial or total incongruity. On the anteroposterior radiograph the first metatarsal is displaced medially, while any combination of the lateral four metatarsals is displaced laterally. Sagittal displacement also occurs in conjunction with coronal displacement.

## Anatomy

The tarsometatarsal joint consists of the five metatarsal bones, three cuneiforms, and the cuboid. The medial three metatarsals articulate individually with one of the three cuneiforms. The cuboid articulates with the fourth and fifth metatarsals. The second metatarsal is the longest of all metatarsals, and the

second cuneiform is the shortest of the cuneiforms. This produces an indentation in the line of the cuneiforms into which the long second metatarsal fits.[82] Lenczner et al[84] emphasize that the stability of the second metatarsal base is the key to the structure of the tarsometatarsal joint. The second metatarsal has a broader dorsal surface and a narrow ventral surface, which makes this bone resemble the keystone of a Roman arch in shape, position, and function (Fig. 8-10).[10,84] Because of its recessed position between the medial and lateral cuneiforms, the second metatarsal articulates with all three cuneiforms.[16] Cain and Seligson[16] also report that the second metatarsal holds the keystone position of the tarsometatarsal joint and that no significant dislocation of the metatarsals or cuneiforms can occur unless this keystone is disrupted.

Anderson[4] reports that it is rare to see a tarsometatarsal dislocation without fracture of the base of the second metatarsal, and Aitken and Poulson[3] emphasize that only if this recess is unusually shallow can a dislocation occur without a fracture of the second metatarsal. In addition to the stability provided by the bone anatomy, the ligmentous structures of the tarsometatarsal joint are instrumental in instability. The second, third, fourth, and fifth metatarsal bases are bound to each other by transverse ligaments located on both the dorsal and plantar aspects of the joint. The plantar ligaments support the arch and are much stronger than the dorsal ligaments.[25] There is no ligament between the bases of the first and second metatarsals; instead, the four lesser metatarsals are attached primarily to the first cuneiform by an obliquely placed plantar and dorsal ligament. This oblique ligament, termed *Lisfranc's ligament*,[70] is important because it is responsible for avulsion fractures of the base of the second metatarsal so frequently seen in these fracture-dislocations.[4] The oblique Lisfranc's ligament is so placed that when an abduction force is applied to the metatarsus, it results in rupture or avulsion of the ligamentous insertion or fracture of the base of the second metatarsal, which permits lateral dislocation of the foot.[25]

The first metatarsal is secured to the medial cuneiform by ligaments placed in an axial direction. These ligaments permit marked abduction before yielding, and great force is necessary to disrupt their attachments.[25] The insertion of the anterior tibial tendon on the medial aspect of the proximal first metatarsal and the peroneus longus tendon into the lateral aspect of the proximal first metatarsal are both factors adding to the security of the first metatarsal cuneiform joint.

The structures on the sole of the foot, including the plantar fascia, the intrinsic foot muscles, and the

TYPE A: TOTAL INCONGRUITY

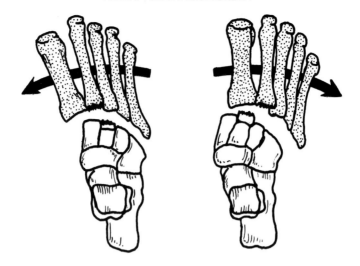

TYPE B: PARTIAL INCONGRUITY

Medial

Lateral

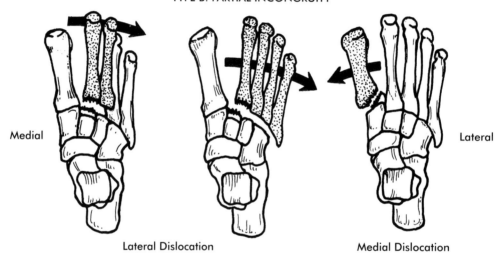

Lateral Dislocation

Medial Dislocation

TYPE C: DIVERGENT

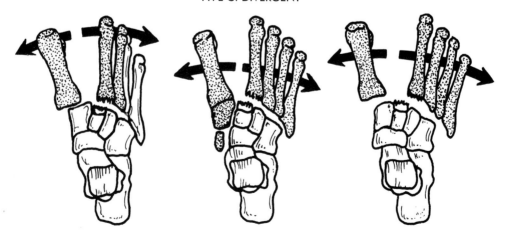

Partial Displacement

Total Displacement

**Fig. 8-9.** Classification of the Lisfranc fracture-dislocation. (Adapted from Hardcastle PH et al: Injuries to the tarsometatarsal joint: incidence, classification and treatment, *J Bone Joint Surg* 64B:349, 1982.)

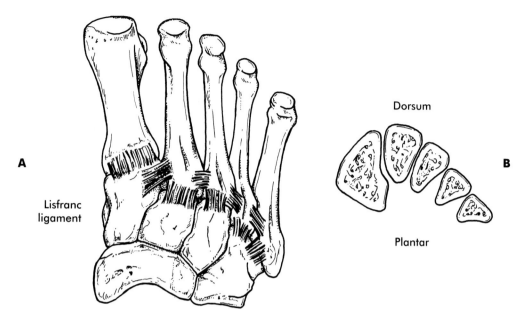

**Fig. 8-10. A,** The base of the second metatarsal is mortised between three cuneiforms. The second, third, and fourth metatarsals are connected to each other by dorsal and plantar transverse ligaments. There is no transverse ligament between the bases of the first and second metatarsals. The lateral four metatarsals are attached to the first cuneiform by the obliquely directed Lisfranc's ligament. **B,** Transverse section of the metatarsals. Dorsum of second metatarsal is wider than the plantar aspect.

stronger plantar tarsometatarsal ligaments, make plantar dislocation unlikely. On the other hand, the soft tissue overlying the dorsal aspect of these joints is rather scant.[3,4] These anatomical facts are responsible for displacement being most always dorsal and lateral.[13]

Finally, the location of the junction of the dorsalis pedis artery with the plantar arterial arch at the proximal end of the space between the first and second metatarsals places this artery at risk for injury with any type of tarsometatarsal dislocation.[34]

### Mechanism of injury

The forces responsible for tarsometatarsal dislocation can be classified as direct and indirect.* A direct force such as a truck running over the foot or a heavy weight dropped directly on the foot[82] results in plantar dislocation[66,82,107] of the metatarsal bases. Secondary medial or lateral displacement may occur depending upon the exact nature of the applied force.[62] The mechanism of direct force produces extensive soft tissue damage, and multiple associated fractures may be common.

The application of indirect force can also produce tarsometatarsal dislocations.[19,70,129,133] Jumping onto the plantar flexed foot or the application of a force up

*References 53, 62, 66, 70, 82, 107, 133.

through the toes of the equinus positioned foot can also result in the most common displacement, dorsal and lateral.[19] Jeffreys reported two patterns of indirect injury.[70] First, simple lateral dislocation of the forefoot can be produced by pronation of the hindfoot with a fixed forefoot position. Second, a medial dislocation of the first metatarsal cuneiform joint can be produced by supination of the hindfoot with a fixed forefoot; this mechanism is followed by complete dislocation of the forefoot after fracture of the second metatarsal.[70]

Wiley[129] believes the pattern of the fractured metatarsals and the configuration of the tarsometatarsal joint suggest the mechanism involved in producing tarsometatarsal dislocations is either violent abduction or plantar flexion of the forefoot. When the forefoot is violently abducted, the brunt of the force is concentrated on the fixed base of the second metatarsal. As the remaining metatarsals slide en masse, the second metatarsal cannot move until it fractures. If a significant degree of lateral displacement of the metatarsals occurs, the cuboid bone may be crushed. Fractures of the cuboid and second metatarsal bones are therefore pathognomonic signs of this abduction type of tarsometatarsal disruption.[66,129] According to Wiley, plantar flexion injuries[34] occur in two ways. The first mechanism involves a force applied to the heel along the axis of the foot when the toes are fixed

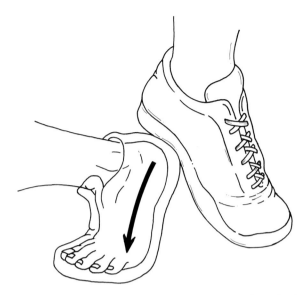

Fig. 8-11. Patient's foot is fixed on the ground with the metatarsophalangeal joints plantar flexed. Another player falls on the heel of the flexed foot.

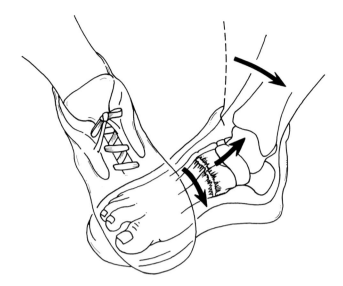

Fig. 8-12. The forefoot is fixed by another player's foot. The proximal foot and ankle are hyperextended, resulting in anterior lateral subluxation or dislocation at Lisfranc's joint.

and was described in the early literature as occurring when cavalrymen were thrown from their horses. Adelaar[2] describes a mechanism common in today's football and rugby competition in which the plantar-flexed foot is planted on the ground and struck from a posterior direction by an opposing player. He describes a similar injury occurring in the performing arts when the loaded foot collapses in the extreme pointe position.[2] This mechanism of injury is also frequent in sports, especially football, when a player falls on the heel of another player whose foot is fixed on the ground in plantar flexion (Fig. 8-11). Coming down to a plantar-flexed foot puts increased stress on the tarsometatarsal joint and leads to later problems. This is also the mechanism of injury seen in the Lisfranc stress fractures in female ballet dancers due to standing en pointe.[97] The entire joint complex may dislocate with or without associated fractures. Associated rotation at the time of application of this plantar flexion force can result in various combinations of associated fractures.[54,70] Another mechanism, common in athletics, is a violent hyperextension of the lower leg, ankle and mid foot on a fixed forefoot. This results in anterior lateral subluxation or dislocation of the Lisfranc's joint (Fig. 8-12).

Plantar flexion of the foot is commonly noted in motor vehicle accidents, a situation far more common in today's society.[70] In this instance the ankle is in a plantar-flexed position and the foot becomes part of a long lever arm consisting of the entire lower leg. With the lower leg and foot in the same linear axis, a force applied to the end of the foot is transmitted up this axis. If the line of this force is dorsal to the tarsometa-

tarsal joint, the weak dorsal ligament of the joint disrupts as the force increases.

Finally, Wilson demonstrated tarsometatarsal injuries can result from eversion, inversion, and plantar flexion.[133] Forefoot eversion (pronation) produces two stages of tarsometatarsal injury.[133] The first stage is medial dislocation of the first metatarsal bone alone (the so-called isolated dislocation). The second stage, produced by more eversion, consists of medial dislocation of the first metatarsal and dorsolateral dislocation of the four lesser metatarsal bones (the "divergent dislocation"). Forefoot inversion (supination) also produces two stages of injury. The stage I injury consists of dorsolateral dislocation of up to four lesser metatarsal bones. The second stage consists of dorsolateral dislocation of all five metatarsal bones. Finally, pure plantar flexion force without rotation produces variable fracture patterns.

In summary, these injuries are not the result of simple inversion, eversion, or plantar flexion mechanisms. They result from a combination of these forces plus rotation along the axis of the foot. Therefore the injuries may occur with or without fracture, depending upon the twisting forces simultaneously applied.[53] The importance in understanding these various mechanisms of injury is that at times the dislocation may have spontaneously reduced and the only clue to the extent of the injury may be the fracture pattern of the tarsal and metatarsal bones.[53]

### Diagnosis

In two groups of patients injuries to the tarsometatarsal joints may be overlooked. First, in multiply injured patients with severe trauma to other organ systems, closed injuries of the forefoot frequently go undiagnosed.[4,10,13] In less severely displaced subluxations, clinical and roentgenographic findings may be subtle and go unrecognized. More importantly, simple sprains of the tarsometatarsal joints with or without minimal widening between the first and second metatarsal bases occur, and their recognition is *essential* for proper treatment.[24]

The signs and symptoms in tarsometatarsal dislocation vary greatly depending upon the degree of displacement.[4] Spontaneous reduction is not unusual and can complicate the diagnosis.[4]

The patient usually presents complaining of severe pain in the midpart of the foot and at times relates of a feeling of paresthesia.[4,53] The patient complains of the inability to bear weight on the foot.[13] Swelling and associated deformity of the foot are obvious in complete dislocation.[6,89,103,104] The deformity of the foot consists of forefoot equinus, forefoot abduction, and prominence of the medial tarsal area.[73] Giannestras and Sammarco[53] report that swelling of the foot may occur as soon as 2 hours following the injury. If the injury is seen early before swelling, shortening and displacement of the forefoot may be noticeable.[4,10,53] There is diffuse tenderness across the tarsometatarsal joint, and marked pain is experienced upon passive motion.[4,10] In the case of subluxation of the Lisfranc joint or diastasis between the first and second metatarsal bases, point tenderness may be the only clinical finding. In complete dislocation the dorsalis pedis pulse may or may not be palpable.[53] Both Gissane[54] and Groulier and Pinaud[60] reported cases of tarsometatarsal dislocation requiring amputation.

### Roentgenographic evaluation

Radiographs taken in three planes—anteroposterior, lateral, and 30-degrees oblique—are essential to diagnose the initial displacement of subtle diastasis between the first and second metatarsal bases and to assess whether the reduction is anatomic.[53,62] Granberry and Lipscomb[59] reported that in only 8 of 25 cases were tarsometatarsal dislocations not associated with significant fractures. LaTourette et al[82] report fractures of the base of the second metatarsal, consisting of either a large or small fragment, are present in 90% of all tarsometatarsal dislocations. Aitken and Poulson[3] report that fractures of the base of the second metatarsal and compression fractures of the cuboid are the most common fractures associated with tarsometatarsal dislocations. Due to the possibility that a fracture-dislocation has spontaneously reduced and due to the existence of subluxations in which the dislocation is not complete, roentgenographic hints

that suggest tarsometatarsal injury are important to note. A fractured base of the second metatarsal with any displacement should suggest an injury to the Lisfranc joint.[53] Myerson[102] described a small bone fragment—representing an avulsion fracture of the medial base of the second metatarsal or lateral base of the first metatarsal—as a clue to this injury. They used the term *fleck sign* and found it was radiographically evident in 90% of their patients with tarsometatarsal injuries. Cain and Seligson[16] report avulsion of the medial pole of the navicular suggests a tarsometatarsal joint injury, and Schiller and Ray suggest the presence of an isolated medial cuneiform dislocation should also suggest the presence of an unrecognized (perhaps spontaneously reduced) tarsometatarsal injury.[116] Coker and Arnold[24] suggest that a fracture of the base of the second metatarsal, a fracture of a cuboid, and the loss of a few degrees of varus of the first metatarsal are all clues that a tarsometatarsal dislocation has occurred. If one suspects a spontaneously reduced dislocation by the presence of such associated fractures, or by residual subluxation of the tarsometatarsal joint, further evaluation by comparative roentgenographs is essential. If this does not clarify the pathology, stress roentgenographs using an anesthetic is essential to evaluate the injury.

Anderson[4] emphasized evaluation of the relationship of the metatarsal bases with the cuneiforms and cuboid, not only in detecting subluxations of this joint, but also in evaluating the quality of reduction. Giannestras and Sammarco[53] stated that the lateral two or three metatarsals tend to be somewhat variable in their relation to the lateral cuneiform and cuboid, and that this relationship is less reliable in diagnosing dislocations.[53] In 1975 Foster and Foster[46] reviewed the roentgenographs of 200 feet. They found the most consistent relationship at the tarsometatarsal joint was the alignment of the medial edge of the base of the second metatarsal with the medial edge of the second cuneiform on frontal or oblique views. They thought that a space between the first and second metatarsal was, of itself, not evidence of a dislocation unless there was a step-off at the base of the second metatarsal and second cuneiform (Fig. 8-13). Although the medial aspect of the base of the fourth metatarsal is usually aligned with the medial edge of the cuboid, these authors found a slight step-off (1 to 2 mm) in several cases without injury. They found that the base of the first metatarsal usually aligns with the lateral edge of the first cuneiform but that variations occur, particularly when the diameter of the metatarsal base is smaller than that of the medial cuneiform. The authors stressed that the base of the third metatarsal usually aligns with the medial aspect of the third cuneiform, but this junction may be

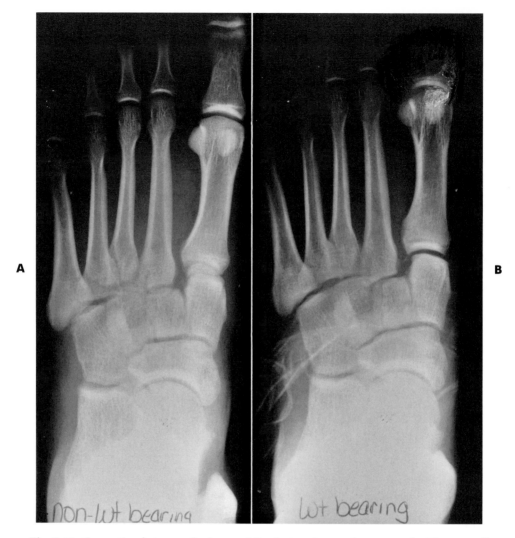

**Fig. 8-13.** Separation between the bases of the first and second metatarsals. The step-off at the base of the second metatarsal and second cuneiform confirms a Lisfranc joint subluxation. Weight-bearing films are essential. **A,** Non–weight-bearing radiographs. **B,** Weight-bearing radiograph (note increase in step-off).

difficult to see on routine views. Foster and Foster[46] also emphasized that the position of the fifth metatarsal is often difficult to assess.

Stein[120] reported in 1983 that when all four lateral metatarsals move as a group, dislocation can be readily appreciated. However, he stressed that it was not unusual to see intermetatarsal ligamentous disruption. In these instances, evaluation of the position of only one metatarsal could lead to a missed diagnosis. Stein[120] therefore believes the clinician must assess the anatomic position of all five metatarsal shafts as they articulate with the tarsal bones. He reviewed 100 radiological studies of the foot and observed the following constant anatomic relationships:

1. The medial border of the fourth metatarsal always forms a continuous straight line with the medial border of the cuboid on the medial oblique view (Fig. 8-14).
2. The intermetatarsal space between the third and fourth metatarsals is continuous with the intertarsal space between the lateral cuneiform and the cuboid. Therefore the lateral border of the third metatarsal shaft forms a straight line with the lateral border of the lateral cuneiform.
3. On the medial oblique view the intermetatarsal space between the second and third metatarsals is continuous in a straight line with the intertarsal space between the lateral and middle cuneiforms (Fig. 8-14).

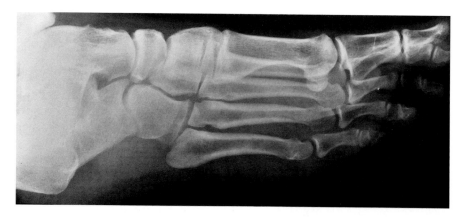

**Fig. 8-14.** Medial oblique view of the foot. The medial border of the cuboid and fourth metatarsal form a continuous line. The lateral border of the third metatarsal forms a continuous line with the lateral border of the third cuneiform. The intermetatarsal space between the second and third metatarsals is continuous with the intermetatarsal space between the middle and lateral cuneiforms.

4. On the anteroposterior view the medial border of the second metatarsal forms a continuous straight line with the medial border of the middle cuneiform (Fig. 8-15).
5. Therefore the intermetatarsal space between the first and second metatarsals is continuous with the intertarsal space between the medial and middle cuneiform.
6. The first metatarsal aligns itself with a medial cuneiform medially and laterally (Fig. 8-15).

Stein stressed that these relationships are constant regardless of the rotation of the foot when the roentgenographs are taken.

Stein also emphasized that it is difficult to assess the position of the fifth metatarsal in relationship to the cuboid. However, the fourth and fifth metatarsals almost always move as a unit in their relationship to the cuboid, even if there is a disruption of the intermetatarsal ligaments between the third and fourth metatarsals. Therefore an evaluation of the position of the fourth metatarsal is usually satisfactory to assess the position of the fifth.[120]

Evaluation of lateral weight-bearing radiographs is critical, especially in patients with a diastasis of the bases of the first and second metatarsals. Faciszewski et al[43] found the measurement of the distance between the plantar surfaces of the medial cuneiform and the fifth metatarsal base on the weight-bearing lateral radiograph was a reliable indicator of how much flattening of the longitudinal arch had occurred. Normally the medial cuneiform is dorsal to the base of the fifth metatarsal. With flattening of the longitudinal arch, these relationships become reversed, with the medial cuneiform plantar to the fifth metatarsal base.

Foster[47] reported the normal talometatarsal angle from the lateral weight-bearing radiograph measured up to 10 degrees.

**Treatment**

The goal of treatment of fracture-dislocations of the tarsometatarsal joints is the restoration of a painless and stable plantigrade foot.[58] Geckeler[51] emphasized that unless reduced early and completely, these injuries cause permanent pain and disability. Although there have been reports of minimal symptoms following minimal or no treatment and persistent subluxation,[3,15,70,84] most recent authors emphasize that reduction of the dislocation is essential for a good result.* Key and Conwell[78] stress that an anatomical reduction is a prerequisite for a painless functioning foot.[78]

In complete dislocation or residual subluxation, closed reduction should be attempted as soon as possible.[58] If manipulation is carried out immediately, the reduction may be accomplished easily, unless a chip fracture interferes with the reduction.[19,20] Cain and Seligson[16] carefully outlined the technique of manipulative reduction of these injuries. The first step is to restore the length of the foot. Cain and Seligson[16] accomplish this by manually pulling on the metatarsals while the heel is fixed. Once the length is restored, the second metatarsal is reduced by direct pressure into its mortise, thereby reestablishing the transverse arch of the midfoot.[16] Collett et al[25] also emphasize the importance of applying uniform traction as an essential part of the reduction. They recommend the use of woven wire traps (Chinese finger traps) placed

*References 7, 10, 19, 31, 43, 53, 58, 59, 101.

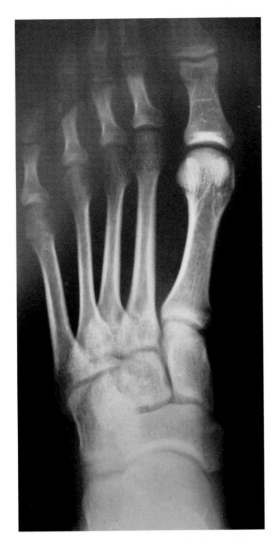

**Fig. 8-15.** Anteroposterior view of the foot. The medial border of the second metatarsal forms a continuous straight line with the medial border of the middle cuneiform. The intermetatarsal space between the first and second metatarsals is continuous with the intertarsal space between the medial and middle cuneiforms. The first metatarsal is aligned with the medial cuneiform medially and laterally.

cast application to be certain that the reduction and the percutaneous pin fixation are accurate. Bassett also recommends Kirschner wire (K-wire) stabilization to prevent displacement after initial reduction.[10] Foster and Foster[46] believe that if anatomic or near anatomic alignment is achieved by closed means, then cast immobilization can be used. They recommend percutaneous K-wire fixation only in cases of unstable reduction.

Following successful reduction with or without percutaneous fixation, the patient is placed in a short-leg cast. Cassebaum[19] recommends non–weight bearing for 6 to 8 weeks following reduction. Loss of reduction may also develop when weight bearing is initiated too early.[13] Adelaar has experienced good results using percutaneous wires with no loss of the reduction if the wires are kept in place 6 to 8 weeks. The patient is placed in a non–weight-bearing cast for 3 months. Following this, a semirigid full-length orthotic with metatarsal support is used for a year.

After closed manipulation, a careful roentgenographic evaluation ascertains that an anatomic reduction has been obtained. Collett et al[25] emphasize that the reduction must be anatomic on the anteroposterior, lateral, and oblique views since the dislocation occurs in all three planes. Evaluation of the relationship of the base of the metatarsals to the cuneiform and cuboids as outlined in the section, Roentgenographic Evaluation, is essential. Wilson[133] found that of 14 patients who had undergone a closed reduction and were subsequently treated conservatively, only 1 had an anatomical reduction; in half the patients a residual displacement of 5 mm or more was present. This stresses the importance of an accurate roentgenographic evaluation of the closed reduction.

Anderson,[4] Wilson,[133] and Myerson et al[101] recommend open reduction and K-wire internal fixation in cases in which an anatomic closed reduction is not obtained. Mauldin[93] advocates immediate open reduction with cross screw fixation. A straight medial incision extends over the medial cuneiform, extending 3 cm distal to the first tarsometatarsal joint. The anterior tibialis tendon must be identified and retracted. A second incision is centered over the second tarsometatarsal joint. The second and third metatarsal bases are held reduced as a guide pin is passed from the superomedial border of the medial cuneiform across the base of the second metatarsal and into the third metatarsal base. In a divergent type of fracture dislocation, the base of the first metatarsal is then reduced and provisionally stabilized with another guide wire. This is passed from the medial border of the base of the first metatarsal, crosses underneath the previously placed guide wire, through the middle cuneiform, and into the lateral cuneiform. Care

over the toes. The patient is placed prone with the foot projecting beyond the end of the table. Anderson[4] also recommends the use of Chinese finger traps applied to the toes to obtain traction. Once the metatarsals are out to length, manipulation of the metatarsals into their proper position is performed. Fitte and Garacotche[44] also use traction, obtained with pins through the metatarsals and calcaneus.

Anderson,[4] Hardcastle et al,[62] Myerson et al,[101] and Adelaar[2] believe that, although most of these dislocations can be reduced closed, they are unstable. In patients in whom the reduction is not stable, they recommend percutaneous pin fixation to maintain the reduction. Roentgenographs should be taken before should be taken to start the guide wire at least 1.0 cm from the joint line so as not to split the base of the first metatarsal on screw placement. An intraoperative radiograph confirms correct location of the guide wires. Sequentially a cannulated drill and a 4.0-mm cannulated Richards self-tapping screw of appropriate length are directed over each guide wire in the sequence in which the guide wires were placed. Securing the second and third metatarsal bases usually stabilizes the fourth and fifth metatarsals.

Postoperatively patients are non–weight bearing in a fracture boot for 8 weeks, followed by 4 weeks of weight bearing to tolerance. Postoperative rehabilitation includes removing the fracture boot daily and using the toes to pick up objects. The hardware is removed electively after 12 weeks postoperatively through the medial incision, when there is radiographic and clinical evidence of union.

Faciszewski et al[43] recommends basing treatment on the weight-bearing lateral radiograph. Patients without flattening of the longitudinal arch are treated non–weight bearing in a short-leg cast for 6 weeks, followed by a short-leg walking cast for 2 weeks. Patients with flattening of the longitudinal arch on their standing radiograph are treated with open reduction and internal fixation with either K-wires or screws. These authors found no relationship between residual diastasis of the first and second metatarsals and the functional result. However, patients with flattening of the longitudinal arch on the lateral weight-bearing radiograph had poor functional results.

### Irreducible dislocations

Tarsometatarsal fracture-dislocations irreducible by closed means have been reported by several authors.[29,40,90] Lowe and Yosipovitch,[90] Holstein and Joldersma,[67] and DeBenedetti et al[29] report the reduction was blocked by a slip of the tibialis anterior tendon trapped between the medial and middle cuneiform. Engber and Roberts,[40] Ballerio,[9] and Huet and Lecoeur[68] report that a superiorly dislocated peroneus longus tendon may act as an obstruction to reduction. Open reduction to remove the trapped tibialis anterior or peroneus longus tendon is the treatment of choice.[29,40]

Lenczner et al[84] noted the avulsed fragment may act to prevent an anatomic reduction of the metatarsal base within the cuneiform mortise, resulting in persistent subluxation of the metatarsal. If the avulsion fracture remains attached to Lisfranc's ligament and cannot be displaced by closed manipulation to allow the metatarsal base access to the mortise, the fragment should be excised at open reduction.

Geckeler[51] believed it was nearly impossible to reduce dislocations of the tarsometatarsal joint by manipulation and therefore recommended operative treatment. Wilson[133] also found manipulative reduction not dependable and recommended, unless anatomical reduction was obtained, open reduction and fixation with Kirschner pins. Anderson[4] also recommended open reduction and internal fixation with Kirschner pins in cases in which an anatomic closed reduction was not obtained. Granberry and Lipscomb[59] also recommend open reduction and internal fixation if an anatomic reduction was not obtained by closed means. Additionally, they suggested fusion of the involved joints in patients who required open reduction.

Del Sel in 1955[31] recommended primary open reduction and temporary internal fixation by percutaneous wires in patients with tarsometatarsal fracture dislocations. He recommended the use of an incision in the first interosseous space with evacuation of the blood clot located there. In some cases a second incision was necessary to reduce the second and third metatarsals. He recommended debridement of bits of cartilage, soft tissue, and bone from the tarsometatarsal joint and then stabilizing the reduction using percutaneous K-wires. The wires were left in place for 2 to 4 weeks. After the wires were removed, the patients were encouraged to walk in a below-the-knee cast. Tondeur[124] also advised open reduction and internal fixation of tarsometatarsal dislocations.

Wright[134] recommends longitudinal incisions on the dorsum of the foot for open reduction. Wippula[130] also recommends the use of a longitudinal incision between the first and second metatarsals on the dorsum of the foot. He found that when the first and second metatarsals were reduced, the remainder of the metatarsals easily fell into place. He also used K-wire fixation from the metatarsals into the tarsal bones for stability.

Arntz et al[7] reported multiple problems with K-wire fixation including pin migration, infection of pin tracts, and loss of reduction. Because of these difficulties, they recommend open reduction of fracture and fracture dislocations of the tarsometatarsal joint followed by temporary internal fixation using AO screws. Exposure is achieved through one or more longitudinal incisions. The capsules of the tarsometatarsal joints are opened through a single dorsal incision. Comminuted interarticular fragments are reduced when possible, and smaller irreducible fragments are excised. Once a precise reduction of each tarsometatarsal joint has been achieved, a notch is made on the dorsum of the metatarsal approximately 15 to 20 mm distal to the joint.

A drill bit 3.2 mm in diameter or smaller is then

used to make a hole beginning in the proximal edge of the notch, directing it across the base of the metatarsal into the body of the respective cuneiform. A 4.0-mm diameter screw or malleolar screw is used to fix the joint with slight compression while holding the reduction anatomically. According to Arntz et al, when the first metatarsal cuneiform joint had been reduced and stabilized, there was simultaneous reduction of the second metatarsal, which was stabilized in a similar manner. When the third metatarsal is also dislocated, a second dorsal incision is made between the third and fourth metatarsal and the third metatarsal cuneiform joint similarly stabilized. Once the third metatarsal cuneiform joint is stabilized, the fourth and fifth metatarsal joints usually are fully reduced. Occasionally a single screw is placed through a small stab incision across the base of the fifth metatarsal into the cuboid. Postoperatively patients are treated by partial weight bearing for 6 weeks. They are then placed in a weight-bearing cast and full weight bearing is allowed for the initial 4 to 6 weeks. Internal fixation was maintained until x-rays showed evidence of osseous union. In their series the screws were removed an average of 16 weeks following injury. There was no evidence of redisplacement or recurrent subluxation when radiographs were compared that had been made postoperatively, after removal of the screws, and at final follow-up. The authors report they had patients with apparently healed dislocations displace following the removal of K-wires at 6 weeks following fixation. For these reasons, they recommend leaving the screws in place for a minimum of 12 weeks.

According to Arntz et al, fixation of the tarsometatarsal joints with AO screws had no apparent influence on the development of arthritic change in the affected tarsometatarsal joints. They found no discernible radiographic differences between adjacent joints, some of which had been stabilized with screws and others which had not. Arntz et al believed that the tarsometatarsal joints — because of their normally limited range of motion — tolerated this method of stable internal fixation well. In their opinion injury to the articular cartilage and failure to achieve and maintain an anatomic reduction proved to be the most important factors in the development of posttraumatic arthritis.

## Results

Aitken and Poulson[3] reported that although posttraumatic arthritis and ankylosis of the tarsometatarsal joints were common, they were not a source of discomfort and disability in the majority of their patients. Indeed, they did not see the need for a tarsometatarsal fusion in their patients at follow-up.

Myerson[102] found that degenerative changes were found in almost every patient following tarsometatarsal dislocation, but that there was a low level of correlation between the degree of degenerative changes and clinical results. Similarly Brunet and Wiley[15] reported that despite various treatment methods, foot comfort usually progressed to a stable level by about 1.3 years after injury. They reported that neither the initial fracture type nor treatment had any apparent bearing on the subsequent function and found no correlation between radiographic assessment of the injury and the patient's symptoms. Almost 80% of their patients were able to return to their original occupation, and the majority were pain-free. Brunet and Wiley believe that the relative absence of pain — even with persistent gross subluxation and radiographic evidence of advanced arthritis — may be secondary to a stable ankylosis or to disruption of sensory fibers of the torn capsular and ligamentous structures of the joint. On the contrary, LaTourette et al[82] found that all patients complain of some degree of discomfort in the foot following tarsometatarsal injury. Additionally, the majority of patients complained of swelling. Hesp et al[65] in 1984 reviewed 22 cases with 52 months of follow-up. A significant number of their patients developed late degenerative arthritis of the tarsometatarsal joint. They believe the severity of the initial injury was the determining factor in late degenerative arthritis. Faciszewski et al[43] found no relationship between persistent diastasis between first and second metatarsals and fractures of the foot.

Goossans and DeStoop[56] reported 35% of their patients developed degenerative arthritis following tarsometatarsal dislocation. Three of their patients underwent tarsometatarsal arthrodesis and all had good results and returned to work. Johnson and Johnson[72] reported a Dowell graft arthrodesis technique used in 15 patients with posttraumatic degenerative arthritis after tarsometatarsal fracture dislocation. Sangeorzan et al[115] reported 15 patients who, following fracture dislocation of the tarsometatarsal joint, had persistent pain requiring arthrodesis. The patients complained of pain and progressive flatfoot deformity with forefoot abduction. The authors described a technique involving exposing Lisfranc's joint, denuding articular cartilage, reduction of the dislocation and fixation using lag screws. The authors recommend that, when significant persistent displacement is present, reduction should be performed before arthrodesis. The authors reported good-to-excellent results in 70% of their patients. Poor reduction, a delay in treatment, and injuries occurring in the workplace all portend a poor prognosis following tarsometatarsal dislocations. Arthrodesis for persistent pain following subtle injury to the Lisfranc joint provides a pain-free joint, but the ability to participate in athletics is limited.

Obtaining and maintaining an anatomic reduction is believed to be of major importance in avoiding the degenerative changes that may require surgery at a later date.[53] LaTourette et al[82] evaluated their results using gait analysis by foot switches attached to the sole of the patient's shoes.[27,92,113] They concluded anatomic reduction and early ambulation produce better results. Myerson[102] concluded that the major determinant of unacceptable results was the quality of the initial reduction. According to these authors, open anatomic reduction and internal fixation using K-wires yielded the best results. Wilson,[133] too, found the most critical factor in preventing late deformity, stiffness, and degenerative arthritis was an anatomical reduction obtained by either closed or open means. Wilppula[130] demonstrated that, although an anatomical result was no guarantee of a symptom-free foot, in general, a good anatomical result usually produced a good functional result. Additionally, Wilppula[130] reported that symptoms of degenerative arthritis in the tarsometatarsal joint tended to subside gradually during several years of follow-up. He found no need for arthrodesis as a salvage procedure in his patients, although he suggested that early arthrodesis might have accelerated their recovery. Wilppula also found limitation of motion in the foot was present in half his patients and suggested that intensifying the mobilizing exercises during treatment could reduce this disability. According to Adelaar, although anatomic reduction does produce the best results, forefoot stiffness, unequal metatarsal plantar pressure, and intrinsic contractures may still produce a symptomatic foot particularly when sympathetic dystrophy complicates these severe crushing injuries.

Lenczner et al[84] reported that the majority of their poor results were secondary either to failure to obtain an adequate reduction or failure to maintain the reduction of the tarsometatarsal injury. This stresses the importance of stable fixation after reduction to prevent redislocation during the period of immobilization.[10] Arntz et al[7] believed that the results following tarsometatarsal dislocations were most dependent upon the accuracy of the reduction and the presence of associated osteochondral fractures in the tarsometatarsal joint. Finally, Jeffreys[70] emphasizes that although accurate reduction is essential to prevent long-term disability, the late development of osteoarthritis may be determined by the damage sustained by the articular cartilage at the time of the injury. Therefore in certain cases osteoarthritis may develop in spite of the method of treatment selected.

### Author's preferred method of treatment

The importance of early diagnosis and treatment of injuries to the tarsometatarsal joints cannot be overemphasized. Anteroposterior, oblique, and lateral roentgenographs will demonstrate frank dislocation of the tarsometatarsal joints. However, careful evaluation of roentgenographs of the foot is essential to detect the subtle signs of a subluxation of the tarsometatarsal joint or complete tarsometatarsal dislocation that has spontaneously reduced. When the clinical examination reveals tenderness at the tarsometatarsal joint, a full roentgenographic evaluation of the joint, including lateral weight-bearing roentgenographs, is essential. In cases in which such injury is suspected, I use stress roentgenographs, possibly with an anesthetic, to determine the degree of instability.

In complete dislocation, if the patient's medical condition or skin damage over the dislocation prevent open reduction, I proceed to closed reduction. In my experience the earlier a reduction is attempted, the more likely an anatomic reduction will be obtained by closed methods.

Traction is obtained with the patient supine by suspending the leg with Chinese finger traps applied to the toes. A counterweight is placed over the ankle. Once the tarsometatarsal joints have been restored to length by traction, manipulation in the dorsal plantar plane is performed. Roentgenographic evaluation is then performed to ascertain the quality of the reduction. Anatomic reduction of the relationship of each of the metatarsals to their respective cuneiform or cuboid is demanded. If such a reduction is obtained, I use two percutaneous K-wires, one from the first metatarsal into the medial cuneiform and the second from the fifth metatarsal into the cuboid to stabilize the dislocation. The question of whether a closed reduction is stable is not considered in determining whether K-wire fixation is needed. In my opinion all these injuries, which were dislocated initially, require K-wire stabilization. In patients with minor degrees of subluxation of the tarsometatarsal joint reduced by closed means, K-wire fixation is reserved only for those in whom cooperation with the postreduction regimen is questionable.

Following reduction and stabilization, the foot is placed in a short-leg fracture boot for 4 weeks with toe-touch weight bearing. The toes are left free at the end of the cast to encourage exercises of the metatarsophalangeal joints. After 4 weeks, when the swelling is decreased, the fracture boot is removed to allow range-of-motion exercises. Partial weight bearing is allowed. The fracture boot and the pins are removed at 12 weeks. At this point the foot is placed in a good shoe with a longitudinal arch support for an additional 9 to 12 months.

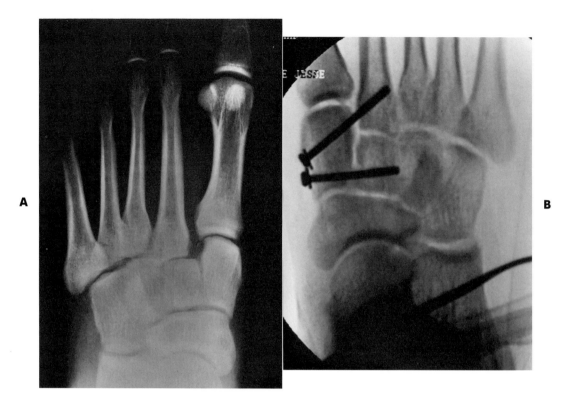

**Fig. 8-16. A,** Diastasis of Lisfranc's joint in a high school football player. **B,** Open reduction and stable internal fixation using AO screws.

If skin and medical conditions permit, I prefer to proceed with open reduction and internal fixation. In my experience the best results are obtained with an anatomic reduction. The most predictable way for me to obtain an anatomic reduction and allow secure fixation for 12 weeks is through open reduction and internal fixation. I have used both K-wire and screw fixation and prefer the latter. Difficulty achieving anatomic reduction through closed reduction and percutaneous pinning has led to this protocol. At the time of open reduction, the reduction must be anatomic in all three planes. This is often difficult to do by closed means with the foot in finger traps. The transverse "Roman arch" at the base of the metatarsals as well as the contralateral talometatarsal angle must be reconstituted during open reduction.

I prefer an incision over the first tarsometatarsal joint. Subsequent parallel longitudinal incisions are used, usually between the third and fourth metatarsals, to expose the remainder of the tarsometatarsal joint. Usually debridement of small articular cartilage and osseous fragments is necessary to effect the reduction. In patients in whom there is a gross amount of swelling at the time of open reduction, interosseous decompression fasciotomies are performed between each of the metatarsals in an effort to decrease fibrosis. The cross screw fixation technique[93] or straight lag

compression technique of Arntz et al[7] give equally good results. In patients with gross swelling at the time of open reduction, interosseous decompression fasciotomies are performed between each of the metatarsals. Postoperatively the limb is placed in a short-leg fracture boot and elevated. When edema allows, usually after 48 hours, the patients start toe-touch weight bearing for 8 weeks. After the soft tissues have quiesced and sutures are removed at 2 weeks, the patient can take the fracture boot off several times during the day to perform active range of motion and pick up objects with the toes. After 8 weeks the patient progresses to weight bearing to tolerance. After 12 weeks patients are allowed to wear a crepe-soled shoe with an arch support. When radiographs and clinical examination show evidence of fracture union, the hardware is removed, usually at 14 to 16 weeks.

In athletes with subtle injury to Lisfranc's joint with diastasis of the first and second metatarsal bases, I prefer open reduction and internal fixation using screw fixation (Fig. 8-16). Even though some authors report no relationship between function and persistent diastasis in the general population, in my experience persistent diastasis in athletes has adversely affected performance. Following open reduction patients are in a partial weight-bearing cast for 6 weeks followed by a weight-bearing cast for 4 weeks.

The internal fixation is removed at 12 weeks, and the athletes are fitted with arch supports for their shoes.

In my experience early mobilization and an early exercise program help reduce edema and speed the return of patients to their normal activities. It is not uncommon for patients to complain of persistent aching in the tarsometatarsal joint for prolonged periods, despite an anatomic reduction. Good arch support and stiff-soled shoe are used to control these symptoms.

## REFERENCES

1. Acker JH, Drez D: Nonoperative treatment of stress fractures of the proximal shaft of the fifth metatarsal: jones fracture, *Foot Ankle* 7:152, 1986.
2. Adelaar RS: *The treatment of tarsometatarsal fracture dislocation.* In *AAOS Instructional Course Lectures,* vol 34, 1990, p 141.
3. Aitken AP, Poulson D: Dislocations of the tarsometatarsal joint, *J Bone Joint Surg* 45A:246, 1963.
4. Anderson LD: Injuries of the foot, *Clin Orthop* 122:18, 1977.
5. Arangio GA: Proximal displaced fractures of the fifth metatarsal (Jones fracture): two cases treated by cross pinning with review of 100 cases, *Foot Ankle* 3:293, 1983.
6. Arenberg AA: Vyvikhi v sustave lisfranka (dislocation of Lisfranc's joint), *Vestn Khir* 102:126, 1969.
7. Arntz CJ, Veith RG, Hansen SJ Jr: Fractures and fracture-dislocations of the tarsometatarsal joints, *J Bone Joint Surg* 70A:173, 1988.
8. Ashurst APC: Divergent dislocation of the metatarsus, *Ann Surg* 83:132, 1926.
9. Ballerio A: Un caso raro di Lussazione tarso metatarsale isolata, *Chir Organi Mov* 38:286, 1953.
10. Bassett FH: Dislocations of the tarsometatarsal joints, *South Med J* 57:1294, 1964.
11. Battey MA: The lesser metatarsal stress fracture as a complication of the Keller procedure, *J Am Podiatr Assoc* 70:182, 1980.
12. Bernstein A, Stone JR: March fracture: a report of three hundred and seven cases, and a new method of treatment, *J Bone Joint Surg* 26:743, 1944.
13. Blodgett WH: *Injuries of the forefoot and toes.* In Jahss MH, editor: *Disorders of the foot,* vol 2, Philadelphia, 1982, WB Saunders.
14. Brown DC, McFarland GB: Dislocation of the medial cuneiform bone in tarsometatarsal fracture-dislocation, *J Bone Joint Surg* 57A:858, 1975.
15. Brunet JA, Wiley JJ: The late results of tarsometatarsal joint injuries, *J Bone Joint Surg* 69B:437, 1987.
16. Cain PR, Seligson D: Lisfranc's fracture-dislocation with intercuneiform dislocation: presentation of two cases and a plan for treatment, *Foot Ankle* 2:156, 1981.
17. Carp L: Fracture of the fifth metatarsal bone, with special reference to delayed union, *Ann Surg* 86:308, 1927.
18. Carr JB, Hansen ST, Benirschke SK: Surgical treatment of foot and ankle trauma: the use of indirect reduction techniques, *Foot Ankle* 9:176, 1989.
19. Cassebaum WH: Lisfranc fracture–dislocations, *Clin Orthop* 30:116, 1963.
20. Chapman MW: *Fractures and dislocations of the ankle and foot.* In Mann RA, editor: *DuVries surgery of the foot,* ed 4, St Louis, 1978, CV Mosby.

21. Cherkes-Zade DI: Pepelomy-vyvikhi v sustave lisfranka (fracture-dislocation of the Lisfranc's joint), *Vestn Khir* 103:102, 1969.
22. Christopher F: Fractures of the fifth metatarsal, *Surg Gynecol Obstet* 37:190, 1923.
23. Clancy WG Jr: Lower extremity injuries in the jogger and distance runner, *Phys Sports Med* 2:47, 1974.
24. Coker TP Jr, Arnold JA: *Sports injuries to the foot and ankle.* In Jahss MH, editor: *Disorders of the foot,* vol 2, Philadelphia, 1982, WB Saunders.
25. Collett HS, Hood TK, Andrews RE: Tarsometatarsal fracture dislocations, *Surg Gynecol Obstet* 106:623, 1958.
26. Crenshaw AH: *Delayed union and nonunion of fractures.* In Edmonson AS, Crenshaw AH, editors: *Campbell's operative orthopaedics,* ed 6, St Louis, 1980. CV Mosby.
27. Curry CL: Stride characteristics of normal adults, Master's thesis, USC School of Physical Therapy, March 1976.
28. Dameron TB: Fractures and anatomical variations of the proximal portion of the fifth metatarsal, *J Bone Joint Surg* 57A:788, 1975.
29. DeBenedetti MJ, Evanski PM, Waugh TR: The unreducible Lisfranc's fracture, *Clin Orthop* 136:238, 1978.
30. DeCoster T, Alvarez R, Trevino S: External fixation of the foot and ankle, *Foot Ankle* 17:40, 1986.
31. Del Sel JM: The surgical treatment of tarsometatarsal fracture-dislocations, *J Bone Joint Surg* 37B:203, 1955.
32. DeLee JC, Farney WC: Incidence of injury in Texas high school football, *Am J Sports Med* 20:575, 1992.
33. DeLee JC, Evans JP, Julian J: Stress fracture of the fifth metatarsal, *Am J Sports Med* 11:349, 1983.
34. DePalma A: *The Management of Fractures and Dislocations,* vol 2, Philadelphia, 1959, WB Saunders.
35. Detlefsen M: Die luxation im Lisfrancschen gelenk als typischi verletzung des Montorrad fahrers, *Beitr Orthop Traumatol* 15:242, 1968.
36. Devas M: *Stress fractures,* Edinburgh, London, New York, 1975, Churchill Livingstone.
37. Drez D Jr et al: Metatarsal stress fractures, *Am J Sports Med* 8:123, 1980.
38. Dukowsky J, Freeman BL: Fracture dislocation of the articular surface of the third metatarsal head, *Foot Ankle* 10:43, 1989.
39. Easton ER: Two rare dislocations of the metatarsals at Lisfranc's joint, *J Bone Joint Surg* 20:1053, 1938.
40. Engber WD, Roberts JM: Irreducible tarsometatarsal fracture-dislocation, *Clin Orthop* 168:102, 1982.
41. Engh CA, Robinson RA, Milgram J: Stress fractures in children, *J Trauma* 10:532, 1970.
42. English TA: Dislocations of the metatarsal bone and adjacent toe, *J Bone Joint Surg* 46B:700, 1964.
43. Faciszewski T, Burks RT, Manaster BJ: Subtle injuries of the Lisfranc joint, *J Bone Joint Surg* 72A:1519, 1990.
44. Fitte M, Garacotche I: Luxation-fracture de l'articulation de Lisfranc, *J Chir* 56:367, 1940.
45. Ford LT, Gilula LA: Stress fractures of the middle metatarsals following the Keller operation, *J Bone Joint Surg* 59A:117, 1977.
46. Foster SC, Foster RR: Lisfranc's tarsometatarsal fracture-dislocation, *Radiology* 120:79, 1976.
47. Foster SC: Lisfranc tarsometatarsal fracture dislocations, *Radiology* 21:988, 1981.
48. Frieberg AH: Infraction of the second metatarsal bone, a typical injury, *Surg Gynecol Obstet* 19:191, 1914.
49. Funk FJ: Tarsometatarsal fracture-dislocations, closed (Lisfranc): early diagnosis and treatment, presented at AOA Third International Symposium: "Musculoskeletal Trauma," San Francisco, May 17-21, 1982.

50. Garcia A, Parkes JC: *Fractures of the foot.* In Giannestras NJ, editor: *Foot disorders: medical and surgical management,* ed 2, Philadelphia, 1973, Lea & Febiger.

51. Geckeler EO: Dislocations and fracture-dislocations of the foot: transfixion with Kirschner wires, *Surgery* 25:730, 1949.

52. Giannestras NJ: Shortening of the metatarsal shaft in the treatment of plantar keratosis, *J Bone Joint Surg* 40A:61, 1958.

53. Giannestras NJ, Sammarco GJ: *Fractures and dislocations in the foot.* In Rockwood CA Jr, Green DP, editors: *Fractures,* vol 2, Philadelphia, 1975, JB Lippincott.

54. Gissane W: A dangerous type of fracture of the foot, *J Bone Joint Surg* 33B:535, 1951.

55. Goldstein LA, Dickerson RC: *Atlas of orthopaedic surgery,* St Louis, 1974, CV Mosby.

56. Goossens M, DeStoop N: Lisfranc's fracture-dislocations: etiology, radiology and results of treatment, *Clin Orthop* 176:154, 1983.

57. Gould N, Trevenio S: Sural nerve entrapment by avulsion fracture of the base of the fifth metatarsal bone, *Foot Ankle* 3:153, 1981.

58. Graham J, Waddell JP, Lenczner E: Tarsometatarsal (Lisfranc) dislocation, *J Bone Joint Surg* 55B:666, 1973.

59. Granberry WM, Lipscomb PR: Dislocation of the tarsometatarsal joints, *Surg Gynecol Obstet* 114:467, 1962.

60. Groulier P, Pinaud JC: Les luxations tarsometatarsiennes (a propor de dix observations), *Rev Chir Orthop* 56:303, 1970.

61. Hansen ST: Severe trauma to the forefoot: initial management, Presented at AOA Third International Symposium: "Musculoskeletal Trauma," San Francisco, May 17-21, 1982.

62. Hardcastle PH et al: Injuries to the tarsometatarsal joint: incidence, classification and treatment, *J Bone Joint Surg* 64B:349, 1982.

63. Heck CV: Fractures of the bones of the foot (except the talus), *Surg Clin North Am* 45:103, 1965.

64. Heckman JD: *Fractures and dislocations of the foot.* In Rockwood CA, Green DP, editors: *Fractures,* Philadelphia, 1984, JB Lippincott, p 1808.

65. Hesp WLEM, VanderWerken C, Goris RJA: (Lisfranc's) dislocations: fractures and/or dislocations through the tarsometatarsal joints, *Injury* 15:261, 1984.

66. Hillegass RC: *Injuries to the midfoot: a major cause of industrial morbidity.* In Bateman JE, editor: *Foot science,* Philadelphia, 1976, WB Saunders.

67. Holstein A, Joldersma RD: Dislocation of the first cuneiform in tarsometatarsal fracture-dislocation, *J Bone Joint Surg* 32A: 419, 1950.

68. Huet P, Lecoeur P: Sur 4 cas de luxation tarsometatarsienne, *Acad Chir Mem* 72:124, 1946.

69. Irwin CG: Fractures of the metatarsals, *Proc R Soc Med* 31(part 2): 789, 1938.

70. Jeffreys TE: Lisfranc's fracture-dislocation. A clinical and experimental study of tarso-metatarsal dislocations and fracture-dislocations, *J Bone Joint Surg* 45B:546, 1963.

71. Johnson VS: *Treatment of fractures of the forefoot in industry.* In Bateman JE, editor: *Foot science,* Philadelphia, 1976, WB Saunders.

72. Johnson JE, Johnson KA: Dowel arthrodesis for degenerative arthritis of the tarsometatarsal Lisfranc's joints, *Foot Ankle* 6:243, 1986.

73. Jones R: Fracture of the base of the fifth metatarsal bone by indirect violence, *Ann Surg* 35:697, 1902.

74. Jones R: Fractures of the fifth metatarsal bone, *Liverpool Med Surg J* 42:103, 1902.

75. Kavanaugh JH, Brower TD, Mann RV: The Jones fracture revisited, *J Bone Joint Surg* 60A:776, 1978.

76. Kelikian H: *Hallux valgus, allied deformities of the forefoot and metatarsals,* Philadelphia, 1965, WB Saunders.

77. Key JA, Conwell HE: *The management of fractures, dislocations and sprains,* ed 3, St Louis, 1942, CV Mosby.

78. Key JA, Conwell HE: *The management of fractures, dislocations and sprains,* ed 6, St Louis, 1956, CV Mosby.

79. Klenerman L: *The foot and its disorders,* Oxford, 1976, Blackwell Scientific.

80. Klenerman L: *The foot and its disorders,* ed 2, Oxford, London, Edinburgh, Boston, Melbourne, 1982, Blackwell Scientific.

81. Lapidus PW, Guidotti FP: Immediate mobilization and swimming pool exercises in some fractures of foot and ankle bones, *Clin Orthop* 56:197, 1968.

82. LaTourette G et al: *Fractures and dislocations of the tarsometatarsal joint.* In Bateman JE, Trott AW, editors: *The foot and ankle,* New York, 1980, B C Decker.

83. Lehman RC et al: Fractures of the base of the fifth metatarsal distal to the tuberosity: a review, *Foot Ankle* 7:245, 1987.

84. Lenczner EM, Waddell JP, Graham JD: Tarsal-metatarsal (Lisfranc) dislocation, *J Trauma* 14:1012, 1974.

85. Levy JM: Stress fractures of the first metatarsal, *Am J Roentgenol* 130:679, 1978.

86. Lewin R, editor: *The foot and ankle,* Philadelphia, 1940, Lea & Febiger.

87. Lichtblau S: Painful nonunion of a fracture of the 5th metatarsal, *Clin Orthop* 59:171, 1968.

88. Lindholm R: Operative treatment of dislocated simple fracture of the neck of the metatarsal bone, *Ann Chir Gynaecol Tenn* 50:328, 1961.

89. London PS: Major injuries of the foot, *J Bone Joint Surg* 58B:385, 1976.

90. Lowe J, Yosipovitah Z: Tarsometatarsal dislocation: a mechanism blocking manipulative reduction, *J Bone Joint Surg* 58A:1029, 1976.

91. Mann, Personal communication, 1980.

92. Manter JT: Distribution of compression forces in joints of the human foot, *Anat Rec* 96:313, 1946.

93. Mauldin D: Personal communication.

94. McKeever FM: Fractures of the tarsal and metatarsal bones, *Surg Gynecol Obstet* 90:735, 1950.

95. McKeever FM: *Injuries of the forefoot.* In *American Academy of Orthopaedic Surgeons Instructional Course Lectures,* vol 2, Ann Arbor, 1944, JW Edwards, p 120.

96. Meurman KOA: Less common stress fractures in the foot, *Br J Radiol* 54:1, 1981.

97. Micheli LJ, Sohn RS, Solomon R: Stress fractures of the second metatarsal involving Lisfranc's joint in ballet dancers, *J Bone Joint Surg* 67A:1372, 1985.

98. Morrison GM: Fractures of the bones of the feet, *Am J Surg* 38:721, 1937.

99. Morrissey EJ: Metatarsal fractures, *J Bone Joint Surg* 28:594, 1946.

100. Moseley HF: Traumatic disorders of the ankle and foot, *Clin Symp* 17:29, 1965.

101. Myerson MS et al: Fracture dislocations of the tarsometatarsal joints: end results correlated with pathology and treatment, *Foot Ankle* 6:225, 1986.

102. Myerson M: Acute compartment syndromes of the foot, *Bull Hosp Jt Dis Orthop Inst* 47:251, 1987.

103. Narat JK: An unusual case of dislocation of metatarsal bones, *Am J Surg* 6:239, 1929.

104. O'Donoghue DH: *Treatment of injuries to athletes,* ed 3, vol 1, Philadelphia, 1976, WB Saunders.

105. Omer GE, Pomerantz GM: Principles of management of acute injuries of the foot, *J Bone Joint Surg* 51A:813, 1969.

106. O'Rahilly R: A survey of carpal and tarsal anomalies, *J Bone Joint Surg* 35A:626, 1953.

107. O'Regan DJ: Lisfranc dislocations, *J Med Soc N J* 66:575, 1969.

108. Pearson JB: Fractures of the base of the fifth metatarsal, *Br Med J* 1:1052, 1962.

109. Peltier LF: Eponymic fractures: Robert Jones and Jones's fracture, *Surgery* 71:522, 1972.

110. Perriard M, Deterle J, Jeannet E: Les lesions traumatiques recentes comprises entre les articulations de Chopart et de Lisfranc, incluses, *Z Unfallmed Berufskr* 63:318, 1970.

111. Pritsch M et al: An unusual fracture of the base of the fifth metatarsal bone, *J Trauma* 20:530, 1980.

112. Quenu E, Kuss G: Etude sur les luxations du metatarse, *Rev Chir* 39:1, 1909.

113. Rousek R: Stride characteristics of normal adults, Master's thesis, USC School of Physical Therapy, November, 1976.

114. Sammarco GJ: *Biomechanics of the foot.* In Frankel VH, Nordin M, editors: *Basic biomechanics of the skeletal system*, Philadelphia, 1980, Lea & Fibiger, p 193.

115. Sangeorzan BJ, Veith RG, Hansen ST: Salvage of Lisfranc's tarsometatarsal joints by arthrodesis, *Foot Ankle* 4:193, 1990.

116. Schiller MG, Ray RD: Isolated dislocation of the medial cuneiform bone—a rare injury of the tarsus, *J Bone Joint Surg* 52A:1632, 1970.

117. Shereff MJ: *Fractures of the forefoot.* Instructional Course Lectures, AAOS, vol 29, 1990, p 133.

118. Sisk TD: *Fractures.* In Edmonson AS, Crenshaw AH, editors: *Campbell's operative orthopaedics*, ed 6, vol 1, St Louis, 1980, CV Mosby.

119. Speed K: *Fractures and dislocations*, ed 2, Philadelphia, 1928, Lea & Febiger.

120. Stein RE: Radiological aspects of the tarsometatarsal joints, *Foot Ankle* 3:286, 1983.

121. Stewart IM: Jones's fracture: fracture of base of fifth metatarsal, *Clin Orthop* 16:190, 1960.

122. Stone MM: Avulsion fracture of the base of the fifth metatarsal, *Am J Orthop Surg* 10:190, 1968.

123. Taussig G, Hautier S: Les fractures-luxations de l'articulation de Lisfranc, *Ann Chir* 23:1131, 1969.

124. Tondeur G: Un cas de luxation-fracture tarsometatarsienne, *Acta Orthop Belg* 27:286, 1961.

125. Torg JS et al: Fractures of the base of the fifth metatarsal distal to the tuberosity: classification and guidelines for nonsurgical and surgical management. (Accepted for publication by *J Bone Joint Surg*.)

126. Tountas AA: Occult fracture-subluxation of the midtarsal joint, *Clin Orthop* 243:195, 1988.

127. Turco VJ, Spinella AJ: Tarsometatarsal dislocation—Lisfranc injury, *Foot Ankle* 2:362, 1982.

128. Wharton HR: Fractures of the proximal end of the fifth metatarsal bone, *Ann Surg* 47:824, 1908.

129. Wiley JJ: The mechanism of tarso-metatarsal joint injuries, *J Bone Joint Surg* 53B:474, 1971.

130. Wilppula E: Tarsometatarsal fracture dislocation, *Acta Orthop Scand* 44:335, 1973.

131. Wilson PD: Fractures and dislocations of the tarsal bones, *South Med J* 26:833, 1933.

132. Wilson ES Jr, Katz FN: Stress fractures. An analysis of 250 consecutive cases, *Radiology* 92:481, 1969.

133. Wilson DW: Injuries of the tarso-metatarsal joints: etiology, classification and results of treatment, *J Bone Joint Surg* 54B:677, 1972.

134. Wright PE: *Dislocations.* In Edmonson AS, Crenshaw AH, editors: *Campbell's operative orthopaedics*, vol 1, St Louis, 1980, CV Mosby.

135. Young JK: Fracture of the proximal end of the fifth metatarsal bone, *Ann Surg* 47:824, 1908.

136. Zelko RR, Torg JS, Rachun A: Proximal diaphyseal fractures of the fifth metatarsal—treatment of the fractures and their complications in athletes, *Am J Sports Med* 7:95, 1979.

137. Zogby RB, Baker B: A review of nonoperative treatment of Jones fracture, *Am J Sports Med* 15:304, 1987.

# Chapter 9

# Arthritic, metabolic, and vascular disorders

**James L. Beskin**

An *athlete* is defined as one who engages in exercises of physical agility and strength.[7] From the physician's perspective, this includes a number of individuals not readily identified with the Olympic-class athlete's physique. Most of today's "athletes" are everyday working people whose goal is to maximize their abilities in their chosen activity. Many simply want to feel better and live healthier lives. Not surprisingly many patients with chronic debilitating diseases turn to the highly promoted benefits of exercise to maximize their function and improve their life-styles.

The athlete's foot should first be considered as the human foot. Athletes who have been healthy are not immune from disease; likewise, individuals with chronic illness are not precluded from exercise and sports. With more and more people seeking physical conditioning as a means of self-improvement, the health care community must expand its understanding of diseases that may affect the athlete. There are clearly some diseases that are improved by exercise. Others, such as diabetes, may result in higher morbidity when they are not identified and the exercise regimen modified accordingly. Ankylosing spondylitis, gout, AIDS, and many other diseases may present later in life and would not generally prevent an athlete from achieving a high level of function before symptoms occur. Many of these diseases exhibit their initial manifestations in the foot. The physician knowledgeable of these entities will be best able to distinguish the underlying pathology from injury in the athlete.

## ARTHRITIDES

One of the most common complaints among athletes is a painful or swollen foot. How then can mechanical wear and tear be distinguished from an underlying inflammatory disorder? The process begins by taking a careful history. Questions should help determine whether the symptoms are directly related to the exercise activity. It is important to discover if there has been any change in the type or intensity of training and whether the patient has experienced similar episodes in the past. If the athlete presents with a recurring problem, it is again important to differentiate a serendipitous relationship to exercise. Are the symptoms limited to a discrete area of the foot or are multiple joints involved? Is there bilateral or symmetric involvement? When symptoms include multiple joints, tendons, or ligaments of the feet or other areas of the body, a more diffuse process must be considered.

Another important factor in distinguishing injuries from disease is determining how long the problem has been present, as well as its response to treatment. Most mechanical or overuse injuries should respond to rest and rehabilitative exercises. An underlying inflammatory disease, such as psoriasis, could perpetuate symptoms from Achilles tendinitis or plantar fasciitis beyond the normal expected recovery.

In addition to pertinent past medical problems, the family history and social history should be explored. The patient's family history may reveal diseases with a genetic predisposition such as gout or rheumatoid arthritis. Risk factors for sexually transmitted diseases

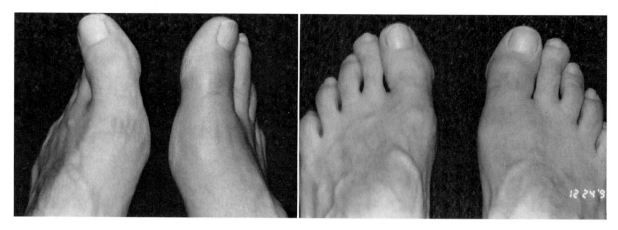

**Fig. 9-1.** Great toe with gout.

such as Reiter's syndrome and AIDS are also important since they often exhibit early manifestations in the foot. Tick-mediated Lyme disease should also be considered in patients with arthralgias and occupational or recreational exposure to the outdoors.

**Classification and evaluation of disease**

Synovitis—or inflammation of the normal synovial membrane—present in all diarthrodial joints, is the hallmark of arthritis. Synovial tissue is composed of several types of cells with specialized functions to maintain joint homeostasis. These functions include the production of nutrients necessary for cartilage metabolism and protective immune responses. The redness and swelling associated with synovitis are nonspecific findings that can be associated with mechanical, infectious, crystal-induced, autoimmune, or other etiologies resulting in inflammation of the joints.

Another finding often associated with the arthritides is enthesopathy, the process of focal inflammation at the site of ligament, tendon, or joint capsule attachment to bone. Enthesopathy is frequently accompanied by joint stiffness and pain, as well as reactive bone formation evidenced by "spurs." Enthesopathy must be distinguished from the more common overuse injuries and tendinitis.

Common clinical features are important in identifying diseases resulting in musculoskeletal inflammation. On physical examination, the specific pattern of inflammation helps to pinpoint the underlying pathology. For example, symmetric involvement of the metatarsophalangeal (MP) joints is suggestive of an immune-mediated process such as rheumatoid arthritis or systemic lupus erythematosus. Raynaud's phenomenon is also a common finding in this group and may be indicative of an autoimmune or collagen vascular disease as well. On the other hand, isolated swelling of one or two of the lesser toes resulting in a sausage-like appearance, or dactylitis, is highly suggestive of a seronegative disorder such as psoriatic arthritis. This group of patients is also more likely to suffer from an enthesopathy, whereas rheumatoid arthritis and collagen vascular diseases most often result in synovitis of the joint. Similarly, gout has clinical peculiarities that help with its identification. (Fig. 9-1). Its notable predilection for the first MP joint in middle-aged males should not, however, exclude it from consideration in other inflammatory manifestations about the foot.

Laboratory studies play an important role in classifying and evaluating patients suspected of having inflammatory arthritis. Seropositive results indicate the presence of rheumatoid factor, which is most commonly associated with rheumatoid arthritis. However not all rheumatoid arthritis patients are seropositive, and conversely, false-positive results occur in healthy people. Further, other collagen vascular diseases such as lupus and scleroderma may develop a seropositive response to testing.

Seronegative disorders are characteristically negative for rheumatoid factor testing. As a group these include all other forms of arthritis, including the spondyloarthropathies, crystal-induced arthritis, and infectious arthritis. Additional laboratory methods are necessary to distinguish these groups.

The human lymphocyte antigen (HLA) and other genetic markers have proven useful in identifying patients at risk for certain diseases. HLA-B27 has a definite association with the spondyloarthropathies such as ankylosing spondylitis, Reiter's syndrome, inflammatory bowel disease, and psoriasis; HLA-DR2 is associated with systemic lupus and HLA-DR4 with rheumatoid arthritis.[4]

Antinuclear antibodies (ANAs), anti-DNA antibodies, antiphospholipid antibodies, and other immunologic assays are indicated to isolate some of the other seronegative disorders seen in the collagen vascular diseases. These include lupus, scleroderma, dermatomyositis, polymyositis, and the vasculitic disorders.

Routine laboratory studies are needed as well. A complete blood cell count and sedimentation rate, along with aspiration of the affected joint for synovial fluid analysis, should be performed in most circumstances. These basic studies are often the best means to distinguish between infectious and crystal-induced arthritis.

X-ray studies are important to assess the location and degree of bone involvement. Characteristic "pencil in cup" erosions of the digits as well as "bone spurs" from reactive enthesopathy are helpful in evaluating seronegative spondyloarthropathies. Tophus formation may be evident in long-standing gouty arthritis, and subchondral calcification may give clues to calcium pyrophosphate crystal disease. Juxtaarticular osteopenia, erosions, and narrowing of the articular spaces are suggestive of rheumatoid arthritis.

Finally, one should consider HIV testing in athletes in whom risk factors have been identified. These risk factors include not only homosexual and bisexual behavior, but the more prevalent unprotected heterosexual experiences with multiple partners. As we gain more experience in treating HIV and AIDS, it is becoming increasingly evident that the foot will provide an opportunity to diagnose a significant number of patients. One of the early features of HIV infection is inflammatory enthesopathy that frequently begins in the foot. Other manifestations include nail onychomycosis, plantar warts, flare-ups of psoriasis, and neuropathy. Kaposi's sarcoma, often acquired by AIDS patients, may also present in the foot of infected patients.

It is beyond the scope of this text to provide a detailed analysis of each of the many rheumatologic entities that may affect the foot. It is useful, however, to categorize the groups of diseases with similar patterns of presentation and treatment. The box on this page lists many of the inflammatory arthritides found in the foot.

**Treatment**

Optimal treatment of the inflammatory process is based on an accurate diagnosis. Much of the destructive behavior of these diseases can be limited with proper medical management. In severe cases it is advisable to consult with a rheumatologist.

Though most of the nonsteroidal antiinflammatory drugs (NSAIDs) have a beneficial effect on these disorders, several trials of the different classes of NSAIDs for efficacy and tolerance are usually required to obtain optimal results. Indomethacin and phenylbutazone have proven especially useful in patients with enthesopathies. The judicious use of injectable

---

**Inflammatory arthritides found in the foot**

***Spondyloarthropathies (seronegative)***

Reiter's syndrome
Ankylosing spondylitis
Psoriatic arthritis
Inflammatory bowel disease

***Collagen vascular diseases (seropositive or seronegative)***

Rheumatoid arthritis
Lupus
Scleroderma
Dermatomyositis/polymyositis
Vasculitic syndromes
 Polyarteritis nodosa
 Henoch-Schönlein purpura
 Raynaud's disease

***Crystal-induced (seronegative)***

Gout
Chondrocalcinosis

***Infectious arthritis (seronegative)***

***Miscellaneous inflammatory diseases (seronegative)***

AIDS
Lyme disease
Sarcoidosis
Rheumatic fever

---

steroids in the small joints or plantar fascia ligament may also be rewarding. However, extreme caution should be exercised in using steroids around tendons because rupture may ensue. Methotrexate, systemic steroids, gold salts, and other potentially toxic treatment protocols are best left to the rheumatologist's discretion.

Traditional orthotic management should be explored as well. Enthesopathy of the Achilles tendon or plantar fascia ligament is usually improved by mechanically unloading it with a soft heel lift with shock-absorbing qualities. Similarly, posterior tibial tendinitis often responds to a medial arch support with a one-quarter- to three-eighths-inch medial heel wedge. Metatarsal lifts and inserts made of the softer Plastizote materials may help better distribute stress from inflamed joints of the forefoot. Adding rigid "turf toe" liner to the shoe may also help unload painful MP joints by limiting forefoot mobility in the shoe during push-off.

Surgical options are usually reserved for significantly painful deformities, such as bunions and hammertoes, which make shoe fitting difficult and add risk of skin breakdown during increased levels of activity. Rarely, tendon exploration and synovectomy may be necessary to avoid impending rupture. When tendon function is compromised, as often occurs at the posterior tibial tendon, repair and augmentation with a tendon transfer is advisable. Isolated joint debridement or arthrodesis may be necessary where long-standing synovitis or articular damage has occurred.

## METABOLIC BONE DISEASE

Metabolic bone diseases represent generalized disorders of the skeleton resulting from multiple chemical and hormonal factors. The effect on bone results from an imbalance in remodeling activity or a defect in matrix mineralization. In general, metabolic bone diseases represent an uncommon cause of dysfunction in the athlete's foot. However, because of the foot's weight-bearing demands, relatively minor alterations in bone quality may result in dysfunction and injury.

A common example is an older female with osteoporosis and recurrent stress fractures who wants to remain active in sports. To properly advise this individual about recreational options, it is vital to thoroughly evaluate the osteopenia, as many causes are treatable. The patient should be evaluated for parathyroid dysfunction, vitamin D deficiency, and other hormonal imbalances before the problem is attributed to the more common postmenopausal osteoporosis. Even this latter form of osteoporosis is treatable to the extent of minimizing the risk of further deterioration. The box at right lists the major causes of osteopenia that should be considered in evaluating a patient with diminished bone density and stress fractures.

Routine blood studies should include levels of serum calcium, phosphorus, and alkaline phosphatase; other useful parameters include urinary calcium and phosphorus excretion and parathormone assay. When indicated, bone densitometry studies should be obtained to evaluate the patient's relative risk of further injury, as well as to document future changes and response to treatment.

Other generalized conditions such as diabetes may not have a direct effect on bone, but because of compromised vascular function or neuropathy, the soft tissues and underlying bone may be at risk. Malperforans ulcers, osteomyelitis, Charcot's arthropathy, as well as the more common skin dermatophytoses are not rare in active diabetics. Long-standing diabetics are also more prone to develop osteoporosis and stress fractures than normal individuals. The box on p. 129 lists conditions associated with diabetes that may have consequences in their foot care.

---

**Potential causes of osteopenia**

***Osteoporosis***

Senile
Postmenopausal
Regional migratory or transient
Idiopathic osteoporosis in young men

***Osteomalacia***

Vitamin D deficient
X-linked vitamin D–resistant
Hypophosphatasia
Antacid-induced
Calcium deficiency
Renal osteodystrophy

***Endocrinologic***

Hyperthyroidism
Hyperparathyroidism
Acromegaly
Hypercortisolism
Diabetes
Hypogonadism
Pregnancy

***Drug-induced***

Steroids
Anticonvulsants
Heparin

***Deficiency states***

Malnutrition
Calcium deficiency
Scurvy

***Miscellaneous***

Chronic liver disease
Alcoholism
Gastrointestinal malabsorption disease
Chronic pancreatitis
Chronic renal disease
Mastocytosis
Congenital osteogenesis imperfecta

---

Rather than being excluded from sports, diabetics should be encouraged to participate. Many potentially beneficial effects of exercise, including glucose control, apply to diabetics. However the care of their feet requires careful screening and evaluation of potential problems. Most important is recognizing underlying neuropathy or vascular insufficiency. This is easily accomplished during the office examination by sensory testing to pinprick and Semms Weinstein monofilaments. Diminished pulses should also undergo further evaluation with Doppler flow studies. Recognizing problems and alerting diabetics to seek

---

**Potential manifestations of diabetes in the foot**

Osteomyelitis
Septic arthritis
Autonomic neuropathy
Neuroarthropathy
Vascular angiopathy
Gout
Pseudogout
Osteoporosis
Hyperkeratosis
Dermatophytoses
Joint stiffness/deformity

---

care promptly for changes in their feet is exceedingly important. Early intervention can minimize the consequences of an underlying infection or neuropathic arthropathy.

When foot structure is relatively normal and sensation is preserved, standard athletic shoes are usually satisfactory for diabetics. Replacement of the shoe or liner with custom-molded materials is advisable if callus formation or bony prominences increase the risk of skin breakdown. Professional care to shave callosities, as well as to provide routine periodic evaluation of an active diabetic's feet, is prudent.

Finally, consideration of the beneficial and adverse metabolic effects of vitamin usage in athletes is necessary. The water-soluble vitamins include B complex and C. The fat-soluble vitamins include A, D, E, and K. The water-soluble vitamins are characterized by limited storage capacity and are lost through urinary excretion, whereas the fat-soluble vitamins have a larger reserve capacity because they are stored in fat and liver tissue.

In general, athletes are more likely than nonathletes to use some form of nutritional supplement.[1] This—along with the possibility that food intake may be altered for weight reduction—increases the potential for aberrant vitamin dosages.

Few if any benefits have been documented in athletic performance associated with supplemental vitamin consumption.[1] However, some adverse conditions related to excess vitamin consumption may present as foot pathology.

Several potential problems associated with vitamin excess have been established. Megadoses of vitamins may have direct toxic effects or may adversely alter other concurrent diseases. They may also result in dependency states or interact with other drugs and vitamins.[2] Niacin taken in doses of over 3 g/day has been associated with vasomotor flushing, peptic ulcers, and hepatotoxity. This dose is also known to

compete with uric acid excretion and may precipitate gouty arthritis.

Vitamin $B_6$, or pyridoxine, is known to cause irreversible toxicity resulting in sensory neuropathy with doses over 2 g/day. Findings are typically in the lower extremities and consist of unsteady gait and numb feet. Biopsies have demonstrated axonal degeneration in affected nerves.

Hypervitaminosis A may result in cortical hyperostosis and arthralgias when ingested in doses of 60,000 U/day. Elevations of serum calcium levels and birth defects have also been related to excessive doses of vitamin A. Similarly vitamin D toxicity may result in elevated serum calcium levels, as well as associated ectopic calcium deposition in soft tissues.

Vitamin C dependency has been reported with doses as low as 200 mg/day and "rebound scurvy" has occurred after withdrawal from such levels of chronic ascorbic acid intake.[2] In elevated doses, vitamin C has also been shown to reduce absorption of vitamin $B_{12}$ and may reduce the accuracy of "chemsticks" in evaluating glucose control in diabetics.

These and other potentially adverse effects of excess vitamin intake warrant our understanding of their role in patients' care. Although the less common vitamin deficiencies may be clearly detrimental, too much of a good thing should be avoided.

## PERIPHERAL VASCULAR DISORDERS

Many patients with vascular diseases present with signs and symptoms evident at a site distal to the anatomic location of the pathology. Since the majority of the vessels in the lower limb either terminate or originate in the foot, it is not surprising that the foot is most often affected by circulatory problems. Peripheral vascular disorders are best categorized according to the functional and anatomic roles of the vessels (i.e., arteries, veins, and lymphatics).

### Arterial disease

Arterial diseases usually result in reduction of blood flow to the foot. Most commonly, this is an occlusive process involving the vessel itself or from mechanical obstruction of the vessel lumen by foreign material. The most common cause of occlusion is atherosclerosis and associated embolic atheromatous plaques.[5] These problems are not as common in younger athletes but can present in middle-aged or older active people as painful claudication, skin discoloration, swelling, or chronic slow-healing wounds. Other conditions, such as diabetes or hyperlipidemia, may predispose individuals to atherosclerosis and its associated sequelae at an early age despite physical conditioning. Early detection by examination, cholesterol screening, and vascular studies minimizes long-term complications. A program of continued exercise activity to enhance collateral vascularization is to be encouraged.

Two conditions affecting the popliteal artery should be considered in evaluating claudication in young athletes: popliteal artery entrapment syndrome and adventitial cystic disease of the popliteal artery. Popliteal artery entrapment syndrome has a male predilection of 15:1 and typically presents by the second or third decade. The onset of symptoms frequently occurs after an episode of intense exercise. Symptoms are described as cramping in the calf and foot, often associated with paresthesias and numbness. The underlying pathology is an anomalous course of the popliteal artery that is medial to the medial head of the gastrocnemius. By passing around the muscle, it is subject to tension from muscle contraction or muscle hypertrophy. The diagnosis can be made clinically in some patients by identifying diminished pulses when the foot is maximally dorsiflexed or during resisted plantar flexion. Arteriography is the most reliable means to confirm the diagnosis. Optimal treatment for symptomatic patients is surgical release of the offending muscle and mobilization of the artery.

Adventitial cystic disease of the popliteal artery generally affects males in their fourth or fifth decade. The disease results in cystic swelling within the adventitia of the artery, similar to a ganglion. The cyst is thought to be indolent in its development, but the onset of symptoms is typically abrupt. The patient presents with sudden claudication and absent pedal pulses in an otherwise healthy-appearing limb. Diagnosis is made by arteriography and ultrasonography. Treatment is based on removal or decompression of the cyst. Current techniques favor CT-guided aspiration of the cyst in properly selected patients.[2]

Several temperature-related conditions may affect arterial flow to the foot. Raynaud's phenomenon is manifested by pallor and cyanosis of the digits in response to cold exposure or emotional stress. During a typical episode, the digits become pale, with sharp demarcation from the area of normal color proximally. It can present at any age but is most common in women between 20 and 40 years old. The etiology is unknown. Raynaud's patients frequently complain of chronically cold hands and feet and may demonstrate some cyanosis of the tips of the digits when examined between attacks. When associated with other diseases, such as scleroderma, it is referred to as *Raynaud's phenomenon.* When it is primary, it is called *Raynaud's disease.*

The prognosis for Raynaud's patients is generally good. For athletes requiring exposure to the outdoors during winter months, protective clothing is usually sufficient. Some of the commercially available sock and shoe warmers may prove useful as well. In severe cases preferred pharmacologic treatment includes the use of calcium antagonists (e.g., nifedipine). Alpha-adrenergic blockers and vasodilators may also be helpful.

Another cold temperature related condition that may affect the foot during outdoor activities is chilblain or pernio—an inflammatory disorder of skin induced by cold that most often affects women in their second or third decade. The lesions appear as bluish-red edematous areas of the skin in the lower extremities. Patients typically report symptoms of itching and burning. With repeated exposure, the lesions may become chronic and ulcerative. Healing generally occurs during the warmer months but often leaves a permanent area of pigmentation.

Frostbite occurs from freezing of the tissues and resultant vascular injury (Fig. 9-2). Results of treatment vary from full recovery to gangrene, depending on the degree of injury. Long-term sensitivity to cold with vasospasm and Raynaud's phenomenon are frequent sequelae of frostbite.

Erythromelalgia is a rare disorder, usually involving the feet, in which paroxysmal vasodilatation, erythema, and burning pain are brought on by exposure to heat. The etiology may be primary or it may be secondary to concomitant diseases such as diabetes, hypertension, venous insufficiency, or myeloproliferative disorders. Erythromelalgia should be suspected when the patient's subjective complaints of erythema and burning pain are associated with an objective elevation in skin temperature. It often starts out as a mild discomfort mimicking neuropathy, but may slowly progress to the point where patients are severely disabled. Treatment is usually directed toward avoiding excessive heat; flare-ups are treated with cold packs and elevation. Pharmacologic use of vasoconstrictive agents and β-adrenergic blockers has been recommended for severe cases.

### Venous disease

Most of the pathologic sequelae from venous diseases develop in the lower extremities. Problems may occur in one or a combination of the three subcomponents of the leg's venous system—that is, the superficial saphenous system, the deep vein system, and the communicating veins.

Thrombophlebitis, or intravascular coagulation, is usually related to the three factors identified in Virchow's triad: venous stasis, injury to the vein wall, or a hypercoagulable state. Direct trauma from contact sports, limited activity after injury or elective surgery, as well as a previous history of phlebitis, may make some individuals prone to develop this potentially

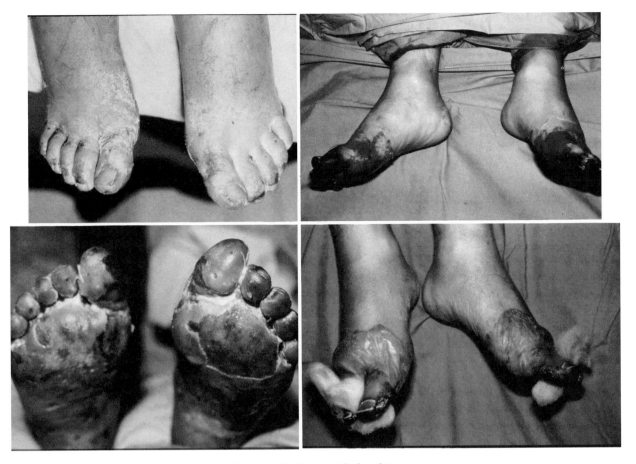

**Fig. 9-2.** Patients with frostbite.

serious complication. Unexplained swelling in the lower extremities should always raise the suspicion of possible thrombophlebitis.

Evaluation is directed at identifying whether the process involves the deep or superficial venous system. Tender, red, palpable cords in the subcutaneous tissues suggest superficial venous involvement. However, because of the risk of potentially fatal emboli if the deep venous system is involved, definitive studies are usually indicated. Currently available noninvasive testing such as duplex ultrasonography provides approximately 90% diagnostic accuracy. Invasive venography studies should be reserved for inconclusive results by other methods.

Treatment is based on the extent of the involvement. Superficial phlebitis generally responds to a program of rest, elevation, and warm compresses, and does not, in itself, pose any immediate risk of mortality. When appropriate, the treatment program may be supplemented with NSAIDs or antibiotics. Deep venous thrombosis carries the threat of potentially fatal consequences and thus requires the immediate institution of bed rest and anticoagulation therapy. Such treatment reduces the likelihood of

thrombus propagation and lessens the risk of emboli.

Varicose veins are prominent, tortuous, abnormally distended veins that occur in approximately 20% of adults. They are five times more common in women and are often associated with a family history of varicosities.[5] Congenitally absent or defective valves are the usual underlying cause of varicose veins. Obstruction of outflow from venous thrombosis or pregnancy may also precipitate varicosities.

Normally calf muscle contractions serve to "pump" blood up the venous gradient, with intact valves preventing backflow. When the superficial valves are incompetent, pooling blood distends the veins and leads to further compromise of remaining valve function. When athletes with varicose veins exercise, as much as 25% of the outflow may be trapped in a circular pattern between the superficial and deep system.[3] Surprisingly, this large amount of trapped outflow has not been shown to have an effect on exercise tolerance. Patients with venous insufficiency do, however, often complain of heaviness and tightness in the lower limbs with exercise. Exercise may greatly increase the degree of venous congestion and produce a deep-seated discomfort known as "venous claudication." As the condition progresses, the deep and perforator system valves may fail, resulting in chronic edema, dermatitis, and stasis ulcers. Treatment is aimed at reducing venous backflow with use of supportive elastic stockings and selected surgical removal of varicose veins.

## Lymphatic disease

Another source of edema in the lower extremities is dysfunction of the lymphatic system. The lymph vessels serve as conduits to return lymph fluid back to the venous system through the thoracic duct at the left jugular vein. The interposed lymph nodes perform immunologic and filtering functions for the advancing lymph fluid. The lymphatic channels, which normally follow the venous tree, are susceptible to many of the same extrinsic forces that affect the venous system. These include trauma, mechanical obstruction from tumors, surgical removal of lymph nodes, fibrosis from radiation therapy, and venous hypertension. Rarely, filarial infection may be the source of lymphatic dysfunction in individuals who have been exposed to the tropics.

The well-known but poorly understood problem of primary lymphedema is related to aberrant development or function of the lymphatic system. This condition is most common in women and is frequently unilateral. Manifestations may be evident at birth but usually appear not later than age 40. When suspected, the diagnosis may be confirmed with a radioisotope lymphogram and contrast lymphangiography. Treatment is directed toward reducing edema with elevation, support stockings, and in some instances, use of diuretics. Reducing the risk of infection by practicing good hygiene is also important. Chronic lymphedema predisposes patients to skin infections, which may in turn exacerbate fibrosis and obstruction of lymph flow. Rarely, surgical debulking of subcutaneous tissues may become necessary in advanced cases.

**Case Study 1.** A 22-year-old man presented with pain and swelling in his right great toe for over 2 years. He had previously been active in a variety of competitive high school and recreational sports that were abandoned because of pain. Swelling was chronic and limited to the first toe area. There was no history of injury or other joint problems. His medical history and family history were reported to be completely negative.

Examination revealed an enlarged right first toe with painful, limited range of motion of the interphalangeal (IP) joint (Fig. 9-3). The MP joint, lesser toes, and remaining foot examination were otherwise normal. X-ray studies demonstrated reactive bone and osteolysis at the first toe IP joint (Fig. 9-4). Additional questioning and examination revealed a small 3-mm patch of scaly skin over the triceps area of his

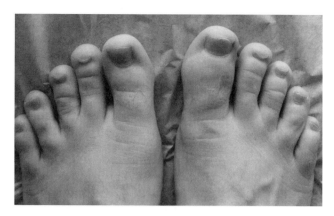

**Fig. 9-3.** Enlarged right first toe with painful, limited range of motion of IP joint.

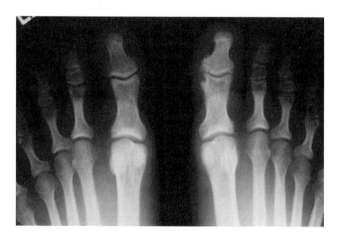

**Fig. 9-4.** X-rays demonstrating reactive bone and osteolysis at the first toe IP joint.

left arm. Further evaluation by a dermatologist confirmed the diagnosis of psoriasis and psoriatic arthritis of the first toe. Improvement occurred shortly after initiating treatment with indomethacin.

## REFERENCES

1. Alhadeff L et al: Toxic effects of water soluble vitamins, *Nutr Rev* 42:33, 1984.
2. Bergan JJ: *Adventitial cystic disease of the popliteal artery.* In Rutherford RB, editor: *Vascular surgery,* ed 3, Philadelphia, 1989, WB Saunders.
3. Bjordal RI: Simultaneous pressure and flow recordings in varicose veins of the lower extremity, *Acta Chir Scand* 136:309, 1970.
4. Jahss MH: Foot and ankle pain resulting from rheumatic conditions, *Curr Opin Rheumatol* 4:233, 1992.
5. Kontos HA: *Vascular diseases of the limbs.* In Wyngaarden JB, Smith LH, Bennett JC, editors: *Cecil textbook of medicine,* ed 19, Philadelphia, 1992, WB Saunders, p 355.
6. Mendelson RA: *Vitamins and exercise.* In Torg JS, Welsh RP, Shepherd RJ, editors: *Current therapy in sports medicine,* Toronto, 1990, BC Decker, p 182.
7. *Webster's third new international dictionary of the English language, unabridged,* Springfield, MA, 1981, Merriam-Webster.

# Chapter 10

# Dermatologic, infectious, and nail disorders

**James S. Lillich**

The skin and nails of the foot are subject to a wide range of traumatic and environmental abuses in athletics, predisposing the foot to numerous types of dermatologic afflictions. Many times these are passed over by the physician as being insignificant. However the sports medicine physician should be aware that any of these disorders can cause significant alterations in performance and can lead to more serious secondary problems. This chapter addresses the more common conditions that may affect athletes, regardless of their sport.

## TRAUMATIC CONDITIONS
### Friction blisters

Friction blisters are one of the most common injuries to athletes. When shearing forces are rapidly applied to the skin, a dyshesion occurs intradermally, or between the epidermal and dermal layers, causing a localized accumulation of fluid or blood.[5] These effects are exaggerated in the athletic shoe due to its hot, humid environment and even more if the shoe is ill-fitting.[23]

Prevention of blister formation is attained by decreasing the friction forces between the shoe and the skin. Careful fitting of athletic shoe wear[4] to relieve pressure over bony prominences and to prevent sliding or pistoning of the foot is important. Runners should also try switching to a more forgiving surface such as grass or cinders to allow more sliding motion of the shoe to help decrease friction buildup.[27] Athletes with chronic blistering problems should always wear socks with their shoes. The socks act as an interface to dissipate shear stresses between the shoe and the skin. If the socks are too large, bunching up will occur and may aggravate the problem. A well-fitted, absorbent sports-specific sock or two pairs of socks with a thinner pair next to the skin are advisable.[7] Foot powders are useful for drying the interdigital spaces. Greasy ointments may be of some preventative value in minimizing friction over bony prominences.

Once a blister has formed, most feel that draining the blister is beneficial in reducing pain and preventing further spread of the entrapped fluid from the periphery. The overlying skin should be left intact to act as a protective membrane as long as possible to increase healing time.[11] Padding, such as moleskin, can be applied with an adherent over the blister until proper healing occurs.[6]

### Black heel

Patients may present with peculiar blue or black discolorations along the posterolateral hindfoot (Fig. 10-1). This condition has been appropriately named "black heel" or talon noir. It is usually seen in adolescent or young adult athletes.[48] Black heel is rarely symptomatic and many times is brought to the attention of the physician due to concerns that it may represent a more serious problem such as a pigmented neoplasm (i.e., melanoma).[4] Lesions are composed of multiple minute punctate petechiae in the intradermal layers,[20] resulting from shearing forces applied to the heel during sports that involve sudden stops such as basketball, football, lacrosse, tennis, and jogging.[48]

The lesion will spontaneously resolve with the

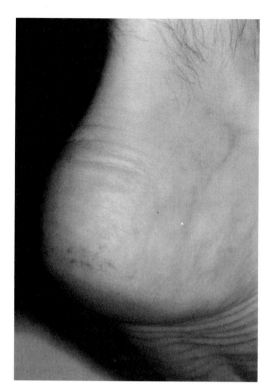

**Fig. 10-1.** Talon noir or "black heel" in a 23-year-old male runner.

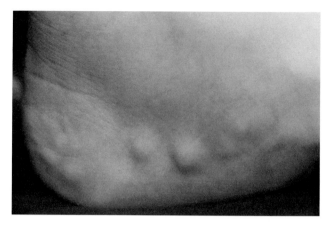

**Fig. 10-2.** Multiple large piezogenic papules displayed along the medial border of a 28-year-old aerobic instructor.

cessation of the sport. Sport-specific shoes with padded or cushioned heels may help prevent talon noir.[24] Other treatment is rarely necessary.

### Piezogenic papules

Peculiar subcutaneous herniations of fat in the medial or lateral plantar heel pad are relatively common in older patients and are termed *piezogenic papules.*[21] These are usually asymptomatic and require no treatment. However in younger individuals involved in long-distance running (Fig. 10-2) or various other sports involving repetitive heel contact, these lesions can become highly painful[43] and seriously hinder performance. These may be secondary to inflammatory changes in the deeper dermal layers.[39] Surgical treatment is not indicated, but cushioning the heel or application of a heel cup affords some relief. Corticosteroid injections into the painful area should be avoided due to a weakening of the supportive collagen matrix within the dermal layers.

### Frostbite

Hypothermic injuries are most commonly manifested in the distal extremities due to the body's efforts to vasoconstrict peripheral vessels and shunt blood to maintain core body temperature. Prolonged exposure to cold is the usual underlying cause regardless of which sport is involved. In addition, when the foot is

exposed to wind and moisture, the effects can be multiplied due to the insulating power of the surrounding sock or shoe.[30]

During the initial onset of hypothermia, athletes may experience some increasing amounts of pain in the more distal aspect of the foot. However, as frostbite progresses, this may gradually lessen due to a change in the sensitivity of the sensory nerves. Thus many times the onset of frostbite goes unrecognized. Cessation of pain and the onset of a warm pleasant feeling within the foot is a reliable warning sign for the initial onset of frostbite.[14] Once this occurs, the condition is relatively irreversible. The initial appearance of frostbite of the foot is usually manifested in the toes, where the skin becomes blanched and has a waxy appearance.[14] Tissue necrosis occurs due to a combination of the freezing of extracellular water, disruption of the cellular membrane due to intracellular ice crystal formation,[3] and ischemic necrosis secondary to a vasoconstrictive response in the involved areas.

Classification of hypothermic injury initially was divided into frostnip or frostbite. Frostnip or superficial frostbite involved only the skin and the tissue layers immediately below it. Deep frostbite involved the skin and subcutaneous layers and could be extensive enough to involve the muscle and bone.[4]

A more appropriate classification is that of Orr and Fainer,[31] who divide hypothermic injuries into four degrees, which are helpful in determining the appropriate treatment course and prognosis for the injury. A first-degree frostbite usually involves only a sloughing of the superficial skin layers. A second-degree frostbite usually reveals extensive blistering and edema in the skin, which develop into a black eschar within approximately 2 to 4 weeks. The underlying subcutaneous tissue is undamaged and after the eschar sloughs, healing of the skin usually progresses without the need for grafting. Third-degree frostbite involves more extensive injury to the subcutaneous tissues. A thickened, black eschar will appear. Healing is greatly prolonged, and skin grafting of the underlying areas may be necessary. In fourth-degree frostbite, there is extensive involvement of the underlying tissues such as the muscle and bone. This may require extensive debridement and, in severe cases, may require amputation. Whatever the degree of frostbite, debridement should be delayed until a clear demarcation line is seen between viable and nonviable tissue.

The initial treatment of frostbite is a rapid rewarming of the foot. However, this should not be performed until it is known that there is no further chance for subsequent cold exposure, since this can cause further injury to the tissues.[36] Rewarming the foot should occur through the use of a water bath that is approximately 38° C to 44° C.[45]

Others have found that the initial use of hyperbaric oxygen has been beneficial in decreasing the extent of the tissue injury.[15,45] The extremities should be elevated to decrease edema, and massage of the foot should be avoided since this may induce further skin injury due to mechanical trauma.[45]

As mentioned earlier, surgical debridement should be delayed as long as possible to avoid damage to early epithelization.[46] However, if eschar becomes constricting, then escharotomy may be necessary. Cold intolerance and hypersensitivity are not uncommon in patients who have previously suffered a frostbite injury.

Prevention of frostbite injuries is basically common sense. The appropriate outerwear for maintaining core temperature lessens the shunting mechanism from the extremities and thus lessens the chance of frostbite injury to the foot. Keeping the foot dry as possible is important since water can significantly decrease the insulating properties of most clothing.[30] Constrictive socks and shoe wear should be avoided to maximize circulation. Also, vapor barriers such as brushed knit nylon, laminated with urethane film worn close to the skin helps to slow heat loss and lower moisture production by the foot.[14] These suggestions are especially important in athletes who have a preexisting vascular disease such with Raynaud's disease, smoking history, or diabetes.

## INFLAMMATORY INFECTIOUS DISORDERS
### Tinea pedis

Of the many infections that may affect the foot in athletes, tinea pedis is by far the most common, thus the term "athletes foot." It is usually seen in adult male athletes and is relatively uncommon in women and children.[8] It usually involves the intertriginous spaces of the foot (Fig. 10-3). Clinical studies have

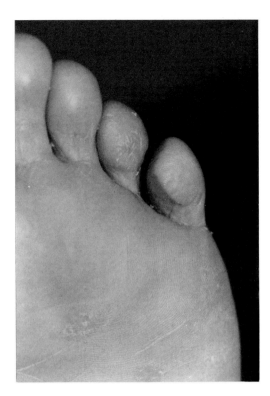

**Fig. 10-3.** Intertriginous tinea pedis.

shown that the fourth interspace is the usual initial point of the infection. Intertriginous tinea pedis normally begins along the plantar aspect of this web space and proceeds to the undersurface of the toes and occasionally to the dorsum of the toes and more posterior aspects of the midfoot and hindfoot. The persistent moist environment present within the athlete's shoe appears to be the main predisposing cause for tinea infections.[33]

During the early phases of the infections, a superficial whitish scaling of the skin may be noted and the patient may be relatively asymptomatic (Fig. 10-4). They may complain of itching or burning, especially after a sports activity. In this stage the infection normally is due to dermatophytes alone. However, more commonly, maceration of the tissues within the intertriginous areas allows for a secondary bacterial superinfection.[25] Most of the more severe cases are related to this, not to the initial dermatophyte involvement. Resnick et al believe that the moist environment in showers and locker rooms serves as a reservoir for dermatophyte infections, and that the incidence of tinea pedis is higher in those who use the showers on a regular basis.[24,34] The most common fungal organisms are *Trichophyton mentagrophytes* and *T. rubrum.*[8,21] Other than the clinical presentation and symptoms, an important diagnostic tool is the "wet mount," performed from skin scrapings. This is usually performed with a #15 scalpel blade. Several

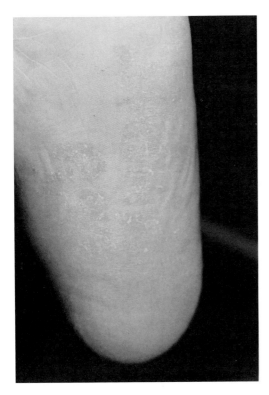

**Fig. 10-4.** Early tinea pedis in a young athlete.

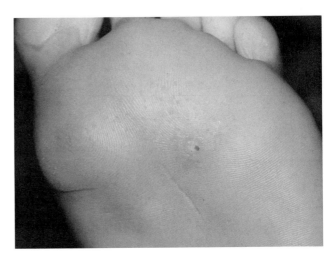

**Fig. 10-5.** Plantar wart that has been pared shows the center petechial hemorrhages.

scales are scraped onto a slide, and then 10% potassium hydroxide and a coverslip are applied over this. The slide is then gently heated and can be examined immediately or may need to be examined the next day. This can reveal the presence of the *Trichophyton* organism with branching hyphae and mycelia.[21] These can be difficult to differentiate if the examiner is not experienced, and consultation with a dermatologist may be necessary.

Once the offending organism has been identified, treatment involves the use of topical antifungals, the most effective of which contain miconazole, tolnaftate, haloprogin, or clotrimazole. Many of these can be found in over-the-counter preparations. In cases suspected of bacterial superinfection, the use of topical astringents may be necessary such as aluminum chloride solution, potassium permanganate, and silver nitrate.[21] A 30% aluminum chloride solution is beneficial, since it also is capable of drying the web spaces rapidly.[24] In more severe cases antibiotics by mouth may be necessary.

Due to the nature of this infection, recurrence is common.[24] Aeration of the foot is important and can be accomplished by having the athlete wear a more absorbent type of sock made of cotton and avoiding synthetic materials. Shoes should be left in a well-ventilated area to aid proper drying in between sporting activities and, if necessary, alternating shoe wear may be beneficial. Drying powders containing

tolnaftate have also been shown to decrease the incidence of infection.[26]

### Contact dermatitis

Contact, or shoe, dermatitis is relatively uncommon but can be mistakenly identified as a tinea infection.[7] It is normally the result of an allergic reaction to a material within the athlete's shoe or sock. The eruption usually occurs on the dorsum of the foot, or toes, which helps to differentiate it from tinea infection. The offending agents within the shoe usually are rubber components.[34,42] Confirmation is normally obtained through observing local skin reactions to a patch test containing the offending agent.[21] Many workers believe that the moist environment of the athletic shoe is necessary in the production of the dermatitis and, if the foot is kept relatively dry, contact dermatitis would not happen.[13,16]

Treatment involves changing to shoe wear that does not contain the offending material.[24] If an appropriate type of shoe wear cannot be found, the liberal use of absorbent dusting powers may allow the individual to use the same shoe without dermatitis erupting.[13]

### Plantar warts

Plantar warts are a common and, many times, painful condition affecting both athletes and nonathletes alike. An increased incidence of plantar warts in athletes may be due to the moist environment of the shoe.[34] This may be difficult to differentiate from hyperkeratosis on the plantar aspect of the foot. However the wart characteristically shows small petechial hemorrhages (Fig. 10-5) present within the core of the wart when it is pared.[28] Also, plantar warts do not occur over the metatarsal heads, but proximal or distal to them. Another characteristic finding is that plantar warts are usually painful to pinch from the margins, whereas the callus is usually tender to direct pressure.[11]

Treatment in athletes is difficult due to the disability usually associated with treatment.[24] Paring of the wart may give temporary relief, but elimination of the wart can be accomplished only through more aggressive types of treatment. Current treatment modes are numerous and vary greatly from local injections[8,21,34] around the wart to surgical debridement.[11,22,25] I believe that direct elimination of the wart using electrocautery or liquid nitrogen followed by curettement is most beneficial. If one has the availability of a laser, vaporization with this apparatus also gives good results. Surgical excision of the wart should be avoided except in extreme cases, since this may leave a painful scar along the plantar aspect of the foot. For those individuals who are more wart-prone, drying powders and absorbent socks should be used to eliminate the moist environment.[24]

## ANATOMIC ABNORMALITIES
### Hyperhidrosis

Idiopathic hyperhidrosis, although relatively rare, can present a perplexing problem for both weekend sportsmen or competitive athletes. Excessive sweating is usually manifested in the soles, axillae, and palms.[37] The provoking stimuli is usually emotional, but physical exercise accounts for approximately 13% of cases.[1] It bears mentioning since the excessive moisture produced within the shoe can be a serious problem for athletes. The moist environment macerates the skin, causing significant problems with blistering and infectious disorders such as tinea pedis.

Most patients find layering of socks and dry powders to be of little benefit. Treatment can be initiated by the sports physician through the use of a topical solution of 20% aluminum chloride (hexahydrate) and anhydrous ethyl alcohol (Drysol), which is applied to the sole of the foot at bedtime and is then removed the following morning.[47] Treatment is continued daily for 10 days, then maintenance therapy continues on a once-weekly basis. For cases not controlled by this method, a dermatologist should be consulted for further treatment.

### Hyperkeratosis

Corns and calluses run the gamut of symptoms in athletes. One can safely say that examination of any athlete's foot would reveal at least one area of callused skin. Although both corns and calluses consist of circumscribed plaques of hyperkeratosis induced by intermittent friction or shearing trauma,[49] the under-

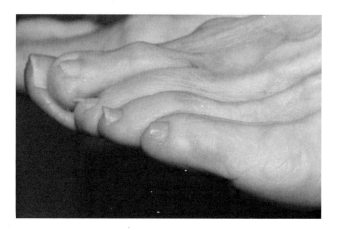

**Fig. 10-6.** Hard corn of the fifth toe.

lying causes and treatment vary and are thus discussed separately.

### Corns (clavus, heloma durum)

These lesions can be broken down into two basic varieties. The *hard corn* is usually seen on the lateral aspect of the proximal interphalangeal joint of the small toe (Fig. 10-6) or over the dorsum of the second, third, or fourth toes at the proximal or distal interphalangeal joint level. Those seen at the proximal interphalangeal joint are many times associated with the hammer, or claw toe deformity, or in the case of the small toe, a slight medial rotational deformity. Those occurring at the distal interphalangeal joint are usually seen in association with a mallet toe deformity.

Corns are caused by two different agents. The intrinsic agent is the osseous condyle underneath and the extrinsic agent is the toe box of the shoe.[9] The skin is caught in between these, and hypertrophies secondary to friction created between the two results in the thickening of the keratin layer of the skin. These lesions are usually well demarcated, avascular, and painful to direct pressure. If improper fitting of the shoe or obvious anatomic abnormalities are not seen, examination of the athletic shoe may reveal a prominent seam causing the corn.

Conservative treatment involves paring the corn with a #15 scalpel blade and/or regular buffing with a pumice stone. Topical agents and salicylate plasters should be avoided. Careful selection of shoe wear to provide a more roomy toe box is also indicated.

*Soft corns (tyloma molle)* refer to keratoses present between the toes where moisture helps to soften and macerate the lesion.[29] These may become relatively large and may also contain areas of central ulceration. Most commonly they are seen between the lesser toes (Fig. 10-7) and are a result of interdigital incongruity secondary to deformities of the toe or prominent condyles of the interphalangeal joints.[17] Conservative treatment involves debridement of the loose skin followed by padding of the interdigital area with foam spaces, lamb's wool, or moleskin. A different brand or size of athletic shoe wear providing a roomier toe box is also desirable.

Surgical treatment for either hard or soft corns usually involves correction of the underlying toe deformity or excision of the prominent bony condyle. (These procedures are discussed in Chapter 16.)

### Calluses

Calluses of the feet are a common problem in the general population and can occur in various portions of the plantar aspect of the foot. Each callus is generated by excessive localized pressure either from abnormal anatomic intrinsic factors or from factors such as improperly fitting shoes.[9] One of the more menacing callus problems for athletes is the intractable plantar keratosis (IPK). This lesion is usually highly painful and is localized to the area under one or more metatarsal heads.[28] If untreated, they can significantly alter the athlete's running gait, which in turn may lead to further injury.

When examining the foot, one should make particular note of the size, density, and location of the IPK. Punctate, hard keratoses usually represent an abnormal prominent plantar condyle on the metatarsal (Fig. 10-8). More diffuse IPKs are caused by abnormalities of the distal plantar metatarsal alignment.[10] If one or more metatarsals are plantar flexed in relation to the other, then typically a large diffuse callus will be present under those receiving the most plantar pressure (Fig. 10-9).

Treatment of these lesions works to relieve the thickness of the keratotic lesion and also decrease the intrinsic plantar pressure from the overlying metatarsal head. Paring the callus with a scalpel blade or regular filing with a callus file or pumice stone can give sufficient relief alone as long as it is continued on a regular basis. Salicylate plasters help to soften the lesion and also reduce pain but should be used cautiously. A metatarsal pad placed strategically on the insole of the shoe or incorporated into a molded foot orthosis appears to work best in reducing pain and preventing rapid reformation of the keratosis.[10,12,19]

If athletes continue to experience pain despite appropriate conservative treatment, or they do not wish to participate in regular callus care, surgical treatment is necessary. This usually involves planing of the plantar aspect of the metatarsal head, or metatarsal osteotomy. These procedures are discussed elsewhere in this book.

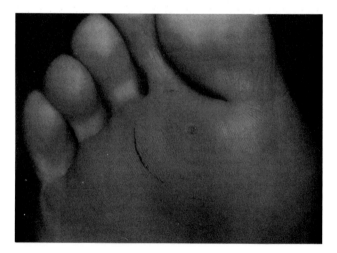

**Fig. 10-8.** Punctate intractable plantar keratosis.

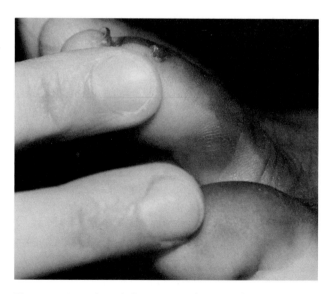

**Fig. 10-7.** Interdigital clavus or "soft corn" along the lateral aspect of the proximal interphalangeal joint of fourth toe.

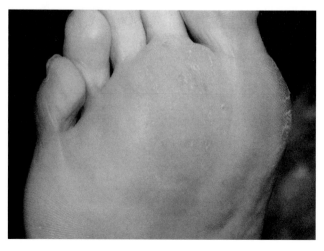

**Fig. 10-9.** Diffuse intractable plantar keratosis.

Other more unusual calluses occur on the sides of the heel and forefoot and are commonly referred to as "pinch calluses" (Fig. 10-10). These are usually a result of poorly fitted shoe wear. If the lesions become painful, paring the callus, or regular use of a pumice stone along with change in shoe wear is often the only treatment necessary.

## NAIL DISORDERS
### Onychomycosis

A common nail affliction is the dermatophyte infection known as *tinea unguium.* In the early stages the nail usually becomes slightly discolored and loses its luster. Most commonly this involves the distal ridge of the nail along the nail folds. The nail then gradually thickens and becomes more distorted with

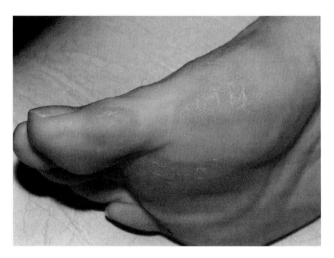

Fig. 10-10. Pinched callus.

infolding of the medial and lateral ridges (Fig. 10-11). Subungual keratinous debris forms.[2] Usually tinea unguium is the most symptomatic when involving the great toenail; this can be particularly problematic for many athletes due to the rubbing of the nail across the dorsum of the toe box of the shoe, which causes pain in the distal aspect of the hallux. This can result in a subungual hematoma or paronychial bacterial super-infection.

Treatment of this condition is most frustrating to both the patient and treating physician. Numerous topical agents are now available, but for the most part offer little chance of clearing the underlying problem. Oral griseofulvin can offer a cure to some individuals. However, the drug must be taken for many months until the complete nail regrowth cycle has taken place. Griseofulvin also has been associated with numerous side effects including hepatic dysfunction, headaches, gastrointestinal upset, and photosensitivity.[40]

Overall, the best and safest results are usually obtained by frequent, careful nail debridement. This involves frequent filing or buffing of the dorsal aspect of the nail to decrease the thickness and rigidity of the nail. Careful trimming of the distal, medial, and lateral ridges help prevent impaction of the nail into the nail folds and subsequent bacterial infection. Increasing the height of the toe box within the athletic shoe is also beneficial, but is rarely an option that can be exercised.

### Onychocryptosis

Another common problem seen in many patients, but of particular interest in athletes, is the ingrown

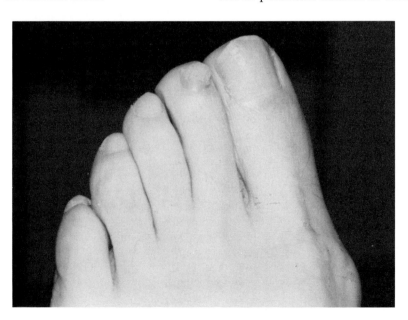

Fig. 10-11. Onychomycosis of the second toenail.

**Table 10-1.** Onychocryptosis

| Stage | Characteristics | Treatment |
|---|---|---|
| I | Normal nail plate but broken or improperly trimmed | Proper nail trimming<br>Warm soaks<br>Topical antibiotic ointment |
| II | Nail plate deformity<br>Excessive granulation tissue buildup over the nail<br>Hypertrophy of the nail fold | Debridement of the nail and granulation tissue<br>Oral antibiotics, soaks |
| III | Grossly deformed, incurvated nail<br>Abundant granulation tissue over and under the nail<br>Purulent drainage<br>Multiple failed conservative treatments | Surgical ablation of the offending nail margin and skin fold<br>Oral antibiotics |

toenail. Many times this small lesion can cause a great deal of pain and make sporting events miserable. The etiology of this condition is either hereditary or secondary to anatomic abnormalities, such as discrepancies between nail plate and nail bed widths, and incurvated nail plate, or subungual exostosis.[2] Numerous other precipitating factors include excessive moisture, poor nail care, and trauma—all of which are evident in athletes. Involvement of the great toe is by far more common than the lesser nails. Medial and lateral margins are equally involved.[22]

There are various classifications of ingrown toenails, with the main emphasis based on the difference between normal and abnormal nail plate anatomy.[2,21,22,36] This should be determined on the initial evaluation by carefully examining the margins of the nail. This can usually be accomplished without the need for a local injection of anesthetic. A small cotton ball or pledget soaked with 2% lidocaine solution is applied over the granulation tissue for approximately 10 to 15 minutes. The granulation tissue is gently pushed away from the nail plate to expose the ingrown margin. A small pair of needle-tip forceps are used to raise the remaining nail fold. This usually gives the physician adequate visualization of the offending nail plate margin. One should be aware of the continuity and shape of the nail, areas of granulation tissue, subungual collections of debris or pus, and hypertrophy of the nail folds—all of which are important in the decision process for treatment.

Conservative treatment in athletes is preferable, especially in those whose nail plate is relatively normal. In cases of recurrent infection and/or nail plate abnormalities, surgical treatments offer substantial benefit. After the initial evaluation of the nail and the patient's history is evaluated, one can develop an appropriate treatment rationale. Table 10-1 briefly describes the treatment corresponding to the following three stages of the disease.

*Stage I* — Conservative treatment is usually suc-

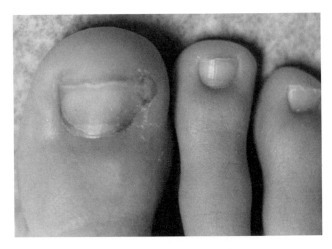

**Fig. 10-12.** Onychocryptosis, mild form, stage I.

cessful. These patients usually display relatively normal nail plate anatomy, but due to improper trimming, nail trauma, or an ill-fitting pair of shoes, a small spike of nail protrudes into the surrounding nail fold and starts the inflammatory process in motion (Fig. 10-12). One should carefully trim the spike to leave a smooth margin. The patient then soaks the foot twice a day for 20 to 30 minutes in lukewarm soapy water. Following this, the nail fold is gently pushed back away from the nail plate margin, using a cotton swab or cuticle pusher. Antibiotic ointment is then applied in the groove. This is continued until the inflammation, swelling, and tenderness have resolved, usually within 4 to 5 days. Sports are participated in as tolerated, and oral antibiotics are rarely needed. The patient should be counseled on proper nail trimming to help prevent recurrence.

*Stage II* — These patients present with excessive granulation tissue formation along the nail fold (Fig. 10-13). This is frequently seen in recurrent infections secondary to nail plate deformity. The granulation tissue, or "proud flesh," is friable and may extend

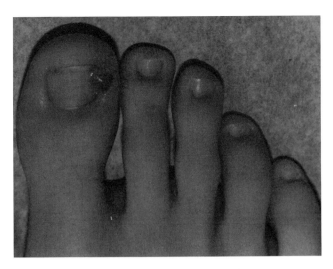

**Fig. 10-13.** Onychocryptosis, moderate form, stage II.

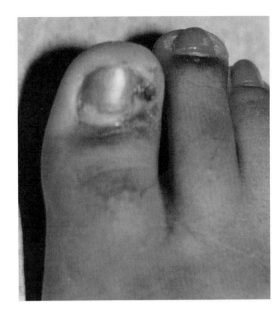

**Fig. 10-14.** Onychocryptosis, severe form, stage III.

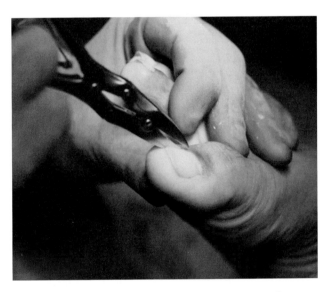

**Fig. 10-15.** Resection of later incurvated nail plate.

under the nail plate. Significant hypertrophy of the nail fold is usually present along with paronychia.[2] Treatment is carried out using a local digital anesthetic using a 1% or 2% lidocaine solution. The offending nail margin is debrided and slightly beveled from a proximal to distal direction, but care should be taken to avoid creating any spikes in the more proximal aspect of the nail plate. All granulation tissue should be exposed and cauterized with silver nitrate or electrocautery. Oral antibiotics and daily soaks are beneficial until the paronychia resolves. Careful trimming of the nail along with mobilization of the nail fold away from the plate as previously described help prevent recurrence. Surgical ablation is necessary in some cases, as described under stage III lesions. Simple avulsion of the nail should be avoided since recurrences are common.[22]

*Stage III* — The grossly deformed, incurvated nail in this stage presents as the obvious offending agent. Abundant granulation tissue overgrowing a nail subungually is usually present (Fig. 10-14). Marked purulent or foul-smelling drainage is noted and cellulitis may extend to the side and distal tip of the toe. Conservative treatment has been tried in the past but has been unsuccessful. Trimming of the nail is usually difficult. These sports enthusiasts present with a frustrating history of multiple recurrences, or incomplete relief of the problem since the onset, despite regular treatment. Surgical ablation of the incurvated nail plate matrix and skin fold offers the best remedy for this stage.[18] To relieve the acute inflammation and infection, conservative treatment is generally advisable. This involves soaks twice a day, along with oral antibiotics and cessation of sports for at least 1 week before surgical intervention.

Ablation is performed under a digital block with 1% lidocaine and 25% bupivacaine (Marcaine) mix-

ture in a 50:50 ratio. A small Penrose drain is used as a tourniquet at the base of the toe. The incurvated nail plate is gently elevated with a small dental Freer elevator to the germinal core. It is then cut straight from distal to proximal so that the incurvated areas can be removed (Fig. 10-15). A deep wedge is then excised to remove the nail recess germinal matrix along the plantar and dorsal aspect of the proximal nail fold (Fig. 10-16). Curettement and/or electrocautery are then used to thoroughly debride any remaining tissue and provide hemostasis. The wound is closed with interrupted nylon sutures (Fig. 10-17). The patient is allowed to remove the dressing after 2 days. Bathing the foot can then be started along with

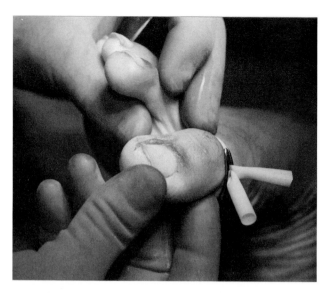

**Fig. 10-16.** Deep wedge resection of lateral nail fold and germinal matrix.

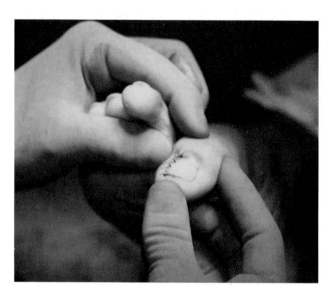

**Fig. 10-17.** Reapproximation of new lateral nail fold and plate.

cleansing the wound with hydrogen peroxide and application of antibiotic ointment and a small Band-aid. Sutures are removed in 10 to 14 days. Sports may begin at that time and progress as tolerated. I found this procedure to have an excellent satisfaction rate, especially with athletes. It can be combined to remove both medial and lateral nail folds at the same time.

Only in severe cases should whole-nail ablation (a Zadik or a Thompson-Terwilliger procedure) be performed in athletes. My experience is that in athletes, these procedures leave a deformed distal tuft of the toe that is not only cosmetically displeasing but is uncomfortable in many types of athletic shoe wear.

A note should be made of the phenol ablation

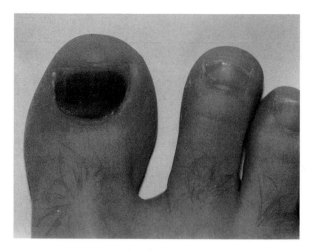

**Fig. 10-18.** Subungual hematoma.

procedures. Although these require less soft tissue excision and less postoperative discomfort,[44] the recurrence rate of these procedures is undesirable, especially when used in the more severe stage III cases.[22]

### Subungual hematoma (tennis toe, jogger's toe, or skier's toe)

This traumatic injury is associated with a number of sports, thus the multiple names attached to the condition. It results from hemorrhages and accumulation of blood between the nail plate and nail bed (Fig. 10-18). Most common in the great toe, it can occur in the second toe, especially if it exceeds the length of the other toes.[41] The most common cause is the dyshesion of the nail plate from the underlying nail bed as a result of repeated abrupt contact of the distal end of the nail with the anterior aspect of the shoe.[4,38] Many times the hemorrhage is not initially apparent, and discoloration may not present for several days to weeks. The nail may initially present with a rather pale, blanched appearance, but will progress to a blue to black discoloration.

Prevention is attained through attention to shoe wear that has adequate room in the toe box both anteriorly and dorsally over the nails. More aggressive trimming of the nail also may help to prevent recurrence.[21] Once the hematoma has been identified, acute relief can be obtained by draining the pooled blood with a trephine or needle cautery through the dorsum of the nail plate. This helps prevent delay in nail regrowth and secondary dystrophy, which may result from excessive pressure of accumulated blood from the matrix.[2]

### REFERENCES

1. Adar R et al: Palmar hyperhidrosis and its surgical treatment: a report of 100 cases, *Ann Surg* 186:34, 1977.
2. Baran R, Dawber RPR, editors: *Disease of the nails and their management*, Boston, 1984, Blackwell Scientific.

3. Barber FA et al: Cold injury, *Surg Rounds Orthop* 2:31, 1988.
4. Basler RSW: Skin injuries in sports medicine, *J Am Acad Dermatol* 21:1257, 1989.
5. Basler RSW: Skin lesion related to sports activity, *Prim Care* 103:479, 1983.
6. Baxter DE: Running injuries of the forefoot, *Med J St Joseph Hosp Houston* 17:42, 1982.
7. Benda C: Stepping into the right sock, *Phys Sports Med* 19:125, 1991.
8. Bluefarb SM: *Scope monograph of dermatology,* Kalamazoo, MI, 1976, Upjohn.
9. Brahms MA: Common foot problems, *J Bone Joint Surg (Am)* 49(A):1653, 1967.
10. Brainard BJ: Managing corns and plantar calluses, *Phys Sports Med* 10:61, 1991.
11. Cortese TA Jr et al: Treatment of friction blisters, *Arch Dermatol* 97:717, 1968.
12. Cracchiolo A: Office practice: footwear and orthotic therapy, *Foot Ankle* 2:242, 1982.
13. Fisher AA: *Contact dermatitis,* Philadelphia, 1986, Lea & Febiger.
14. Frey C: Frostbitten feet, *Phys Sports Med* 20:67, 1991.
15. Gage AA et al: Experimental frostbite and hyperbaric oxygenation, *Surgery* 66:1044, 1969.
16. Gaul LE, Underwood GB: Failure of modern footwear to meet body requirements for psychic and thermal sweating, *Arch Dermatol Syphil* 62:33, 1950.
17. Gillett HG: Interdigital clavus: predisposition is the key factor of soft corns, *Clin Orthop* 140:103, 1979.
18. Heifetz CJ: Ingrown toenail: a clinical study, *Am J Surg* 38:298, 1937.
19. Holmes GB Jr, Timmerson L: A quantitative assessment of the effect of metatarsal pads on plantar pressures, *Foot Ankle* 11:141, 1990.
20. Houston SD, Knox JM: Skin problems related to sports and recreational activities, *Cutis* 19:487, 1977.
21. Jahss MH: *Disorders of the foot,* Philadelphia, 1982, WB Saunders.
22. Johnson K: *Surgery of the foot and ankle,* New York, 1989, Raven Press.
23. Joy RJT et al: The effect of prior heat acclimatization upon military performances in hot climates, *Mil Med* 129:51, 1964.
24. Levine N: Dermatologic aspects of sports medicine, *J Am Acad Dermatol* 3:415, 1980.
25. Leyden JJ, Kligman AM: Interdigital athlete's foot, *Arch Dermatol* 114:1466, 1978.
26. Leyden JJ, Kligman AM: Aluminum chloride in the treatment of symptomatic athlete's foot, *Arch Dermatol* 111:1004, 1975.
27. Lillich JS, Baxter DE: Common forefoot problems in runners, *Foot Ankle* 7:145, 1986.
28. Mann RA, Duvries HL: Intractable plantar keratosis, *Orthop Clin North Am* 4:67, 1973.
29. Margo MK: Surgical treatment of conditions of the fore part of the foot, *J Bone Joint Surg (Am)* 49(A):1665, 1967.
30. Mikelionis J: Mountains, snow and skin, *Cutis* 20:346, 1977.
31. Orr KD, Fainer DC: Cold injuries in Korea during the winter of 1950-51, *Medicine* 31:177, 1952.
32. Reichel M, Laub DA: From acne to black heel: common skin injuries in sports, *Phys Sports Med* 20:111, 1992.
33. Reinhardt JH et al: Experimental human *Trichophyton mentagrophytes* infections, *J Invest Dermatol* 63:419, 1979.
34. Resnik SS, Lewis LA, Cohen BH: The athlete's foot, *Cutis* 20:351, 1977.
35. Roach JJ: Coping with killing cold, *Phys Sports Med* 3:34, 1975.
36. Ross WR: Treatment of the ingrown toenail, *Surg Clin North Am* 49:1499, 1969.
37. Sams WM Jr, Lynch P, editors: *Principles and practice of dermatology,* New York, 1990, Churchill Livingstone.
38. Scher RK: Jogger's toe, *Int J Dermatol* 17:719, 1978.
39. Schlappner LA et al: Painful and nonpainful piezogenic pedal papules, *Arch Dermatol* 106:729, 1972.
40. Schumacher M, editor: *Physicians desk reference,* ed 46, Montvale, NJ, 1992, Medical Economics Data, p 2090.
41. Scioli M: Managing toenail trauma, *Phys Sports Med* 20:107, 1992.
42. Shatin H, Reisch M: Dermatitis of the feet due to shoes, *Arch Dermatol Syphil* 69:651, 1954.
43. Shelley WB, Rawnsley HM: Painful feet due to herniation of fat, *JAMA* 205:308, 1968.
44. Shepherdson A: Nail matrix phenolization: a preferred alternative to surgical excision, *Practitioner* 219:725, 1977.
45. Washburn B: Frostbite, *N Engl J Med* 266:974, 1962.
46. Weatherley-White RC et al: Experimental studies in cold injury: 3. Observations on the treatment of frostbite, *Plast Reconstr Surg* 36:10, 1965.
47. White JW Jr: Treatment of primary hyperhidrosis, *Mayo Clin Proc* 61:951, 1986.
48. Wilkinson DS: Black heel: a minor hazard of sport, *Cutis* 20:393, 1977.
49. Wilkinson DS: *Textbook of dermatology,* ed 2, vol 1, Boston, 1986, Blackwell Science, p 589.

# Anatomic Disorders in Sports

# Chapter 11

# Ankle injuries

**Pamela F. Davis**
**Saul G. Trevino**

Acute ankle injuries are one of the most common problems encountered in sports medicine. The incidence of ankle injuries in the general population has been estimated at one inversion injury per 10,000 persons per day.[8,64,76] In a study of West Point cadets, 30% of the cadets had suffered one inversion sprain over 4 years.[46] Acute ankle sprains occur frequently in particular sports. Garrick reported that ankle injuries comprised 45% of basketball injuries, 25% of volleyball injuries, and 31% of soccer injuries.[38] Syndesmosis injuries of the ankle occur in as many as 10% of all ankle sprains;[11,17] however, more recently an incidence of syndesmosis sprains of 18% in a professional football team has been noted.[7] Deltoid ligament sprains occur in association with lateral ligament injury ruptures in almost 3% of cases.[15] Because of the frequency of ankle injuries, and the number of structures potentially involved, the sports medicine physician must be well versed in the differential diagnosis as well as be an expert in the evaluation of ankle injuries. Only by knowing precisely what structures are injured can an appropriate treatment regimen be instituted to rapidly return an athlete to his particular sports at his preinjury levels of performance. Unfortunately ankle sprains are not always simple injuries and can result in residual symptoms in 33%[6] to 40%[33] of patients.

## ANATOMY

A potentially critical error in thinking is often made in evaluating ankle injuries. Often one considers only the ankle joint and its ligaments; however, inversion sprains involve two joint complexes: the ankle joint and the subtalar joint. The German language clearly defines this distinction as the "Obersprungelenk" and "Untersprungelenk," which means upper ankle joint and lower ankle joint, respectively. Additionally, although the most common ankle injury is an inversion sprain, the athlete may not remember the precise mechanism of injury; therefore other structures may be involved.

The lateral ankle ligament complex can be divided into three major structures: the anterior talofibular ligament (ATFL), calcaneofibular ligament (CFL), and posterior talofibular ligament (PTFL) (Fig. 11-1). Other structures of importance in the lateral ankle region are the lateral talocalcaneal ligament (LTCL), the ankle syndesmosis and its ligaments, and the subtalar joint with its ligaments.

The ATFL is the most anterior structure. It lies in a horizontal plane traversing from the anterior surface of the distal fibula to the body of the talus just anterior to the lateral malleolar articular surface. The ATFL is intimately involved with the joint capsule and is easy to see in a dissection. If the patient has had repeated injuries, the distinction between ligament and joint capsule is often not visible because of scarring.

The CFL is a taut structure. It lies in a vertical plane directed approximately 90 degrees inferior to the ATFL, although there is wide variation. This ligament is attached on the inferior distal surface of the fibula and descends attaching to a small tubercle on the posterior aspect of the calcaneus. The CFL spans the so-called upper and lower ankle joints and is not intracapsular. It is intimately attached to the capsule and to the peroneal sheath on its undersurface. Thus with complete tears of the CFL, there is communication between the ankle joint and peroneal tendon sheath. In evaluating lateral ligament injuries, peroneal sheath injections verify injury to the CFL by

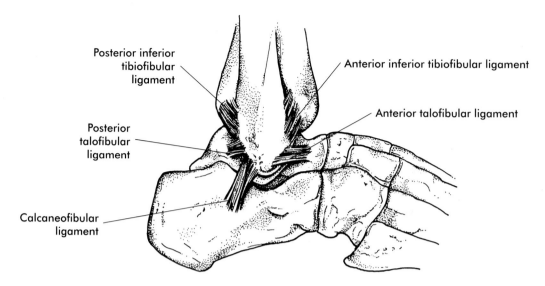

**Fig. 11-1.** Lateral ligaments of the ankle. The composite of ligaments of the syndesmosis and the four ligaments of the ankle joint.

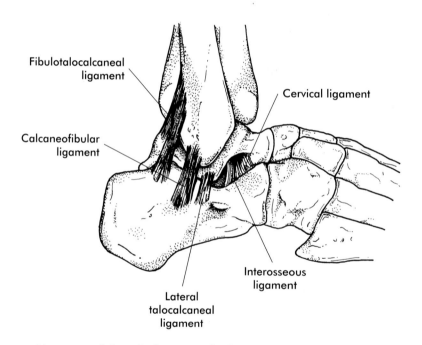

**Fig. 11-2.** Ligaments of the subtalar joint. The five primary and secondary stabilizers of the subtalar joint. The calcaneofibular ligament is the main primary stabilizer of the subtalar joint, not the interosseous or cervical ligaments.

documenting extravasation of dye from the peroneal sheath into the ankle joint.[5]

The PTFL originates from the posterior aspect of the fibula and attaches on the posterior surface of the talus, the posterolateral tubercle of the talus, and the os trigonum when present. It is the strongest ligament of the three lateral ankle ligaments and is least likely to be injured in the common ankle sprain.

The subtalar joint has two major ligaments: the cervical ligament and the interosseus talocalcaneal ligament (Fig. 11-2). The cervical ligament is the strongest ligament of the subtalar joint. It originates on the calcaneus posterior to the anterior tuberosity in the sinus tarsi and inserts on the talar neck. The interosseus talocalcaneal ligament originates from the calcaneus anteromedial to the posterior facet and inserts on the medial aspect of the inferior surface of the body of the talus.

A smaller ligament, the LTCL, may be torn by an inversion injury of the ankle. The LTCL is a small

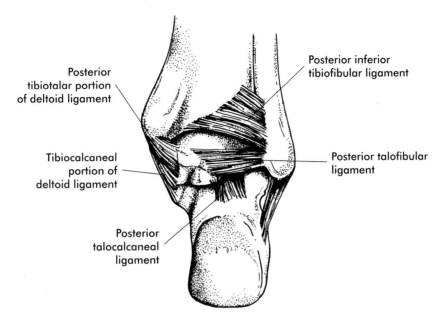

**Fig. 11-3.** Posterior view of ankle ligaments.

structure that spans the lateral aspect of the subtalar joint (talocalcaneal joint). It originates from the lateral process of the talus and courses just anterior and parallel to the CFL. Due to its small size, the LTCL is difficult to distinguish from the lateral talocalcaneal capsule. The LTCL is a secondary restraint to subtalar instability.

Syndesmosis sprains are frequently confused with common inversion sprains. The syndesmosis consists of the anterior and posterior inferior tibiofibular ligaments, the interosseus ligament, and the interosseus membrane. The syndesmosis is an extremely strong structure; however, it is frequently injured in external rotation injuries of the ankle.[7,44] The syndesmosis is one of the initial structures to be damaged in either a supination-eversion injury or a pronation-eversion injury as described by Lauge-Hansen.[56-59]

The deltoid ligament on the medial aspect of the ankle is the medial collateral ankle ligament. It is composed of two portions: the superficial and the deep layers. The superficial deltoid ligament originates on the medial malleolus and inserts in multiple locations from the navicular, most anteriorly to the sustentaculum tali of the calcaneus posteriorly (Fig. 11-3). The deep deltoid arises from the medial malleolus and inserts on the medial aspect of the talus. The deep deltoid is a shorter thicker ligament and it is the primary ligamentous restraint of lateral talar motion.

## MANAGEMENT OF ACUTE INVERSION INJURIES
### Mechanism of injury

Ankle inversion injuries most commonly occur when the ankle is plantar flexed because the ankle is

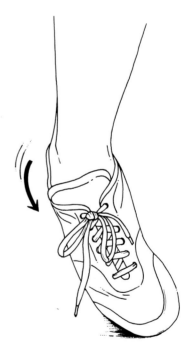

**Fig. 11-4.** Plantar flexion inversion injury, causing the ankle to invert and adduct. (Redrawn with permission from Renström PAFH, Kannus P: Management of ankle sprains, *Oper Techn Sports Med*, vol 2, no 1, 1994.)

in its loose pack position (position of least bony stability). The basketball player landing on another player's foot from a jump is a good example. Another example of a plantar flexion inversion injury is the cross-country runner who steps on a tree root, causing the ankle to invert (Fig. 11-4). Usually the ATFL is torn

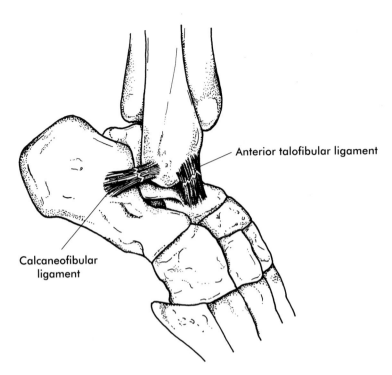

**Fig. 11-5.** Plantar flexion inversion injury, causing the ankle to invert and tear the anterior talofibular ligament and the calcaneofibular ligament.

first, followed by the CFL (Fig. 11-5). The PTFL is an extremely strong structure and is rarely injured with simple inversion ankle injuries; if injured, it signifies that the ankle has more likely been dislocated. Generally the CFL tears when there is a greater varus component of the inversion force. An isolated CFL tear occurs when a varus force is applied to the neutral or dorsiflexed ankle. Injury to the anterior portion of the deltoid ligament frequently occurs with injuries producing complete tears of the ATFL and PTFL. Thus tenderness medially over the anterior deltoid ligament is a clue to a severe ankle sprain.[44]

### Prevention

Taping has been shown to decrease the incidence of injury in basketball players.[37] Ankle taping is effective in preventing extremes of ankle motion,[60] but loses 40% of its effectiveness after 10 minutes of playing.[73] Laced ankle stabilizers are more effective than taping in preventing ankle injuries in football players.[74] Frequently patients with significant mechanical instability can still function when these braces are worn in stress situations such as sports. In addition to prophylactic bracing or strapping, exercises such as Achilles tendon stretching[46] and peroneal muscle strengthening and proprioception exercises also contribute to decreasing the incidence of ankle injuries.

### Diagnosis

History and physical examination are the keys to diagnosis of ankle sprains. A patient generally reports an ankle injury that may have occurred by any number of mechanisms. Clear elucidation of the mechanism of injury helps in making the proper diagnosis. Inversion and eversion injuries of the ankle should be differentiated. As discussed later in this chapter, eversion injuries can lead to syndesmosis injury, deltoid ligament injury, or posterior tibial tendon injury—all of which need specific treatment that is very different from the treatment for inversion injuries. The plantar flexion inversion injury accompanied by a sudden onset of pain after an audible "pop" is suggestive of a serious lateral ligament injury. Inability to bear weight followed by marked ecchymosis and a subsequent feeling of giving way during ambulation also point to significant ligamentous pathology. One should inquire for a history of previous ankle injury on the affected or unaffected side and delineate what treatment has been given. Athletes who have suffered multiple lateral ankle ligament injuries may be candidates for early operative intervention. A thorough physical examination facilitates diagnosis of subtle but significant pathology; thus imprecise diagnosis leading to inadequate or inappropriate treatment is avoided. However, even with an excellent physical examination, it is frequently difficult to distinguish between a moderate or severe sprain without using expensive diagnostic measures. Therefore rather than performing a complete workup on every moderate to severe ankle sprain initially, the athlete should be immobilized and treated as if the injury is severe. If pain and tenderness improve more rapidly

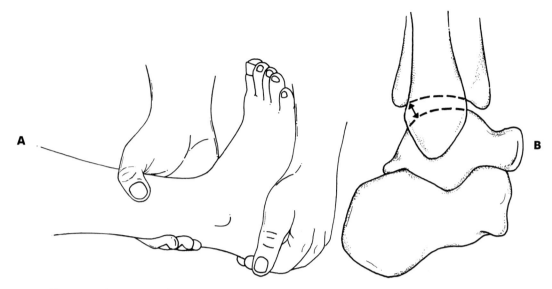

**Fig. 11-6. A,** Anterior drawer test. **B,** From the anterior drawer stress radiograph, one can determine anterior talar displacement by measuring the shortest distance between the most posterior articular surface of the tibia and the talar dome. (**A** and **B,** Redrawn with permission from Renström PAFH, Kannus P: Management of ankle sprains, *Oper Techn Sports Med,* vol 2, no 1, 1994.)

than expected for a severe injury, the rehabilitation program can be accelerated and no harm has been done. The golden opportunity for examination of an injured ankle is immediately following the injury. As swelling occurs after injury, the specificity of palpable tenderness decreases. The location of maximal tenderness and swelling is the best clue in finding which specific ligament or other structures are injured. Establishing a routine examination facilitates arriving at the correct diagnosis and avoiding omittance. First, establish the areas of maximal tenderness for location of probable ligament damage. A complete examination includes palpation of the ATFL, CFL, PTFL, and syndesmosis. Other structures that should be included for evaluation are the calcaneocuboid joint, posterior tibial and peroneal tendons, fifth metatarsal base and shaft, and medial and lateral malleoli. Of course, tenderness over the bony structures indicates a possible fracture and radiographs should be obtained.

Special tests complete the routine examination. The anterior drawer[1] and talar tilt tests are manual stress tests to evaluate the competence of the ATFL and CFL, respectively. The anterior drawer test is performed with the patient sitting with the knee flexed 90 degrees (Fig. 11-6). Patients have a tendency to extend the knee, which alters the resistance for translation of the talus on the tibia; therefore the examiner should make sure the patient is relaxed. With the heel grasped and pulled forward, a posterior force is placed on the tibia. Visible dimpling over the anterolateral aspect of the ankle, the so-called "suction sign," signifies incompetence of the ATFL. When

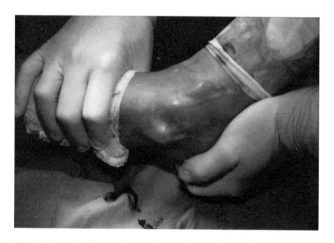

**Fig. 11-7.** Suction sign. The suction sign is demonstrated with the anterior drawer maneuver. A grade III sprain is demonstrated by a suction sign anterior to the fibula.

examining the patient with an acute injury, there may be effusion and so much swelling that the suction sign is not apparent (Fig. 11-7). In this setting the examiner also relies on the quality of the endpoint felt when performing the anterior drawer test. A soft endpoint accompanied by increased excursion of the talus suggests a complete rupture in the ligament. A partial ligament tear is suggested if excursion of the talus is slightly increased, and there is a moderate to firm endpoint.

The second manual stress test of the ankle ligaments is the talar tilt test (Fig. 11-8). To perform this test, the examiner supports the medial aspect of the tibia in one hand and the opposite hand is placed on the lateral aspect of the heel. The ankle is positioned at 0 degrees of dorsiflexion and the examiner inverts the heel forcibly. Normally excursion of the talus is limited and there is a firm endpoint. An increase in talar tilt accompanied by lateral dimpling indicates damage to the CFL. A soft endpoint indicates a complete rupture. In acute cases an anesthetic may be used to decrease involuntary guarding by the patient and improve validity of the anterior drawer and talar tilt tests. Some examiners prefer to perform both the anterior drawer and talar tilt tests with the ankle slightly plantar flexed; however, this is controversial.

The peroneal tendon should be examined for subluxation or dislocation. Test for subluxation by placing the foot in a dorsiflexed or everted position, then have the patient resist inversion. With damage to the peroneal retinaculum, subluxation or dislocation of the tendons is observed. If peroneal tendon subluxation or dislocation is diagnosed, immobilization for 6 weeks is indicated. As a matter of completeness, the Thompson test to rule out Achilles tendon rupture[88,89] should be performed. The test is performed after positioning the patient prone with the foot off the examination table, then squeezing the gastroc-soleus complex. The normal finding is passive plantar flexion when the gastroc-soleus muscle belly is squeezed. Absence of plantar flexion of the foot is indicative of a ruptured Achilles tendon. Frequently patients present to the physician with a misleading history of a presumed ankle inversion sprain, when in reality the Achilles tendon has been ruptured. If the patient is most tender over the extensor digitorum brevis muscle, one must suspect injury to the calca-

neocuboid joint. Injury of the calcaneocuboid joint includes fracture of the anterior process of the calcaneus or damage to the bifurcate ligaments (lateral calcaneonavicular ligament and medial calcaneo-cuboid ligament). The calcaneocuboid joint is tested by stabilizing the hindfoot and stressing the forefoot in adduction and abduction.

Not uncommon are traction injuries to the superficial peroneal nerve and sural nerve. If these nerves have been injured, they are tender on palpation. Traction injuries of these nerves can lead to a prolonged recovery.[68] The occasional patient may develop severe reflex sympathetic dystrophy, which markedly impacts recovery.

Several tests may be performed to rule out syndesmosis injury. (See the section, Management of Ankle Syndesmosis Injuries.)

Plain radiographs of the ankle including anteroposterior, lateral, and mortise views are required in the evaluation of moderate and severe ankle injuries to rule out fractures and diastasis of the ankle joint. Commonly associated fractures seen on the routine three-view series are osteochondral fractures of the talus, lateral process fractures of the talus, fractures of the anterior process of the calcaneus, and of course, medial or lateral malleolus fractures. If physical examination suggests fracture of the fifth metatarsal, an anteroposterior and oblique view of the foot should be ordered (lateral view of the foot may be included on the lateral view of the ankle as a matter of routine). After routine review of the radiographs for possible fractures, the mortise view should be evaluated for widening of the tibiofibular clear space, which indicates a syndesmosis tear with diastasis.[42] On the lateral x-ray observe for the presence of an os peroneum, a sesamoid bone located within the peroneus longus tendon that rides in the groove of the cuboid. Proximal migration or fracture of the os peroneum is evidence of rupture of the peroneus longus tendon. If initial radiographs are interpreted as normal and the patient returns on follow-up visit not doing well, the ankle series should be repeated. Evidence of an osteochondral fracture, such as increased density of the medial or lateral corners of the dome of the talus, often appears late.

Stress radiographs are particularly helpful for evaluating young athletes with an acute injury or any patients with chronic instability of the ankle. In acute ligament injuries, stress radiographs are recommended if a grade III injury is suspected because of a history of a snap or a pop at the time of injury; physical findings of ecchymosis over the lateral ankle and/or hindfoot; or tenderness of the anterior aspect of the deltoid ligament, with more severe tenderness of the lateral ligaments.[82] This is because elite athletes with

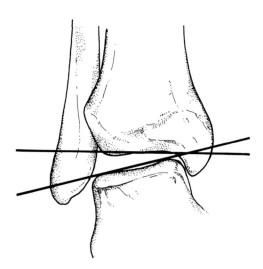

**Fig. 11-8.** Talar tilt test. (Redrawn with permission from Renström PAFH, Kannus P: Management of ankle sprains, *Oper Techn Sports Med*, vol 2, no 1, 1994.)

documented severe mechanical instability may be candidates for early surgical intervention. The most commonly used stress tests are the anterior drawer and talar tilt tests. These studies may be performed manually or with the aid of a stressing jig such as the TELOS device (Austin and Associates, Falston, MD 21047). This device produces standardized studies by applying a specified 150-N force. Using a stress device, Karlsson found that anterior translation of the talus of 10 mm and talar tilt of 9 degrees or greater reliably indicated mechanical ankle instability.[50]

Other radiographic tests that have been used in the past to document lateral ankle ligament injury include ankle arthrography and peroneal tenography.[5,10,31,72] Because of current treatment regimens and the availability of magnetic resonance imaging (MRI), these invasive radiographic tests are rarely performed.

MRI accurately demonstrates acute lateral ankle ligament injury by the presence of periarticular hemorrhage and edema, an irregular or wavy contour, and discontinuity of ligaments.[79,93] Associated soft tissue pathology such as deltoid ligament and peroneal tendon injury is also identified by MRI.[79] This modality is valuable in identifying elongated or redundant ligaments that occur in chronic sprains. Because of the expense, MRI is usually reserved for the evaluation of chronic undiagnosed problems.

## Classification

Ligament injuries fall into a three-grade classification system that applies to any joint. The classification system is based on pathology, function, and instability. Grade I injuries have stretching of the ligament without macroscopic tear, and the joint is considered stable on testing. The patient's functional ability is not impaired. Grade II, a moderate injury, consists of a partial macroscopic tear and mild to moderate instability. There is moderate swelling and tenderness, and the patient's functional ability is compromised. The grade III sprain is a severe injury due to complete rupture of the ligament, resulting in marked swelling and ecchymosis and instability of the joint.

Problems arise in applying the general three-grade classification system to the ankle joint because it limits itself to injury of a single ligament. Broström has shown that 20% of inversion ankle injuries involve both the ATFL and CFL.[9,13,14] A classification system specific to the ankle should address multiple ligament injuries as well as more complex injuries. In complex injuries not only are ankle ligaments injured, but the peroneal complex as well as bony structures also may be compromised. The peroneal tendons and sheath are frequently damaged in inversion injuries.[25,28] The extensor retinaculum and periosteal attachments on the fibula are also commonly disrupted and contribute to the morbidity of lateral ankle injuries. It is not uncommon for avulsion or osteochondral fractures to occur with inversion injuries. For these reasons, a comprehensive classification system for inversion sprains is proposed (Table 11-1).

In the comprehensive classification system, no changes are proposed for grades I and II. However the grade III classification is expanded to be more precise. Grade IIIa indicates a complete tear of the ATFL. Grade IIIb indicates a complete tear of the ATFL and the CFL. Grade IIIc indicates complete tears of the ATFL and CFL with peroneal complex damage. Grade IIIc is subdivided into two types. Grade IIIc type 1 involves an interstitial tear of the peroneal tendon. Grade IIIc type 2 involves peroneal subluxation or dislocation. An additional grade of injury is added in this proposed classification. Grade IVa signifies an

**Table 11-1.** Proposed classification system

| Grade | Pathology | Instability |
|-------|-----------|-------------|
| I | Stretch | None |
| II | Partial tear | Mild to moderate |
| IIIa | Complete tear of ATFL | Positive anterior drawer test |
| IIIb | Complete tear of ATFL and CFL | Posterior anterior drawer and talar tilt tests |
| IIIc1 | Complete tear of ATFL and CFL: Peroneal tendon tear | Positive anterior drawer and talar tilt tests Peroneal tendon stable in groove but tender to palpation |
| IIIc2 | Complete tear of ATFL and CFL: Peroneal tendon subluxation or dislocation | Positive anterior drawer and talar tilt tests Peroneal tendon subluxation or dislocation with resisted eversion and dorsiflexion |
| IVa | Complete tear of ATFL and CFL: Avulsion fraction of fibula | Positive anterior drawer and talar tilt tests |
| IVb | Complete tear of ATFL and CFL: Osteochondral fracture of talus | Positive anterior drawer and talar tilt tests |
| IVc | Complete tear of ATFL and CFL: Lateral process fracture of talus | Positive anterior drawer and talar tilt tests |

avulsion fracture of the fibula. A Grade IVb injury includes the two ligament tears plus an osteochondral fracture of the talus. A Grade IVc injury is the combination of ATFL and CFL tears with a fracture of the lateral process of the talus.

This proposed classification system helps to encompass the full spectrum of lateral ankle injuries. In addition to classifying the ligament injuries, it includes peroneal complex injuries and associated fractures. Approaching the inversion ankle sprain with a comprehensive classification system enables the practitioner, especially the nonspecialist, to avoid overlooking commonly associated injuries. When associated injuries of the tendons or fractures are present, routine protocols designed for treatment of simple ligament injuries need modification. Often it is in the patient's best interest to refer complex inversion injuries to a musculoskeletal specialist for consultation or treatment.

### Functional rehabilitation

The goal of treatment and rehabilitation of all ankle injuries is to prevent chronic functional instability. More severe injuries (severe grades II and III) are more likely to develop residual instability than less severe injuries (grade I). Because of the potential for prolonged morbidity and disability associated with chronic instability, severe injuries should be identified and treated appropriately. Chronic functional instability is associated with mechanical instability and peroneal weakness. Traction neuropathy of the superficial peroneal nerve or sural nerve may also contribute to functional instability of the ankle. Patients with complete ligament tears need a longer period of immobilization and subsequent protection by bracing or taping.[24] Because patients, especially highly motivated athletes, want to return to play as soon as possible, physicians must design a treatment regimen that provides protection to promote tissue healing, but allows rehabilitation with strengthening and proprioception exercises as soon as possible.

Functional treatment (early controlled mobilization) initially consists of using ice, compression, and elevation of the injured ankle, followed by a period of immobilization and rest to limit the extent of injury and allow soft tissue healing to begin. The length of immobilization depends on the severity of the ligament injury. Following immobilization, exercises emphasizing peroneal and dorsiflexor strengthening and Achilles tendon stretching are begun. Agility and endurance exercises, as well as proprioception retraining, completes the rehabilitation program.

Currently the literature supports functional treatment as the treatment of choice for grades I, II, and even III lateral ligament injuries of the ankle.[16,24,33,48]

Functional treatment returns patients to their normal activity quicker than operative repair[20,30] and does not subject them to the additional trauma and possible complications inherent in operative treatment. A review of 12 prospective, randomized studies* comparing surgical treatment with nonoperative treatment showed that early controlled mobilization was definitely the treatment of choice for acute lateral ankle ligament injuries.[48] In the cost-benefit analysis of functional treatment versus operative treatment, functional treatment achieves excellent results for the majority of patients without the expense of hospitalization, surgery, and treatment of surgical complications. For patients needing elective or delayed repair of the lateral ankle ligaments after functional treatment, results of operative treatment compare favorably with those of primary acute repair.† For these reasons, functional treatment of acute lateral ankle ligament injuries is the treatment of choice.

Contraindications to functional treatment of ankle injuries include the presence of any surgical lesion such as a displaced osteochondral fracture or a large displaced avulsion fragment of the tip of the fibula. The patient who presents with an acute severe ankle sprain combined with a long history of chronic instability and multiple severe sprains despite previous attempts at functional treatment is a candidate for surgery in the acute phase of his injury. Early operative treatment may also be considered for high-level athletes with acute complete tears of the ATFL and CFL. In some surgeons' opinion severe combined medial and lateral ligament injuries are also an indication for early operative intervention.

Functional rehabilitation consists of three phases of treatment.[82] Phase one consists of protection, rest, ice, compression, and elevation (PRICE). The second phase consists of peroneal and dorsiflexor strengthening exercises and Achilles stretching exercises. The third phase consists of functional conditioning with proprioception exercises and agility and endurance training. Progression through the phases depends on the extent of the ligament injury, resolution of pain, and weight-bearing ability of the patient. If the patient develops pain or swelling during any phase of the rehabilitation protocol, the intensity of the program is decreased and physical therapy modalities such as cryotherapy and ultrasound are used to decrease the inflammation and symptoms.

During phase one of the treatment protocol, application of ice three times a day has been shown to be most effective, especially when combined with compression and elevation, in decreasing the amount of

*References 13, 20, 30, 33, 41, 52, 54, 66, 67, 71, 84, 92.
†References 13, 16, 40, 50, 78, 85.

swelling.[21,43,46,86] During phase one the athlete is encouraged to use crutches until weight bearing without discomfort is possible. When weight bearing is comfortable and swelling and tenderness have markedly decreased, the patient progresses to phase two. The patient with a grade I or II ligament injury progresses rapidly from phase one to phase two of the functional treatment protocol. Usually only a splint is used for 1 to 2 days, and the patient is allowed to progress to phase two as soon as full weight bearing is tolerated comfortably. For the patient with a grade III ligament injury, a splint is applied initially followed by casting for at least 3 weeks. Immobilization of the ankle in maximal dorsiflexion and some eversion[81] reduces the ankle joint and promotes apposition[24] of the torn ends of the ligaments for healing. During the period of immobilization, isometric exercises are prescribed to limit the amount of muscle atrophy secondary to immobilization.[75] After immobilization the patient progresses to phases two and three, just as do patients with grade I or II injury.

Phase two of the functional rehabilitation program is based on strengthening the peroneal and dorsiflexor muscles of the ankle.[82] Decreased dorsiflexion range of motion of the ankle, as well as weakness of the peroneal muscles, is associated with persistent complaints of functional instability and pain.[3,35] Dorsiflexion range of motion is increased by Achilles tendon stretching, which has been shown to decrease the incidence of ankle sprain.[63] Plantar flexion is rarely a problem after lateral ankle ligament injuries, and increased plantar flexion predisposes the patient to ankle instability. Therefore plantar flexion range-of-motion exercises are deemphasized in the rehabilitation program. Strengthening exercises of the ankle everters and dorsiflexors are performed in an isometric, concentric, and eccentric manner. Isometric exercises are performed by everting or dorsiflexing the ankle against a fixed point of resistance, such as a wall or a piece of furniture. Theraband or surgical tubing is used for resistance when performing concentric and eccentric contractions. A concentric contraction occurs as the muscle is shortened against resistance, and an eccentric contraction occurs as the muscle lengthens when returning to the neutral position. The patient progresses to phase three of the protocol when dorsiflexion range of motion is near normal and no pain or swelling is evident after exercise sessions. Many patients progress rapidly through phase two; however, the strengthening and stretching exercises are continued throughout the rehabilitation program.

In phase three of the functional rehabilitation protocol, reestablishing motor coordination through proprioception exercises, functional conditioning, and endurance training is emphasized. The foundation of proprioception retraining involves coordination exercises done on an ankle tilt board or ankle disc. The incidence of functional instability of the ankle is reduced by incorporating proprioception retraining into the treatment protocol.[35,39,90] The patient progresses through functional activities beginning with brisk walking, then running, then figure-eight running, advancing to hopping, jumping, and cutting. Progression through these activities occurs as confidence in the ankle increases.

The usual functional rehabilitation program lasts 4 to 6 weeks, depending on the extent of the injury, duration of immobilization, and the patient's response to rehabilitation. During phases two and three of the rehabilitation program, some patients with grade I injuries and most with grade II and III injuries should be protected by functional splints such as an Aircast, lace-up braces, or taping. Patients with grade III injuries should be protected for at least 3 to 6 months after returning to sports.[24]

### Surgical treatment

When should surgery be performed for acute lateral ankle ligament injuries and what are the limitations and complications of surgery? In 1966 Broström did a comparison study of the results of surgery versus 3 weeks of casting versus 3 weeks of strapping.[13] In this prospective study the surgical procedure (repair of the torn ATFL) resulted in the least symptoms of instability, 3%. The nonoperative treatments resulted in symptoms of instability in approximately 20% of cases. There was no difference in the results of casting versus strapping. Surprisingly he found no residual symptoms after syndesmosis tears or deltoid tears. Despite results that seemed to favor surgical treatment, Broström concluded that surgery should not be recommended for routine use due to the morbidity and cost of routine surgery. If only 20% of patients treated with nonoperative functional treatment ultimately need surgery, the expense of surgery, exposure to possible surgical complications, and loss of work time resulting from surgery contraindicates operative care for the remaining 80% except in rare cases. Today, when cost-effectiveness is emphasized, functional treatment should be standard care.

In young athletes with complete tears of both the ATFL and the CFL, surgery may be indicated in the acute setting;* however this is controversial. Surgery is indicated for patients with a history of chronic symptoms of lateral ligament instability and recurrent acute severe ankle sprains. A clear indication for surgery is a displaced osteochondral fracture of the talus. A nondisplaced fracture of the talus should be

---

*References 8, 19, 20, 41, 54, 71.

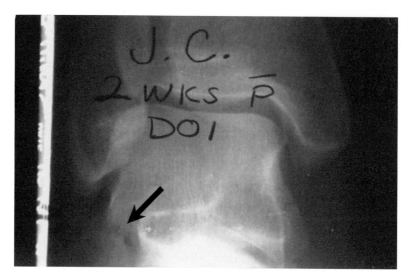

**Fig. 11-9.** Anteroposterior radiograph of the ankle. An arrow points out a probable fracture of the lateral process of the talus.

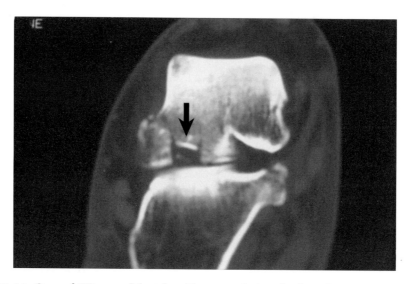

**Fig. 11-10.** Coronal CT scan of the talus. The coronal view displays the posterior subtalar joint. There is a large lateral process fracture, which is displayed laterally. The arrow points to a severe compression fracture associated with this injury.

treated by immobilization in a cast for at least 6 weeks. A large avulsion fracture of the fibula indicates incompetence of the CFL and should be repaired, because this injury frequently leads to chronic symptoms and instability. After weighing the risks and benefits of surgery for acute lateral ankle ligament injury, if surgery is elected, the surgeon may select from a number of nonanatomic ligament reconstructions or anatomic ligament repair. The reader is referred to the section on operative treatment of chronic ankle instability for a discussion of the different types of operative procedures.

**Case Study 1.** A 38-year-old female sustained an ankle sprain when she tripped over a tree stump. Radiographs taken in the emergency room were read as negative for a fracture. Initial treatment was with an elastic bandage and crutches. Due to persistent symptoms, radiographs were repeated by her family practice doctor. These films revealed a fracture of the lateral aspect of the talus.

Initial films were reviewed by the orthopedist, who felt that there was a lateral process fracture due to lateral comminution on the anteroposterior view (Fig. 11-9). The exact details of the extent and pattern of the fracture were visualized best by computed tomography (CT) on coronal sections (Fig. 11-10).

The fracture was treated by open reduction internal fixation with iliac crest bone graft to replace the joint compression fracture. Fixation was achieved with 4-mm cannulated screws (Fig. 11-11, *A* and *B*). Early range of motion was started at 2 weeks with the patient remaining

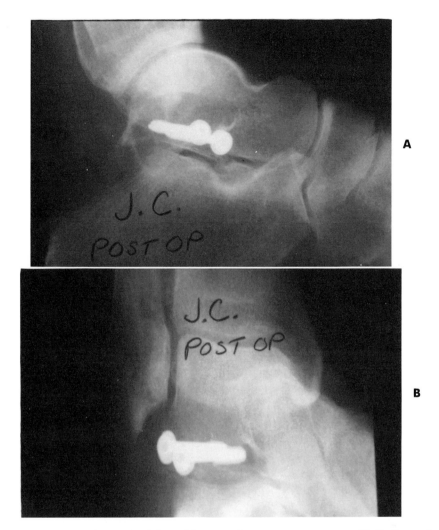

**Fig. 11-11.** Lateral radiograph of the ankle (**A**) and anteroposterior view (**B**). Radiographs of the ankle demonstrate reduction of the lateral process fracture with two cannulated cancellous screws. Note that bone graft was necessary to maintain the reduced compression fracture.

non–weight bearing for 2 months. This case would be considered a grade IVc injury and stresses the importance of the comprehensive classification system.

**Case Study 2.** A 14-year-old world-class gymnast sustained an inversion injury to her left ankle on dismounting from a balance beam. She was still having pain from a prior Lisfranc sprain, which may have predisposed her to improper landing.

Routine radiographs revealed an avulsion fracture of the calcaneus (Fig. 11-12). MRI supported this finding (Fig. 11-13). Stress radiographs revealed a positive drawer test on the left and a bilateral talar tilt of 7 degrees.

A nonathlete could have been treated conservatively, but with her background, surgery was performed. Operative findings revealed the bony avulsion of the insertions of the calcaneofibular ligament. This was reattached with a metal retention suture (Fig. 11-14).

Postoperative management was 4 weeks of immobilization in a cast. Weight bearing was started after the first week.

A stirrup splint was used for further protection after this period. Care must be used to avoid prolonged immobilization in athletes who need to return to full range of motion (e.g., ballet dancers and gymnasts).

**Case Study 3.** A 35-year-old female sustained an inversion injury while running. She was treated for a minor sprain with an elastic wrap and crutches. She was still symptomatic 3 months later.

A consulting orthopedist noted pain along the inferior border of the cuboid without evidence of tenderness or laxity over the lateral ligaments. Radiographs revealed a possible fracture of the os peroneum (Fig. 11-15). The patient was observed and treated conservatively.

One year later the patient continued to have pain in the same location. Repeat radiographs showed widening between the two fracture fragments (Fig. 11-16). At the time of surgery there was a rupture of the peroneus longus tendon with retraction of the tendon medial to the undersurface of the cuboid. The fragment was excised and

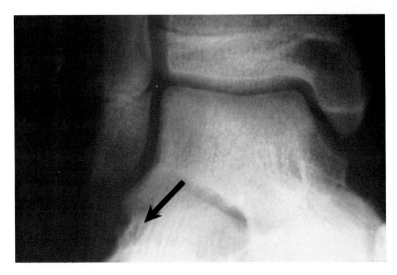

**Fig. 11-12.** Anteroposterior radiograph of the ankle. An arrow points to an avulsion fracture of the calcaneus. This represents an avulsion of the insertion of the calcaneofibular ligament.

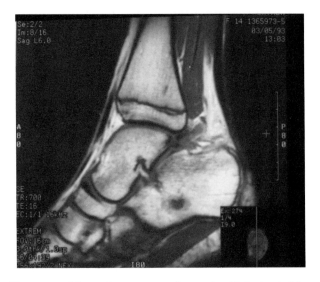

**Fig. 11-13.** Magnetic resonance image (sagittal view). Marrow edema in the middle portion of the calcaneus supports the radiographic findings of an avulsion fracture of the insertion of the calcaneofibular ligament.

the stump of the peroneus longus reattached to the peroneus brevis.

The significance of a fracture of the os peroneum is its intimate relationship to the accompanying peroneus longus. Any widening is indication for surgical repair.

## MANAGEMENT OF CHRONIC LATERAL ANKLE INSTABILITY
### Mechanism of injury

The incidence of chronic symptoms after treatment for acute lateral ankle injuries is approximately 10% to 30%.[2,12,78] Complaints vary but include functional instability (feeling of giving way), frank mechanical instability, recurrent swelling, pain, and stiffness. Ten to twenty percent of patients with acute injuries may later require surgery for chronic functional instability. Ankle instability is categorized as either mechanical or functional. Functional instability, first described by Freeman, is the patient's subjective complaints of giving way in the ankle joint.[34,35] Functional instability occurs with sports activity or during daily activities, such as walking on uneven ground or pivoting to make a sharp turn. Tropp[90] described functional instability as a motion beyond voluntary control, but not exceeding the physiologic range of motion. Causes of functional instability include proprioceptive disorders, pain, and muscle weakness.

Mechanical instability of the ankle is motion beyond the physiologic range of motion. Clinically mechanical instability is demonstrated by the anterior drawer and talar tilt tests. Stress radiographs using manual stress or a stressing jig objectively document the degree of mechanical instability. Unfortunately there is no correlation between the presence of mechanical instability and functional instability.[35] A study by Tropp[90] demonstrated that half of functionally unstable ankles were mechanically stable. The ability to maintain postural equilibrium was reduced in the presence of functional instability but not affected by mechanical instability. Tropp thought that the mechanical and functional instabilities might be parallel phenomena but not necessarily correlated to one another. Functional instability can be successfully treated with coordination exercises using an ankle tilt board.[35,39,90]

The differential diagnosis of chronic lateral ankle instability must be kept in mind. Injury of soft tissues other than the lateral ligaments cause chronic symp-

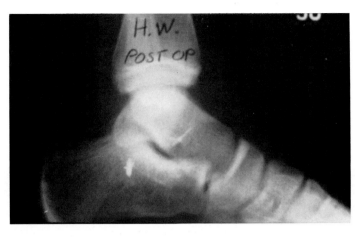

**Fig. 11-14.** Lateral radiograph of the ankle. A metallic hook in the calcaneus was used to reattach the insertion of the calcaneofibular ligament. This tear was the primary tear in this injury.

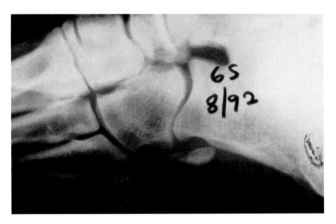

**Fig. 11-15.** Lateral radiograph of the ankle. The os peroneum is identified as a sesamoid bone underneath the sulcus of the cuboid. There is a small separation in the proximal pole of this bone. This sesamoid is buried in the peroneus longus tendon.

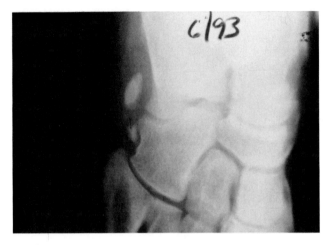

**Fig. 11-16.** Lateral radiograph of the ankle. The os peroneum now has a prominent separation. This finding represents a complete tear of the peroneus longus tendon. Operative findings confirmed this chronic tear with retraction of the distal fragment.

toms that mimic lateral ankle instability. An example is soft tissue impingement in the lateral gutter.[32,94,98] Bassett et al[4] described hypertrophy of the distal fascicle of the anteroinferior tibiofibular ligament that caused talar impingement and abrasion of the talar articular cartilage. Other causes of chronic ankle symptoms include peroneal tendon subluxation, dislocation, or interstitial tear; loose body; tibiotalar or talofibular bony impingement; and traction injuries of the peroneal or superficial peroneal nerves. Similarly, bony pathology including osteochondral fracture of the talus, avulsion fracture of the distal fibula, fracture of the anterior process of the calcaneus, and fracture of the lateral process of the talus may result in chronic symptoms. Any of these conditions may be isolated or associated with ligamentous instability. Other conditions in the vicinity of the lateral ankle that may mimic lateral ligament instability are sinus tarsi syndrome, isolated subtalar instability, or transverse talar instability. A cavovarus foot deformity may also predispose to recurrent instability.[55]

### Diagnosis

Patients with chronic lateral ankle instability usually have a history of significant acute inversion ankle injury. In many cases the acute injury was treated inadequately. The usual complaints on presentation for chronic instability are pain, swelling, feeling of giving way, and recurrent ankle sprains. Some patients complain of stiffness with activity. Many patients relate a history of recurrent inversion injuries that occur when walking on uneven surfaces or descending stairs. The recurrent sprains are accompanied by severe pain that may or may not result in marked swelling or ecchymosis.

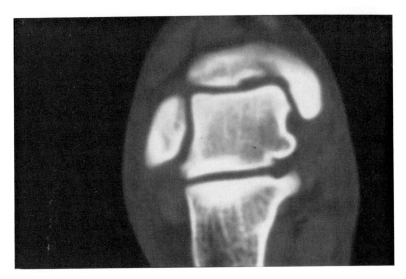

**Fig. 11-17.** CT of the hindfoot (coronal view). A negative CT scan was found in the initial evaluation.

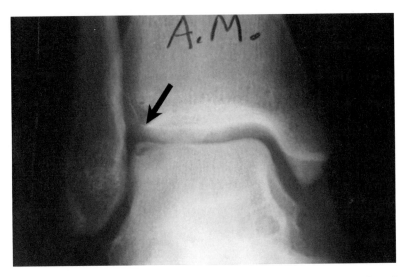

**Fig. 11-18.** Anteroposterior radiograph of the ankle. A classic grade III (Berndt and Hardy) osteochondral lesion is indicated by the arrow. This lesion was found to be completely detached at the time of arthroscopy.

A positive history is supported by clinical examination. There is increased excursion of the talus with anterior drawer and talar tilt testing. Peroneal muscle weakness is associated with functional instability. Mechanical instability is confirmed by the presence of positive anterior drawer and talar tilt stress radiographs. An anterior drawer of 10 mm and a talar tilt of 9 degrees or greater reliably indicates mechanical instability.[50]

Evaluation of patients with chronic ankle symptoms or instability should always include repeat radiographs. Frequently a bone scan for localization of the pathology is indicated. If the bone scan is abnormal, tomography or CT scans will clarify the pathology. MRI is indicated if tendon injury, soft tissue impingement, or avascular necrosis of the talus is suspected.

**Case Study 4.** A 16-year-old cheerleader injured her left ankle when she landed on another cheerleader. Initial radiographs were suspicious for a possible lateral osteochondral fracture, but the subsequent CT scan was negative (Fig. 11-17). The patient did not respond to an aggressive rehabilitation program following casting. She complained 6 months later of snapping and popping in her ankle joint with lateral pain. Repeat radiographs revealed a lateral osteochondral lesion (Fig. 11-18).

Before surgery, stress radiographs measured a 10-mm drawer test (Fig. 11-19). For this reason, both arthroscopy

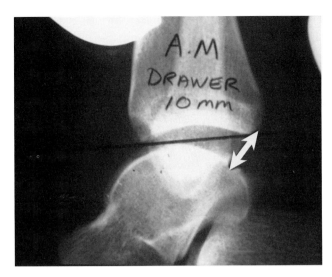

**Fig. 11-19.** Lateral radiograph of the ankle. With anterior stress 10 mm of displacement is measured. This measurement is indicative of significant laxity of the anterior talofibular ligament.

and lateral ligament reconstruction were performed. A modified Broström procedure was used after the osteochondral fragment was removed.

Repeat radiographs are necessary with persistent symptoms, and stress radiographs should be part of the routine examination. Osteochondral defects are frequently associated with residual ankle instability.

### Functional rehabilitation

Rehabilitation of functional instability emphasizes muscle strengthening and proprioception exercises with tilt board or ankle disc. Peroneal muscle strengthening, Achilles tendon stretching, and proprioceptive training exercises are important components of the rehabilitation program. At least 10 weeks of rigorous rehabilitation is suggested for maximal benefit. The results of rehabilitation for combined functional and mechanical instability have not been reported in the literature to our knowledge. Evidently most of these patients are treated operatively. However, patients with documented mechanical instability improve with functional rehabilitation; thus it should be attempted before surgical intervention.

### Surgical treatment

**Soft tissue impingement syndromes.** If anterolateral impingement or talar impingement by the anteroinferior tibiofibular ligament is suspected on physical examination, treatment is initiated with antiinflammatory drugs and aggressive physical therapy. If the patient's symptoms are not improved by aggressive nonoperative treatment, arthroscopic surgery is indicated. In cases of lateral gutter soft tissue impingement, arthroscopic examination reveals proliferative

synovitis and fibrotic scar. The soft tissue consists of hypertrophied synovium and fibrotic scar and is referred to as a "meniscoid lesion."[32,98] Talar impingement by the anteroinferior tibiofibular ligament causes abrasions of the anterolateral talar dome.[4,32] Both the meniscoid lesion and hypertrophy of the distal fascicle of the anteroinferior tibiofibular ligament are visualized and treated with arthroscopy.[4,32]

**Lateral ligament instability.** More than 50 procedures for lateral ligament reconstruction have been described, which probably indicates that a superior method has not been developed. Most procedures have good results on a short-term basis. A clear indication for surgery is the presence of both functional and mechanical instability with failure of nonoperative management. Patient age appears to have little bearing on the outcome of surgery. The lack of a clear definition of instability on stress radiographs has prompted many clinicians to rely on clinical judgment alone. Others continue to use established radiographic criteria in an attempt to redefine these criteria.

Operative procedures are categorized into two groups: anatomic repair (popularized by Broström[13]) and nonanatomic reconstructions.

**Anatomic repair.** Broström believed that direct repair of the lateral ankle ligaments could be performed long after the injury because the ligamentous tissue remained available for repair with the ends encased in scar tissue.[13] His method of repairing the ligaments included imbrication and suture of the torn ends of the ligament or suture of the ligament to bone. Other authors[1,32,46,49] agreed with Broström; however, they noted that the frayed ligament ends are not necessarily easy to find and often have healed together in an elongated fashion. Their recommendation was shortening, imbrication, and repair of the ligament to bone troughs or reinforcement with local tissue. One advantage of anatomic repair is that no normal tissue is sacrificed. Another advantage of anatomic repair of the lateral ligaments is that it does not create a tenodesis effect, which alters ankle and subtalar joint biomechanics. Thus no loss of inversion or subtalar motion results.

Of six clinical series reporting on 460 ankles,* 87% to 95% of the patients had good to excellent outcomes for a 2- to 6-year follow-up. The largest single series[49] consisted of 152 ankles with an average follow-up of 6 years and 87% good to excellent results. Of the 140 patients involved in sports, 120 were able to return to their sport at their preinjury level of activity. There was not deterioration of the surgical results over time. For 16 of the 20 patients with a fair or poor outcome,

*References 1, 8, 32, 46, 49, 94.

three factors were consistently present: history of at least 10 years of instability before surgery, generalized joint hypermobility, and reconstruction of the ATFL alone.

Currently the senior author's (SGT) technique of anatomic ligament repair is a modification of the Broström procedure[14] and parallels the technique described by Karlsson et al[51] (Fig. 11-20, *A, B,* and *C*). The technique is described. A posterolateral incision is made behind the fibula and extended toward the sinus tarsi area. The placement of the incision behind the fibula is cosmetically acceptable and allows access to the CFL for reconstruction. A skin flap is elevated over the anterior aspect of the fibula, with care being taken not to damage the sural nerve, its communicating branch, or any branches of the superficial peroneal nerve. The inferior retinaculum is identified, mobilized, and tagged for possible later reconstruction. The extensor tendons are mobilized medially. A longitudinal incision is made in the anterolateral aspect of the capsule, leaving a cuff of the capsule and ATFL attached to the fibula. The ATFL is not specifically identified because it is usually encased in capsular scar tissue. The CFL is identified through a small incision in the peroneal sheath. Care is also taken to identify the peroneal tendons and inspect for interstitial tear. A trough is made in the surface of the fibula at the origin of the ATFL. The anterior capsule and ATFL is repaired to the bone through three drill holes in the prepared trough with #O-PDS suture. The CFL is repaired to its insertion on the calcaneus in a similar manner. Ankle motion and stability are checked to confirm adequate tension of the repaired ligaments and presence of physiologic range of motion.

Postoperatively the patient is immobilized in a splint for the first week and then placed in a short-leg walking cast for an additional 5 weeks. Athletes who require full plantar flexion for their sports, such as gymnasts and ballet dancers, are immobilized for a total of only 4 weeks. Following casting, an ankle brace is worn to limit inversion. The postoperative rehabilitation program is the same as that described for functional treatment of acute lateral ligament injuries. After the patient returns to sports, he is protected from reinjury by taping, ankle corset, or a pneumatic stirrup splint. Reusable ankle braces or splints provide considerable savings over taping; therefore, unless one has funding for a personal trainer and large amounts of tape, braces are now more commonly used.

**Nonanatomic reconstructions.** Nonanatomic reconstructions predominantly use either a split portion or complete section of the peroneus brevis tendon. The Watson-Jones (Fig. 11-21),[95] Evans,[29] and Chrisman-Snook[18] procedures have been the most

popular techniques of lateral ligament reconstruction. Reconstruction techniques using the plantaris tendon,[2,53] partial Achilles tendon,[83,87] or free autogenous graphs such as a toe extensor or fascia lata[27] have been reported.[6] Excellent-to-good results are achieved in over 90% of patients for reconstructive procedures.[77] However, due to the nonanatomic nature of the reconstructions, decreased inversion and subtalar motion are common postoperatively.

The Watson-Jones procedure is performed by sectioning the peroneus brevis tendon and directing it from posterior to anterior through a tunnel in the distal fibula, then through a tunnel in the neck of the talus, then back through a second drill hole in the fibula. The Watson-Jones technique reconstructs the ATFL more effectively than the CFL. In a review of surgical treatment of chronic lateral ankle instability by Peters et al,[70] it was concluded that the most common complication of the Watson-Jones procedure was restricted range of dorsiflexion and inversion motions (10% to 30% of cases). A long-term follow-up study of the Watson-Jones procedure[91] revealed residual instability or insecurity and positive anterior drawer stress radiographs in 66% of cases.

The Evans procedure, a simplification of the Watson-Jones procedure, was originally performed by directing the transected peroneus brevis tendon through a drill hole in the distal fibula, then suturing the tendon back to the musculotendinous junction in an overlapped fashion (Fig. 11-22). The Evans procedure reconstructs neither the CFL nor the ATFL but functions as a result of the two. Therefore the talus is not restricted from subluxing anteriorly with plantar flexion of the ankle. Orava et al[69] noted a 50% incidence of radiographically proven increased anterior drawer following the Evans procedure. Peters et al[70] reviewed 11 clinical series (360 ankles) and found that overall stability was restored in 90% to 100% of patients and 80% to 95% of patients had good or excellent results. Complications of the Evans procedure include up to 4% incidence of neuroma and up to 30% incidence of restricted inversion.[70] Late follow-up by Karlsson et al[49] revealed that 50% of patients had fair or poor results because of pain and instability, and 40% of the patients who returned to sports ceased to participate due to recurrent ankle symptoms.

The Chrisman-Snook modification of the Elmslie procedure[27] is performed by using a split portion of the peroneus brevis tendon to reconstruct the ATFL and CFL (Fig. 11-23). This modification was believed to be an improvement because half the peroneus brevis tendon was used instead of fascia lata. Peters et al[70] reviewed four clinical series (100 ankles) and found that stability was restored in 95%, and 90% of

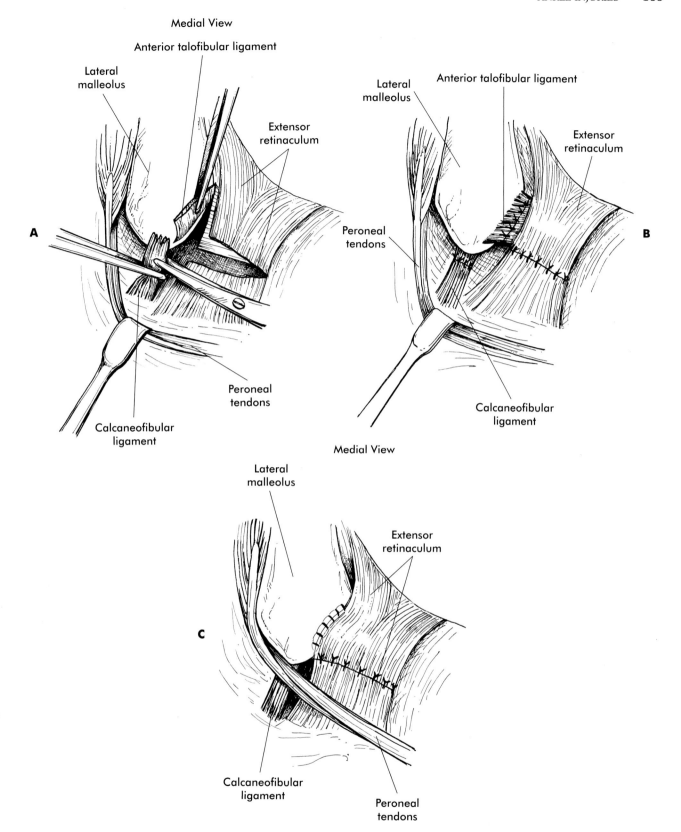

**Fig. 11-20. A,** Modified Broström technique. Trimming the calcaneofibular ligament. **B,** Modified Broström technique. Shortening and reattachment of attenuated anterior talofibular ligament and calcaneofibular ligament. **C,** Modified Broström technique. Suture of extensor retinaculum over repair. (**A, B,** and **C,** Redrawn with permission from Renström to Trevino S: *Management of ankle sprains.* In *Operative techniques in sports medicine,* vol 2, no 1, Philadelphia, 1994, WB Saunders.)

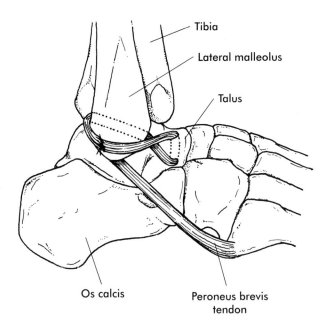

Fig. 11-21. Modified Watson-Jones procedure. (Redrawn with permission from Renström PAFH, Kannus P: Management of ankle sprains, *Oper Techn Sports Med,* vol 2, no 1, 1994.)

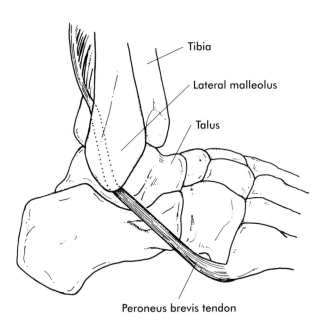

Fig. 11-22. Modified Evans procedure. (Redrawn with permission from Renström PAFH, Kannus P: Management of ankle sprains, *Oper Techn Sports Med,* vol 2, no 1, 1994.)

the patients had good to excellent results. Complications noted in Peters' review included neuromas in 16% or less, decreased dorsiflexion in 20%, and decreased inversion in all patients. Snook, Chrisman, and Wilson reported a 10-year follow-up of 48 patients

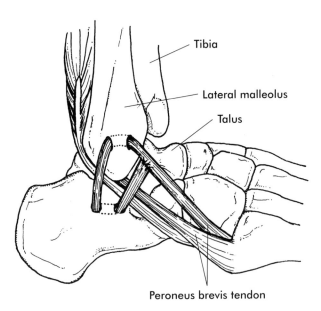

Fig. 11-23. Chrisman-Snook modification of the Elmslie procedure. (Redrawn with permission from Renström PAFH, Kannus P: Management of ankle sprains, *Oper Techn Sports Med,* vol 2, no 1, 1994.)

who had been treated with their procedure.[85] Ninety-eight percent of the patients had good or excellent results. There were only 3 patients with recurrences, all secondary to significant trauma. Chrisman and Snook felt the loss of 20 degrees or less of inversion was inherent to the procedure and did not report it as a complication.

Hortsman et al[45] in a review of lateral ligament reconstructions were surprised to find a high incidence of postoperative pain. Sixty-three percent of patients with a Chrisman-Snook procedure had some degree of pain, although only five percent of the patients described the pain as severe. Eighty-three percent of patients who underwent an Evans repair described some degree of pain. The Chrisman-Snook operation was found to have the lowest incidence of instability, 12%; however, it had the highest incidence of loss of inversion, 70%. Talar tilt was controlled well with the Chrisman-Snook and Evans procedures, but not with the Watson-Jones procedure. Overall 90% of the patients were satisfied; however, Hortsman believed that the Chrisman-Snook operation had superior results because it was the most anatomic reconstruction.

## MANAGEMENT OF ANKLE SYNDESMOSIS INJURIES
### Mechanism of injury

Typically the athlete does not recall the mechanism by which a syndesmosis injury occurs; however syndesmosis injuries are thought to occur primarily by an external rotation mechanism. Fritchy[36] described a pure external rotation injury in skiers that produced isolated syndesmosis injuries. The tip of the ski catches a slalom post, forcing the ski and ankle rapidly into external rotation while all other motions of the foot and ankle are restricted by the ski boot. Another mechanism by which the syndesmosis may be injured is hyperdorsiflexion.[26,44]

## Diagnosis

Following the acute ankle injury the athlete typically presents with a chief complaint of tenderness over the anterolateral aspect of the ankle just proximal to the joint line, the area of the syndesmosis. There is usually minimal swelling or tenderness in the areas of the lateral ligaments unless the examination has been delayed and dependent swelling has occurred. It is not unusual to find that the athlete has some tenderness over the medial aspect of the ankle, specifically in the anterior portion of the deltoid ligament. The "squeeze test" is a provocative test performed by squeezing the fibula to the tibia at the midcalf. In cases of syndesmosis injury, maximal pain will be perceived at the distal tibiofibular syndesmosis. However, if there is a Maisonneuve fracture, maximal tenderness will be perceived at the site of the fracture. After the squeeze test,[44] as a part of the standard ankle physical examination, the anterior drawer and tilt test are performed; however, they are negative. The examiner may grasp the calcaneus and shift the hindfoot medial to lateral on the fixed tibia and in cases of frank diastasis there may be increased medial lateral play, which is abnormal. The external rotation stress test causes pain at the syndesmosis if injury is present. The test is performed by externally rotating the foot on the stabilized leg with the knee flexed to 90 degrees.[7] Unless these two provocative tests for syndesmosis injury are performed, this injury may be missed until the athlete complains of continued symptoms beyond the period of normal healing for lateral ligament injuries. Typically ankle syndesmosis injuries result in prolonged morbidity and probably a higher incidence of residual symptoms when compared with lateral ligament injuries. An athlete suspected of having a syndesmosis injury must undergo a radiographic evaluation. Bony avulsion fragments from the anterior tubercle or posterior tubercle of the tibia have been reported to occur in 10% to 50% of cases of syndesmosis injuries.[7,36] The relationship of the fibula to the tibia should also be evaluated. An excellent review of the radiographic evaluation of the tibiofibular syndesmosis has been done by Harper and Keller.[42] They defined criteria for determining whether a normal tibiofibular relationship was present. The three criteria were as follows: (1) tibiofibular clear space on anterior and mortise views less than 6 mm, (2) tibiofibular overlap on the anteroposterior view greater than 6 mm, and (3) tibiofibular overlap on the mortise view greater than 1 mm. Of these criteria the width of the tibiofibular clear space on both the anteroposterior and mortise views was the most reliable criteria for detecting early syndesmotic widening. If a patient is suspected of having a syndesmosis injury, but measurements on routine views are negative for diastasis, stress radiographs taken while external rotation and abduction forces are being applied to the ankle can reveal occult diastasis.[26] Bone scans have also been used to identify syndesmosis injuries and ankle injuries without fracture or frank diastasis.[62] The bone scan is positive if increased focal activity is observed in the area of the anterior tibiofibular ligament and interosseous membrane. CT scan and MRI may be indicated to diagnose syndesmosis injuries.[22,36,61] However, because of the expense and need for expertise in interpreting these tests, they are not recommended for routine evaluation of suspected syndesmosis injuries.

## Treatment

Partial, isolated syndesmosis tears should be treated nonoperatively, provided that there is no widening of the distal tibiofibular joint space and no osseous avulsion on radiographs.[36] Immobilization in a walking cast for 2 to 6 weeks followed by rehabilitation and taping upon return to play is an acceptable regimen. If frank or occult ankle diastasis is diagnosed on plain or stress radiographs, surgical management is indicated. Repair of the anterior tibiofibular ligament by direct suture or fixation of the avulsion fragment, as well as temporary fixation of the distal tibiofibular syndesmosis with a syndesmosis screw, is recommended.[36] During the syndesmosis screw fixation, the ankle should be held in maximal dorsiflexion and the screw should be placed approximately 1 to 2 cm proximal to the tibiofibular ligaments. Postoperatively a short-leg non–weight-bearing cast is applied. Partial weight bearing is allowed at 3 to 4 weeks postoperatively. Immobilization for 6 to 8 weeks is recommended. Unprotected full weight bearing is allowed after the syndesmosis screw is removed at 8 to 12 weeks. Prolonged morbidity following ankle syndesmosis injuries is most commonly due to mild to moderate stiffness. Patients may also complain of mild to moderate pain, swelling, and, rarely, a mild limp, although heterotopic ossification at the syndesmosis is a frequent sequela of syndesmosis injuries; in the absence of frank synostosis, long-term results are not affected by heterotopic ossification.

If tibiofibular synostosis occurs, symptomatic athletes will begin to complain of pain during the push-off phase of running at 3 to 12 months postinjury. Frank synostosis disrupts the normal tibiofibular rotational movement and proximal distal migration of the fibula.[65,80] Clinical evaluation usually reveals decreased dorsiflexion of the ankle. If the athlete remains symptomatic, surgical excision of the synostosis is indicated only after the synostosis has matured.[65] Interoperatively meticulous hemostasis should be obtained, and postoperative immobilization in a short-leg non–weight-bearing cast for 3 weeks is recommended.[65] Upon removal of the cast, active range-of-motion and strengthening exercises are begun. Despite excellent surgical technique, the recurrence rate of frank synostosis is high.[96]

## MANAGEMENT OF DELTOID LIGAMENT INJURY
### Mechanism of injury

The deltoid ligament may be injured in severe inversion injury in up to 10% of cases. In these cases the deltoid ligament injury is of secondary importance; therefore the ankle is treated by functional rehabilitation for lateral ligament injuries. When the deltoid ligament injury is the primary injury, it usually occurs by an eversion or external rotation mechanism or by a straight abduction mechanism. Severe forces usually are required to injure the strong deep deltoid ligament. An example of a possible mechanism of injury is the case of an athlete landing a jump with the foot in abduction and the heel in valgus, leading to increased stresses on the deltoid ligament.[19]

### Diagnosis

Typically the patient with a deltoid ligament injury recalls the specific injury, if a ligament has been torn, the patient hears or feels a pop on the medial side of the ankle. Immediate pain and subsequent swelling ensues. Although pain and swelling may be maximal on the medial aspect of the ankle, it is always important to do a complete foot and ankle lower-leg examination to rule out associated injuries such as lateral ligament injury, Maisonneuve fibular fracture, or ankle syndesmosis injury. To complete the evaluation on the medial aspect of the ankle, one should evaluate the function of the posterior tibial and flexor muscles. Although extremely rare, tibial and saphenous nerve traction injuries should be ruled out.

Radiographic evaluation should begin with anteroposterior, lateral, and mortise views of the ankle. Associated fracture or ankle diastasis is identified with these plain views. If these radiographs are negative and physical examination is suggestive of a ruptured deltoid ligament, a valgus talar tilt stress radiograph can be obtained. No amount of talar tilt on valgus stress is normal. If stress radiographs are negative, and the patient has been treated conserva-

tively and remains symptomatic, an MRI may reveal the pathology. In the presence of complete rupture of the deltoid ligament, an avulsion fragment of the medial malleolus is present.

### Treatment

The treatment of deltoid ligament ruptures depends upon the associated injuries. The usual principles for treatment of ankle fractures or ankle diastasis is followed. In cases of isolated deltoid ligament rupture, immobilization in a short-leg walking cast initially followed by functional rehabilitation is recommended.

Chronic medial instability of the ankle is uncommon.[47] The patient may have undergone functional treatment after deltoid injury was diagnosed or the diagnosis may have been never made and therefore appropriate treatment not initiated. If the appropriate diagnosis and treatment had not been made previously, the patient with chronic deltoid insufficiency should be treated with a functional rehabilitation program because the symptoms may be decreased and made tolerable. After failure of a conservative program, surgery to stabilize the medial ankle may be considered. If the tissue of the deep and superficial deltoid ligaments is of acceptable quality, direct imbrication of the ligaments may be performed.[23] If the residual deltoid ligament tissues are inadequate, tendon graft is performed. A splint posterior tibial tendon graft using the anterior portion of the posterior tibial tendon and directing it through a bone tunnel in the medial malleolus was described by Wiltberger.[97] Repair of a deltoid ligament avulsion injury by using a Kessler-type suture through the deltoid ligament into two drill holes in the medial malleolus has also been described.[47] Postoperatively 2 weeks of immobilization in a non–weight-bearing short-leg cast followed by 4 weeks of immobilization in a cast-brace is recommended. During the period of cast-bracing, patients are allowed to perform active range-of-motion exercises out of the cast-brace and are allowed to ambulate with weight bearing as tolerated. Six weeks postoperatively patients may begin weight bearing with a free ankle hinge brace, strengthening exercises are begun. This rehabilitation protocol is similar to that recommended by Jackson.[47]

**Case Study 5.** A 26-year-old male presented to an orthopedic surgeon 2 weeks after injuring his left ankle while playing basketball. He landed on another player's foot while coming down from a jump, sustaining an eversion injury. He was seen in the emergency room 2 hours after the injury where radiographs were negative for a fracture. He was treated with ice and crutches only. The patient had a history of at least five previous left ankle injuries, all of which were described as inversion injuries.

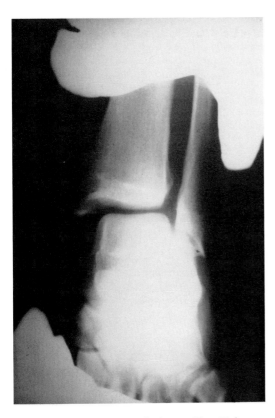

**Fig. 11-24.** Anterior view of the ankle. Valgus stress intraoperatively reveals significant laxity of the deep deltoid ligament.

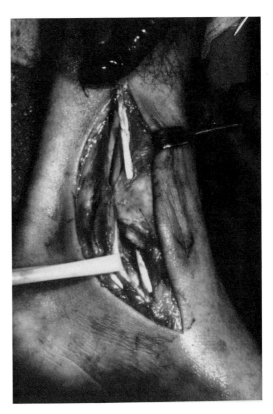

**Fig. 11-25.** Intraoperative reconstruction of the deltoid ligament. Half the posterior tibial tendon is used to augment the deficient deltoid ligament and protect against valgus stress.

Examination 2 weeks after the injury revealed marked swelling over the medial aspect of the ankle and maximal point tenderness inferior and posterior to the medial malleolus. There was also slight tenderness over the ATFL. The posterior tibial tendon was palpable, but dysfunctional, as the patient could not plantar flex and invert the foot simultaneously. The anterior drawer test was positive. Radiographs revealed an old avulsion fracture of the medial malleolus and osteophytes of the anterior ankle. The patient was immobilized in a short-leg cast and reevaluated 2 weeks later. The examination was suggestive of a posterior tibial tendon injury; however, deltoid ligament injury was also possible. Therefore an MRI was obtained to delineate the pathology. The MRI was suggestive of posterior tibial tendon pathology due to the presence of a large amount of peritendinous fluid, and a deltoid ligament tear was thought to be less likely by the radiologist. The patient was taken to surgery for medial ankle exploration. With the patient anesthetized, but before making an incision, valgus stress radiographs were obtained, which demonstrated a talar tilt of 7 degrees opening medially, confirming medial ankle instability (Fig. 11-24). The posterior tibial tendon was found to be intact without evidence of interstitial degeneration or tearing. The portion of the deltoid ligament was found to be avulsed from its attachment on the talus. Therefore reconstruction using the anterior one-third of the posterior tibial tendon was performed (Fig. 11-25). A section of posterior tendon was passed through a drill hole in the

medial malleolus doubled back on itself and secured to the insertion point on the talus with a Statek and 2-0 PDS suture. Before reconstructing the deep deltoid ligament, a loose bone fragment was removed from within the deltoid ligament. Postoperatively the patient was immobilized for 8 weeks in a short-leg cast. Weight bearing was allowed 1 month postoperatively. Physical therapy was initiated after the cast was removed and consisted of range-of-motion, strengthening, and proprioception retraining.

### REFERENCES

1. Anderson KJ, Lecocq JF, Lecocq EA: Recurrent anterior subluxation of the ankle, *J Bone Joint Surg* 34A:853, 1952.
2. Anderson ME: Reconstruction of the lateral ligaments of the ankle using the plantaris tendon, *J Bone Joint Surg* 67A:930, 1985.
3. Balduini FC et al: Management and rehabilitation of ligamentous injuries to the ankle, *Sports Med* 4:364, 1987.
4. Bassett FH III et al: Talar impingement by the anteroinferior tibiofibular ligament: a cause of chronic pain in the ankle after inversion sprain, *J Bone Joint Surg* 72A:55, 1990.
5. Black HM, Brand RL, Eichelberger MR: An improved technique for the evaluation of ligamentous injury in severe ankle sprains, *Am J Sports Med* 6:276, 1978.
6. Bosien WR, Staples OS, Russell SW: Residual disability following acute ankle sprains, *J Bone Joint Surg* 37A:1237, 1955.
7. Boytim MJ, Fischer DA, Neuman L: Syndesmotic ankle sprains, *Am J Sports Med* 19:294, 1991.
8. Brooks SC, Potter BT, Rainey JB: Treatment for partial tears of

the lateral ligament of the ankle: a prospective trial, *Br Med J* 282:606, 1981.

9. Broström L: Sprained ankles: I—Anatomic lesions in recent sprains, *Acta Chir Scand* 128:483, 1964.

10. Broström LL SO, Lindvall N: Sprained ankles: II—Arthrographic diagnosis of recent ligament ruptures, *Acta Chir Scand* 129:485, 1965.

11. Broström L: Sprained ankles: III—Clinical observations in recent ligament ruptures, *Acta Chir Scand* 130:560, 1965.

12. Broström L, Sundelin P: Sprained ankles: IV—Histological changes in recent and chronic ligament ruptures, *Acta Chir Scand* 132:248, 1966.

13. Broström L: Sprained ankles: V—Treatment and prognosis in recent ligament ruptures, *Acta Chir Scand* 132:537, 1966a.

14. Broström L: Sprained ankles: VI—Surgical treatment of chronic ligament ruptures, *Acta Chir Scand* 132:551, 1966b.

15. Bruns J, Dahmen G: Involvement of the inner malleolus and deltoid ligament in supination trauma of the ankle joint, *Aktuel Traumatol* 17:209, 1987.

16. Cass JR et al: Ankle instability: comparison of primary and delayed reconstruction after long-term followup study, *Clin Orthop* 198:110, 1985.

17. Cedell C: Ankle lesions, *Acta Orthop Scand* 46:425, 1975.

18. Chrisman OD, Snook GA: Reconstruction of lateral ligament tears of the ankle: an experimental study and evaluation of seven patients treated by a new modification of the Elmslie procedure, *J Bone Joint Surg* 51A:904, 1969.

19. Clanton TO, Schon LC: Athletic injuries to the soft tissues of the foot and ankle. In Mann RA, Coughlin MJ, editors: *Surgery of the foot and ankle*, ed 6. St Louis, 1993, Mosby, p 1128.

20. Clark BL, Derby AC, Power GRI: Injuries of the lateral ligament of the ankle. Conservative vs operative repair, *Can J Surg* 8:358, 1965.

21. Cote DJ et al: Comparison of three treatment procedures for minimizing ankle sprain swelling, *Phys Ther* 68:1072, 1988.

22. DenHartog B et al: The role of magnetic resonance imaging in evaluating chronic ankle pain after sprain, presented at the American Orthopaedic Foot and Ankle Society Meeting, Boston, July 27, 1991.

23. DuVries HL: Reconstruction of the medial collateral (deltoid) ligament. In Inman VT, editor: *DuVries' surgery of the foot*, St Louis, 1973, Mosby–Year Book, p 477.

24. Drez D et al: Nonoperative treatment of double lateral ligament tear of the ankle, *Am J Sports Med* 10:197, 1982.

25. Eckbert WR: Acute rupture of the peroneal retinaculum, *J Bone Joint Surg* 58A:670, 1976.

26. Edwards GS, DeLee JC: Ankle diastasis without fracture, *Foot Ankle* 4:305, 1984.

27. Elmslie RC: Recurrent subluxations of the ankle joint, *Ann Surg* 100:364, 1934.

28. Escalas F, Figueras JM, Merino JA: Dislocation of the peroneal tendons, *J Bone Joint Surg* 62A:451, 1980.

29. Evans DL: Recurrent instability of the ankle—a method of surgical treatment, *Proc R Soc Med* 46:343, 1953.

30. Evans GA, Hardcastle P, Frenyo AD: Acute rupture of the lateral ligament of the ankle: To suture or not to suture? *J Bone Joint Surg* 66B:209, 1984.

31. Evans GA, Frenyo SD: The stress-tenogram in the diagnosis of ruptures of the lateral ligament of the ankle, *J Bone Joint Surg* 61B:347, 1979.

32. Ferkel RD et al: Arthroscopic treatment of anterolateral impingement of the ankle, *Am J Sports Med* 19:440, 1991.

33. Freeman M: Instability of the foot after injuries to the lateral ligament of the ankle, *J Bone Joint Surg* 47B:669, 1965.

34. Freeman MAR: Treatment of ruptures of the lateral ligaments of the ankle, *J Bone Joint Surg* 47B:661, 1965.

35. Freeman MAR, Dean MRE, Hanham IWF: The etiology and prevention of functional instability of the foot, *J Bone Joint Surg* 47B:679, 1965.

36. Fristchy D: An unusual ankle injury in top skiers, *Am J Sports Med* 17:282, 1989.

37. Garrick JG, Requa RK: Role of external support in the prevention of ankle sprains, *Med Sci Sports Exer* 5:200, 1973.

38. Garrick JM: The frequency of injury, mechanism of injury, and epidemiology of ankle sprains, *Am J Sports Med* 5:241, 1977.

39. Gauffin H, Tropp H, Odenrick P: Effect of ankle disk training on postural control in patients with functional instability of the ankle, *Int J Sports Med* 9:141, 1988.

40. Gould N, Seligson D, Gassman J: Early and late repair of lateral ligament of the ankle, *Foot Ankle* 1:84, 1980.

41. Gronmark T, Johnsen O, Kogstad O: Rupture of the lateral ligaments of the ankle: a controlled clinical trial, *Injury* 11:215, 1980.

42. Harper MC, Keller TS: A radiographic evaluation of the tibiofibular syndesmosis, *Foot Ankle* 10:156, 1989.

43. Hocutt JE et al: Cryotherapy in ankle sprains, *Am J Sports Med* 10:316, 1982.

44. Hopkinson WJ et al: Syndesmosis sprains of the ankle, *Foot Ankle* 10:325, 1990.

45. Hortsman JK, Kantor GS, Samuelson KM: Investigation of lateral ankle ligament reconstruction, *Foot Ankle* 1:338, 1981.

46. Jackson DW, Ashley RD, Powell JW: Ankle sprains in young athletes: relation of severity and disability, *Clin Orthop* 101:201, 1974.

47. Jackson R, Wills RE, Jackson R: Rupture of the deltoid ligament without involvement of the lateral ligament, *Am J Sports Med* 16:541, 1988.

48. Kannus P, Renstrom P: Current concepts review: treatment for acute tears of the lateral ligaments of the ankle, *J Bone Joint Surg* 73A:305, 1991.

49. Karlsson J et al: Reconstruction of the lateral ligaments of the ankle for chronic lateral instability, *J Bone Joint Surg* 70A:581, 1988.

50. Karlsson J et al: Surgical treatment of chronic lateral instability of the ankle joint, *Am J Sports Med* 17:268, 1989.

51. Karlsson J et al: Lateral instability of the ankle treated by the Evans procedure: a long term clinical and radiological follow-up, *J Bone Joint Surg* 70B:476, 1988.

52. Klein J et al: Operative or conservative treatment of recent rupture of the fibular ligament in the ankle: a randomized clinical trial, *Ufallchirug* 91:154, 1988.

53. Kelikian H, Kelikian AS: *Disorders of the ankle*, Philadelphia, 1985, WB Saunders.

54. Korkala O et al: A prospective study of the treatment of severe tears of the lateral ligament of the ankle, *Int Orthop* 11:13, 1987.

55. Larsen E, Angermann P: Association of ankle instability and foot deformity, *Acta Orthop Scand* 61:136, 1990.

56. Lauge-Hansen N: Fractures of the ankle: analytic historic survey as the basis of new experimental, roentgenologic and clinical investigations, *Arch Surg* 56:259, 1948.

57. Lauge-Hansen N: Fractures of the ankle: II—Combined experimental-surgical and experimental-roentgenologic investigations, *Arch Surg* 60:957, 1950.

58. Lauge-Hansen N: Fractures of the ankle: III—Genetic roentgenologic diagnosis of fracture of the ankle, *Am J Roentgenol* 71:456, 1954.

59. Lauge-Hansen N: Fractures of the ankle: IV—Clinical use of genetic roentgen diagnosis and genetic reduction, *Arch Surg* 64:488, 1952.

60. Laughman RK et al: Three-dimensional kinematics of the taped ankle before and after exercise, *Am J Sports Med* 8:425, 1984.

61. Linsjo U et al: Computed tomography of the ankle, *Acta Orthop Scand* 50:797, 1979.
62. Marymont JV, Lynch MA, Henning CE: Acute ligamentous diastasis of the ankle without fracture, *Am J Sports Med* 14:407, 1986.
63. McCluskey GM, Blackburn TA, Lewis T: Prevention of ankle sprains, *Am J Sports Med* 4:151, 1976.
64. McCulloch PG et al: The value of mobilisation and non-steroidal anti-inflammatory analgesia in the management of inversion injuries of the ankle, *Br J Clin Pract* 29:69, 1985.
65. McMasters PE: Treatment of ankle sprain: observations in more than five hundred cases, *JAMA* 122:659, 1943.
66. Moller-Larsen F et al: Comparison of three different treatments for ruptured lateral ankle ligaments, *Acta Orthop Scand* 59:564, 1988.
67. Niedermann B et al: Rupture of the lateral ligaments of the ankle: operation or plaster cast? A prospective study, *Acta Orthop Scand* 52:579, 1981.
68. Nitz AJ, Dobner JJ, Kersey D: Nerve injury and grade II and III ankle sprains, *Am J Sports Med* 13:177, 1985.
69. Orava S et al: Radiographic instability of the ankle joint after Evans repair, *Acta Orthop Scand* 54:734, 1983.
70. Peters JW, Trevino SG, Renstrom PA: Chronic lateral ankle instability, *Foot Ankle* 12:182, 1991.
71. Prins JG: Diagnosis and treatment of injury to the lateral ligament of the ankle: a comparative clinical study, *Acta Chir Scand Suppl* 486:1, 1978.
72. Raatikainen T, Mikko P, Puranen J: Arthrography, clinical examination, and stress radiograph in the diagnosis of acute injury to the lateral ligaments of the ankle, *Am J Sports Med* 20:2, 1992.
73. Rarick GL et al: The measurable support of the ankle joint by conventional methods of taping, *J Bone Joint Surg* 44A:1183, 1962.
74. Rovere GD et al: Retrospective comparison of taping and ankle stabilizers in preventing ankle injuries, *Am J Sports Med* 16:228, 1988.
75. Rozier CK, Elder JD, Brown M: Prevention of atrophy by isometric exercise of a casted leg, *J Sports Med* 19:191, 1979.
76. Ruth CJ: The surgical treatment of injuries of the fibular collateral ligaments of the ankle, *J Bone Joint Surg* 43A:229, 1961.
77. St. Pierre R et al: A review of lateral ankle ligamentous reconstruction, *Foot Ankle* 3:114, 1982.
78. Sammarco GJ, DiRaimondo CV: Surgical treatment of lateral ankle instability syndrome, *Am J Sports Med* 16:501, 1988.
79. Schneck CD, Mesgarzadeh M, Bonakdarpour A: MR imaging of the most commonly injured ankle ligaments, *Radiology* 184:507, 1992.
80. Scranton PE, McMaster JH, Kelly E: Dynamic fibular function, *Clin Orthop* 118:76, 1976.
81. Smith RW, Reischl S: The influence of dorsiflexion in the treatment of severe ankle sprains: an anatomical study, *Foot Ankle* 9:28, 1988.
82. Smith RW, Reischl S: Treatment of ankle sprains in young athletes, *Am J Sports Med* 14:465, 1986.
83. Solheim LF, Denstad TF: Chronic lateral instability of the ankle: a method of reconstruction using the Achilles tendon, *Acta Orthop Scand* 51:193, 1980.
84. Sommer HM, Arza D: Functional treatment of recent ruptures of the fibular ligament of the ankle, *Int Orthop* 13:157, 1989.
85. Snook GA, Chrisman OD, Wilson TC: Long-term results of the Chrisman-Snook operation for reconstruction of the lateral ligaments of the ankle, *J Bone Joint Surg* 67A:1, 1985.
86. Starkey JA: Treatment of ankle sprains by the simultaneous use of intermittent compression and ice packs, *Am J Sports Med* 4:142, 1976.
87. Storen H: A new method for operative treatment of insufficiency of the lateral ligaments of the ankle joint, *Acta Chir Scand* 117:501, 1959.
88. Thompson TC: A test for rupture of the tendo Achilles, *Acta Orthop Scand* 32:461, 1992.
89. Thompson TC, Doherty JH: Spontaneous rupture of the tendon of Achilles: a nonclinical diagnostic test, *J Trauma* 2:126, 1962.
90. Tropp H: Functional instability of the ankle joint. Medical Dissertation No. 202, pp 1-92, Likoping University, Linkoping, Sweden. Linkoping, VTT-Grafiska, 1985.
91. Van der Rijt AJ, Evans GA: The long term results of Watson-Jones tenodesis, *J Bone Joint Surg* 66B:371, 1984.
92. Van Moppens FI, vand den Hoogenband CR: Diagnostic and therapeutic aspects of inversion trauma of the ankle joint, Thesis, University of Maastricth, The Netherlands, Utrecht/Antwerpen, Bohn, Scheltema and Holkema, pp 1-166, 1982.
93. Verhaven EFC et al: The accuracy of three-dimensional magnetic resonance imaging in the diagnosis of ruptures of the lateral ligaments of the ankle, *Am J Sports Med* 19:583, 1991.
94. Waller JF: Hindfoot and midfoot problems in the runner. In Mack RP, editor: *Symposium on the foot and leg in running*, St Louis, 1982, CV Mosby, p 64.
95. Watson-Jones R: Recurrent forward dislocation of the ankle joint, *J Bone Joint Surg* 34B:519, 1952.
96. Whiteside LA, Reynolds FC, Ellsasser JC: Tibiofibular synostosis and recurrent ankle sprains in high performance athletes, *Am J Sports Med* 6:204, 1978.
97. Wiltberger BR, Mallory TM: A new method for the reconstruction of the deltoid ligament of the ankle, *Orthop Rev* 1:37, 1972.
98. Wolin I, Glassman F, Sideman S: Internal derangement of the talofibular component of the ankle, *Surg Gynecol Obstet* 91:193, 1950.

# Chapter 12

# Disorders of the subtalar joint

**Marion C. Harper**

Disorders of the subtalar joint in athletes may be divided into several major categories. The first is that group of abnormalities reflecting some injury either recent or remote to the articular surface. These injuries—which may lead to some degree of arthrosis—commonly involve three anatomic areas: the anterosuperior process of the calcaneus, lateral process of the talus, and posterior process of the talus.

The second category involves a congenital or developmental anomaly of the joint architecture presenting symptomatically following skeletal maturation. The most notable example would be a tarsal coalition as discussed elsewhere in this text.

A final group of disorders involves the functional sequelae of some degree of ligament insufficiency, typically posttraumatic, in the hindfoot. This may result in the syndrome usually termed *subtalar instability*.

## POSTTRAUMATIC OSSEOUS DISORDERS
### Fractures of the anterosuperior process of the calcaneus

**Anatomy and mechanism of injury.** The anterosuperior process of the calcaneus, although somewhat variable in its exact configuration, is a discrete, easily identifiable structure on both gross and radiographic examination of the foot (Fig. 12-1). Perhaps best described as a saddle-shaped promontory usually slightly overhanging the adjacent cuboid and calcaneocuboid joint, this structure has largely been misunderstood in terms of its anatomic ramifications. Classifying fractures of this process as nonarticular, as has commonly been done, ignores the fact that this

promontory articulates inferiorly with the cuboid as a portion of the calcaneocuboid joint. In addition, the medial aspect of the process superiorly commonly articulates with the inferior portion of the talar neck as the relatively short narrow anterior facet of the talocalcaneal joint (Fig. 12-1). Thus fractures of the anterosuperior process of significant size may involve both the subtalar and calcaneocuboid joints.

Another pertinent aspect of the anatomy in this region, particularly as it relates to the etiology of fractures of this process, is the associated ligamentous support. Key ligaments attaching to this structure include the superficial layer of the inferior extensor retinaculum, the cervical (anterior interosseous talocalcaneal) ligament, and the bifurcate ligament with its calcaneocuboid and calcaneonavicular components (Fig. 12-2). All probably play a role in causing the common avulsion fracture of the superior portion of the process typically associated with inversion plantar flexion injuries. The other fracture pattern involving this structure involves a compression force applied across the calcaneocuboid joint in association with forceful abduction of the foot. This so-called "nutcracker" injury, which usually results in extensive comminution of the calcaneocuboid joint with relative sparing of the subtalar joint, is not discussed in this section.

**Diagnosis.** Fractures of the anterosuperior process of the calcaneus should be suspected in anyone having sustained an inversion injury, particularly if pain and swelling are most severe in an area several centimeters anterior and slightly below the lateral malleolus. This area corresponds to the superior

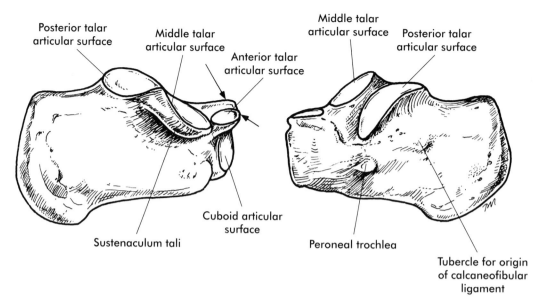

**Fig. 12-1.** Anterosuperior process of the calcaneus *(long arrow)*, including the anterior facet of the subtalar joint *(small arrow)*.

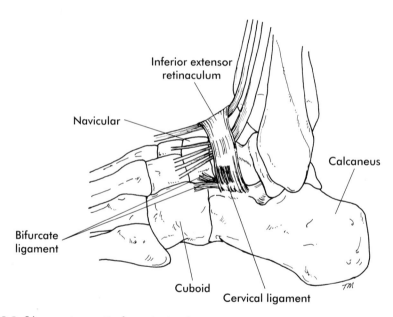

**Fig. 12-2.** Ligamentous attachments to the anterosuperior process of the calcaneus, including the inferior extensor retinaculum, bifurcate ligament, and cervical ligament.

aspect of the calcaneocuboid joint and is somewhat more inferior and anterior than that associated with the usual ankle sprain. The common association of these avulsion fractures with inversion injuries, plus the fact that this injury is often misdiagnosed as a ligament disruption, has led to the term *sprain fracture.*

Radiographically these fractures usually are not visible on routine anteroposterior (AP) radiographs of the foot, but occasionally can be seen on the lateral view. The best projection is an oblique view that avoids overlapping of the anterosuperior process with the talar neck. If questionable, AP and lateral tomograms have been used successfully to define the fracture pattern and degree of articular involvement. Computed tomography (CT) using sagittal and coronal slices also offers an excellent way to evaluate this injury.

**Treatment.** To determine the optimal treatment, either tomograms or a CT scan should be well

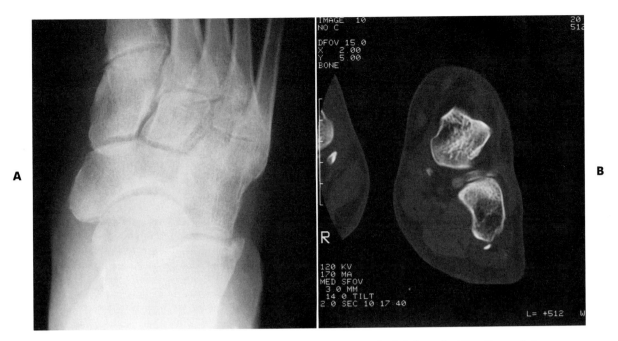

**Fig. 12-3.** A 30-year-old female with a twisting injury to the left foot. **A,** AP radiograph is interpreted as revealing a small avulsion fracture off the lateral calcaneus. **B,** CT scan demonstrates significant involvement of the calcaneocuboid joint.

scrutinized to assess the size of the fracture fragments, degree of comminution, and extent of articular involvement. Depending upon these factors, the basic decision is between nonoperative and operative treatment. Although no specific guidelines are available, the consensus is that small fractures with only mild displacement and little joint involvement should be treated nonoperatively, typically with a removable ankle support or in a cast. In cases where the fracture fragment is large, displaced, and has a significant articular component, consideration should be given to surgical treatment. A longitudinal incision over the superior aspect of the calcaneocuboid joint allows excellent exposure of both the fragment and articular surface. The choice then becomes one of fragment excision or open reduction and internal fixation. The former is simpler and perhaps more definitive, with the latter having appeal if the fragment can be reduced anatomically and held well with K-wires. With either form of treatment, an effort should be made to initiate a program of midfoot and hindfoot motion as soon as feasible.

With either form of treatment, one must also accept the possibility of lingering symptoms and eventual arthrosis. Degan et al, reporting the results of conservative treatment, relate that the average time for recovery was 10 months, with less than half of their patients being pain-free at follow-up.[8] Only limited reports are available as to the results of open reduction and internal fixation. The other surgical option (i.e., excision of the fragment) for the patient with long-term pain and disability is generally satisfactory.[8,15] A final choice for the individual with significant arthrosis is an arthrodesis, usually involving the calcaneocuboid joint (see Case Study 1).

**Case Study 1.** A 30-year-old female fell, sustaining a twisting injury to the left foot with resultant lateral pain, swelling, and ecchymosis. Initial radiographs were interpreted as revealing only a small "chip" fracture off the lateral calcaneus anteriorly (Fig. 12-3, A). The diagnosis of a foot sprain with a small associated avulsion fracture was made, and the patient was treated with crutches and elastic support. Because of persistent lateral pain, a CT scan was obtained 6 months postinjury. This study revealed a fracture of the anterosuperior process of the calcaneus with significant involvement of the calcaneocuboid joint (Fig. 12-3, B). The patient declined surgery and to date remains moderately symptomatic while wearing an ankle-foot orthosis (AFO) intermittently.

### Fractures of the lateral process of the talus

**Anatomy and mechanism of injury.** The lateral process of the talus is the wedge-shaped lateral portion of the talar body as it extends from the inferior aspect of the fibulotalar articulation to the undersurface of the talus (Fig. 12-4). This structure therefore incorporates two articular surfaces: the fibulotalar recess or lateral gutter of the ankle joint and the posterior facet of the subtalar joint.

The most notable ligament attaching to the lateral process is the lateral talocalcaneal, a structure of variable strength and presence[13] and not particularly important in providing stability for the hindfoot.

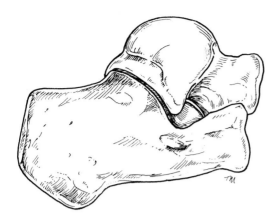

**Fig. 12-4.** Lateral process of the talus.

Although various mechanisms of injury have been offered for this fracture, the most popular theory is one of inversion and dorsiflexion resulting in a compressive force being delivered to the lateral talus.

**Diagnosis.** As with fractures of the anterosuperior process of the calcaneus, both the mechanism of injury and clinical findings are similar to those seen with a typical lateral ankle sprain. Thus this fracture should be observed for in all patients treated for inversion injuries of the ankle. Because the tenderness and swelling are in the same area as occurs with disruptions of the anterior talofibular and calcaneofibular ligaments, the key to early diagnosis is a thorough evaluation of the initial radiographs. Fractures of the lateral process can usually be seen to some degree on a routine ankle series, particularly on the mortise view. If unclear, an oblique view with the extremity internally rotated 45 degrees and the foot in equinus may be optimal. If still in doubt, AP and lateral tomograms will usually show the fracture well, although the definitive study is usually the CT scan, particularly if appropriate cuts are made through this region.

**Treatment.** The key determinants in the treatment of fractures of the lateral talar process are the size of the fragment, the degree of comminution, and the extent of involvement of the subtalar and lateral ankle joints.

Relatively small fractures with slight displacement and limited articular disruption may be treated with 4 to 6 weeks of casting. For larger, displaced fractures with significant articular involvement, operative intervention is indicated. Through an anterolateral approach along the anterior and inferior aspect of the fibula, the ankle joint is entered and the lateral process well visualized. If the fracture fragment is large enough to allow secure internal fixation with K-wires or small screws, this approach is reasonable. If, however, comminution is significant, the fragments should be excised. With either operative approach,

motion of both the ankle and subtalar joints should be instituted early. For patients not seen until fracture healing has begun or with a symptomatic nonunion, excision of the fragment is usually the treatment of choice.

As regards prognosis, the earlier the diagnosis is made and treatment begun, the better the eventual outcome.[9,22,24] Even nondisplaced fractures with optimal treatment, however, can result in chronic symptoms,[22,24] and this information should be related to the patient early on. In many cases this appears to relate to arthrosis of the subtalar joint (see Case Study 2).

**Case Study 2.** A 29-year-old male fell, sustaining an injury to the right foot and ankle. Swelling and ecchymosis was noted both medially and laterally about the hindfoot and ankle. Initial radiographs were interpreted as revealing small avulsion fractures off the lateral talus and medial malleolus (Fig. 12-5, *A*). Following 5 weeks in a short-leg cast, he developed disabling pain about the lateral ankle and hindfoot, most notable when walking on uneven ground. Physical examination 6 months postinjury revealed tenderness just below the tip of the lateral malleolus with some restriction of subtalar motion. A CT scan confirmed the presence of a large displaced fracture of the lateral process of the talus with early arthrosis of the subtalar joint (Fig. 12-5, *B*). Surgical removal of the fragment resulted in moderate improvement in pain, although at final follow-up, the patient was still using a posterior polypropylene AFO intermittently.

### Fractures of the posterior process of the talus

**Anatomy and mechanism of injury.** The posterior process of the talus is made up of the posteromedial and posterolateral tubercles, with the latter being larger and more prominent (Fig. 12-6). Separating these two structures is the groove for the flexor hallucis longus tendon. The superior aspect of the posterolateral tubercle is extraarticular as regards the ankle joint, in contrast to the inferior surface, which is part of the posterior facet of the subtalar joint. The posteromedial tubercle is largely extraarticular for both joints. As regards ligamentous attachments, the most notable ligament inserting on either tubercle is the posterior talofibular ligament attachment laterally.

The most confusing anatomic feature in this region is the os trigonum, an accessory ossicle found in association with the posterolateral tubercle. This occurs as a separate ossicle in approximately 10% of patients and as a trigonal process or elongated lateral tubercle in as many as 50%.[5] Representing an accessory center of ossification either separate from or fused to the lateral process, this structure in the former configuration may be difficult to distinguish from a fracture.

The two mechanisms of injury for this fracture offered in the literature are both forced plantar flexion

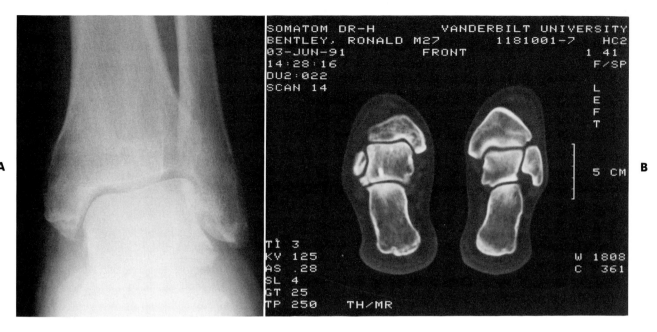

**Fig. 12-5.** A 29-year-old male who injured his right foot in a fall. **A,** Initial mortise radiograph of the ankle is read as showing small avulsion fractures of the talus and medial malleolus. **B,** CT scan 6 months postfracture reveals a large displaced fracture of the lateral process of the talus.

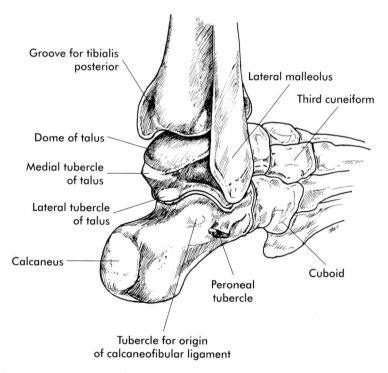

**Fig. 12-6.** Posterior process of the talus as made up of the posterolateral and posteromedial tubercles separated by the groove for the flexor hallucis longus tendon. (From Harper MC: Stress radiographs in the diagnosis of lateral instability of the ankle and hindfoot, *Foot Ankle* 13:435, 1992.)

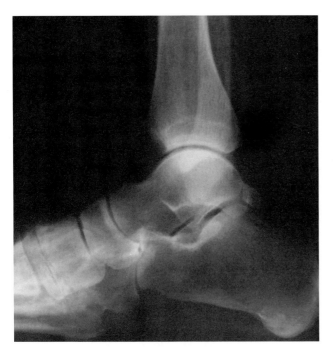

**Fig. 12-7.** Typical os trigonum.

and dorsiflexion of the ankle. In the former, impingement of the posterior plafond against the posterolateral process occurs, whereas in the latter, the posterior talofibular ligament may create an avulsion injury.

**Diagnosis.** For this injury the history and physical examination are highly important. For example, a fracture should be associated with an incident wherein significant force has been expended across the ankle. In contrast, a history of repetitive lower-energy stress associated with the onset of symptoms would suggest an inflammatory process involving an os trigonum. An example of the latter would be a posterior impingement or os trigonum syndrome wherein this structure is repeatedly compressed — for example, in a ballet dancer assuming pointe or demipointe position.[17] In either case, pain is usually posterior and aggravated by both ankle and subtalar motion.

On physical examination, swelling, tenderness, and ecchymosis may be present anterior to the Achilles tendon about the posterior talus. Pain should occur with plantar flexion and dorsiflexion of both the ankle and great toe.

Radiographically the posterior talus is best seen on the lateral view. An os trigonum may vary markedly in size and configuration but typically will appear as a small oval or three-sided ossicle contiguous with the posterior talus. The margins should be smooth and the interval between the talus and the ossicle uniform in width (Fig. 12-7). A fracture of the posterolateral process in contrast usually has irregular margins at

the fracture site, with the fracture interval less than uniform in appearance. In either case an articular surface with subchondral bone for the subtalar joint may be evident on the fragment. If unclear the definitive study is either lateral tomography or a CT scan using sagittal cuts.

To make this diagnosis more difficult yet, there is an apparent clinical entity wherein the fibrocartilaginous connection between the talar body and an os trigonum is injured but not completely disrupted. The clinical picture for this disorder is much the same as that seen with the posterior impingement or os trigonum syndrome. With even tomography failing to show an anatomic separation, diagnosis would depend upon a bone scan, which should reveal increased uptake in this area. A bone scan may also be indicated in distinguishing an occult fracture from an asymptomatic accessory ossicle.

**Treatment.** Once again, the treatment for a fracture of the posterolateral talar process depends upon the size of the fragment, the extent of comminution, and the degree of displacement. Small fractures with limited displacement and incongruity of the subtalar joint may be managed with approximately 6 weeks of casting. Large fragments, in contrast, should prompt strong consideration for surgery, especially if displaced to any degree. This may be done through a posterolateral approach, with care being taken to stay medial to the sural nerve. When exposed, the choice will be between open reduction and internal fixation with K-wires or small screws versus simple excision of the fragment. With instability not being an issue and the latter being much simpler, excision is probably the treatment of choice for most fractures. Certainly in cases of either delayed diagnosis or delayed union, this would appear to be the case. In addition, an os trigonum that remains chronically inflamed despite a significant period of rest and even casting may need to be excised.

**Case Study 3.** A 29-year-old male fell, injuring his right foot. Tenderness, swelling, and ecchymosis were noted posterior to the malleoli both medially and laterally. Initial radiographs revealed an apparent fracture of the posterior talus (Fig. 12-8, *A*) but the patient failed to return for follow-up until 6 months later when lateral tomograms confirmed the presence of a nonunion of a fracture of the posterolateral process (Fig. 12-8, *B*). Excision of the fragment was carried out, but because of increasing pain and arthrosis involving the subtalar joint, a subtalar arthrodesis was done 2 years postfracture.

### Posttraumatic ligamentous disorders

**Anatomy and mechanism of injury.** The key ligamentous structures stabilizing the subtalar joint extend from the superficial aspect of the sinus tarsi and

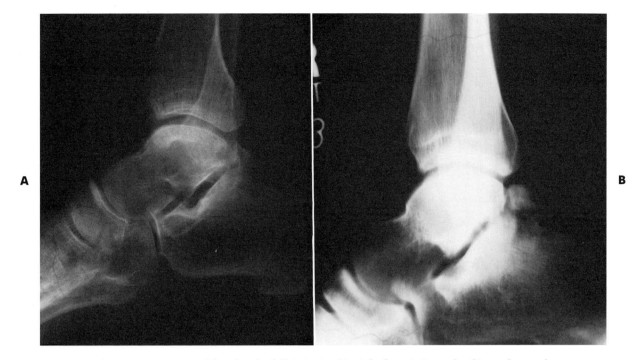

**Fig. 12-8.** A 29-year-old male who fell, injuring his right foot. **A,** Lateral radiograph reveals a fracture of the posterior talar process. **B,** Lateral tomogram performed 6 months later demonstrates a large fracture of the posterolateral tubercle.

hindfoot to deep within the tarsal canal. Proceeding from lateral to medial, they are the superficial layer of the inferior extensor retinaculum, the calcaneofibular ligament, the deep layer of the extensor retinaculum, the cervical ligament, and the interosseous talocalcaneal ligament.[13] Any or all may be disrupted as an inversion injury increases in severity from a relatively mild lateral sprain to a transient subtalar dislocation. Thus it is reasonable to expect the lateral instability syndromes that may follow severe or repetitive inversion injuries to encompass some degree of excessive mobility of the calcaneus beneath the talus. The difficulty has been and remains the detection and quantification of this probable instability.[7]

Inversion of the hindfoot as a component of supination in the gait cycle has been studied by a number of workers. All have emphasized the rotational motion necessary through the subtalar joint to allow the foot to progress from a position of pronation to supination and accommodate the associated internal and external rotation of the tibia. Wright et al found the average subtalar rotation during stance phase to be 6 degrees.[26] Manter emphasized the screwlike motion of the subtalar joint estimating 1.5 mm of displacement of the talus over the calcaneus for each 10 degrees of subtalar rotation.[21]

The stabilizing effect of the calcaneofibular ligament, as well as other ligamentous structures in the sinus and canalis tarsi on hindfoot inversion, has been

demonstrated by several investigators.[14,17,18,20,25] Considering that the calcaneofibular ligament is known to be commonly disrupted with the more severe inversion injuries, it appears reasonable to believe that some degree of excessive mobility of the calcaneus beneath the talus plays a role in patients relating symptoms of chronic instability. This concept is supported by the observation that patients with clinical instability commonly have unimpressive ankle stress radiographs and yet may be helped by surgical repairs that limit supination.[1,7,12,16,19]

**Diagnosis.** The definitive diagnosis of subtalar instability remains somewhat elusive, probably relating both to difficulty in visualizing this joint and appreciating an increase in rotational movement therein. Because division of the calcaneofibular ligament in cadaver specimens has been noted to cause gaping-open of the joint laterally,[14,20] an effort was made initially to detect this opening effect via stress AP tomography.[2] This technique, however, has proven to be technically difficult and of little clinical value.[7] More recently, efforts have focused on the so-called stress Broden view. With this technique, the extremity is positioned as for a Broden view of the hindfoot with the leg internally rotated 45 degrees, the foot in equinus, and the x-ray beam focused on the sinus tarsi at an angle of 30 to 40 degrees off the vertical.[3] The posterior facet of the subtalar joint is then well visualized, and any lateral opening during inversion stress noted. This

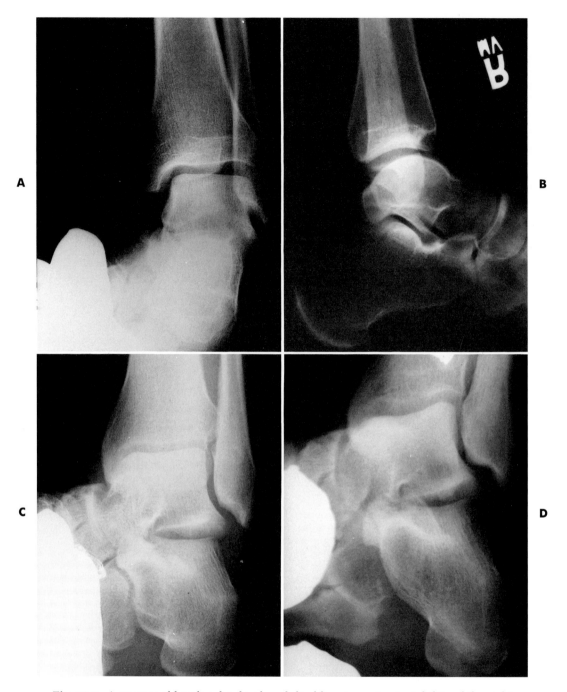

**Fig. 12-9.** A 41-year-old male who developed disabling inversion instability of the right foot and ankle following a lateral "ankle sprain." **A** and **B**, Stress radiographs of the ankle demonstrate only slight talar tilt and 3 mm of excessive anterior talar excursion. Stress Broden views of both the symptomatic right foot **(C)** and the asymptomatic left foot **(D)** reveal approximately equal apparent divergence of the articular surfaces of the subtalar joint. (From Harper MC: Stress radiographs in the diagnosis of lateral instability of the ankle and hindfoot, *Foot Ankle* 13:435, 1992.)

technique, however, also appears to have some inherent difficulty in that patients with instability symptoms commonly exhibit some apparent divergence of the articular surfaces on both symptomatic and asymptomatic sides, as will randomly selected asymptomatic patients.[12]

The diagnosis of this syndrome thus remains somewhat circumstantial. It should be considered likely in the individual with symptoms of inversion instability, who demonstrates on clinical examination or stress radiography of the ankle relatively unimpressive findings. This patient usually relates a history of one or more severe inversion injuries. The subjective complaint will primarily be instability with pain and swelling occurring secondarily as versus the chronic pain patient wherein the foot and ankle may "give way" after pain has occurred. On physical examination, one may be able to appreciate some subtle increase in hindfoot inversion. There may be evidence of generalized ligamentous laxity. The key diagnostic feature, however, is usually a history of recurrent disabling instability.

**Treatment.** As with ankle instability, which may often indeed be associated with this syndrome and thus comprise in many patients a combination of ankle and subtalar instability, initial therapeutic efforts should involve lower-leg strengthening, especially the peroneal muscles and proprioceptive retraining. Some external support such as a stirrup ankle brace may be indicated as well. If symptoms persist, however, surgical reconstruction should be considered. In athletes one would like to eliminate what may often be excessive mobility at both the ankle and subtalar joint while not restricting the motion necessary for normal biomechanics of the foot. In the past this has been a cause of failure of repairs using the peroneal tendons, particularly regarding excessive restriction of inversion. A repair that attempts to tighten the pertinent anatomic restraints in their normal orientation should have the best prospect for achieving this goal. Two of the repairs based on this concept are those described by Broström in 1966[4] and Ahlgren and Larsson in 1989.[1] In the former, a curved incision is made along the anterior and inferior margin of the lateral malleolus. Both the anterior talofibular and calcaneofibular ligaments are identified, usually in a somewhat elongated or thinned configuration. Intervening scar is excised and the ligament ends freshened. A repair is then done with the foot and ankle in neutral. If necessary, a portion of the inferior extensor retinaculum can be mobilized and overlapped as described by Gould.[10] Four to six weeks of cast immobilization is followed by a rehabilitation program.

In the second repair, an L-shaped incision is made over the distal and posterior lateral melleolus. A distally based flap of periosteum incorporating the proximal attachments of the anterior talofibular and calcaneofibular ligaments is carefully elevated from the distal malleolus. The exposed malleolar tip is decorticated and the flap advanced proximally 3 to 5 mm and sutured to bone through drill holes with the foot in eversion. This is again followed by 6 weeks of casting. Both of these techniques yield a high percentage of satisfactory results in terms of relief of instability symptoms with minimal loss of normal mobility (see Case Study 4).

**Case Study 4.** A 41-year-old male sustained a severe inversion injury to the right foot and ankle associated with marked swelling and ecchymosis. Following treatment with crutches and an elastic wrap, he developed recurrent episodes of "giving way" of the ankle and hindfoot into supination. Physical examination was unremarkable except for an anterior drawer test that was thought to be mildly positive.

Stress radiographs of the ankle revealed only 6 degrees of talar tilt on the AP view (Fig. 12-9, A) with widening of the joint space posteriorly to a distance of 6 mm on the lateral view (Fig. 12-9, B). Stress Broden views of both hindfeet revealed an approximately equal amount of divergence of the articular surfaces of the posterior facet of the subtalar joints (Fig. 12-9, C and D). The instability symptoms were refractory to a peroneal strengthening program plus the wearing of an ankle support. The patient underwent a reconstructive procedure using local tissue, including a portion of the inferior extensor retinaculum. At 1 year follow-up, relief of both instability symptoms and pain was rated as good.

## REFERENCES

1. Ahlgren O, Larsson S: Reconstruction for lateral ligament injuries of the ankle, *J Bone Joint Surg* 71B:300, 1989.
2. Brantigan JW, Pedegana LR, Lippert FG: Instability of the subtalar joint: diagnosis by stress tomography in three cases, *J Bone Joint Surg* 59A:321, 1977.
3. Broden B: Roentgen examination of the subtaloid joint in fractures of the calcaneus, *Acta Radiol* 31:85, 1949.
4. Broström L: Sprained ankles: VI. Surgical treatment of "chronic" ligament ruptures, *Acta Chir Scand* 132:551, 1966.
5. Burman MS, Lapidus PW: The functional disturbances caused by the inconstant bones and sesamoids of the foot, *Arch Surg* 22:936, 1931.
6. Chrisman OD, Snook GA: Reconstruction of lateral ligament tears of the ankle: an experimental study and clinical evaluation of seven patients treated by a new modification of the Elmslie procedure, *J Bone Joint Surg* 51A:904, 1969.
7. Clanton TO: Instability of the subtalar joint, *Orthop Clin North Am* 20:583, 1989.
8. Degan TJ, Morrey BF, Braun DP: Surgical excision for anterior-process fractures of the calcaneus, *J Bone Joint Surg* 64A:519, 1982.
9. Dimon JH: Isolated displaced fracture of the posterior facet of the talus, *J Bone Joint Surg* 43A:275, 1961.
10. Gould N: Repair of lateral ligament of ankle, *Foot Ankle* 8:55, 1987.
11. Hamilton WG: Stenosing tenosynovitis of the flexor hallucis longus tendon and posterior impingement upon the os trigonum in ballet dancers, *Foot Ankle* 3:74, 1982.
12. Harper MC: Stress radiographs in the diagnosis of lateral instability of the ankle and hindfoot, *Foot Ankle* 13:435, 1992.
13. Harper MC: The lateral ligamentous support for the subtalar joint, *Foot Ankle* 11:354, 1991.
14. Heilman AE et al: An anatomic study of subtalar instability, *Foot Ankle* 10:224, 1990.
15. Jahss MH, Kay BS: An anatomic study of the anterior superior process of the os calcis and its clinical application, *Foot Ankle* 3:268, 1983.
16. Johannsen A: Radiological diagnosis of lateral ligament lesion of the ankle, *Acta Orthop Scand* 49:295, 1978.
17. Kjærsgaard-Andersen P, Wethelund J-O, Nielsen S: Lateral talocalcaneal instability following section of the calcaneofibular ligament: a kinesiologic study, *Foot Ankle* 7:355, 1987.

18. Kjærsgaard-Andersen P, Wethelund J-O, Nielsen S: The stabilizing effect of the ligamentous structures in the sinus and canalis tarsi on movements in the hindfoot, *Am J Sports Med* 16:512, 1988.

19. Kristiansen B: Evan's repair of lateral instability of the ankle joint, *Acta Orthop Scand* 52:679, 1981.

20. Laurin A, Ouellet R, St-Jacques R: Talar and subtalar tilt: an experimental investigation, *Can J Surg* 11:270, 1968.

21. Manter JT: Movements of the subtalar and transverse tarsal joints, *Anat Rec* 80:397, 1941.

22. Mukherjee SK, Pringle RM, Baxter AD: Fracture of the lateral process of the talus: a report of thirteen cases, *J Bone Joint Surg* 56B:263, 1974.

23. Sarrafian S: *Anatomy of the foot and ankle*, Philadelphia, 1983, JB Lippincott.

24. Shelton ML, Pedowitz WJ: Injuries to the talus and midfoot. In Jahss MH, editor: *Disorders of the foot*, vol 2, Philadelphia, 1982, WB Saunders.

25. Stephens MM, Sammarco GJ: The stabilizing role of the lateral ligament complex around the ankle and subtalar joints, *Foot Ankle* 13:130, 1992.

26. Wright DG, Desai SM, Henderson WH: Action of the subtalar and ankle-joint complex during the stance phase of walking, *J Bone Joint Surg* 46A:361, 1964.

# Chapter 13

# Diagnostic and operative ankle arthroscopy

**Champ L. Baker, Jr.**
**J. Melvin Deese, Jr.**

## INDICATIONS FOR ARTHROSCOPIC SURGERY OF THE ANKLE

Injuries to the ankle are often diagnosed with an accurate, detailed history and a comprehensive clinical examination. Ancillary tests, such as radiographs, computed tomography (CT) scans, magnetic resonance imaging (MRI), bone scans, and arthrograms, can also be indicated in determining the cause of the patient's problem. However, the diagnosis of intraarticular lesions of the ankle, as in other major joints, is often made only upon direct visualization. Diagnostic and operative arthroscopy, with its shorter rehabilitation time, has proven extremely beneficial in helping athletes with knee, shoulder, and elbow injuries return to competition. In some instances the arthroscope can also assist the surgeon to complete the diagnosis and provide therapeutic treatment for traumatic disorders of the ankle.

Arthroscopy was first performed by the Japanese in 1918.[12] The first experimental use of the arthroscope in America was reported by Burman in the early 1930s.[5] Although the Japanese described a method of arthroscopic examination of the ankle in 1939,[14] it was not until the early 1970s that the standard portals were described and the first clinical experience with ankle arthroscopy was reported. Over the last several years, many authors have published their results of arthroscopic treatment of a wide variety of ankle disorders.* At this time the indications for ankle arthroscopy appear fairly clear. In athletes there are

three major indications for diagnostic and operative arthroscopy:

1. Removal of distal anterior osteophytes that develop following impaction injuries, especially in jumping sports
2. Diagnosis and operative treatment of loose bodies in the ankle—in particular, loose bodies from osteochondritis dissecans or transchondral talar dome fractures
3. Evaluation and treatment of posttraumatic synovitis of the ankle—in particular, anterolateral impingement.

Although there are other uses for the arthroscope, such as treatment of the arthritic ankle, use of the arthroscope in athletes has specific and limited application. At this time the arthroscope is not used to treat ligamentous instability in the ankle.

## OPERATIVE TECHNIQUE AND SETUP

Ankle arthroscopy is a surgical procedure performed with strict antiseptic control in the operating room with a local, regional, or general anesthetic. General anesthesia is most commonly used because it allows complete muscle relaxation and assures an optimal operative environment.

The position of the patient is determined by the surgeon; however, most surgeons prefer having the patient supine with the leg held loosely in a knee holder or placed over a bolster so that the knee can be flexed 90 degrees and the ankle draped freely (Fig. 13-1). This position allows the surgeon to either sit or

*References 1, 3, 7, 9, 10, 13.

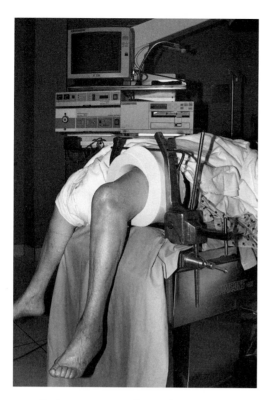

**Fig. 13-1.** Patient positioned on the table before ankle arthroscopy.

stand during surgery and allows access to either the anterior or posterior portals. Other positions are the straight supine position with the knee partly flexed and the foot and ankle free on the table or the decubitus position with the patient on his or her side.

A tourniquet is usually used, depending on the surgeon's preference. The bony landmarks of the ankle, including the medial and lateral malleolus, are outlined with a sterile marking pen. The central dorsalis pedis artery and the saphenous vein are palpated and outlined. The intermediate dorsal cutaneous branch of the superficial peroneal nerve is often outlined on the anterolateral spectrum of the ankle (Fig. 13-2). The ankle joint is marked, and the portals are outlined.

The three standard portals most commonly used for ankle arthroscopy are the anterolateral, anteromedial, and posterolateral portals. The anterior central, posteromedial, and trans Achilles portals are unnecessary and are considered dangerous because of their proximity to neurovascular structures.

### Anterolateral portal

The anterolateral portal is established just lateral to the common extensor tendon and the peroneus tertius tendon at the level of the tibiotalar joint (Fig. 13-3). The intermediate dorsal cutaneous branch of the superficial peroneal nerve courses obliquely across

the ankle and is in close proximity to this portal. Often it can be visualized under the skin and should be avoided to prevent postoperative sensory disturbances.

### Anteromedial portal

The anteromedial portal is established at the level of the tibiotalar joint just medial to the tibialis anterior tendon and lateral to the easily identified saphenous vein (Fig. 13-4).

### Posterolateral portal

An accessory portal may be indicated at times to increase inflow and to allow better evaluation of the posterior chamber when loose bodies are suspected. If it is needed, this portal is established at the level of the tibiotalar joint, lateral to the Achilles tendon, medial to the peroneal tendon, and central to the sural nerve and saphenous vein (Fig. 13-5).

### Distraction

Manual manipulation of the tibiotalar joint for distraction may be all that is needed for visualization of the "loose" ankle joint or the ankle with pathology in the anterior chamber. Most lesions requiring surgical intervention in athletes are located anteriorly, and manual or noninvasive distraction is adequate for visualization of the joint. If the athlete's ankle is tight, a posterior loose body or a posteromedial talar dome lesion can be difficult to reach, and some form of distraction may be needed.

Invasive pin distraction involves the lateral placement of pins into the tibia above and into the calcaneus below the joint and the use of a mechanical distractor to increase the joint space. If the distractor is placed on the medial side, it is in the tibia and talus (Fig. 13-6). However this type of distraction is thought to be disadvantageous when used in athletes. The drill holes in the distal tibia can serve as a stress riser, and a prolonged period of postoperative mobilization or protection may be necessary to prevent fracture of the tibia. When treating athletes in which the arthroscope is intended to facilitate rehabilitation, mechanical distractors may prove to do just the opposite.

Several methods of noninvasive distraction can be easily employed. The most commonly used method is straight manual distraction in which gravity and the surgeon's or assistant's hand pulls the joint apart (Fig. 13-7). The Kerlix Yates-Grana loop is a semicontrolled method of ankle distraction in which a gauze loop is used to distract the joint (Fig. 13-8).

Both the 4-mm, 30-degree angled arthroscope and the smaller 2.7-mm arthroscope (Fig. 13-9) provide excellent pictures in the ankle. In general, the larger arthroscope is preferred because it provides a larger,

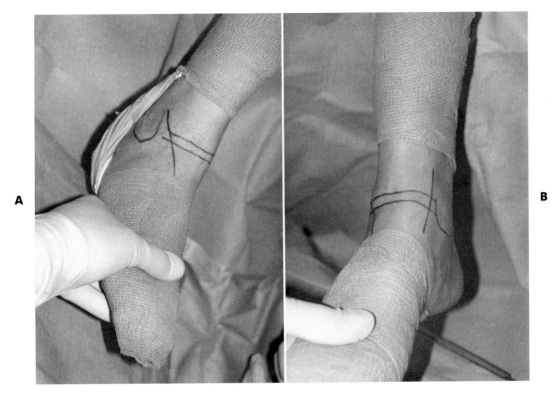

**Fig. 13-2. A,** Outline of lateral bony landmarks and peroneal nerve. **B,** Outline of medial bony landmarks and great saphenous vein.

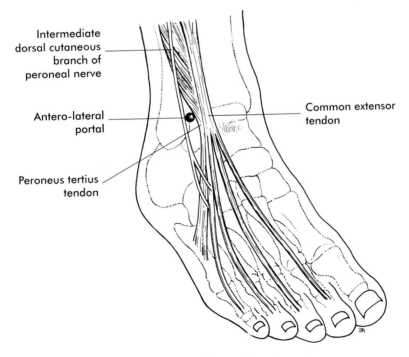

Intermediate dorsal cutaneous branch of peroneal nerve

Antero-lateral portal

Peroneus tertius tendon

Common extensor tendon

**Fig. 13-3.** Location of anterolateral portal.

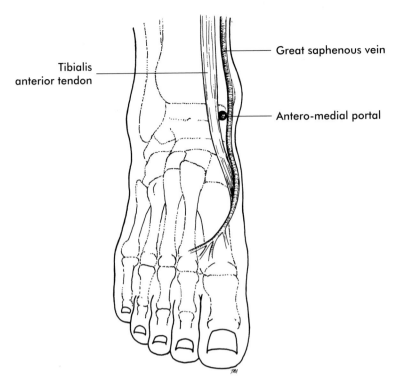

**Fig. 13-4.** Location of anteromedial portal.

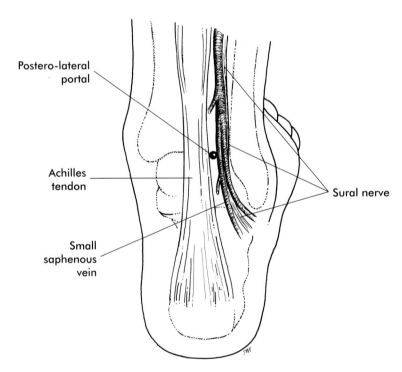

**Fig. 13-5.** Location of posterolateral portal.

clearer picture on the television monitor, and it has greater resistance to bending. The smaller 2.7-mm arthroscope provides a good picture and better visualization of the tight corners where the larger arthroscope is usually unable to pass. A television monitor and video recording equipment are routinely used for visualization and documentation of intraarticular disorders.

The surgeon may choose to use a pump to aid in distraction of the joint and improve irrigation flow.

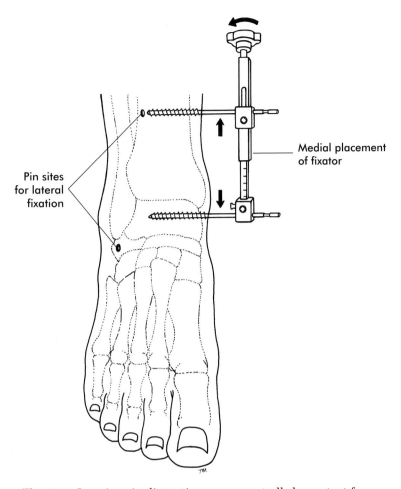

**Fig. 13-6.** Invasive pin distraction uses a controlled, constant force.

Standard instruments include probes, curettes, clamps, and motorized shavers and burrs.

### Arthroscopic technique

The patient is placed in the supine position on the operating table, and the end of the table is lowered allowing the knee to be flexed. The lower leg is prepared and draped with a sterile sleeve and is allowed to hang free over the end of the table. After the landmarks are identified and marked with a sterile pen, the tourniquet is inflated.

An 18-gauge needle is inserted through the anterolateral soft tissues into the joint, and 20 to 30 ml of irrigating solution is injected to distend the joint (Fig. 13-10). Removal of the stylet of the needle to confirm backflow ensures that the joint is distended. A #11 blade knife is used to incise the skin, and a hemostat is used to spread the soft tissues and move the sensory nerves out of the way (Fig. 13-11). Use of a cannula system is best because it allows more than one portal to be used simultaneously without losing position. Cannulas without side portals should be used in the ankle to prevent extrava-

sation of fluid. A dull trocar is placed through the cannula and inserted through the anterolateral portal into the joint. The capsule of the joint is thin, and entry into the joint is easily obtained. After fluid coming through the cannula confirms the presence of the trocar in the joint, the arthroscope can be inserted into the joint.

Next an 18-gauge needle is inserted into the anteromedial portal. Its proper placement is ensured by viewing the entry on the television monitor (Fig. 13-12). Again, a stab incision is made in the skin, and soft tissues are spread by a hemostat. A second cannula is then brought through the anteromedial portal. The opposite portal can be used for a probe or for a secondary inflow cannula.

Systematic examination of the joint is then carried out as the arthroscope is directed from the anterolateral chamber to visualize the distal fibula and tibiotalar articulation to the anterolateral portion of the joint. Next the surgeon looks across the tibiotalar joint to the inner margin of the medial malleolus (Fig. 13-13). By moving the arthroscope, the entire medial mortise can be seen. The arthroscope can then be switched to the anteromedial portal to complete the examination, looking from medial to lateral. Depending on the patient's preoperative symptoms and clinical examination, the sites of suspected lesions are the anterolateral joint where the talus articulates with the distal tibia and the inner margin of the fibula. This is a common site for the development of thickened, fibrotic soft tissue, the so-called meniscoid lesion. This area of impingement commonly produces symptoms in the patient with posttraumatic persistent synovitis. The anterolateral surface of the talus, as well as the posteromedial talar dome, are the most common donor sites for softening fibrillation or frank separation of chondral fractures of the talus. These surfaces must be observed and probed. The ankle is manually distracted and brought into maximal dorsiflexion and plantar flexion to allow the surgeon to visualize and probe these areas completely.

Next the surgeon visualizes the distal anterior tibia and the corresponding area on the anterior talus as the foot is brought into forced dorsiflexion. An increased bony buildup on the distal tibia and the dorsal talus may be the site of lesions related to "kissing exostoses."

Loose bodies may be free-floating in the joint. The surgeon must look and palpate posteriorly in an attempt to induce loose bodies to float to the anterior

chamber where they can be more easily grasped and removed.

### Postoperative course

Operative arthroscopy of the ankle in athletes is performed as an outpatient procedure. After completion of the procedure, the entry wounds are either sutured with a single stitch or covered with a Band-aid. A bulky sterile wrap is applied, and the patient is returned to the recovery room. Ice is used to minimize

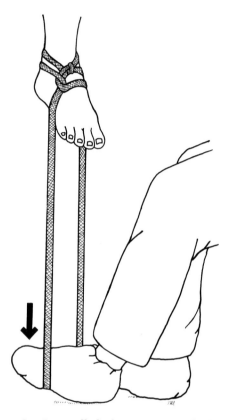

**Fig. 13-8.** Semicontrolled distraction method of Yates-Grana in which a loop of gauze dressing is held by the surgeon's foot.

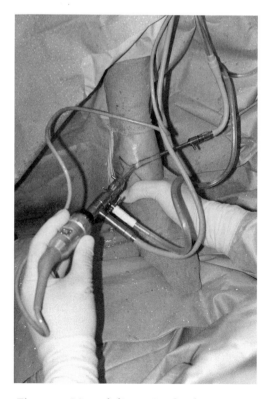

**Fig. 13-7.** Manual distraction by the surgeon.

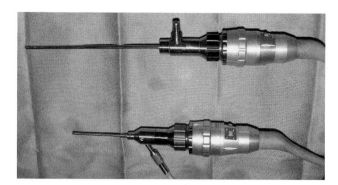

**Fig. 13-9.** A 4-mm, 30-degree angled arthroscope *(top)*. A 2.7-mm, 30-degree angled arthroscope *(bottom)*.

swelling. In the immediate postoperative period, the patient begins active-assistive range-of-motion exercises and resistive exercises. Initially weight bearing is protected until full motion is returned. Depending on the status of the articular surface, the patient may then begin unprotected weight bearing.

Patients are allowed to progress in their rehabilitation program after they achieve painless, full range of motion, and return of strength without swelling.

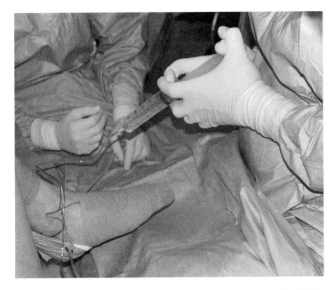

**Fig. 13-10.** An 18-gauge needle is used to introduce fluid for distension.

## Complications

Complications associated with ankle arthroscopy range from 10% to 15%.[11] These complications include sensory disturbances from either temporary or permanent damage to the sensory cutaneous nerve on the lateral aspect of the ankle. This damage can be avoided by proper marking of the nerve preoperatively and use of hemostats to spread soft tissues.

If the foot is largely dependent following the procedure, persistent swelling and drainage can lead to postoperative infection. Several measures should be taken at the completion of the procedure to avoid these problems. The surgeon should elevate the patient's leg postoperatively and place a protective wrap on the ankle, as well as ensure that there are no frank arterial bleeders. The tourniquet should be deflated to assure that hemostasis is achieved before wrapping the ankle. In addition, the use of noninvasive distractors is recommended for athletes, because drilling across the distal tibia or through the calcaneus can serve as a stress riser for fracture. It also lessens the chance for pin tract infection.

## SPECIFIC INDICATIONS IN THE ATHLETE
### Arthroscopic treatment of anterior osteophytes in the ankle

**Case Study 1.** A 21-year-old female collegiate all-American gymnast presented with a history of pain associated with her floor routine and dismounts from the vault. Although she was able to successfully complete her senior

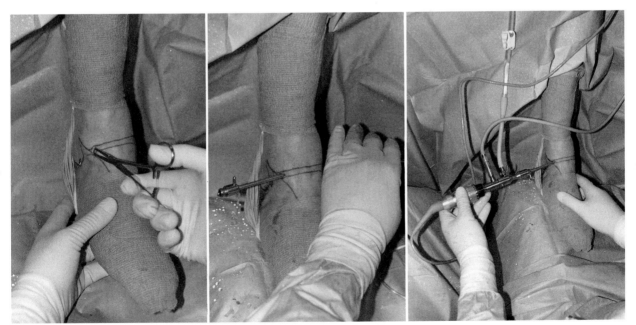

**A**                                                                                                    **B, C**

**Fig. 13-11. A,** A hemostat spreads the portal to avoid nerve damage. **B,** The cannula is introduced (note backflow fluid). **C,** The arthroscope with irrigation and camera attachment is introduced through the anterolateral portal.

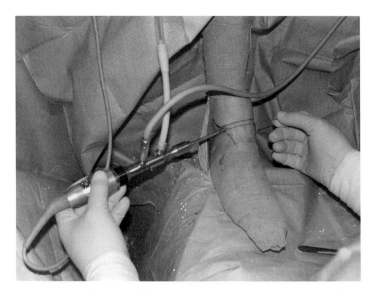

**Fig. 13-12.** A needle is used for the placement of the anteromedial portal.

year, arrangements were made for the floor routine and vaulting to be eliminated from her schedule when her ankle was severely symptomatic. Radiographs confirmed the presence of an anterior talar spur. Following her collegiate career, and as workouts were increased in preparation for the Olympic trials, her symptoms precluded adequate training.

We elected to approach the spur arthroscopically. The lesion was easily seen through an anterolateral portal and consisted largely of an anterior talar osteophyte that was raised, well-rounded, and consistent with chronic irritation. Using the motorized abrader, the bony protuberance was removed without difficulty. The area was smoothed, and passive dorsiflexion showed no contact at the tibiotalar articulation. The patient maintained partial weight bearing for 2 weeks and returned to gymnastics within 4 weeks. She has not experienced further difficulty with her ankle for the past 5 years.

**Diagnosis.** Osteophytes projecting from the anterior portion of the tibia or the talus can develop in the ankle. The growth can be osseous or cartilaginous and can cause impingement during forced dorsiflexion of the ankle. These osteophytes are the result of repeated localized trauma to the athlete's foot as it is subjected to repetitive and prolonged forced dorsiflexion. The osteophyte can develop from an injury or a sudden forceful trauma.[9] Runners, dancers, gymnasts, and high jumpers are prone to develop this type of sports-related injury. The articular cartilage covering the end of the talus and the distal tibia receives the blow as a shock absorber. When the jumping athlete lands and his body weight forces the foot into dorsiflexion, the localized area of stress can cause damage to the articular surface. This surface may fissure and crack and, as nature attempts to heal the damage, a protuberance may develop that can be a chronic source of pain.

With the development of the localized osteophyte or spur, motion is limited, jumping and running sports exacerbate the patient's symptoms, and even going up and down stairs can become a problem. In most cases normal gait is not affected. Symptoms are present only when the osteophyte acts as an irritant and may be related to an increase in activity.

Examination may reveal puffiness around the anterior ankle joint with pain on forced dorsiflexion, and there may be limitation of motion compared with the contralateral ankle. The marked area of tenderness over the osteophyte often can be palpated on either the anterior talus or the distal anterior tibia. At times, both the distal tibia and the anterior talus can develop spurs and present as "kissing exostoses."

If a history of pain on landing is provided by the running or jumping athlete, the diagnosis can be readily made. Plain radiographs usually show the osteophyte on a lateral view (Fig. 13-14). Weight-bearing lateral views may be taken to show the contact point. Although further studies are usually not needed, CT arthrography may be indicated in patients with symptoms, such as those of an anterior spur, to rule out talar lesions or to look for loose bodies that may have developed secondary to the contact area.

The treatment is usually symptomatic. An effort is made to increase the flexibility of the ankle and improve range of motion, which helps to decrease swelling and other symptoms. Rest is beneficial; however, the symptoms often recur when the patient returns to the jumping activity. Nonsteroidal antiinflammatory medications and local treatments, such as heat and ultrasound, provide temporary relief only.

Surgical removal of the spur with abrasion of the area is the treatment of choice. Arthroscopic evalua-

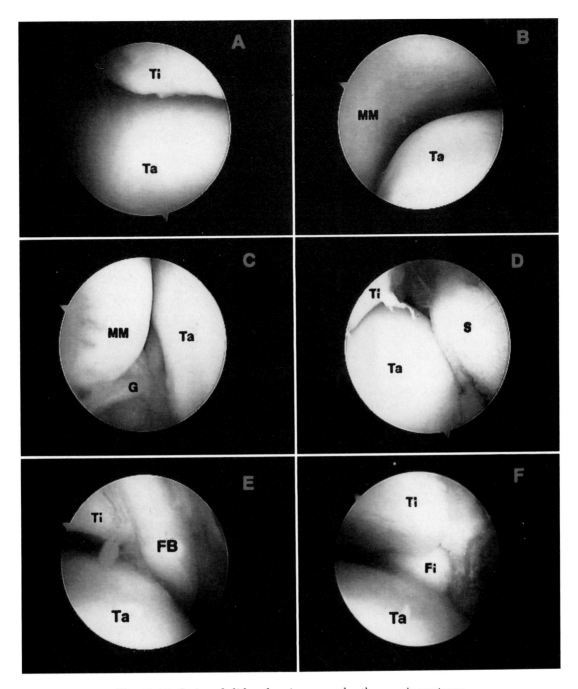

**Fig. 13-13.** Series of slides showing normal arthroscopic anatomy.

tion to identify the spur and then debridement has been a successful method of treating this lesion.[9]

Preoperative planning reveals the location of the spur as either anterior on the tibia or on the talus. Standard anterolateral and anteromedial portals are used, and the instruments are placed in the portal closest to the lesion. The initial examination may identify the lesion, although increased synovial proliferation of the joint secondary to repeated trauma often obscures the spur. If so, a limited synovectomy should be carried out. The arthroscope is first placed in the anterolateral portal with the shaver in the anteromedial portal, and synovial tissue in the anteromedial chamber is debrided. The instruments are then reversed in the portals to clean out the anterolateral chamber and the lateral gutter. A probe may be needed to palpate the anterior distal tibia or look more distally over the talus to view the bony protuberance. With forced dorsiflexion, the point of contact can often be readily identified.

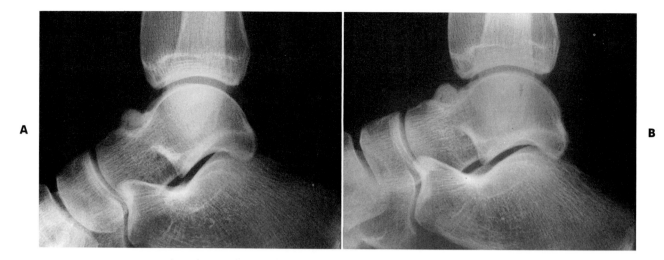

A

B

**Fig. 13-14. A,** Anterior talar osteophyte with the ankle in neutral position. **B,** Anterior osteophyte with the ankle in forced dorsiflexion.

A variety of instruments can be used to remove the mass. Initially a ring curette may be indicated to remove the height of the spur, whereas larger spurs may be removed by a small straight or curved osteotome. Once the osteophyte has broken loose, a clamp is brought in through the opposite portal to remove the bone fragment. A motorized shaver is used to remove soft tissue from around the spur, and either a soft tissue resector or a burr can be used to abrade the area and remove the remainder of the bone. A small arthroscopic burr may be used for this. It is important to reshape the anterior tibia or talus to its original contour, although with excessive abrasion, the surface may become concave. Radiographs can be taken intraoperatively to confirm adequate removal of the osteophyte.

Postoperatively the patient is maintained on a non–weight-bearing regimen until full motion is restored. At that time the patient progresses to gait, running, and ultimately a return to jumping sports. Usually 6 to 8 weeks is required for full return to jumping athletics.

### Arthroscopic treatment of transcondylar talar dome fractures of the ankle

**Case Study 2.** This 20-year-old male member of a collegiate tennis team presented with complaints of catching and popping in both ankles. The patient related a history of repeated ankle sprains over several years but did not have complaints of giving way or instability of his ankles. Clinical examination revealed an increased varus laxity of both ankles with mild swelling and puffiness around the ankles. There was tenderness to palpation over the anterolateral joint line and over the talus with the foot held in inverted plantar flexion. Stress radiographs revealed a 10-degree varus tilt and a negative anterior drawer bilaterally.

A separated osteochondral fragment was seen in the anterolateral aspect of the talus of both ankles.

Because of his symptoms, this scholar athlete was unable to continue playing. He underwent arthroscopic evaluation of his left ankle with removal of loose fragments and debridement and curettement of the donor site. He was then placed in an aggressive rehabilitation program for stretching, strengthening, and proprioceptive exercises.

A similar procedure was performed on the contralateral leg 2 months after the initial procedure. Following his rehabilitation the patient resumed competitive tennis 2 months after the second procedure. He has remained asymptomatic for 3 years.

Loose bodies in the ankle were first called **osteochondritis dissecans** by Kappis in 1922, as cited in Berndt and Harty. Berndt and Harty,[4] in the late 1950s, began using the term *transchondral talar dome fractures* to describe posttraumatic medial and lateral talar lesions. They were able to reproduce these fractures in the laboratory and were the first to use the term *transchondral fractures,* which is specific to both the traumatic etiology of the lesions and to the anatomical locations. Four stages of fracture were produced in the laboratory with lateral lesions produced by inversion and dorsiflexion of the ankle, and medial lesions were produced by inversion and plantar flexion with external rotation of the tibia on the talus (Figs. 13-15 and 13-16).

The classification of transchondral fractures ranges from stage I, a small area of compression of subchondral bone, to stage IV, a displaced osteochondral fracture. Patients often have a history of trauma, although the injury may have occurred several weeks or months before presentation. The diagnosis is rarely made acutely, and often symptoms do not occur until several weeks or months after the injury. Symptoms

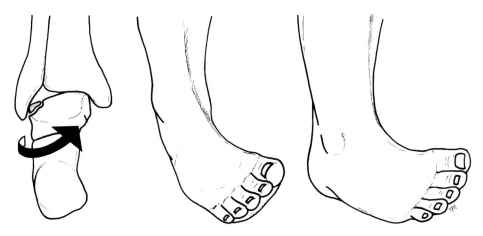

**Fig. 13-15.** Dorsiflexion and inversion mechanism produces a lateral talar dome fracture.

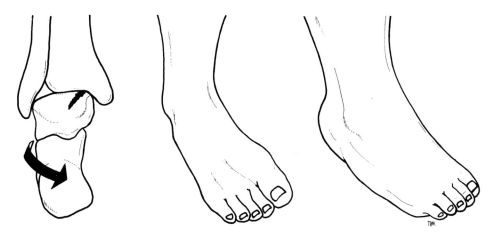

**Fig. 13-16.** Plantar flexion and inversion mechanism produces a medial talar dome fracture.

usually include pain with weight bearing and catching, snapping, and intermittent swelling in the ankle. Clinical examination may reveal tenderness over the anteromedial or anterolateral joint line, and there may be an increase in both anterior drawer and varus stress. Effusion may be present, although the patient may exhibit surprisingly few clinical signs.

Routine anteroposterior, lateral, and mortise x-ray views often demonstrate the lesion's anterolateral or posteromedial location (Fig. 13-17). Tomography may be beneficial (particularly in the lateral projection) in locating the posterior lesion, and CT scans help to reveal the size and precise location of the loose body. MRI also can be helpful in delineating these lesions.

Nonsurgical treatment is recommended for stage I and stage II lesions. Initially stage III and stage IV lesions can be treated nonsurgically with protective mobilization (e.g., splints) and partial weight bearing with progression to full weight bearing, depending on the patient's symptoms. Rehabilitative exercises directed at regaining full range of motion and strength are then initiated. The decision to operate is based on the patient's clinical picture and failure to respond to

nonsurgical treatment. Continued pain, catching, and the inability to participate in sports are the primary surgical indications in patients with a stage III or stage IV lesion.

Before the advent of arthroscopy, removal of loose bodies by arthrotomy was the procedure of choice. Lateral lesions were easily found through an anterolateral approach; however, posteromedial osteophytes often required a more complicated approach and a medial malleolar osteotomy was needed for adequate exposure to the lesion. Arthroscopy is an excellent means of dealing with these talar lesions and preventing the potential complications and morbidity of an open procedure or an osteotomy.

The standard arthroscopic setup and portals are used. The arthroscope is placed in the anteromedial portal, and a probe is inserted through the anterolateral portal. With dorsiflexion and plantar flexion of the ankle, the anterolateral lesion can usually be seen at the anterior lip of the tibiotalar articulation. Most lesions are soft, and the cartilage is fibrillated. The flap can be easily lifted and removed. A ring curette is then used for curettement of the bed, and a motorized

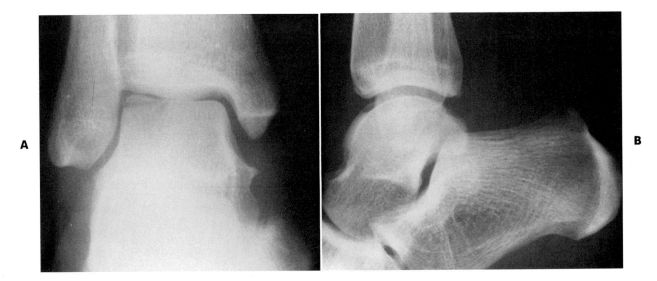

**Fig. 13-17. A,** AP radiograph showing an anterolateral talar dome fracture. **B,** Lateral view of an anterolateral talar dome fracture.

shaver or burr may be used to abrade the bone down to bleeding subchondral bone. This usually allows enough bleeding from small vessels that drilling of the bed with K-wires or a drill is not needed.

Posteromedial lesions can be more difficult to reach, particularly in a tight ankle. In these instances invasive distraction with pins through the distal tibia and the os calcis may be needed. Protective mobilization is required following insertion of pins. However since patients must remain on non–weight-bearing status for several weeks after the debridement of a lesion on an articular surface, invasive distraction does not slow their rehabilitation.

Regardless of the type of distraction used, the posteromedial lesion can best be seen through the anterolateral portal with the probe inserted through the anteromedial portal. The ankle is placed in marked plantar flexion to allow the lesion, which usually lies along the medial edge of the talus, to be seen. Medial lesions are more likely to be seated in the crater and can be lifted with the probe or curette. As with treatment of lateral lesions, the bed is abraded or drilled to promote bleeding.

Postoperatively, the patient begins range-of-motion exercises and remains non–weight bearing until the swelling subsides and painless range of motion is achieved. The patient can usually begin partial weight bearing and resume full weight bearing within 6 months. Excellent-to-good results can be expected in 70% to 90% of patients with transchondral talar dome fractures that are treated arthroscopically with partial synovectomy, debridement of chondral lesions, removal of loose fragments, curettage abrasion, or drilling.[3,13] These results are even more rewarding when compared with the previous method of treatment of these lesions, the arthrotomy or medial malleolar osteotomy.

**Arthroscopic treatment of ankle impingement**

**Case Study 3.** A 19-year-old collegiate baseball pitcher was involved in a motor vehicle accident and sustained trauma to his right hip. He also had complaints of discomfort in his left ankle. He had a contusion of the soft tissues of the hip, which responded rapidly to nonoperative treatment. However 3 weeks after the accident, he developed catching and popping in his left ankle with pain on weight bearing. Radiographs were negative, and the patient was placed on antiinflammatory medication and a strengthening and stretching rehabilitation program for his left ankle with appropriate bracing. Two months after the injury, this right-handed pitcher was unable to resume pitching. He experienced discomfort in his left ankle as he came down on it during the follow through of his pitching motion.

Arthroscopic examination of the ankle revealed a large hypertrophic synovial band that appeared to be trapped between the tibia and talus when his foot went into forced dorsiflexion. No other abnormalities were noted. A limited synovectomy was performed using an arthroscopic motorized shaver system. The patient's symptoms abated quickly, and he returned to pitching without symptoms in 4 weeks. The patient pitched during the next season with no difficulty related to his ankle.

Arthroscopy has proven highly beneficial in the treatment of soft tissue injuries around the ankle following trauma.[7,8,10,11] The development of anterior osteophytes, loose bodies, or osteochondral fracture fragments in the ankle can be readily identified on radiographs. A more difficult diagnosis is one in which persistent synovitis and fibrotic lesions develop in the anterolateral aspect of the ankle after trauma. Patients may have a stable ankle and negative radiographs after nonsurgical treatment but have persistent complaints of intermittent catching, swelling, and pain. Entrapment of the synovium, particularly the anterolateral tibiotalar articulation, may be producing the symptoms. Wolin described this fibrotic enlargement in the lateral aspect of the ankle as a meniscoid type of scar tissue, and he recommended open excision and arthrotomy. Although the true meniscoid-type picture is rare, entrapment of synovial tissue, fibrotic meniscoid tissue, or impingement of accessory bands, particularly in the lateral aspect of the ankle, have been reported with increasing frequency over the last several years.[2,7,10] Recognition of these lesions increased with the advent of ankle arthroscopy. Anterolateral ankle impingement is a well-described syndrome that occurs in athletes and can hinder performance.

Patients usually have a history of a blow or twisting injury to the ankle that does not result in a ligamentous laxity and was thought to be no more than a minor sprain. Regardless of the treatment, whether immobilization or functional mobilization, discomfort may persist in the anterolateral portion of the ankle, particularly with weight bearing and forced dorsiflexion of the ankle. Localized swelling can occur if the patient presents with discomfort of the anterolateral aspect of the ankle and complains of pain with weight bearing. Radiographs, tomography, and CT scans are usually normal. MRI may show an increase of soft tissue mass in the anterolateral aspect of the ankle but is not uniformly reliable for diagnosis of this entity.

Initial treatment is nonsurgical and consists of stretching of the Achilles tendon, strengthening of the anterior tibial and peroneal musculature, and appropriate protective braces or splints. Nonsteroidal antiinflammatory medications can help, and a local steroid injection at the site of tenderness may diminish the pain and be effective in eliminating the symptoms. However patients who have failed a 3-month or longer course of treatment and have continued to be disabled are candidates for arthroscopic evaluation and probable synovectomy.

The standard arthroscopic setup and instrumentation is used. After the arthroscope is introduced through the anterolateral portal and established through the anteromedial portal, evaluation of the anterior chamber of the ankle is carried out. Invasive distraction is not usually necessary. A minimal synovectomy may be needed initially to decompress the anterior chamber and better visualize the articulation of the talus on the tibia in flexion. Entrapment-

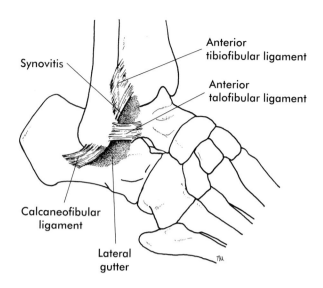

**Fig. 13-18.** Area of soft tissue entrapment of the anterolateral ankle and lateral gutter.

type lesions are most often found in the anterolateral aspect of the ankle in the region of the talofibular articulation (Fig. 13-18). An accessory ligament presents as a space-occupying lesion in this area, running from the distal tibia to the talus. It is thought to be a variant of the meniscoid-type lesion, which also occurs here.

With the arthroscope in the anteromedial portal, a motorized shaver is inserted through the anterolateral portal, and a partial synovectomy of the anterolateral joint is carried out. Care is taken to decompress the anterolateral gutter, as well as clean out the chamber from the talus proximal to the tibia. Inspection is performed for softening of cartilage, talar dome fractures, loose bodies, as well as for talar or tibial spurs. The spurs can be removed at this time.

A tourniquet is usually used for this procedure, but it can be deflated so that individual bleeders can be cauterized with an arthroscopic Bovie to prevent hemarthrosis and recurrence of fibrosis of the synovium in this area.

Following the synovectomy, efforts are made to decrease postoperative swelling and recurrent synovitis. The portals are sutured, and a bulky pressure wrap is applied. The patient is instructed to keep the leg elevated and compressed for the first 48 hours following surgery. If inspection of the wound at that time reveals minimal swelling, the patient is allowed to begin an active-assistive range-of-motion and strengthening program and touch-down weight bearing. The patient progresses to partial and full weight bearing as motion and strength return. After 10 to 14 days, during which the patient is partially disabled, athletes can resume light agility drills.

Results of arthroscopic decompression have been

uniformly good to excellent in 80% to 90% of carefully selected patients in whom true abnormalities exist. Alleviating symptoms by this arthroscopic approach has been particularly successful in running athletes, such as soccer players and basketball players.

## REFERENCES

1. Andrews JR, Previte WJ, Carson WG: Arthroscopy of the ankle: technique and normal anatomy, *Foot Ankle* 6:29, 1985.
2. Baker CL, Graham JM: Current concepts in ankle arthroscopy, *Orthopedics* 16:1027, 1993.
3. Baker CL, Andrews JR, Ryan JB: Arthroscopic treatment of transchondral talar dome fractures, *J Arthroscop Rel Surg* 2:82, 1986.
4. Berndt AL, Harty M: Transchondral fractures (osteochondritis dissecans) of the talus, *J Bone Joint Surg* 41A:988, 1959.
5. Burman MS: Arthroscopy of direct visualization of joints: an experimental cadaver study, *J Bone Joint Surg* 13:669, 1931.
6. Chen YC: Arthroscopy of the ankle joint. In Watanabe M, editor: *Arthroscopy of small joints*, Tokyo, 1985, Igaku-Shoin, p 104.
7. Ferkel RD et al: Arthroscopic treatment of anterolateral impingement of the ankle, *Am J Sports Med* 19:440, 1991.
8. Ferkel RD, Fischer SP: Progress in ankle arthroscopy, *Clin Orthop* 240:210, 1989.
9. Hawkins RB: Arthroscopic treatment of sports-related anterior osteophytes in the ankle, *Foot Ankle* 9:87, 1988.
10. Martin DF, Curl WW, Baker CL: Arthroscopic treatment of chronic synovitis of the ankle, *Arthroscopy* 5:110, 1989.
11. Martin DF et al: Operative ankle arthroscopy. Long-term followup, *Am J Sports Med* 17:16, 1989.
12. O'Connor RL: *Arthroscopy*, Kalamazoo, 1977, Upjohn.
13. Parisien JS: Arthroscopic treatment of osteochondral lesions of the talus, *Am J Sports Med* 14:211, 1986.
14. Parisien JS: Arthroscopy of the ankle: state of the art, *Contemp Orthop* 5:21, 1982.

# Chapter 14

# Plantar heel pain

**Glenn B. Pfeffer**

Plantar heel pain is one of the most common foot problems in the athlete. Sports requiring running and jumping place repetitive stress on the heel and create an overuse syndrome with chronic inflammation. Often it is difficult to determine the exact etiology of the heel pain as several different underlying problems can present in a similar fashion. The complex anatomy of the heel requires one to differentiate among several potentially pathologic structures that lie within a few square centimeters. The ability to effect a cure correlates with the precision of the diagnosis.

Focal causes of plantar heel pain include:

1. Fat pad atrophy
2. Plantar fascial rupture
3. Heel pain syndrome (HPS)
4. Plantar fasciitis
5. Tendinitis of the flexor hallucis longus, flexor digitorum longus, or both
6. Nerve entrapment: *(a)* tarsal tunnel syndrome, *(b)* first branch of the lateral plantar nerve
7. Stress fracture of the calcaneus
8. Tumor

In differentiating these diagnoses, a comprehensive physical examination and medical history are essential. The history should include the patient's general medical condition, exact location and duration of pain and whether it radiates, and relationship of pain to athletic activity—particularly those requiring running and jumping. The runner's symptoms may be further aggravated by hill running and sprinting. Many athletes are able to work out despite the pain, only to have it recur with increased severity when they are through. Radiculopathy in the L5-S1 distribution should be considered in a patient with back pain and a peripheral neuropathy ruled out when heel pain is diffuse and bilateral. The seronegative spondyloarthropathies should be considered in a patient with bilateral heel pain.[8] Chronic pain at rest is an unusual presentation for plantar heel pain, and a tumor of the calcaneus may be the etiology.

## THE FAT PAD

The heel pad cushions the foot with each heel strike. A healthy middle-aged man has a gait velocity of approximately 82 m/minute and a cadence of 116. This rate results in 58 heel strikes per minute with a force of up to 110% of body weight. A sprinter does not place a direct increased stress on the heel, but a middle- or long-distance runner may generate a force of up to 200% of body weight. Considering timing, impact forces, and average heel pain area (23 cm), the loading pressure of a 70-kg man is approximately 9.3 $kg/cm^2$ when running.

Anatomic studies of the human heel pad have identified structural specialization capable of meeting these high impacts.[11] The anatomy of the heel pad was first described by Tietze in 1921.[24] He emphasized the specialized anatomy of the heel pad, with elastic adipose tissue organized as spiral-formed fibrous tissue septa anchored to one another, the calcaneus, and the skin. Designed to resist compressive loads, the tissue septa are U-shaped or comma-shaped fat-filled columns with a vertical orientation. The septa are reinforced internally with elastic transverse and diagonal fibers that connect the thicker walls and separate the fat into compartments or cells. The thickness of the heel pad is the most important factor in determining the stresses seen in the tissues beneath it.[10] After the age of 40 the adipose tissue usually begins to gradually deteriorate, with the insidious loss

Plantar aponeurosis

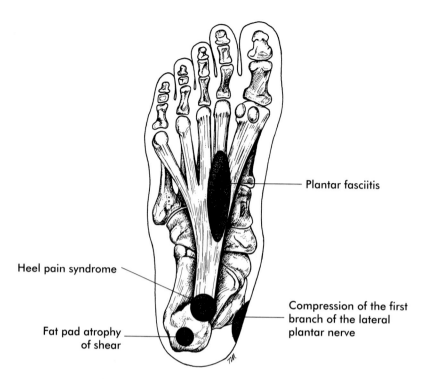

Plantar fasciitis

Heel pain syndrome

Compression of the first
branch of the lateral
plantar nerve

Fat pad atrophy
of shear

**Fig. 14-1.** Focal causes of plantar heel pain.

of collagen, elastic tissue, water, and overall thickness of the heel pad. The result is an inescapable softening and thinning in the heel pad and a concomitant loss of shock absorbency. Some patients experience these changes earlier.

An athlete with heel pain secondary to fat pad atrophy usually complains of diffuse plantar heel discomfort aggravated by sports on harder surfaces, such as a basketball court or cinder track. By clinical examination the patient has soft, flattened heel pads that allow easy palpation of the calcaneal tubercles. Compression of this area by the examiner duplicates the symptoms, with pain maximal over the central weight-bearing portion of the heel pad. There is no radiation of the pain, and the plantar fascia is not tender. The area of maximal tenderness is proximal and central on the heel (Fig. 14-1). There is no surgical treatment for this condition, and the athletic patient's symptoms are best treated with a cushioned heel cup and a shock-absorbent sneaker. A plastic heel cup that elevates the heel may be helpful both by protecting the painful area and by shifting some of the weight bearing more anteriorly. Swimming or biking usually does not aggravate this condition.

## HEEL PAIN SYNDROME

The most common site for plantar heel pain is where the plantar fascia and intrinsic muscles arise

from the medial calcaneal tuberosity on the antero-medial aspect of the heel[23] (Fig. 14-1). During sports activities, particularly long-distance running, the plantar fascia places repetitive traction upon this area. The plantar fascia arises predominantly from the medial calcaneal tuberosity and inserts distally through several slips into the plantar plates of the metatarsophalangeal joints, the flexor tendon sheaths, and the base of the proximal phalanges of the digits.[9,19] When the metatarsophalangeal joints are dorsiflexed with running or jumping, the inelastic plantar fascial fibers place traction on the calcaneus.[9]

Over time, microtears can occur in the plantar fascia near the medial calcaneal tuberosity. A repara-tive inflammatory response develops, along with continued traumatic fatigue in the fascia. Surgical biopsy specimens of the origin of the plantar fascia in athletes with chronic heel pain reveal collagen necro-sis, angiofibroblastic hyperplasia, chondroid metapla-sia, and matrix calcification. Periostitis of the medial calcaneal tuberosity frequently occurs in conjunction with degenerative changes in the plantar fascia, causing a positive delayed technetium-99 bone scan in the majority of painful heels.[28]

Because of the close proximity of the medial calcaneal tuberosity and the origin of the plantar fascia, it is not possible to differentiate clinically a fascial or bony source of an athlete's pain. Both

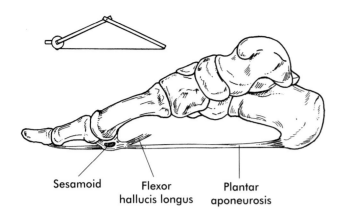

Sesamoid    Flexor              Plantar
            hallucis longus     aponeurosis

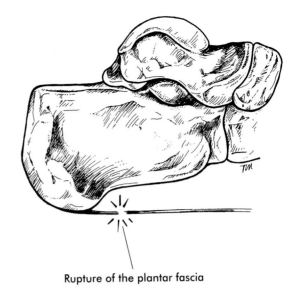

Rupture of the plantar fascia

**Fig. 14-3.** Rupture of plantar fascia.

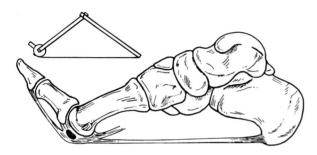

**Fig. 14-2.** Windlass mechanism.

structures are usually involved; thus HPS is the best description for a heel that is painful in this area.[23] Patients may have local soft tissue swelling and focal tenderness over the medial calcaneal tuberosity directly and the plantar fascia distally for several millimeters. The examiner frequently must apply a considerable amount of pressure to localize the painful area. Interestingly patients almost never have increased pain or duplication of symptoms with passive dorsiflexion of the toes, which causes traction on the plantar fascia by the Windlass mechanism (Fig. 14-2). Associated tightness of the Achilles tendon is commonly seen with this condition, because limited ankle dorsiflexion places increased stress on the plantar fascia.

HPS is insidious in onset and is most frequently seen as an overuse condition of long-distance runners.[22] In athletes with an acute onset of symptoms, rupture of the plantar fascia should be considered[14] (Fig. 14-3). Rupture is much less common than chronic HPS and can easily be differentiated on the basis of physical examination and history. A palpable defect in the plantar fascia is present when a rupture occurs. An old partial rupture of the plantar fascia can present with a palpable nodularity in the fascia near the medial calcaneal tuberosity.

Athletes with HPS usually experience symptoms during the first minutes of walking, especially in the

morning when first out of bed. The pain gradually decreases. Discomfort is intensified by athletic activity, especially jumping or running. Some athletes have symptoms only during periods of prolonged running. It is not unusual for athletes to complain of heel pain that occurs only during the first few miles of a workout. No clear correlation between HPS and pes planus or pes cavus has been established. A positive correlation with obesity exists, although most athletic patients do not have this concern. A lateral x-ray of the heel will exclude a stress fracture or tumor of the calcaneus. Even among high-performance athletes, a stress fracture is extremely rare.

Leg lengths should always be examined when evaluating athletes with chronic heel pain. If one leg is longer than the other, often there is a history of repeated injury to the shorter leg. Heel pain is more frequently seen in the shorter leg and may be treated effectively with an appropriate lift. A functional short-leg syndrome can result from running on the same tilt of road or in the same direction on the track. In both instances, after many miles of training, one heel will be more stressed than the other. By using both sides of the road or intermittently changing directions on a training track, stress between both heels can be equalized.

The cornerstone of conservative treatment in athletes is modification in training. Mileage reduction, alternating activities, work reduction, and shortened workouts should be considered.[15] Low-resistance cycling and swimming pool running are effective cardiovascular activities that are usually not stressful to the heel. Oral antiinflammatory agents, contrast baths, ice massage, and soft-soled shoes or sneakers are also used. If the athletic patient has Achilles

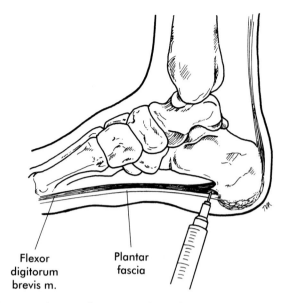

**Fig. 14-4.** A steroid injection from the medial side of the heel. To avoid steroid-induced atrophy of the fat pad, the solution is injected deep into the plantar fascia. The heel spur arises within the origin of the flexor digitorum brevis muscle.

*Flexor digitorum brevis m.*

*Plantar fascia*

tightness, tendon and plantar fascia stretching exercises should be instituted. A shock-absorbent heel cup is also an appropriate first line of treatment. Low dye taping and a one-eighth-inch medial heel wedge may be added in an attempt to reduce the stress on the plantar fascia. A molded plastic ankle-foot orthosis with the ankle fixed in 5 degrees of dorsiflexion may also be indicated. Using this technique, Wapner et al had a 79% success rate after an average of 4 months of splint use.[27] In refractory cases a short-leg cast for 6 weeks followed by a custom-made orthosis may help break a painful cycle.

In athletes with refractory symptoms, a steroid injection is often beneficial. Care should be taken to inject the steroid deep to the plantar fascia so as not to cause atrophy of the fat pad. A medial approach of the injection is best used so the steroid can be spread along the broad origin of the plantar fascia. The needle is walked across the anterior border of the calcaneus just deep to the plantar fascia, thereby avoiding the plantar nerves (Fig. 14-4). Multiple steroid injections may predispose the athletic patient to plantar fascia rupture and should be avoided.[21] The majority of patients respond to these conservative measures. A patient may have some persistent symptoms for up to 6 months, but only 4 to 6 weeks will usually be lost from training or competitive athletics if treatment is started early.

Historically the calcaneal spur was of great importance in the treatment of heel pain. In 1963, however, Tanz demonstrated that only 50% of patients with

plantar heel pain had a heel spur and that 16% of nonpainful heels also had a heel spur.[25] Rubin and Whitten determined that same year that only 10% of patients with heel spurs were symptomatic.[18] Two years later Lapidus and Guidotti showed that the successful treatment of heel pain was not contingent upon the surgical removal of a heel spur and concluded that plantar calcaneal spurs "do not cause the painful heel, as they have been postulated."[13] Subsequent studies have determined that the heel spur arises deep to the plantar fascia in the non–weight-bearing substance of the flexor brevis muscle.

In those few patients who fail prolonged conservative treatment, surgical release of the plantar fascia should be considered. Every attempt, however, should be made to avoid this procedure in competitive athletes. Release of the plantar fascia may have a detrimental effect on function. A recent study demonstrated a change both in arch height and the ratio of arch height to arch length following a plantar fascia release.[6] A less energetic pattern of walking following a plantar fascia release was also seen. Further, if the plantar fascia is divided surgically, increased compressive forces are transmitted to the dorsal aspect of the midfoot, with decreased flexion forces on the metatarsophalangeal joint complex.[19] These changes can lead to dorsal midfoot pain and metatarsalgia postoperatively (Fig. 14-5).

### Surgical technique

Plantar fascia release may be performed using a regional anesthetic with intravenous sedation and a standby general anesthetic. An ankle block is highly useful, using a 1:1 solution of 0.25% bupivacaine hydrochloride (Marcaine) and 1% lidocaine, both without epinephrine.

An oblique incision is begun along the inferomedial aspect of the heel, just anterior to the calcaneus where the inferior abductor fascia joins the medial plantar fascia (Fig. 14-6). This incision is planned anterior to the medial calcaneal branch of the posterior tibial nerve, avoiding inadvertent division of the nerve and the formation of a painful postoperative neuroma. Care should be taken to search for this nerve branch during the operative approach as its course can be more anterior than expected.

Using blunt dissection, the medial edge of the plantar fascia origin is easily visualized. Isolate the fascia from the adipose tissue, which lies inferiorly, and the fascia of the abductor hallucis muscle, which lies superiorly. If necessary, the incision can be extended a few centimeters transversely across the non–weight-bearing aspect of the sole.[26] A Freer elevator is used to isolate the plantar fascia along its origin on the calcaneus. The plantar fascia will often

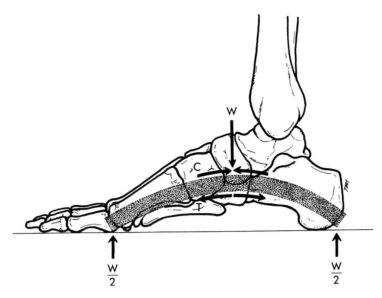

**Fig. 14-5.** If the plantar fascia is divided surgically, there are increased compressive forces transmitted to the dorsal aspect of the midfoot, and decreased flexion forces on the metatarsophalangeal joint complex.

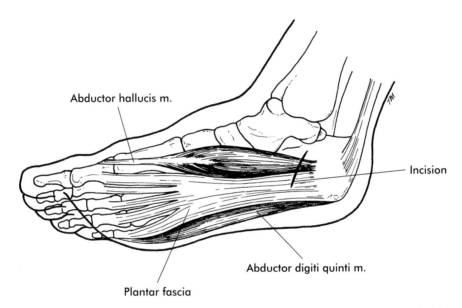

**Fig. 14-6.** Incision used to release the plantar fascia. The incision may be extended along the non—weight-bearing aspect of the foot.

be thickened in this area from chronic inflammatory changes. Heavy tenotomy scissors are then used to divide the plantar fascia as it arises from the calcaneus. Any degenerated portions of the plantar fascia should be excised. If a heel spur is present in the origin of the flexor brevis muscle, it can be easily removed using a small osteotome and rongeur. Care should be taken not to remove cortical bone of the calcaneus and thereby create a stress riser. A microreciprocating rasp works well for both gross

reduction and final smoothing of the calcaneal surface. Protect the first branch of the lateral plantar nerve (nerve to the abductor digiti quinti), which runs across the heel just deep to the heel spur and the flexor brevis muscle. If a tourniquet is used, it should be deflated and hemostasis obtained. A bulky compression dressing is used, and the patient is allowed to bear weight as tolerated with crutches. If bilateral plantar fascial releases are performed, a short-leg weight-bearing cast should be used for 2

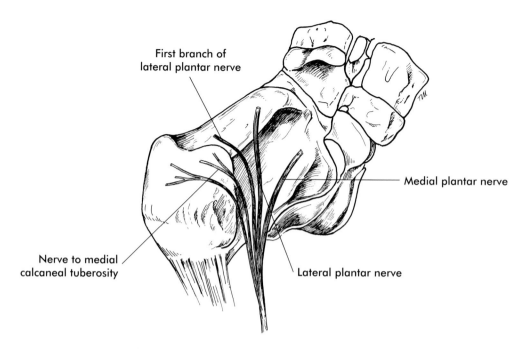

First branch of
lateral plantar nerve

Medial plantar nerve

Nerve to medial
calcaneal tuberosity

Lateral plantar nerve

**Fig. 14-7.** First branch of the lateral plantar nerve.

weeks, both to promote wound healing and to facilitate ambulation.

Minimal incision surgery is not recommended for release of the plantar fascia. Direct visualization of the plantar fascia is required to gain an adequate release, and inadvertent division of the medial calcaneal sensory nerve can easily occur when an incision of 1 cm or less is used.

## ENTRAPMENT OF THE FIRST BRANCH OF THE LATERAL PLANTAR NERVE

One of the most commonly overlooked causes of chronic plantar heel pain in the athlete is entrapment of the first branch of the lateral plantar nerve[1,2,12] (Fig. 14-7). The first branch innervates the periosteum of the medial calcaneal tuberosity, the long plantar ligament, and the abductor digiti quinti and flexor brevis muscles.[17] Entrapment of the nerve accounts for approximately 20% of chronic heel pain. Entrapment occurs as the nerve changes from a vertical to a horizontal direction around the medial plantar aspect of the heel (Fig. 14-8). The exact site of compression is between the heavy deep fascia of the abductor hallucis muscles and the medial caudal margin of the medial head of the quadratus plantae muscle (Fig. 14-9). Athletes who spend a significant amount of time on their toes such as sprinters, ballet dancers, and figure skaters are prone to entrapment of the first branch of the lateral plantar nerve by the well-developed abductor hallucis. The medial calcaneal nerve branches that innervate the plantar medial aspect of the heel pass superficial to the abductor hallucis muscle and are not involved with entrapment of the first branch. Another potential site of entrapment of the first branch is where the nerve passes just distal to the medial calcaneal tuberosity.[12] Inflammation and spur formation in the origin of the flexor brevis muscle can produce sufficient swelling to cause compression of the nerve against the long plantar ligament (Fig. 14-10). The inflammatory changes of HPS can therefore predispose to chronic entrapment of the nerve.

The diagnosis of entrapment of the first branch of the lateral plantar nerve is made on clinical grounds. It is therefore incumbent on the examiner to differentiate first branch entrapment from other more common causes of heel pain (Fig. 14-11). Early morning pain is not as prominent with nerve entrapment, which tends to cause pain more at the end of the day or after prolonged activity. The pathognomonic sign of entrapment of the first branch of the lateral plantar nerve is maximal tenderness where the nerve is compressed between the taut deep fascia of the abductor hallucis muscle and the medial caudal margin of the quadratus plantae muscle. Chronic inflammation of the plantar fascia may predispose to entrapment of the first branch of the lateral plantar nerve. The patient may therefore have some tenderness over the proximal plantar fascia and medial calcaneal tuberosity. Without maximal tenderness over the course of the nerve on the plantar medial aspect of the foot, however, the diagnosis of entrapment should not be made (Fig.

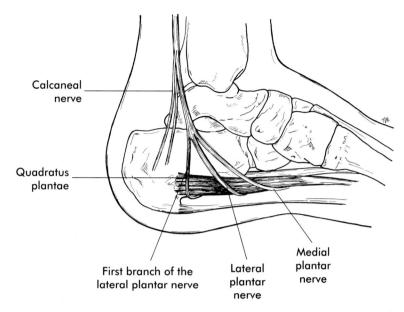

Fig. 14-8. Entrapment of the first branch of lateral plantar nerve occurs as the nerve changes direction from vertical to horizontal around the medial plantar aspect of the heel.

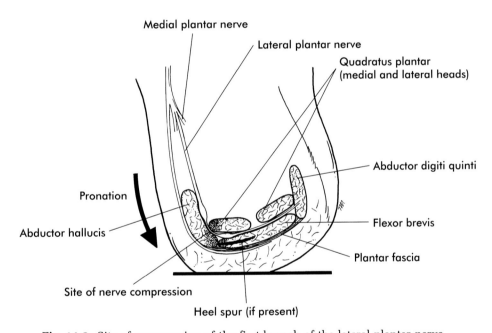

Fig. 14-9. Site of compression of the first branch of the lateral plantar nerve.

14-1). Some patients may have paresthesias elicited with pressure over the nerve at the entrapment site, although this does not occur commonly. Entrapment of the isolated medial plantar nerve, "jogger's foot," occurs more distally at the level of the navicular tuberosity and should not be confused with entrapment of the first branch of the lateral plantar nerve more proximally.

Motor weakness in the abductor digiti quinti muscle may on occasion be detected, although no cutaneous sensory deficit occurs. Electromyography and nerve conduction studies are not yet consistent in diagnosing entrapment of the first branch of the lateral plantar nerve.[20] Measurement of nerve conduction slowing across the site of entrapment is technically demanding and denervation potentials in the intrinsic foot muscles may only rarely occur because of the possible dynamic nature of this particular compression neuropathy. A comparison may be drawn to the diagnosis of a posterior interosseous nerve entrapment in the upper extremity.

Treatment for athletes with entrapment of the first branch of the lateral plantar nerve is similar to that of

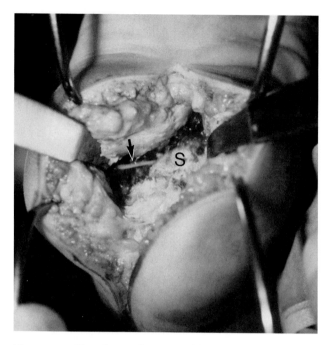

**Fig. 14-10.** The plantar fascia is retracted. The first branch of lateral plantar nerve is exposed *(arrow).* A large heel spur is marked *(S).* (From Kenzora JE: The painful heel syndrome: an entrapment neuropathy, *Bull Hosp Joint Dis* 47:178, 1987.)

HPS, with rest, nonsteroidal antiinflammatory agents, contrast baths, ice massage, physical therapy, and steroid injection serving as the foundation for conservative care. A shock-absorbent viscoelastic heel insert will also help decrease inflammation in the area. In athletic patients with excessive pronation, especially long-distance runners, a nonrigid mediolongitudinal arch support can decrease compression of the nerve.

In 1984 Baxter and Thigpen presented the first large clinical series of patients treated operatively for entrapment of the first branch of the lateral plantar nerve.[2] Twenty-six patients with 34 involved heels underwent operative decompression; 82% of the patients experienced complete relief of their symptoms. In 1992 Baxter and Pfeffer published a series of 69 heels in 53 patients with chronic heel pain who had surgical release of the first branch of the lateral plantar nerve.[1] The average duration of heel pain symptoms was 23 months. No patient had less than 6 months of conservative treatment before surgery. The average duration of preoperative conservative treatment was 14 months. Postoperatively 61 heels (89%) had excellent or good results. The average follow-up was 49 months. Approximately half the patients in Baxter's second study developed heel pain as a result of a sports activity, usually long-distance running. Other activities included aerobics, basketball, volleyball, and tennis. Eighty-five percent of this group had good or excellent results from surgery. The mean

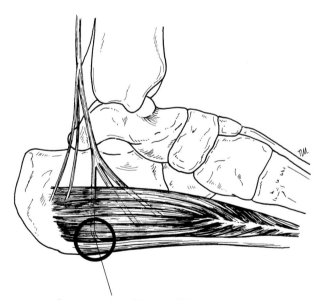

Entrapment of nerve to the abductor digiti quinti m. between deep fascia of the abductor hallucis m. and the medial caudal margin of the quadratus plantae m.

**Fig. 14-11.** Entrapment of nerve to the abductor digiti quinti.

recovery time of the athletic subgroup to resumption of sports activities was 3 months. This amount of time was not considered excessive given the mean of 23 months of preoperative symptoms.

### Surgical technique

The surgical approach to release the first branch of the lateral plantar nerve should be from the medial side of the heel. The patient is supine on the operating table. No tourniquet is required, although an ankle tourniquet can be used. A 4-cm oblique incision is made on the medial heel over the proximal abductor hallucis muscle. The incision is centered over the course of the first branch of the lateral plantar nerve. The medial calcaneal sensory nerve branches are not encountered as they course posterior to the incision. Care is taken, however, to preserve any aberrant branches.

The superficial fascia of the abductor hallucis is divided with a #15 blade and the muscle is retracted superiorly using a Ragnell retractor. A section of deep fascia of the inferior abductor hallucis is removed directly over the area where the nerve is compressed between this taut fascia and the medial border of the quadratus plantae muscle. A small portion of the medial plantar fascia may be removed to facilitate exposure and clearly define the plane between the deep abductor fascia and the plantar fascia. The deep fascia of the abductor hallucis is then divided from inferior to superior to sufficiently free the nerve from entrapment. If present, a heel spur is removed, using a Freer elevator to protect the nerve that runs superiorly. The abductor hallucis muscle belly and its superficial fascia are left intact. A plantar fascia release is not performed unless the patient has been symptomatic over the plantar aspect of the medial calcaneal tuberosity and direct visualization provides evidence of pathology in the proximal portion of the plantar fascia.

At the end of each case, a small hemostat is used to palpate along the course of the nerve to make sure it is free from any adhesions proximally or distally. The wound is closed with interrupted horizontal mattress nylon sutures. No subcutaneous sutures are used. A bulky dressing is placed. Patients are allowed to bear weight in a postoperative shoe as tolerated and to gradually return to sports activities after 3 to 4 weeks.

A plantar heel spur forms in the insertion of the flexor brevis muscle on the calcaneus. The first branch of the lateral plantar nerve courses from medial to lateral directly above this muscle. Although it is unlikely that a heel spur is a direct mechanical cause of plantar heel pain, inflammation in the area of the spur is a theoretical source of compression of the first branch of the lateral plantar nerve as it passes above

the spur. A heel spur, if present, should therefore be excised. Care should be taken when excising the spur to protect the first branch of the lateral plantar nerve. The plantar fascia should not be divided so as to preserve its biomechanical advantage during sports activities.

### TARSAL TUNNEL SYNDROME

Another nerve entrapment capable of producing chronic heel pain is tarsal tunnel syndrome. Posttraumatic adhesions, bony spurs, chronic inflammation, benign tumors, and varicosities can all cause compression of the posterior tibial nerve within the tarsal tunnel. Excessive pronation in a long-distance runner may predispose to tarsal tunnel syndrome by placing repeated stress on the structures on the medial side of the heel. Hindfoot varus, in association with excessive pronation, may also be associated with tarsal tunnel syndrome.

The salient clinical feature of tarsal tunnel syndrome is direct focal tenderness over the nerve as it passes beneath the flexor retinaculum. Percussion of the nerve in this area will reproduce the patient's symptoms, which can include pain, burning, or tingling on the plantar aspect of the foot. Subjective numbness of the toes may occur, although objective decreased sensibility is rarely demonstrated. Some patients may complain of proximal radiation of their symptoms. Electromyography and nerve conduction studies can be helpful in making a diagnosis. A normal study, however, does not exclude the diagnosis of tarsal tunnel syndrome. In general, the plantar heel pain produced by tarsal tunnel syndrome is more diffuse and less focal than that of either HPS or entrapment of the first branch of the lateral plantar nerve. A careful clinical examination should easily distinguish among these three entities.

A medial heel wedge will decrease tension on the nerve. Steroid injection into the tarsal tunnel may also be beneficial but usually produces only transient relief of symptoms. Surgical release of the flexor retinaculum and exploration of the tarsal tunnel can be expected to provide relief of symptoms in 90% of athletic patients. Decompression of both the medial and lateral plantar nerves into the midfoot should be performed in any patient with preoperative tenderness along the course of these nerves (Fig. 14-12). Internal neurolysis of the nerve is rarely indicated.

### PLANTAR FASCIITIS

Tenderness over the plantar fascia in the *midfoot* is a true plantar fasciitis. This condition presents with tenderness over the midportion of the plantar fascia. As opposed to HPS, dorsiflexion of the toes almost always exacerbates the patient's symptoms by the

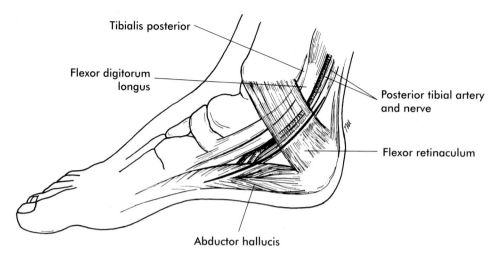

Tibialis posterior

Flexor digitorum longus

Posterior tibial artery and nerve

Flexor retinaculum

Abductor hallucis

**Fig. 14-12.** Decompression of medial and lateral plantar nerves into the midfoot should be performed in any patient with preoperative tenderness along the course of the nerves.

Windlass mechanism stretching the midfascial fibers (Fig. 14-13). There is usually only minimal tenderness over the most proximal fascial fibers, which are painful in HPS. Plantar fasciitis is more frequently seen in sprinters and middle-distance runners who spend more time on their toes during athletic activity.

Tendinitis of the flexor hallucis longus tendon can present with pain in the plantar medial midfoot. This condition can easily be distinguished from plantar fasciitis. Passive dorsiflexion of the great toe aggravates both plantar fasciitis and flexor hallucis longus tendinitis, but resisted flexion of the toe is painful only with involvement of the tendon. Careful palpation with motion of the tendon is usually sufficient to confirm the diagnosis. A painful plantar fibromatosis involving the mid plantar fascia can also be detected by careful examination.

A mediolongitudinal arch support is often not tolerated in a patient with plantar fasciitis because it pushes up on the plantar fascia and increases tension on its fibers. Circumferential taping of the foot with 1-inch adhesive tape applied over a nonadhesive elastic wrap is usually beneficial. Rest, alteration of training, nonsteroidal antiinflammatory agents, ice massage, contrast baths, and physical therapy including ultrasound and plantar fascial stretching are also indicated. A one-eighth-inch medial heel wedge may take tension off the plantar fascia. If these modalities fail, the cornerstone of treatment is the University of California Biomechanics Laboratory (UCBL) orthosis.[4] The theory of the UCBL orthosis is to hold the foot in a position that relieves tension on the plantar fascia. The orthosis accomplishes this reduction in tension by holding the heel in inversion and applying forces

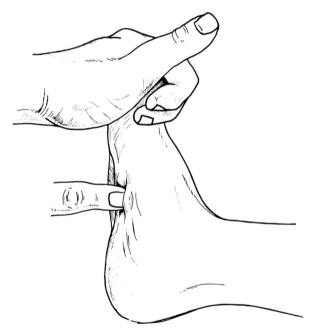

**Fig. 14-13.** Dorsiflexion of the toes causing tension on the plantar fascia. The symptoms of true plantar fasciitis are reproduced with this maneuver.

against the navicular and lateral aspect of the forefoot, without direct pressure on the soft tissue underneath the longitudinal arch. The UCBL insert is usually not helpful in patients with HPS, as the rigid material used in constructing the insert often aggravates the inflamed heel. It is extremely unusual to operate on a patient for true midfoot plantar fasciitis. If prolonged conservative treatment of more than 6 months fails, however, a similar operative approach to that used for HPS is indicated.

## SUMMARY

Ninety-eight percent of patients with heel pain can be treated successfully with conservative treatment. If treatment is begun soon after the onset of symptoms, most athletes can minimize their downtime to 6 weeks or less. Understandably many athletic patients are reluctant to give up or significantly modify their sports activities. They continue to train through the pain and thereby establish a chronic and refractory condition. In those few patients who require surgery, an excellent result can be obtained if the correct diagnosis is made and the surgeon addresses the specific cause of the athlete's plantar heel pain.

**Case Study 1.** A 23-year-old nationally ranked middle-distance runner had chronic heel pain. She failed all conservative treatment including prolonged physical therapy, heel cups, an orthotic device, and shoe modification. She did not want to use a cast. She had maximal tenderness over the medial plantar hindfoot consistent with the diagnosis of entrapment of the first branch of the lateral plantar nerve. Her symptoms had been present for 1 year. Under regional anesthesia she had a surgical release of the deep abductor fascia, freeing up the nerve. Her plantar fascia was left intact. Six weeks later she resumed training with complete relief of pain.

**Case Study 2.** A 44-year-old competitive long-distance runner had 2 years of heel pain consistent with HPS. His mileage had decreased from 80 miles per week to 0. Under regional anesthesia through an oblique medial incision his plantar fascia was released. No heel spur was present. His plantar heel pain gradually resolved over 4 months. He returned to 40+ miles per week.

**Case Study 3.** A 23-year-old male volleyball player was seen for a second opinion regarding chronic heel pain. Surgery had been recommended. The diagnosis was midfoot plantar fasciitis. He wore a rigid plastic orthotic device, which did not help. The orthotic device was discarded and circumferential taping of the midfoot over a nonadherent wrap was begun. He began a program of physical therapy three times a week to stretch the Achilles tendon and plantar fascia and decrease inflammation. A nonsteroidal antiinflammatory agent, ice massage, and contrast baths were also used. His symptoms sufficiently improved so that surgery was not required.

**Case Study 4.** A 24-year-old female long-distance runner had a plantar fascia release. Postoperatively she developed metatarsalgia and dorsolateral midfoot pain. She was seen in consultation after repeated attempts at conservative treatment failed to relieve her midfoot pain. Her plantar heel pain had resolved after surgery. She required 8 weeks of casting to alleviate the midfoot symptoms.

**Case Study 5.** An aerobics instructor was seen for chronic hindfoot pain following a plantar fascia release. A longitudinal incision had been used. A small portion of the medial heel was numb. A neuroma in the superficial medial calcaneal nerve was identified. Symptoms persisted despite two steroid injections into the neuroma. The nerve was resected surgically to its origin within the tarsal tunnel. The patient experienced continued tenderness at the nerve ending. Another patient with a similar problem developed a reflex sympathetic dystrophy that remained refractory to conservative treatment.

## REFERENCES

1. Baxter DE, Pfeffer GB: Treatment of chronic heel pain by surgical release of the first branch of the lateral plantar nerve, *Clin Orthop* 279:229, 1992.
2. Baxter DE, Thigpen CM: Heel pain—operative results, *Foot Ankle* 5:16, 1984.
3. Bordelon RL: Subcalcaneal pain: a method of evaluation and plan for treatment, *Clin Orthop* 177:49, 1983.
4. Campbell JW, Inman VT: Treatment of plantar fasciitis and calcaneal spurs with the UC-BL shoe insert, *Clin Orthop* 103:57, 1974.
5. Cimino WP, Leventen EO: Plantar fasciotomy: treatment of recalcitrant heel pain, presented to AOFAS, Anaheim, 1991.
6. Daly PJ, Kitaoka HB, Chao EYS: Plantar fasciotomy for intractable plantar fasciitis: clinical results and biomechanical evaluation, *Foot Ankle* 13:188, 1992.
7. DuVries HL: Heel spur (calcaneal spur), *AMA Arch Surg* 74:536, 1957.
8. Gerster JC: Plantar fasciitis and Achilles tendinitis among 150 cases of seronegative spondarthritis, *Rheumatol Rehabil* 19:218, 1980.
9. Hicks JH: The plantar aponeurosis and the arch, *J Anat* 88:25, 1954.
10. Jahss MH, Kummer F, Michelson JD: Investigations into the fat pads of the sole of the foot: heel pressure studies, *Foot Ankle* 13:227, 1992.
11. Jahss MH, et al: Investigations into the fat pads of the sole of the foot: anatomy and histology, *Foot Ankle* 13:233, 1992.
12. Kenzora JE: The painful heel syndrome: an entrapment neuropathy, *Bull Hosp Joint Dis* 47:178, 1987.
13. Lapidus PW, Guidotti FP: Painful heel: report of three hundred twenty-three patients with three hundred sixty-four painful heels, *Clin Orthop* 39:178, 1965.
14. Leach R, Jones R, Silva T: Rupture of the plantar fascia in athletes, *J Bone Joint Surg* 60A:537, 1978.
15. Leach RE, Seavey NS, Salter DK: Results of surgery in athletes with plantar facsciitis, *Foot Ankle* 7:155, 1986.
16. Lutter LD: Surgical decisions in athletes' subcalcaneal pain, *Am J Sports Med* 14:481, 1986.
17. Rondhuis JJ, Huson A: The first branch of the lateral plantar nerve and heel pain, *Acta Morphol Neerl Scand* 24:269, 1986.
18. Rubin G, Witton M: Plantar calcaneal spurs, *Am J Orthop* 5:38, 1963.
19. Sarrafian FK: Functional characteristics of the foot and plantar aponeurosis under tibiotalar loading, *Foot Ankle* 8:4, 1987.
20. Schon LC, Glennon TP, Baxter DE: Heel pain syndrome: electrodiagnostic support for nerve entrapment, *Foot Ankle* 14:129-135, 1993.
21. Sellman JR: Plantar fascia rupture associated with corticosteroid injection, Presented at the AOFAS, BANFF, Canada.
22. Snider MJ, Clancy WG, McBeath AA: Plantar fascia release

for chronic plantar fascitis in runners, *Am J Sports Med* 11:215, 1983.

23. Spiegl PV, Johnson KA: Heel Pain Syndrome: which treatments to choose? *J Musc Med* 66, 1984.

24. Tietze A: Ueber den Architektonischen Aurbau des Bindegenebes in der Neuschilchen Fuss-sohle, *Beitr Z Klin Chir* 123:493, 1921.

25. Tanz SS: Heel pain, *Clin Orthop* 28:168, 1963.

26. Ward WG, Clippinger RW: Proximal medial longitudinal arch incision for plantar fascia release, *Foot Ankle* 8:152, 1987.

27. Wapner KL: The use of night splints for treatment of recalcitrant plantar fasciitis, *Foot Ankle* 12:135, 1991.

28. Williams PL et al: Imaging studies of the painful heel syndrome, *Foot Ankle* 7:345, 1987.

# Chapter 15

# Tarsal coalitions

**R. Luke Bordelon**

The syndrome of coalition of the tarsal bones is a significant factor in producing symptoms in athletes because of increased stresses placed upon the foot and ankle due to the lack of normal motion, which results from restriction produced by the coalition.

*Tarsal coalition* is a condition of union of two or more tarsal bones, which may be fibrous, cartilaginous, or osseous. It probably represents a failure of mesenchymal separation rather than fusion of an accessory bone.[6,16,25]

Although the incidence of tarsal coalition may be less than 1% in the general population, this may not be accurate because the medial facet coalition is difficult to identify, and some tarsal coalitions are asymptomatic. In reviewing the families of 31 patients with symptomatic tarsal coalitions, Leonard[18] found that 39% of first-degree relatives had radiographic tarsal coalitions. Thus the actual figure of tarsal coalitions may be closer to 6%.[42] However, the incidence may be less than 1% according to other authors.* Calcaneonavicular coalitions are bilateral in 60% of cases, and talocalcaneal coalitions are bilateral in 50% of cases.[35]

The pathomechanics of the dysfunction of tarsal coalition is restriction of motion of one of the joints of the subtalar joint complex, which acts as a torque converter. This restriction of motion increases the strain on the other joints, thus producing a condition that sets up the cycle of strain, pain, and muscle spasm.[2,20,32,34]

Although tarsal coalition is the most common cause of restriction of motion of the subtalar joint complex, when dysfunction is due to abnormal restriction of motion and pain in this area, one must also consider other causes such as trauma, arthritis, infection, or tumor.[3,31,39]

The general types of coalition are talonavicular, talocalcaneal, and calcaneocuboid. Other coalitions may be present and must be considered if signs and symptoms are suggestive of tarsal coalition, and the standard forms of coalition are not identified.[14,23,25,29,40]

Talonavicular coalition is unusual.[1,2,11] It presents early, perhaps as early as 2 to 3 years of age. It is seen on the anteroposterior, lateral, and oblique views of the foot (Fig. 15-1). This can usually be managed with orthotics and activity restriction, although occasionally a triple arthrodesis may be considered.

Talocalcaneal coalition is a coalition of the medial facet (Fig. 15-2). A routine lateral x-ray may show secondary signs of tarsal coalition such as beaking of the talonavicular joint, blunting and sclerosis of the lateral process of the talus, and narrowing of the posterior facet. The classic view is the axial view of the os calcis.[5,6] However computed tomography (CT) demonstrates this coalition best and should be performed in all cases of suspected coalition of the medial facet.[17,30,36] An abnormal appearance of the medial facet joint with sloping is considered to be consistent with a tarsal coalition. Radionuclide bone scanning has been used to assist in the diagnosis of symptomatic subtalar coalition. It is usually positive when the coalition is symptomatic[8,12,19] (see Case Studies 1, 2, and 3).

The talocalcaneal coalition generally becomes symptomatic between the ages of 8 and 12 years. Examination of the foot reveals absence of motion of the subtalar joint. Motion of the remainder of the foot

*References 5, 6, 9, 18, 35, 42.

207

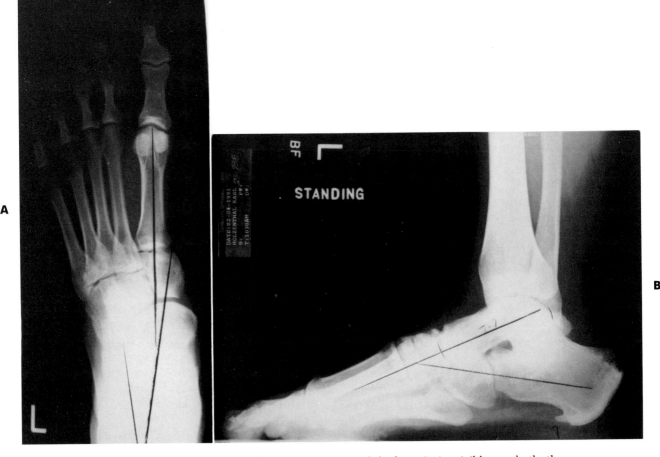

**Fig. 15-1.** Talonavicular coalition seen in an adult foot. It is visible on both the anteroposterior and lateral x-rays.

will vary depending upon whether there is muscle spasm.

**Case Study 1.** A 51-year-old avid golfer had bilateral talocalcaneal coalitions and pain with inversion and eversion limiting recreational activities. A short articulated ankle-foot arthosis (AFO) was molded, fabricated, and fitted. He is wearing the brace 10 to 12 hours a day with relief of pain.

**Case Study 2.** A 12-year-old white female presented with pain in the left foot with increase in pain with increase in activity. Physical examination revealed a structurally normal foot but limitation of motion of the talocalcaneal joint. X-rays (axial view) and CT scan revealed unilateral medial facet coalition. Conservative treatment consisted of a short-leg cast, antiinflammatory medication, and decreased activity. This relieved her pain, but when she returned to basketball, she had an increase in pain and was unable to participate. Surgery was performed consisting of excision of the medial facet coalition. The patient had a good result and was able to resume basketball with only occasional aching after extended use but not enough to prevent participation in a full basketball schedule.

**Case Study 3.** A 12-year-old white male presented with the complaint of difficulty with his feet. His flatfeet were first noted at birth. He had been placed in inserts. He continued to have difficulty, although he was able to perform fairly normal activity until he was about 10½ years of age. He began having increased foot pain and increased deformity.

Examination revealed that the patient had a rigid, abducted, everted foot with peroneal spasm. Structurally, there was gastroc-soleus contracture, and forefoot varus relative to the hindfoot was severe (Fig. 15-3).

X-ray and CT examination revealed a bilateral medial talocalcaneal coalition (Fig. 15-4). The family was advised that he had a talocalcaneal coalition superimposed upon a structural flatfoot deformity, and that this was a severe condition. The suggested procedure was excision of the talocalcaneal coalition, probably followed in 1 year by a correction of the structural flatfoot deformity, with the realization that a triple arthrodesis might have to be performed in this particular case.

Medial talocalcaneal coalitions were resected. He continued to have a rigid foot with limited subtalar motion and limited adduction and inversion. Treatment with casts and

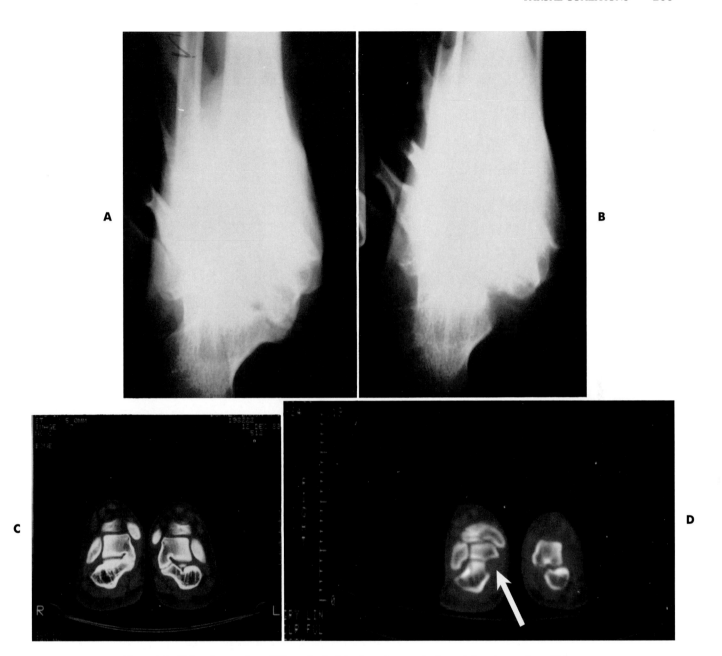

**Fig. 15-2.** Talocalcaneal coalition. **A,** Axial view demonstrates a talocalcaneal coalition. **B,** Axial view following excision of the talocalcaneal coalition. **C,** CT scan demonstrates osseous coalition on one side and fibrous coalition on the other. **D,** CT scan demonstrates postoperative excision of the coalition of the medial facet.

splints and use of orthotics relieved the pain and spasm only temporarily with recurrence of pain and spasm and abnormal position, even with the use of orthotic devices (Fig. 15-5).

Six months after the first surgery, he underwent surgery consisting of correction of the structural deformity of the foot by calcaneal osteotomy and opening wedge osteotomy of the cuboid, triple step cut percutaneous tendo Achilles lengthening, and reefing of the spring ligament and transfer of the anterior half of the posterior tibial distally and lengthening of the peroneus brevis (Fig. 15-6).

This corrected the structural deformity of the foot (Fig.

15-7). The lengthening of the peroneus brevis reduced the abduction deformity due to the peroneus brevis spasm.

He was last seen 2 years postoperatively, when physical examination revealed good motion of the subtalar joint; the only structural abnormality was slight forefoot varus on the left. He was wearing inserts to support the forefoot varus on the left and had resumed normal physical education classes. He was to start football practice. This patient had flatfoot with a tarsal coalition superimposed upon it with tightness of the peroneal tendons. He required peroneus brevis tendon lengthening and structural correction of the flatfoot in order to gain maximal recovery.

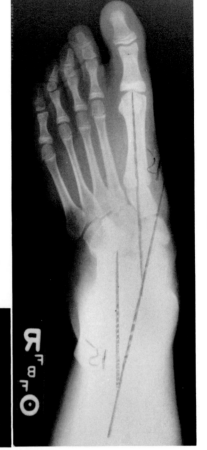

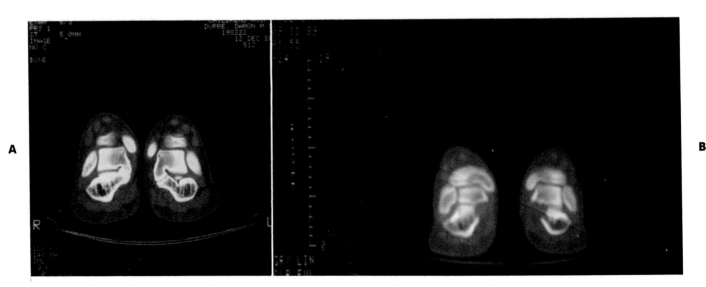

**Fig. 15-3. A,** Preoperative standing lateral view of structural flatfoot with medial talocalcaneal coalition. **B,** Preoperative anteroposterior (AP) view of the foot.

**Fig. 15-4. A,** Preoperative CT scan of the medial talocalcaneal coalition. **B,** Postoperative CT scan of the talocalcaneal coalition.

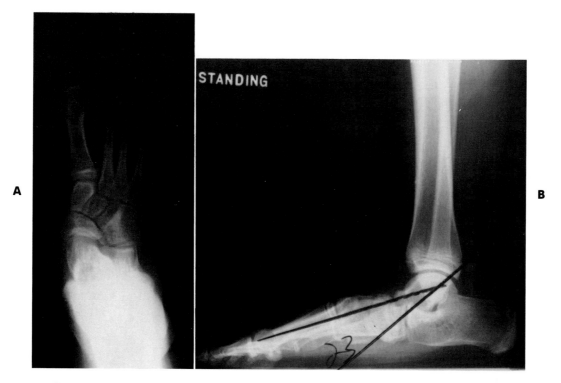

**Fig. 15-5.** Postoperative x-rays (AP and lateral standing views) of excision of medial calcaneal coalition demonstrating that the patient still has flatfoot deformity.

Although the muscle spasm is generally of the peroneals, producing an abducted/everted foot, at times one may have an adducted/inverted foot.[5,6,34,37]

Treatment of the coalition depends upon the age of the patient, symptoms, degree of associated change, and activity level.

If the patient is not symptomatic, treatment is probably not indicated. If the patient is symptomatic, conservative therapy consisting of rest in a short-leg cast, nonsteroidal antiinflammatory medication, and—following the initial period of rest—either an orthotic or a brace to decrease subtalar motion. If this does not suffice to relieve the symptoms and allow the patient full activity, surgical treatment may be considered. In the literature, once a coalition becomes symptomatic and the patient wishes to return to athletic endeavors, conservative treatment is usually not successful.[10,24,34]

Surgical treatment consists of excision of the area of coalition with interposition of a fat graft. Talar beaking is not a contraindication to resection, because this represents a plastic deformation and not a degenerative spur.*

A rigid foot with degenerative changes within the joint is a contraindication to excision of the bar. If a subtalar coalition is symptomatic, the heel is in good

position, and no changes in the talonavicular and calcaneocuboid joints are seen other than beaking, the surgical procedure probably should consist of just fusion of the subtalar joint. With this procedure, the patient may still be able to perform some athletic activities.

## TALOCALCANEAL COALITION
### Surgical procedure for resection of the medial facet (Fig. 15-8)

1. A curvilinear skin incision is made just below the posterior tibial tendon.
2. The posterior tibial tendon is reflected dorsally. The flexor digitorum longus is reflected dorsally or plantarward.
3. The flexor hallucis longus and neurovascular bundle are reflected plantarward.
4. Anterior and posterior parts of the coalition are defined. A hemostat or Keith needle may be used. One should ascertain the anterior and posterior borders to prevent injury to the anterior or posterior facet joints.
5. The coalition is resected with an osteotome, either by removing en bloc or by using a "sliver" technique. The entire coalition should be excised so that normal articular cartilage can be visualized.
6. The subtalar joint is mobilized to ensure that normal motion occurs.

*References 2, 7, 10, 24, 27, 28, 34, 37.

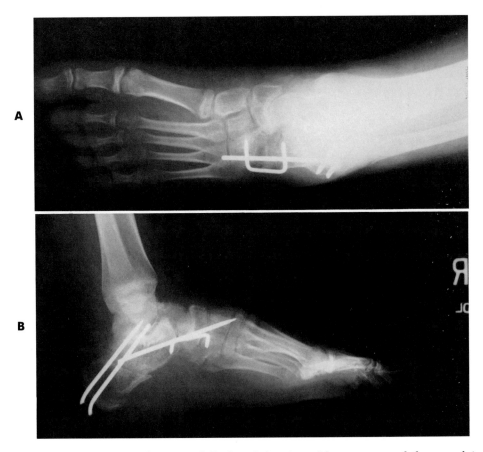

**Fig. 15-6.** Correction of structural flatfoot deformity with osteotomy of the os calcis, osteotomy of the cuboid, reefing of medial structures, and lengthening of the peroneus brevis tendon.

7. Raw surfaces are cauterized with a Bovie and then bone wax is used. A free-fat graft is placed in the area.
8. The wound is loosely closed.
9. The patient is placed in a well-padded postoperative dressing with support from plaster splints.

**Postoperative care**

Elevation is maintained with bathroom privileges for 7 to 14 days until the tendency to swell has subsided. Active motion is started immediately. Immobilization in a splint is used for 10 to 14 days. Weight bearing may be allowed in 4 to 6 weeks if there is good motion and weight bearing does not produce pain or muscle spasm. Once the patient can ambulate without pain and with maintenance of motion, activity is slowly increased. About 6 months is required for return to full activity.

**CALCANEONAVICULAR COALITION**

*Calcaneonavicular coalition* is a union between the anterior part of the os calcis and the navicular. It generally becomes symptomatic between 12 and 16 years of age. The symptoms consist of pain in the foot with increasing activity and limited motion. Some subtalar motion may still be present if there is no spasm of the peroneal tendon. Incomplete coalitions may produce dysfunction of the foot and symptoms misdiagnosed as ankle sprains.[2,38]

The 45-degree oblique radiograph of the foot will best demonstrate a calcaneonavicular coalition (Fig. 15-9). The interval between the calcaneus and the navicular should be carefully evaluated and oblique views taken in different angles to accurately assess the deformity.

Restriction of motion of the subtalar joint from an incomplete coalition may predispose the remainder of the foot to malfunction with repetitive loads. This may be a factor in producing repetitive overuse dysfunctional syndrome such as recurrent fractures of the naviculars. On the lateral view one may see the classical secondary signs of subtalar coalition with beaking of the lateral talocalcaneal joint, broadening and sclerosis of the lateral facet of the talus, and narrowing of the posterior facet.

Oestreich et al[26] described the "anteater nose,"

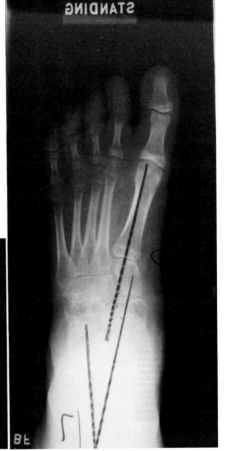

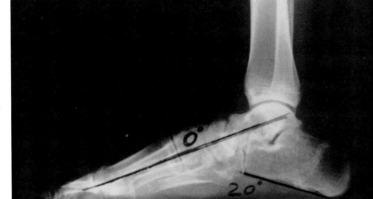

**Fig. 15-7.** Postoperative AP and lateral standing x-rays following surgical correction demonstrating normal position and alignment of bones of the foot.

which is a direct sign of calcaneonavicular coalition as seen on the lateral x-ray film.

CT scanning may be used, but it is not as helpful as in talocalcaneal coalitions.

Treatment depends upon the age of the patient, the symptoms, and degree of associated change. If the patient is asymptomatic, treatment is probably not indicated. If the patient is symptomatic, conservative therapy consisting of rest in a short-leg cast (either ambulatory or nonambulatory), antiinflammatory medication, and orthotics or a brace to decrease subtalar motion may be used. If this is not sufficient to relieve the symptoms and the patient has symptoms with recurrent activity, surgical treatment may be considered. Studies have shown that if a patient becomes symptomatic, the patient may not respond to conservative treatment.[13,24,33]

Surgical treatment consists of excision of the calcaneonavicular coalition with interposition of the extensor brevis.[4-6,13,15,22,40] Talar beaking is not a contraindication to resection of the calcaneonavicular coalition, because this represents a plastic deformation and not a degenerative spur.

However, a rigid foot with degenerative changes within the joints of the subtalar joint complex is a contraindication to excision of the bar. Patients must be told that if the surgical procedure is not successful and they continue to have pain, then a triple arthrodesis may have to be considered.

**Surgical procedure (Fig. 15-10)**

1. An incision is made below the tip of the fibula to allow exposure of the navicular and the anterior part of the os calcis. Care is taken to avoid the sural nerve. A full-thickness skin flap is developed.
2. The origin of the extensor brevis is reflected distally with soft tissue.
3. The calcaneocuboid joint and the sinus tarsi are identified. The calcaneocuboid bar is identified between these two.
4. The coalition is removed by cutting the bar separating it from the navicular and the calcaneus. A rectangular and not trapezoidal portion of bone is removed. Care must be taken to avoid cutting into the calcaneocuboid joint and also to avoid damaging the anterior talocalcaneal joint.

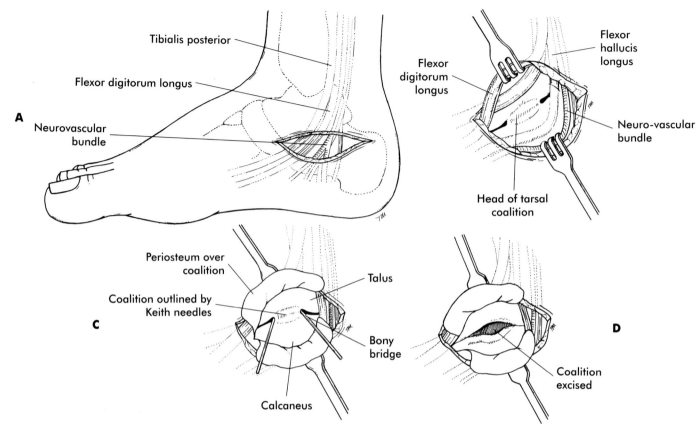

**Fig. 15-8.** Excision of talocalcaneal coalition. **A,** Skin incision. **B,** Reflection of structures dorsally and plantarward to expose the area of coalition. **C,** Outlining the coalition with needles. **D,** Postexcision appearance of the coalition. (From Mann RA, Coughlin MJ, editors: *Surgery of the foot and ankle,* ed 6, St Louis, 1992, CV Mosby. Used by permission.)

5. One must observe the area of the anterior talocalcaneal joint carefully and either completely resect the bone of the calcaneus or leave the joint undisturbed.
6. The foot is mobilized to make sure there is no restriction of motion. If there is, further bone is removed.
7. The bone is cauterized with a Bovie, then bone wax is placed on the raw surfaces. The extensor brevis is placed into the defect. It is secured by sutures holding it to the proximal tissue or by sutures through the foot.
8. The wound is closed in layers. A compression splint is applied.

Postoperatively the patient is maintained non–weight bearing and in a splint for 7 to 10 days with elevation until the swelling has subsided. Active range-of-motion exercises are started immediately. Passive and active range-of-motion exercises are used until there is good active motion. Weight bearing is allowed only after good motion has been obtained, which is usually 4 to 6 weeks postoperatively. If there is recurrence of pain or muscle spasm with activity, the non–weight bearing is used again until there is full range of motion without spasm. Six months is generally required for return to full activity.

## LITERATURE

Elkus[10] described 20 athletes with 26 feet with 15 calcaneonavicular bars, 9 talocalcaneal bars, 1 talonavicular bar, and 1 mixed. The young patient typically presented with vague sinus tarsi pain associated with athletics or minor trauma that was aggravated with increased activity such as hiking, broken field running, sprints, and walking. Often there was a history of repeated ankle sprains. Only 10% of the patients had a marked pronated foot or peroneal shortening. Preoperatively all patients had foot pain and some restriction of subtalar motion. At follow-up the majority of patients had relief of pain, although subtalar motion was variable but increased on average by 15 degrees of inversion and 5 degrees of eversion. If the patient did not respond to conservative

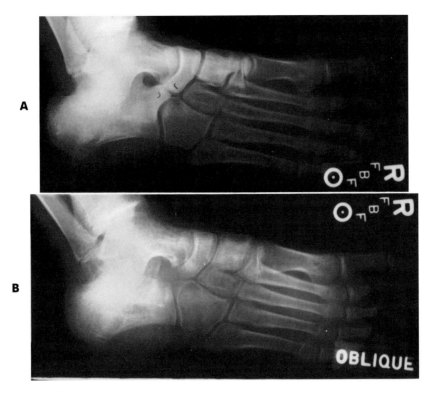

**Fig. 15-9.** Calcaneonavicular coalition. **A,** A 45-degree oblique view of the foot demonstrates the calcaneonavicular coalition. **B,** Postoperative 45-degree oblique view of the foot demonstrates adequate excision of the calcaneonavicular coalition.

measures, including two periods of casting, surgery was considered. Elkus noted that in the eight cases of talocalcaneal coalition with resection, all of the patients experienced improved motion, decreased pain, and a return to athletic activities.

Morgan and Crawford[24] reported on 12 adolescent patients with a diagnosis of tarsal coalition, 8 of whom had calcaneonavicular bars and 4 of whom had talocalcaneal bars. Nonoperative treatment was not successful in any of these cases. Four patients elected not to have surgery, they continued to have difficulty and were unable to participate in sports. Of the 8 patients who had surgery, 7 were able to return to their usual activity and level of competition. One that did not was a 15-year-old with bilateral calcaneonavicular coalitions with arthritic changes. Conservative treatment followed by excision of the bar (even with arthritic changes) in the active adolescent to allow as much motion as possible was recommended. This was recommended with the understanding that if pain and limited motion persisted a triple arthrodesis may be necessary.

Marzano and Alexander[21] reported on the use of a short articulated AFO (a rear-entry short brace with an articulated ankle) for hindfoot disorders with good results (Fig. 15-11). Thirteen percent of these cases involved tarsal coalitions.

O'Neill and Micheli[28] performed a retrospective review of 20 feet in 16 adolescent patients for tarsal coalition. All patients were active in sports and seen in the sports clinic. Ages ranged from 9 to 17 years, with an average age of 13 years, and a follow-up of 5.1 years. The report concerned surgical treatment following failed conservative therapy. All males returned to their previous level of competition in sports, whereas 3 females with 3 feet gave up sports. Combining all 20 feet, 7 were excellent, 12 were good, and 1 was fair. Four had complications, which included 2 neuromas, 1 reflex sympathetic dystrophy, and 1 pseudoarthrosis in the only patient with a bilateral extraarticular arthrodesis. The particular sport performed by the athlete had no effect on the outcome of how the athlete perceived his or her foot. Gymnastics was the principal sport in four patients, and basketball, football, and figure skating were each represented twice. O'Neill and Micheli noted that athletically involved adolescents were not necessarily being diagnosed with tarsal coalitions at an early age versus the nonsports population. They stated that young athletes who underwent resection for tarsal coalition before the onset of degenerative changes could be expected to have an excellent or good outcome and that the presence of talar beaking without other tarsal degenerative changes was not a

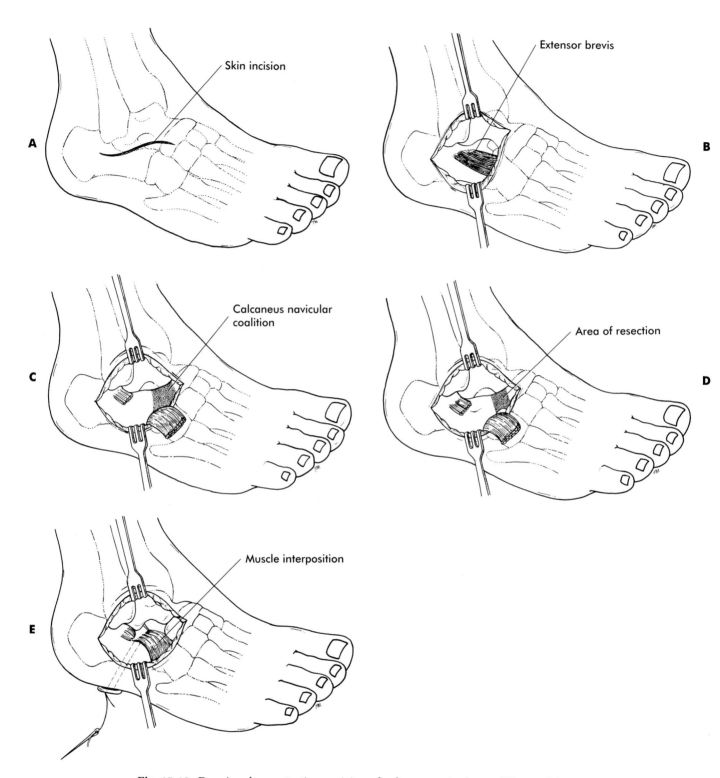

**Fig. 15-10.** Drawing demonstrating excision of calcaneonavicular coalition and interposition of extensor brevis. **A,** Skin incision. **B,** Exposure of the extensor brevis. **C,** Reflection of the extensor brevis forward demonstrates the area of coalition. **D,** Demonstration of the area of coalition to be resected. **E,** Interposition of the extensor brevis muscle. (From Mann RA, Coughlin MJ, editors: *Surgery of the foot and ankle,* ed 6, St Louis, 1992, CV Mosby. Used by permission.)

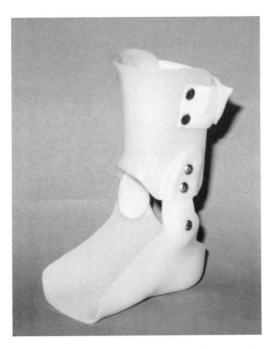

**Fig. 15-11.** Short articulated AFO used to decrease the pain of a tarsal coalition by restricting subtalar motion. (From Marzano R, Alexander I: Short articulated ankle foot orthosis for hindfoot disorders. Paper given at the Summer Meeting of American Orthopaedic Foot and Ankle Society, Napa, Calif, July 1992.)

contraindication to a surgical procedure with resection of the coalition.

Synder et al[38] discussed the relationship of tarsal coalitions to ankle sprains in athletes by reviewing charts and x-rays of individuals who sustained ankle sprains to determine the presence of calcaneonavicular coalitions. They found that some type of calcaneonavicular coalition was present in 63% of 215 patients with 223 ankle sprains. In 130 ankle sprains recorded as occurring directly in athletics, 65% of the x-ray films showed some degree of calcaneonavicular abnormality. Synder et al postulated that if there was some restriction of motion of the hindfoot or midfoot, there would be more trauma exerted on the ankle ligaments, and thus ankle sprain might be more prevalent. However, it should be noted that the diagnosis of calcaneonavicular coalition was made only on x-ray findings and some of these may have been minimal.

## SUMMARY

Tarsal coalitions occur and usually become symptomatic around the time of adolescence. Studies indicate that once the tarsal coalition is symptomatic in an adolescent, it generally does not respond to conservative care. However, conservative care consisting of casting for 3 to 6 weeks, antiinflammatory medication, bracing and/or orthotics should be considered. If the patient desires to return to sports, the best opportunity to try to return to sports is provided by surgical excision of the bar—after which most patients will be able to return to their sports activity.

A person with a symptomatic coalition does not necessarily present with a true rigid peroneal spastic flatfoot. If there is a medial talocalcaneal coalition, the motion of the transverse tarsal joint may be present. If there is a calcaneonavicular coalition, some subtalar joint motion may be possible. This is evidenced by the study of Morgan and Crawford[24] in which only 30% of the patients with a true tarsal coalition had peroneal spasm. In the series of Elkus,[10] only 10% of the patients presented with a marked pronated foot or peroneal shortening.

Although the tarsal coalition is generally well visualized by routine x-rays and CT scan, there are times when limitation of motion of the subtalar joint and persistent pain may continue in the absence of any specific osseous abnormality. In this instance one must consider a fibrous bar. This can occur in the medial talocalcaneal area. An incomplete calcaneonavicular bar may also occur. These are difficult to diagnose. Sometimes a bone scan will reveal an area of increased activity. In difficult cases without any other good answer, exploration may be considered.

In evaluating the patient with pain and limited motion of the subtalar joint, the patient should be evaluated clinically, biomechanically, and structurally in addition to roentgenographically.[2] One may have restricted subtalar motion as a result of peroneal spasm associated with a flatfoot deformity without coalition. One may also see a tarsal coalition associated with a structural deformity (as discussed in Case Study 2). Patients with tarsal coalitions must be divided into those with a tarsal coalition in a structurally normal foot and those with a tarsal coalition in a structurally abnormal foot. In the patient who has a tarsal coalition with a structurally abnormal foot, biomechanical orthotic devices may be necessary to help the foot function more normally following excision of the coalition. In some cases with severe structural abnormalities of the foot such as forefoot varus, heel valgus, and gastroc-soleus contracture, correction of the structural abnormalities may be necessary to produce a normal foot after the bar has been excised. What I have done is to excise the bar, follow the patient conservatively, and 12 months later perform a surgical correction of the structurally abnormal flatfoot.

The beaking seen at the talonavicular joint is generally plastic deformation and not true arthritic change. This beaking is not a contraindication to surgical correction. However some patients will have an abnormally shaped, narrowed, and degenerative posterior subtalar joint. If this is present, this may be a relative contraindication to excision of the bar and may require a fusion.

Since most patients with a tarsal coalition become symptomatic during adolescence, most treatment is directed toward the adolescent with resection of the bar. However sometimes there is a problem with the more mature person who has a tarsal coalition and develops symptoms related to increasing activity. In this scenario conservative treatment may be considered. If the patient continues to have difficulty and is desirous of attempting to continue with the sports activity and there is no narrowing of the joint, consideration may be given to excision of the coalition. One has to realize that a fusion procedure may have to be performed if this does not suffice.

Finally, in evaluating foot and ankle pain, whether in adolescent or mature patients, one must carefully evaluate the position of the components of the foot and the motion of the subtalar joint complex both actively and passively. Incomplete coalitions can produce abnormal forces, which may produce other recurrent abnormalities such as fatigue-type navicular fractures. Every patient who has foot and ankle pain should be carefully evaluated for structural dysfunction of the foot and ankle joint and tarsal coalitions, either obvious or obscure.

## REFERENCES

1. Bonk JH, Tozzi MA: Congenital talonavicular synostosis. A review of the literature and a case report, *J Am Podiatr Med Assoc* 79:186, 1989.
2. Bordelon RL: *Surgical and conservative foot care*, Thorofare, NJ, 1988, Slack.
3. Bower BL, Keyser CK, Gilula LA: Rigid subtalar joint—a radiographic spectrum, *Skeletal Radiol* 17:583, 1989.
4. Chambers RB, Cook TM, Cowell HR: Surgical reconstruction for calcaneonavicular coalition. Evaluation of function and gait, *J Bone Joint Surg (Am)* 64:829, 1982.
5. Cowell HR, Elener V: Rigid painful flatfoot secondary to tarsal coalition, *Clin Orthop* 181:54, 1983.
6. Cowell HR: Tarsal coalition—review and update, *Instr Course Lect* 31:264, 1982.
7. Danielsson LG: Talo-calcaneal coalition treated with resection, *J Pediatr Orthop* 7:513, 1987.
8. Deutsch AL, Resnick D, Campbell G: Computed tomography and bone scintigraphy in the evaluation of tarsal coalition, *Radiology* 144:137, 1982.
9. Drawbert JP et al: Tarsal and carpal coalition and symphalangism of the Fuhrmann type. Report of a family, *J Bone Joint Surg (Am)* 67:884, 1985.
10. Elkus RA: Tarsal coalition in the young athlete, *Am J Sports Med* 14:477, 1986.
11. Ertel AN, O'Connell FD: Talonavicular coalition following avascular necrosis of the tarsal navicular, *J Pediatr Orthop* 4:482, 1984.
12. Goldman AB, Pavlov H, Schneider R: Radionuclide bone scanning in subtalar coalitions: differential considerations, *Am J Roentgenol* 138:427, 1982.
13. Gonzalez P, Kumar SJ: Calcaneonavicular coalition treated by resection and interposition of the extensor digitorum brevis muscle, *J Bone Joint Surg (Am)* 72:71, 1990.
14. Grant AD, Rose D, Lehman W: Talocalcaneal coalition in arthrogryposis multiplex congenita, *Bull Hosp Jt Dis Orthop Inst* 42:236, 1982.
15. Inglis G, Buxton RA, Macnicol MF: Symptomatic calcaneonavicular bars. The results 20 years after surgical excision, *J Bone Joint Surg (Br)* 68:128, 1986.
16. Kawashima T, Uhthoff HK: Prenatal development around the sustentaculum tali and its relation to talocalcaneal coalitions, *J Pediatr Orthop* 10:238, 1990.
17. Lee MS et al: Subtalar joint coalition in children: new observations, *Radiology* 172:635, 1989.
18. Leonard MA: The inheritance of tarsal coalition and its relationship to spastic flat foot, *J Bone Joint Surg* 56B:520, 1974.
19. Mandell GA et al: Detection of talocalcaneal coalitions by magnification bone scintigraphy, *J Nucl Med* 31:1797, 1990.
20. Mann RA: *Surgery of the foot*, ed 5, St Louis, 1986, CV Mosby.
21. Marzano R, Alexander I: Short articulated ankle foot orthosis for hindfoot disorders. Paper given at the Summer meeting of American Orthopaedic Foot and Ankle Society, Napa, California, July 1992.
22. Mitchell GP, Gibson JMC: Excision of calcaneo-navicular bar for painful spasmodic flat foot, *J Bone Joint Surg (Br)* 49B:281, 1967.
23. Miki T et al: Naviculo-cuneiform coalition. A report of two cases, *Clin Orthop* 196:256, 1985.
24. Morgan RC Jr, Crawford AH: Surgical management of tarsal coalition in adolescent athletes, *Foot Ankle* 7:183, 1986.
25. Mosier KM, Asher M: Tarsal coalitions and peroneal spastic flat foot. A review, *J Bone Joint Surg (Am)* 66:976, 1984.
26. Oestreich AE et al: The "anteater nose": a direct sign of calcaneonavicular coalition on the lateral radiograph, *J Pediatr Orthop* 7:709, 1987.
27. Olney BW, Asher MA: Excision of symptomatic coalition of the middle facet of the talocalcaneal joint, *J Bone Joint Surg (Am)* 69:539, 1987. (Published erratum appears in *J Bone Joint Surg (Am)* 69:1111, 1987.)
28. O'Neill DB, Micheli LJ: Tarsal coalition. A follow-up of adolescent athletes, *Am J Sports Med* 17:544, 1989.
29. Pensieri SL et al: Bilateral congenital calcaneocuboid synostosis and subtalar joint coalition, *J Am Podiatr Med Assoc* 75:406, 1985.
30. Pineda C, Resnick D, Greenway G: Diagnosis of tarsal coalition with computed tomography, *Clin Orthop* 208:282, 1986.
31. Pistoia F, Ozonoff MB, Wintz P: Ball-and-socket ankle joint, *Skeletal Radiol* 16:447, 1987.
32. Resnick D: Talar ridges, osteophytes, and beaks: a radiologic commentary, *Radiology* 151:329, 1984.
33. Richards RR, Evans JG, McGoey PF: Fracture of a calcaneonavicular bar: a complication of tarsal coalition. A case report, *Clin Orthop* 185:220, 1984.
34. Scranton PE Jr: Treatment of symptomatic talocalcaneal coalition, *J Bone Joint Surg (Am)* 69:533, 1987.
35. Stormont DM, Peterson HA: The relative incidence of tarsal coalition, *Clin Orthop* 181:28, 1983.
36. Stoskopf CA et al: Evaluation of tarsal coalition by computed tomography, *J Pediatr Orthop* 4:365, 1984.
37. Swiontkowski MF, Scranton PE, Hansen S: Tarsal coalitions: long-term results of surgical treatment, *J Pediatr Orthop* 3:287, 1983.

38. Synder RB, Lipscomb AB, Johnston RK: The relationship of tarsal coalitions to ankle sprains in athletes, *Am J Sports Med* 9:313, 1981.
39. Takakura Y, Tamai S, Masuhara K: Genesis of the ball-and-socket ankle, *J Bone Joint Surg (Br)* 68:834, 1986.
40. Wheeler R, Guevera A, Bleck EE: Tarsal coalitions: a review of the literature and case report of bilateral dual calcaneo-navicular and talocalcaneal coalitions, *Clin Orthop* 177:175, 1981.
41. Wiles S, Palladino SJ, Stavosky JW: Naviculocuneiform coalition, *J Am Podiatr Med Assoc* 78:355, 1988.
42. Wray JB, Herndon CN: Hereditary transmission of congenital coalition of the calcaneus to the navicular, *J Bone Joint Surg* 45A:365, 1963.

# Chapter 16

# Forefoot disorders

Michael J. Coughlin

Metatarsalgia in the athlete can be a debilitating disorder leading to loss of competitiveness or even loss of the ability to participate in a recreational fashion. Forefoot disorders encompass lesser toe abnormalities such as claw toes, hammertoes, mallet toes, and hard and soft corns. More proximally, problems can include intractable plantar keratosis (IPK), bunionettes, neuromas, and metatarsophalangeal (MP) joint capsulitis and instability.

For the athlete, repetitive activities can lead to repeated stress reactions in soft tissues as well as bones and joints. Abrasions and repeated trauma over bony prominences can lead to callus formation and bursitis.

Ideally, avoiding the development of problems through the use of good footwear and proper training practices should be the goal. Many of these problems may develop despite prophylactic care and thus require the intervention of the orthopedic surgeon either conservatively or surgically. When possible, nonsurgical treatment is preferred, leading to a rapid resumption of athletic activity.

The complaint of pain in the forefoot must be differentiated to make a correct diagnosis. The accompanying algorithm (Fig. 16-1) may prove useful in determining the specific forefoot diagnosis when a patient complains of metatarsalgia. Most important is the exact location of pain. In addition, which specific activities increase symptoms and which activities alleviate discomfort? Is the pain dorsal or plantar, medial or lateral? Is there an associated neuritic symptom with the pain? Are enlarged exostoses or prominences associated with pain, swelling, or inflammation?

When a patient complains of metatarsalgia, the initial question on physical examination is, Is there an associated callosity? This can be lateral over the fifth metatarsal head with a bunionette formation. It can be localized to the plantar metatarsal region with an IPK. A callosity may develop over the dorsal distal interphalangeal (DIP) joint (a mallet toe) or the dorsal proximal interphalangeal (PIP) joint (hammertoe). On occasion a patient may complain both of a callosity overlying the PIP joint, as well as beneath the associated metatarsal head. With a concomitant contracture of this toe, the diagnosis of a claw toe is made.

Development of a callus between two toes (a soft corn) or over the lateral aspect of the fifth toe (a hard corn) can be extremely painful.

When a patient complains of metatarsalgia, but there is no callosity present, the patient should be carefully examined for neuritic symptoms. When present, along with other specific symptoms, the diagnosis of an interdigital neuroma is made. When neuritic symptoms are not present, but symptomatic pain is still localized to the forefoot, suspicion of MP joint capsulitis and/or instability is considered. The presence of a positive drawer sign (dorsal plantar instability) or actual malalignment of the involved toe at the MP joint aids in confirming the diagnosis. Although this algorithm is not all-inclusive, and much more goes into the specific diagnostic process than this flow sheet allows, it does offer a method of approaching the athlete with metatarsalgia. Sometimes symptoms overlap, frequently symptoms are vague—and repeated evaluation and physical and radiographic examination are necessary to confirm a diagnosis. The cooperation of patients in defining their symptomatic complaints, and in defining their problem through varying their athletic activity, is highly important. Likewise, their cooperation in modifying activity when conservative management is

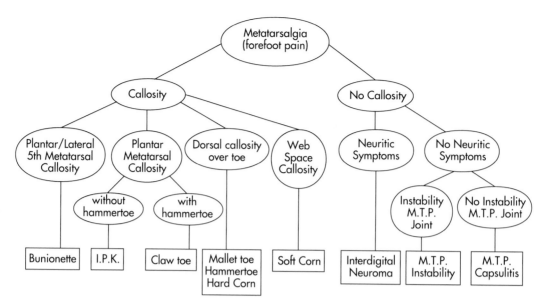

**Fig. 16-1.** Algorithm.

attempted is critical in any successful treatment. When surgery is performed, cooperation in allowing adequate healing to occur before resuming athletic activity is instrumental not only in the recovery process, but also in the avoidance of other associated problems.

## BUNIONETTES

The development of inflammation, an enlarged bursa, or a callus over a prominent fifth metatarsal head may lead a physician to diagnose a bunionette (Fig. 16-2). Just as bunions can present with differing magnitude and different characteristics, so too can a bunionette.[3] A bunionette may appear radiographically as an enlarged fifth metatarsal head (type I). A flare in the metaphysis may cause outbowing of the fifth metatarsal (type II), leading to symptoms, or a widened 4-5 intermetatarsal angle (type III) characteristic of a splayfoot may lead to pain and callus formation (Fig. 16-3).

Initially an athlete may complain of pain directly lateral over the fifth metatarsal head, but the examiner should be aware of plantar symptoms as well. Neuritic symptoms involving the fifth toe may occur due to pressure over the lateral digital nerve to the fifth toe. Complaints of inflammation, blistering, ulceration, or infection may be noted by the athlete.

On physical examination, the aforementioned complaints are usually obvious. Significant callus formation may be observed on the lateral, plantar, or in a lateral plantar position overlying the fifth metatarsal head. Any pronation of the longitudinal arch should be noted as well as any restricted hindfoot motion.

Radiographic evaluation may demonstrate an enlarged metatarsal head, outflaring of the fifth metatar-

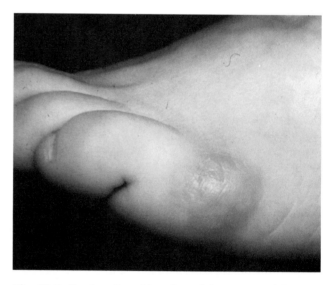

**Fig. 16-2.** Bunionette with enlarged bursa. (Used by permission. Mann RA, Coughlin MJ: In *Keratotic disorders of the plantar skin.* In *Surgery of the foot and ankle,* St Louis, 1993, CV Mosby, p. 443.)

sal metaphysis, or widening of the 4-5 intermetatarsal angle. Abduction of the fifth toe in relationship to the fifth metatarsal head may also be demonstrated.

### Conservative treatment

Early treatment involves attempting to relieve pressure on the underlying bony prominence. Stretching of shoes or obtaining shoes with a soft upper that is more forgiving will relieve overlying pressure. Seams or stitching directly over the bunionette should be avoided. Moleskin applied to a blister may promote healing and protect the area while athletes continue their activities. Altering running and/or training ac-

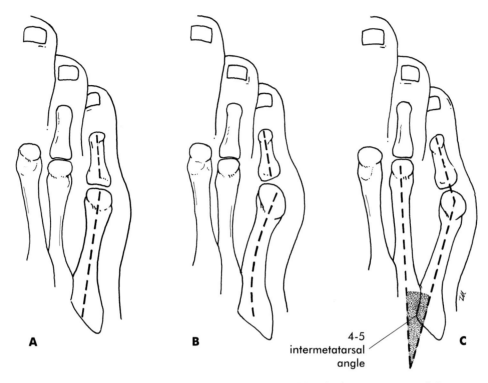

**Fig. 16-3. A,** Bunionette with enlarged fifth metatarsal head. **B,** Bunionette with bowing of metaphysis. **C,** Bunionette with enlarged 4-5 intermetatarsal angle.

tivity may also diminish symptoms. Trimming the callus may significantly relieve symptoms. Physicians may teach their patients how to pare the callus appropriately, and this coupled with a well-placed metatarsal head may allow a return to regular athletic activity.

When athletic activity is significantly impaired even with conservative efforts, surgical intervention may be contemplated (see Case Study 1). Attention must be directed to the location of the callosity for specific osteotomies of the fifth metatarsal direct the metatarsal head in different directions. Minimal surgical intervention is important when treating forefoot callosities. Extensive soft tissue stripping, unsecured osteotomies, and multiple metatarsal osteotomies should all be avoided in athletes. Although they may relieve the painful callosity, the surgery itself may significantly diminish the athletic performance of the patient, and thus be considered unsuccessful. Many procedures are available to surgically treat a bunionette; I have chosen only two surgical procedures as they fulfill the requirement of less surgical exposure, employ internal fixation, and appear better suited to athletes. Again, where possible, conservative treatment should be advocated by the treating physician until obviously it is incompatible with continued athletic function.

**Case Study 1.** A 30-year-old skier developed pain and swelling over the plantar lateral aspect of the fifth metatarsal head. An increased callosity was observed over the plantar lateral aspect of the bunionette. A painful inflamed bursa developed during the middle of ski season that was partially relieved by grinding down the inner aspect of the ski boot overlying the bunionette. Likewise, the area overlying the fifth metatarsal head was relieved in the athlete's everyday footwear by stretching the leather surface.

On physical examination, a normal neurologic and vascular examination was noted. Prominence of the fifth metatarsal head was characterized by a callosity both on the plantar and lateral aspect. Radiographic evaluation demonstrated an enlarged fifth metatarsal lateral condyle.

Conservative care, stretching of shoes, and padding were all recommended.

At the end of ski season, the patient requested surgical treatment. An oblique osteotomy was performed and fixed with Kirschner wires (K-wires). The K-wires were removed 4 weeks after surgery. At 8 weeks following surgery, the osteotomy was healed and the patient began progressive walking that evolved over the ensuing 2 months to jogging and sports activities. The patient skied the following season without symptoms.

**Surgical treatment**

1. The foot is cleansed and draped in the routine fashion. An Esmarch bandage is used to exsan-

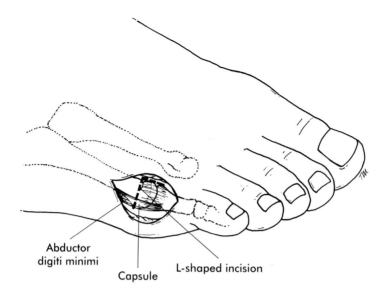

**Fig. 16-4.** An L-shaped capsular incision is used to approach the bunionette.

guinate the foot. The ankle is carefully padded and the Esmarch is used as a tourniquet.

2. A longitudinal lateral incision is centered directly over the bunionette, extending from the midproximal phalanx to 1 cm above the metatarsal head. Care is taken to protect the neurovascular bundles.

3. The MP capsule is detached on the dorsal and proximal aspect and turned downward, exposing the prominent lateral condyle (Fig. 16-4).

4. A sagittal saw is used to resect the lateral condyle in line with the diaphyseal shaft of the fifth metatarsal. (At this point, a decision must be made regarding the type of osteotomy to be performed. For a pure lateral callus, a chevron osteotomy is performed. For a combined plantar lateral callus, a distal oblique osteotomy is performed.)

5A. *Chevron osteotomy*[16,27] — A lateral medial drill hole is placed in the center of the fifth metatarsal head, marking the apex of the chevron osteotomy. A 60-degree angled osteotomy based proximally is directed in a lateral medial plane. The metatarsal head is translated medially and fixed with a percutaneous 0.045 K-wire (Fig. 16-5).

5B. *Distal oblique osteotomy*[4,26] — After exposing the metatarsal head and metaphysis, an oblique osteotomy is performed from a distal lateral to proximal medial direction. The metatarsal head is displaced medially and slightly proximally and is allowed to "raise up" approximately 3 mm to decrease plantar pressure beneath the fifth metatarsal head. The osteotomy is fixed with a percutaneous 0.045 K-wire (Fig. 16-6).

6. Any remaining prominent metaphysis is shaved with the sagittal saw. A drill hole is placed in the dorsal proximal metaphysis, and the capsule is anchored with an interrupted suture. Remaining interrupted sutures are placed to reinforce the capsular repair (Fig. 16-7).

7. The skin is closed in a routine fashion. A gauze and tape dressing is applied and changed on a weekly basis. The patient is allowed to ambulate in a wooden-soled shoe.

8. At 3 weeks the sutures and K-wire are removed.

Athletic activity is increased as swelling and pain diminish. Radiographic confirmation of healing should be present before aggressive activity such as jogging, running, or jumping is commenced.

In general, resolution of the symptomatic bunionette can be achieved with one of the above procedures for type I or type II bunionettes. With a splayfoot and a significantly wide 4-5 metatarsal angle, a diaphyseal midshaft osteotomy may be necessary to achieve more correction.[13] More extensive procedures such as this should be reserved for athletes with significant limitations, as the extensive nature of this surgery may limit postoperative athletic expectations.

## INTRACTABLE PLANTAR KERATOSES

The development of a keratosis beneath one or more of the metatarsal heads is referred to as an *IPK*. A callosity beneath the fifth metatarsal when associated with a bunionette has already been discussed. A callus may be a localized discrete lesion or a diffuse keratotic buildup (Fig. 16-8). Callus formation in athletes is not at all uncommon, and if asymptomatic, rarely requires medical intervention. With significant

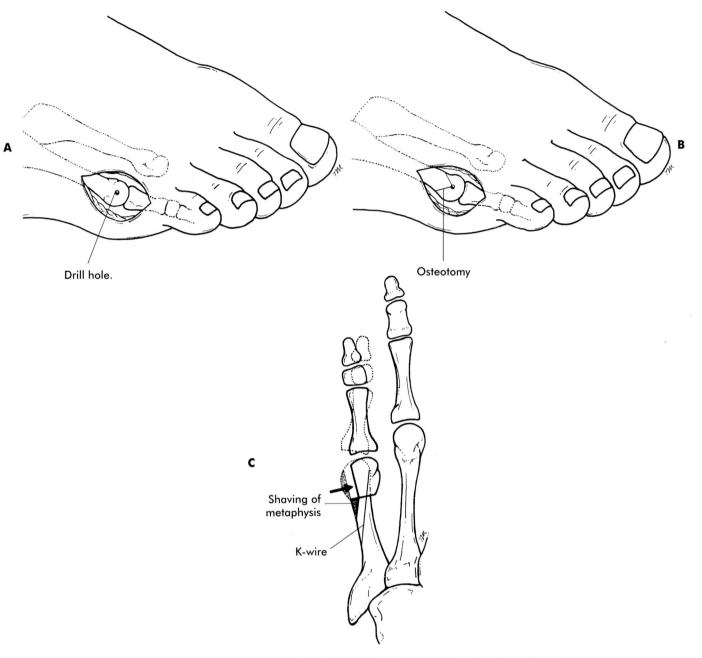

**Fig. 16-5. A,** A drill hole is placed in the center of the metatarsal head and drilled in a lateral to medial direction. **B,** A chevron-shaped osteotomy is based proximally with the apex at the drill hole. **C,** Medial translation of the metatarsal head with K-wire fixation and shaving of the metaphyseal flare (shaded area denotes shaved bone in metaphysis).

buildup, painful symptoms may occur requiring evaluation and treatment.

A diffuse callus may be due to repetitive abrasion associated with athletic activity. It also may be associated with a long second metatarsal or long second and third metatarsal. A discrete callus may occur beneath a single metatarsal head.[20] It is typically associated with an enlarged fibular metatarsal condyle. It is important to distinguish this from a wart

(Fig. 16-9). Although warts (plantar verrucae) typically are not found beneath a metatarsal head, on occasion they can occur in this region and thus must be differentiated from an IPK. Trimming of a wart will uncover end arterials in the lesion characterized by punctate hemorrhages.

Evaluation of the athlete with an IPK involves determining the significance of the symptoms, length of duration, and association, if any, with specific athletic activity. A patient with minimal symptoms requires no treatment.

Radiographic evaluation entails weight-bearing films with markers to determine the exact location of the IPK (a long metatarsal may be associated with an IPK; likewise, a marker may be located directly beneath the fibular condyle of a metatarsal head).

Pressure studies on a Harris mat may also help to define the exact location of increased plantar pressure.

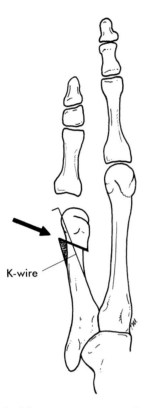

**Fig. 16-6.** Distal oblique osteotomy with K-wire fixation (shaded area denotes shaved bone in metaphysis).

**Conservative treatment**

Conservative treatment revolves around paring the IPK and padding it to relieve the pressure (Fig. 16-10). A patient can be instructed to trim the lesion every 7 to 10 days, and this will significantly relieve discomfort. Placement of a metatarsal pad just proximal to the IPK can transfer pressure to the metatarsal diaphysis and relieve symptoms (see Case Study 2). Custom or prefabricated orthotic devices also can be a significant help in relieving symptoms. Athletes may alter their workout, change sporting activities, change duration or intensity of the workout—all with gratifying results.

**Case Study 2.** A 50-year-old tennis player developed a painful callus beneath the second and third metatarsals. It was a diffusely thickened callus that began to limit his sports activities. On initial evaluation the diffuse callus was trimmed and the patient instructed in how to care conservatively for the IPK. A pumice stone was used to pare the callus. The patient also obtained disposable scalpels to shave his thickened callosity. When he returned for further follow-up, radiographs demonstrated a long second and third metatarsal in relationship to the adjacent metatarsals. A soft pad was placed in his shoe just proximal to the callosity. Between shaving the callosity and padding it, symptoms were completely relieved and he returned to full sports activities. Later a soft orthotic device was fabricated to relieve pressure beneath the second and third metatarsals. These convenient orthotic devices could be moved from shoe to shoe and replaced the temporary soft pads that were used to alleviate his initial symptoms.

When all methods of conservative treatment have been exhausted, surgical intervention may be considered. Caution is advised in considering any metatarsal osteotomy in a high-level athlete. The possibility of delayed union, nonunion, or malunion can significantly impair later athletic activity. The development

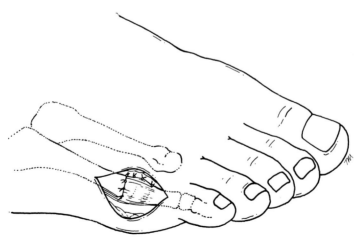

**Fig. 16-7.** L-shaped capsular closure. The dorsal proximal corner may be fixed with a drill hole in the metaphysis to anchor the repair.

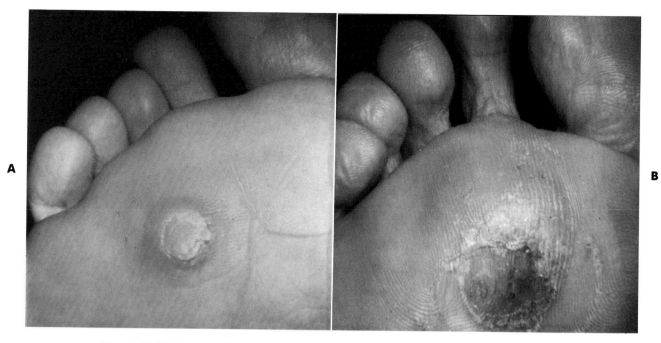

**Fig. 16-8. A,** Discrete callus in a tennis player with an enlarged fibular condyle. **B,** Diffuse callus in a runner. (**A** and **B,** Used by permission. Mann RA, Coughlin MJ: In *Video textbook of foot and ankle surgery,* St Louis, 1991, Medical Video Productions, p. 86.)

of a transfer lesion beneath another metatarsal head is not uncommon. Multiple metatarsal osteotomies are to be discouraged. Likewise, floating metatarsal osteotomies without internal fixation have a high rate of malunion with resultant transfer lesions.

### Surgical treatment: condylectomy[22]

1. The foot is cleansed and draped in a routine fashion. An Esmarch bandage is used to exsanguinate the foot. It is carefully padded at the ankle and used as a tourniquet.
2. A longitudinal incision is centered over the metatarsal head with a "hockey stick" extension into the adjacent interspace. (The extensor tendon may be temporarily released to aid exposure and is repaired at the conclusion of the procedure.)
3. The MP joint capsule is released and the toe is flexed to 90 degrees at the MP joint.
4. A Hoke osteotome is used to osteotomize 25% of the plantar condyle. Care is taken not to fracture the metatarsal head (Fig. 16-11). The condyle is removed.
5. A 0.045 K-wire introduced at the MP joint is driven distally out the tip of the toe. With the MP joint reduced, the pin is driven in a retrograde fashion stabilizing the joint.
6. The extensor tendon (if released) is repaired. The skin is closed in a routine fashion.
7. A gauze and tape dressing is applied and changed

on a weekly basis. The patient is allowed to ambulate in a wooden-soled shoe.
8. At 3 weeks the sutures and K-wire are removed.

Athletic activity is permitted as swelling and pain decrease. The toe is taped in an appropriate position for 6 weeks following surgery.

### Surgical treatment: metatarsal osteotomy

1. The foot is cleansed and draped in a routine fashion. An Esmarch bandage is used to exsanguinate the foot. It is carefully padded at the ankle and used as a tourniquet.
2. A dorsal longitudinal incision is centered over the involved metatarsal.
3A. If a *distal oblique osteotomy*[25] is performed (Fig. 16-12), the cut is directed in a vertical direction. The metatarsal head is displaced upward 3 mm[14] and fixed with a 0.045 K-wire.
3B. If a *vertical chevron osteotomy*[18] is performed (Fig. 16-13), the V-shaped osteotomy is directed in a vertical direction. (This is more stable side to side than a transverse osteotomy.) The metatarsal head is displaced upward 3 mm and fixed with a 0.045 K-wire.
3C. If a *proximal transverse osteotomy*[18] is performed (Fig. 16-14), a dorsal-based wedge is excised. The further proximal the osteotomy is located, the more elevation is achieved with wedge removal. (Care must be taken not to

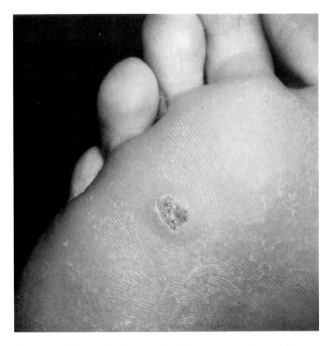

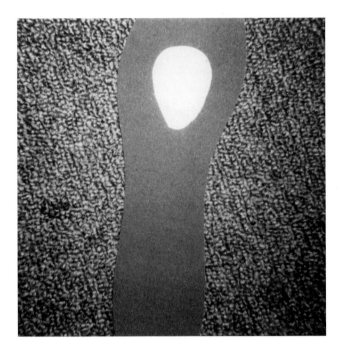

**Fig. 16-9.** A wart is characterized by punctate hemorrhages, which are obvious when the callus is trimmed. (Used by permission. Mann RA, Coughlin MJ: In *Video textbook of foot and ankle surgery,* St Louis, 1991, Medical Video Productions, p. 86.)

**Fig. 16-10.** Padding an IPK often is successful treatment.

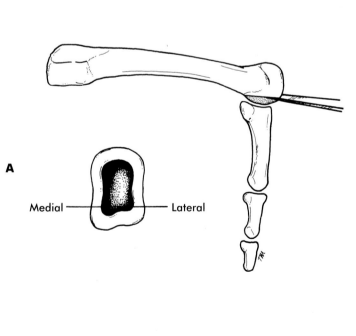

A

Medial —————— Lateral

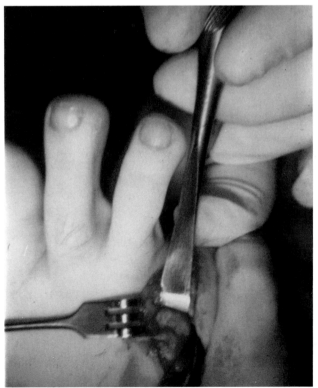

B

**Fig. 16-11. A,** Plantar condylectomy for a discrete IPK. **B,** Interoperative view of plantar condylectomy (one fourth to one third of the plantar metatarsal head is excised).

overcorrect at the osteotomy site.) The wedge may be removed with a sagittal saw or with a small rongeur. Internal fixation is recommended. A screw, pin, or wire loop fixation is used.

4. The wound is closed in a routine fashion. A gauze and tape dressing is applied and changed on a weekly basis. The patient is allowed to ambulate in a wooden-soled shoe.
5. Sutures are removed 3 weeks following surgery. Percutaneous K-wires are removed 3 to 4 weeks following surgery. The forefoot is then strapped with tape and gauze until symptoms remit.
6. Radiographic confirmation of union is important before aggressive athletic activity can be commenced.

Athletic activity is permitted as swelling and pain diminish.

In general, with a plantar condylectomy, satisfactory results are attained for relieving the symptoms of a discrete well-localized IPK.[22] Likewise, a distal osteotomy[18,25] may be efficacious for a similar lesion. A diffuse callus in the athlete is probably best padded and shaved, as a more extensive procedure involving a diaphyseal osteotomy[15] may require prolonged healing time and place the athlete at greater risk for delayed healing, malunion, and transfer metatarsalgia. A proximal closing wedge osteotomy[25]

may be used to elevate a symptomatic long second or third metatarsal. Meticulous attention to the osteotomy and excellent postoperative care are necessary to avoid complications.

## INTERDIGITAL NEUROMAS

An interdigital neuroma may be a source of ill-defined forefoot pain. Located in the second or third intermetatarsal space (IMS), a neuroma is rarely if ever isolated to the first or fourth interspace. Rarely do two simultaneous neuromas occur in the same foot.

Typically an athlete initially describes ill-defined forefoot pain, often exacerbated with running or sports activities, which is relieved by rest or removal of a pair of shoes. Sometimes pain increases with intensity and/or duration of sports activities.

The physical examination includes educating patients regarding which symptoms to watch for. Although ill-defined forefoot discomfort is common, the treating physician needs to help patients define the exact area of pain. With time and education athletes may be able to actually pinpoint the exact area of pain from the dorsal and plantar aspect usually in either the second or third interspace. Neuritic symptoms or numbness in either the second or third common digital nerve distribution may be observed.

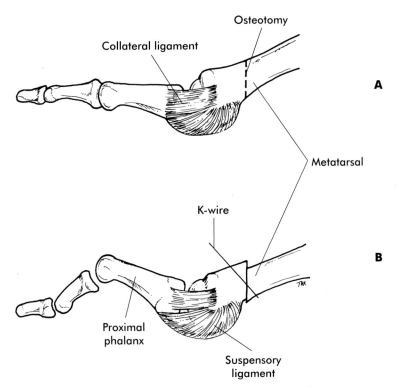

**Fig. 16-12. A,** Distal oblique osteotomy (dotted line shows proposed osteotomy site). **B,** Following displacement and internal fixation with K-wire.

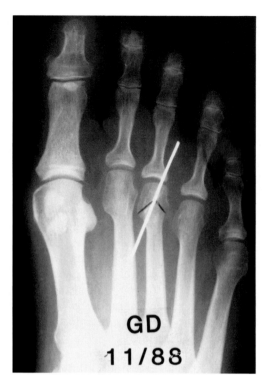

**Fig. 16-13.** Distal chevron osteotomy with internal fixation. (Used by permission. Mann RA, Coughlin MJ: In *Video textbook of foot and ankle surgery,* St Louis, 1991, Medical Video Productions, p. 93.)

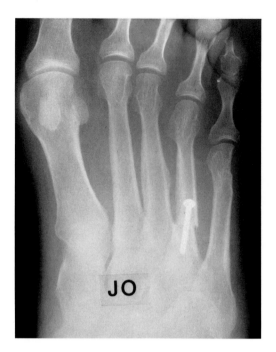

**Fig. 16-14.** Proximal closing wedge osteotomy with screw fixation. (Used by permission. Mann RA, Coughlin MJ: In *Video textbook of foot and ankle surgery,* St Louis, 1991, Medical Video Productions, p. 91.)

On physical examination, care is taken to observe for signs of peripheral neuropathy or vascular insufficiency. The toes are examined for fixed deformity. Any callus or IPK is noted, and the adjacent MP joints are evaluated for pain or instability (see section on Metatarsophalangeal Instability). Palpation of the involved interspace usually elicits pain. Grasping and compression of the transverse arch at the level of the metatarsal heads may elicit a click (Mulder's sign),[24] which occurs when the neuroma subluxates below the metatarsal head and transverse metatarsal ligament (TML).

On occasion, when a patient has difficulty isolating the location of pain, a 1% lidocaine injection may be used to determine the site of pain.[9] During serial office visits 1 week apart, the physician may inject the second IMS, then the third IMS, then the second MP joint, then the third MP joint. The patient is asked to repeat the activity that causes the most discomfort. Within 1 or 2 hours the anesthetic wears off. When temporary relief is achieved with the injection, followed by recurrent symptoms with the "wearing off" of the anesthetic, a diagnosis may be confirmed.

**Conservative treatment**

Early conservative treatment may alleviate symptoms in the athlete. With intermittent symptoms exacerbated by intense athletic activity, or sports of significant duration, a change in the type of activity or its duration may completely relieve symptoms (i.e., a person who jogs 4 miles at a time and develops pain at 2.5 miles may jog for 2 miles and bicycle for 2 to 3 miles and be symptom-free).

Placing a small metatarsal pad just proximal to the symptomatic interspace may relieve symptoms. Change in athletic shoes may also alleviate pain.

When conservative methods including the modification of sports activities have not relieved symptoms, surgical intervention may be considered.[1,21,23]

**Surgical treatment: excision of interdigital neuroma**

1. The foot is cleansed and draped in the usual fashion. An Esmarch bandage is used to exsanguinate the foot. The ankle is carefully padded and the Esmarch is used as a tourniquet.
2. A 2-cm dorsal incision is centered in the involved interspace.
3. The dissection is carried down to the TML (Fig. 16-15).
4. A 2-3 prong Weitlaner retractor is used to distract the adjacent metatarsals and place the TML under tension.
5. The TML is sectioned only when necessary to expose the neuroma and common digital nerve.

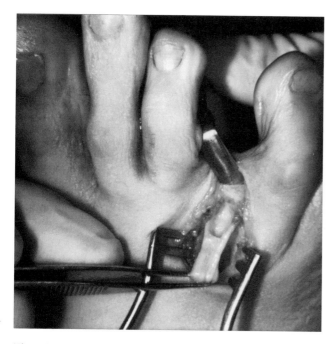

**Fig. 16-15.** Dorsal incision demonstrates a large interdigital neuroma. The transverse metatarsal ligament has been sectioned. (Used by permission. Coughlin, MJ: *Soft tissue afflictions*. In Chapman M, editor: *Operative orthopaedics*, Philadelphia, 1993, JB Lippincott, p. 2289.)

(Sectioning of the TML in the competitive athlete should be avoided if possible.)
6. The nerve is severed distally below the neuroma and then tension is placed upon the proximal nerve. A nerve freer is used to dissect longitudinally to isolate the common digital nerve. With tension on the proximal nerve, a scalpel is used to transect the nerve as proximal as possible in the interspace.
7. The interspace is inspected for any other nerve tissue that may be a cause of pain. The retractor is removed, and the surgical wound is irrigated and closed in a routine fashion.
8. A gauze and tape dressing is applied and changed on a weekly basis, and the patient is allowed to ambulate in a postoperative shoe.
9. Suture removal is carried out 3 weeks following surgery, and a circumferential gauze and tape strapping is continued for 3 more weeks to allow adequate healing of the TML if it was sectioned (Fig. 16-16).

Aggressive walking can be commenced 4 weeks following surgery, with increased activity as pain and swelling permit.

## HARD CORNS AND SOFT CORNS

A hard corn (Fig. 16-17) develops over the lateral aspect of the fifth toe usually due to pressure of the

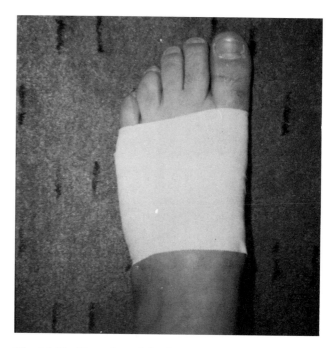

**Fig. 16-16.** Strapping of the foot is continued for 6 weeks postoperatively to promote healing of the transverse metatarsal ligament.

shoe against an underlying exostosis or condyle on the fifth toe. Patients may complain of pain associated with a hypertrophic callus on the lateral aspect of the fifth toe. A soft corn (Fig. 16-18) develops between the toes due to pressure between two adjacent bony prominences. Patient may complain of exquisite pain; maceration sometimes occurs that resembles a mycotic infection. Desiccation of the lesion may then help to distinguish it from an infection.[17]

On physical examination, the obvious callosity occurs overlying a bony prominence. Radiographic evaluation may help to define the location of the lesion (Fig. 16-19).

### Conservative treatment

Padding of the hard corn (Fig. 16-20) may alleviate discomfort. Stretching of shoes overlying the lesion may decrease symptoms. Shaving of the callosity on a frequent basis may diminish the painful symptoms.

With a soft corn, padding of one or both toes with either a foam spacer (Fig. 16-21) or tubular foam gauze often eliminates compression between the two toes. Shaving of the callosity also may be indicated (see Case Study 3). When conservative measures have failed, surgical resection of the involved condyle may eliminate the prominence and alleviate the symptoms.

**Case Study 3.** A 40-year-old jogger developed exquisite pain beneath the fourth and fifth toes. He recognized a macerated area in the fourth web space. It was unclear whether this was a fungus infection or a soft corn.

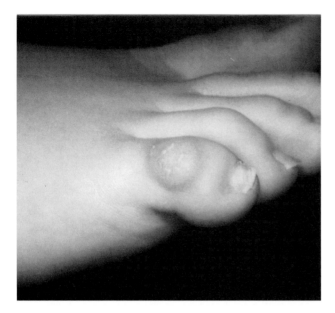

**Fig. 16-17.** Hard corn with keratotic buildup. (Used by permission. Mann RA, Coughlin MJ: In *Video textbook of foot and ankle surgery*, St Louis, 1991, Medical Video Productions, p. 50.)

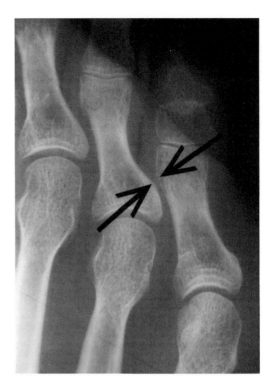

**Fig. 16-19.** Radiograph demonstrating the location of a soft corn. (Used by permission. Mann RA, Coughlin MJ: In *Video textbook of foot and ankle surgery*, St Louis, 1991, Medical Video Productions, p. 51.)

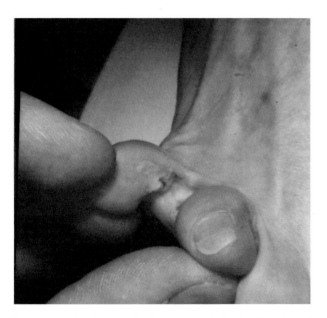

**Fig. 16-18.** A soft corn is demonstrated in the fourth web space, mimicking a mycotic infection. (Used by permission. Mann RA, Coughlin MJ: In *Video textbook of foot and ankle surgery*, St Louis, 1991, Medical Video Productions, p. 51.)

On his initial orthopedic evaluation, radiographs demonstrated impingement between the PIP joint of the fourth toe and the DIP joint of the fifth toe.

Initial treatment used rubbing alcohol applied with a cotton-tipped applicator three times a day to desiccate the area. Then lamb's wool was placed between the toes to pad and alleviate pressure between the two prominent condyles. Later, a foam spacer was placed between the toes and

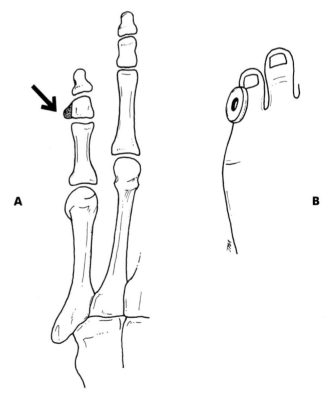

**Fig. 16-20. A,** An underlying exostosis combined with restrictive footwear leads to a hard corn. **B,** A pad may be used to relieve pressure.

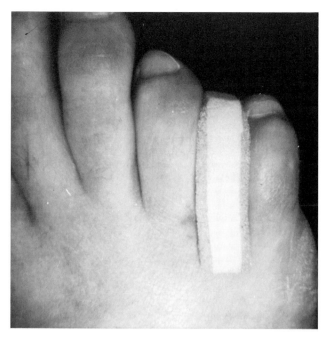

**Fig. 16-21.** A pad is used to relieve pressure in the web space. (Used by permission. Mann RA, Coughlin MJ: In *Video textbook of foot and ankle surgery,* St Louis, 1991, Medical Video Productions, p. 51.)

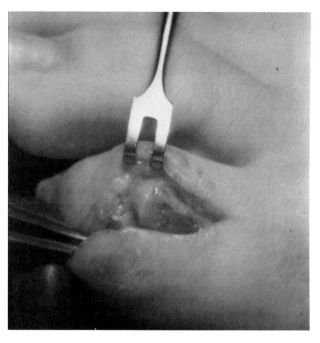

**Fig. 16-22.** A dorsal incision is used for the condylectomy as the treatment for a hard corn. (Used by permission. Coughlin MJ: *Soft tissue afflictions.* In Chapman M, editor: *Operative orthopaedics,* Philadelphia, 1993, JB Lippincott, p. 2223.)

allowed resumption of all jogging activity. No surgery was performed.

### Surgical treatment for hard corns[19]

1. The foot is cleansed and draped in the usual fashion. Often a digital anesthetic block is used, although a foot block may also be considered.
2. A dorsolateral longitudinal incision is centered over the prominent lateral condyle.
3. With sharp dissection, the capsular fibers are peeled off of the condyle.
4. A rongeur is used to remove the prominent condyle, with care taken to leave enough articular surface to retain joint stability (Fig. 16-22).
5. The sharp bony edges are beveled with a rongeur.
6. The capsule is closed with two or three interrupted absorbable sutures.
7. The skin is closed with a running skin closure. A gauze and tape dressing is applied and changed on a weekly basis. The patient is allowed to ambulate in a postoperative shoe.
8. Sutures are removed 3 weeks after surgery. The toe is then taped to the adjacent toe for 4 more weeks to promote stability and avoid injury.

After suture removal, an increase in sports activity can be commenced. Walking and bicycling may be started; running may commence after swelling has sufficiently diminished to allow footwear to fit adequately.

### Surgical treatment for soft corns

1. The foot is cleansed and draped in the usual fashion. Often a digital anesthetic block is used, although a foot block may also be considered.
2. A decision is made whether to treat both lesions on adjacent toes or treat only one. (With a significant lesion on one toe and a minor lesion on the corresponding toe, surgical repair of the larger lesion usually will successfully eliminate the entire problem.) Whether one or both lesions are surgically treated remains the decision of the operating surgeon.
3. A dorsolateral longitudinal incision is centered over the prominent lateral condyle.
4. With sharp dissection, the capsular fibers are peeled off of the condyle.
5. A rongeur is used to remove the prominent condyle, with care taken to leave enough articular surface to retain joint stability (Fig. 16-23).
6. The sharp edges are beveled with a rongeur.
7. The capsule is closed with an interrupted absorbable suture.
8. The skin is closed with a running skin closure. A gauze and tape dressing is applied and changed on a weekly basis. The patient is allowed to ambulate in a wooden-soled postoperative shoe.
9. Sutures are removed 3 weeks after surgery.
10. A small gauze spacer is used between the toes for

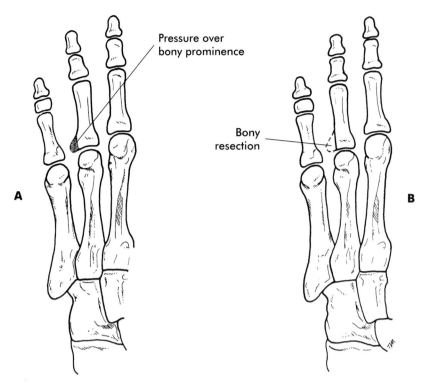

**Fig. 16-23. A,** A soft corn may develop over the base of the proximal phalanx. **B,** Resection of the bony prominence.

another 4 weeks until the surgical incisions have softened. After suture removal, an increase in sports activity can commence. Walking and bicycling may be started. Running may commence after swelling has successfully diminished to allow footwear to fit adequately.

## HAMMERTOES, MALLET TOES, CLAW TOES

Deformities of the lesser toes include both flexible and fixed deformities. Typically callus formation occurs over bony prominences, and at times during athletic activity these areas may become inflamed and painful. A hammertoe (Fig. 16-24) is characterized by a flexion contracture at the PIP joint. Early on, it may present as a flexible deformity that in time may become fixed. With a mallet toe (Fig. 16-25), there is a flexion contracture at the DIP joint. Early on, it may present as a flexible deformity due to tightness of the flexor digitorum longus (FDL) tendon. With time it may become a fixed deformity. A callus may develop dorsally over the DIP joint due to pressure or abrasion from impacting against the toe box. A callus may also develop at the tip of the toe due to pressure against the insole of the shoe.

With a claw toe deformity, typically a flexion contracture develops at the PIP joint with hyperextension at the MP joint. A callosity may develop over the PIP joint; with a long-standing contracture,

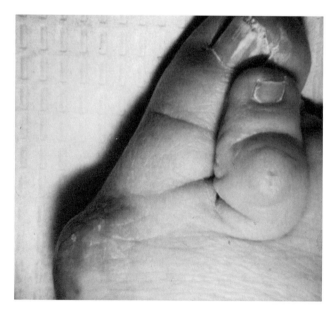

**Fig. 16-24.** Hammertoe deformity. (Used by permission. Mann RA, Coughlin MJ: In *Video textbook of foot and ankle surgery*, St Louis, 1991, Medical Video Productions, p. 40.)

an IPK may develop beneath the metatarsal head. Early on, a flexible contracture may be passively correctable, although with time a fixed contracture may develop.

Subjectively a patient typically complains of pain

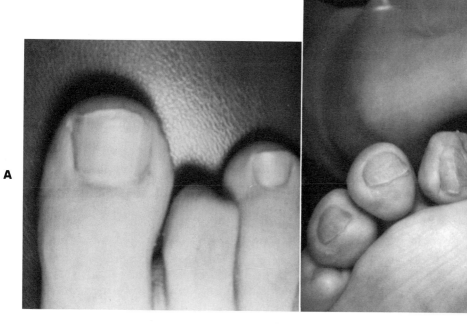

A

B

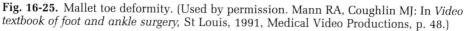

**Fig. 16-25.** Mallet toe deformity. (Used by permission. Mann RA, Coughlin MJ: In *Video textbook of foot and ankle surgery*, St Louis, 1991, Medical Video Productions, p. 48.)

over a prominent callus on the involved toe; occasionally a painful callus will develop at the tip of the toe.

On physical examination, the treating physician observes not only a keratotic buildup over the deformity, but also the attitude of the toe must be examined. The flexibility or rigidity of the deformity may determine the particular surgical repair should it be necessary. The presence of multiple toe deformities, contractures at adjacent joints, and neurologic deficits must be appreciated during the evaluation. With all of these lesser toe deformities, an athlete may complain of blistering, callus formation, swelling, or pain due to a dynamic or static deformity. Occasionally an infection may develop in the overlying tissue.

### Conservative treatment

Conservative care includes relieving pressure over the painful area.[10] The use of roomy footwear will often relieve discomfort in the athlete. Padding often allows return to sports activity. Shaving of painful callosities may temporarily relieve keratotic buildup. Often conservative care will allow an athlete to continue activity, although decreasing the duration or intensity of the workout or changing to a different sporting activity may be necessary on a temporary or permanent basis. When conservative measures do not allow acceptable athletic activity, surgical intervention may be necessary.

### Surgical treatment: hammertoe repair[11]

1. The foot is cleansed and draped in the usual fashion. Usually a digital nerve block is used as an anesthetic.
2. A small Penrose drain may be used as a tourniquet (optional).
3. A dorsal elliptical skin incision is centered over the PIP joint. The incision is carried down to bone with excision of an ellipse of skin, extensor tendon, and capsule exposing the condyles of the proximal phalanx.
4. The collateral ligaments of the PIP joints are severed, enabling the condyles to be delivered.
5. A bone-cutting forceps is used to osteotomize the proximal phalanx in the supracondylar region (Fig. 16-26). The sharp edges are beveled with a rongeur.
6. The articular surface of the middle phalanx is exposed, and a rongeur is used to remove the articular surface (optional).
7. A 0.045 K-wire is introduced at the PIP joint and driven distally, exiting the tip of the toe. Then with the toe reduced to the desired position, the K-wire is driven in a retrograde fashion, stabilizing the hammertoe repair. The pin is bent at the tip of the toe to prevent proximal migration.
8. A gauze and tape dressing is applied and changed on a weekly basis. The patient is permitted to ambulate in a bunion shoe. Sutures and K-wire are removed 3 weeks after surgery.
9. The patient is then instructed to tape the toe to an

adjacent toe for an additional 4 weeks to protect it from injury.

After the K-wire is removed, increased walking activity is performed. Cycling may be allowed. Running or jogging is usually avoided until swelling has diminished (6 to 8 weeks). Often there will be 10 to 15 degrees of motion at the involved joint following adequate healing. Whether an arthrodesis occurs is not of significant concern. Fibrous ankylosis with a small amount of motion is equally acceptable.

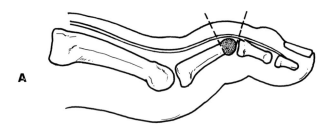

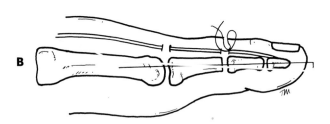

**Fig. 16-26.** Hammertoe repair. **A,** Proposed resection. **B,** K-wire fixation following condylectomy.

## Surgical treatment: early flexible mallet toe repair

1. The foot is cleansed and draped in the usual fashion. A digital block is used for anesthesia. (With an early mallet toe deformity, the toe can be passively corrected to neutral with pressure.)
2. A #11 scalpel blade is introduced on the plantar aspect of the DIP joint and the FDL tendon is released.
3. The incision is closed with an interrupted skin suture.
4. A gauze and tape dressing is applied, and the patient is allowed to ambulate in a postoperative shoe.
5. The sutures are removed 10 days after surgery.

Athletic activity can be resumed rapidly following this procedure with little downtime.

When a fixed mallet toe is corrected, a similar procedure is performed as is carried out for a hammertoe deformity. In this case the procedure is carried out at the DIP joint (Fig. 16-27).[12]

For a hammertoe that can be passively corrected, and has no element of fixed contracture, a flexion tendon transfer may be used. The procedure is technically more difficult than a condylectomy, but leaves the toe more flexible. The FDL tendon is transferred to the dorsum of the proximal phalanx. This procedure removes a deforming force and at the same time makes the FDL a plantar flexor of the proximal phalanx. Whether it is a dynamic transfer or a tenodesis is unclear, but it is a useful procedure for repair of the flexible hammertoe. This procedure is also used for a flexible claw toe and for the unstable MP joint (both discussed later).

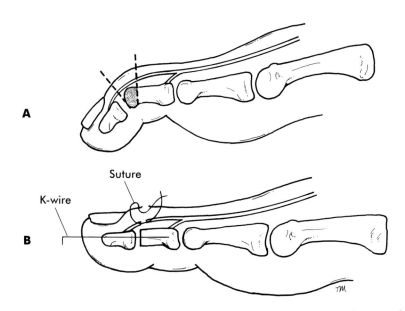

**Fig. 16-27.** Mallet toe repair. **A,** Proposed resection. **B,** K-wire fixation following condylectomy.

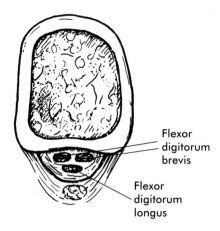

**Fig. 16-32.** Cross section of lesser toe at level of metatarsal head demonstrating flexor digitorum brevis and longus.

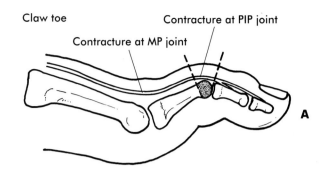

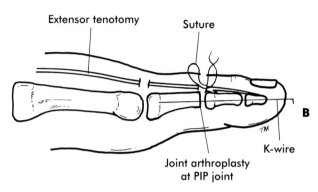

**Fig. 16-33. A,** Claw toe deformity. **B,** Following metatarsophalangeal joint release and extensor tenotomy and PIP joint arthroplasty.

causes such as spasticity, muscular dystrophy, spinal abnormality, and previous trauma (old fractured tibia, old compartment syndrome, etc.).

Many cases may be effectively treated with roomy footwear, padding, and pedicures; however, on occasion an athlete is so symptomatic that surgery is contemplated. Although claw toes frequently involve multiple toes, they have similarities with different stages in the development and treatment of a hammertoe deformity.

Early on, flexible claw toes (although multiple in nature) resemble flexible hammertoes. A flexor tendon transfer of the second, third, and fourth toes may achieve adequate realignment by releasing the contracted FDL tendon and depressing the proximal phalanx through the tendon transfer (see the section on Flexible Hammertoe Repair). Rarely is a flexor tendon transfer performed on the fifth toe. A flexor tenotomy is occasionally performed, although often the fifth toe is asymptomatic.

As a claw toe becomes fixed, a patient may develop symptoms of a hammertoe with callus formation overlying the PIP joint. Because of the fixed dorsiflexion contracture at the MP joint, the toe buckles, depressing the metatarsal head. A plantar callus (IPK) may develop due to increased pressure beneath the metatarsal head. The treating physician needs to remember that the IPK is usually due to the contracted toe rather than to a prominent metatarsal condyle. Correction of the toe deformity often is associated with diminution or resolution of the plantar callosity.

The fixed claw toe resembles a fixed hammertoe, although the claw toe also has a contracture at the MP joint. A PIP joint contracture is surgically repaired (Fig. 16-33) with a condylectomy of the proximal phalanx (see the section on Fixed Hammertoe Repair). Obviously, once the PIP joint contracture has been

corrected, attention must be directed to the MP joint contracture.

### Surgical treatment: metatarsophalangeal soft tissue arthroplasty[5,12]

1. The foot is cleansed in the usual fashion. An Esmarch bandage is used to exsanguinate the foot. The ankle is carefully padded and the Esmarch is used as a tourniquet.
2. An oblique or longitudinal incision is centered over the MP joint.
3. The long extensor tendon is split longitudinally and Z-lengthened.
4. The medial, dorsal, and lateral capsule is completely released to allow reduction of the MP joint. (This requires a significant release in a plantar direction of both collateral ligaments.) When a toe still does not reduce completely following an MP release, there may be adhesions between the plantar capsule and the plantar metatarsal head. These usually can be released with a curved Freer elevator. The toe should be then easily reducible in a dorsal plantar plane.
5. An 0.062 K-wire is used to stabilize the repair. The pin is introduced at the MP joint and driven in a distal direction, exiting the tip of the toe. (When

combined with a hammertoe repair, it is introduced at the PIP joint and driven proximally, exiting the base of the proximal phalanx. It is then driven distally, exiting the tip of the toe.)

6. The pin is then driven in a retrograde fashion, stabilizing the MP joint. The pin is bent at the tip of the toe to prevent proximal migration.

7. The extensor tendon is repaired in a lengthened fashion, and the skin is closed in a routine fashion. A gauze and tape dressing is applied and changed on a weekly basis. The patient is allowed to ambulate in a postoperative shoe.

8. Three weeks following surgery, the K-wire and sutures are removed.

The toe is taped in a corrected position for 4 to 6 weeks. After removal of the K-wire, increased activity is permitted. Walking, cycling, and swimming are allowed. It is wise to progress slowly with the introduction of jogging and running until adequate healing has occurred and swelling has subsided (6 to 8 weeks).

## METATARSOPHALANGEAL JOINT INSTABILITY

Instability of the MP joint can be an extremely difficult diagnosis to make, especially early on when there is a lack of clinical deformity. Typically the second MP joint is the most frequent location of instability, probably due to the longer length of the second ray. In a report on athletes with second MP instability,[6] Coughlin reported 100% of the patients to have an elongated second metatarsal in relationship to adjoining metatarsals. Most likely due to the stress of repeated and prolonged athletic activity, pain without deformity develops in the forefoot.

Typically an athlete initially describes ill-defined forefoot pain often exacerbated by running and sports activities and relieved by rest. Sometimes pain increases with intensity and/or duration of sports activities.

On physical examination, the treating physician needs to initially isolate the exact point of tenderness. With palpation, tenderness is typically elicited over the plantar, medial, or lateral MP capsule. Usually pain is not so pronounced in the third or second intermetatarsal spaces, although it may initially be difficult to differentiate second MP pain from a second IMS neuroma. A critical differentiating finding, however, is that there are no neuritic symptoms in the second or third toes and no numbness associated with capsulitis or instability of the second MP joint. (A second IMS neuroma may occur along with second MP instability; however, this is unusual.)

Capsulitis or inflammation of an MP joint can be associated with systemic or localized arthritis, but

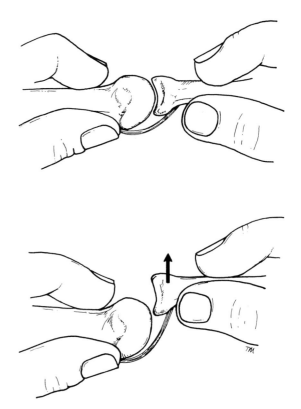

**Fig. 16-34.** A drawer sign is used to detect dorsal plantar instability.

these conditions often involve other MP joints, whereas without a preexisting inflammatory arthropathy, only the second MP joint is usually involved. A drawer sign[2] (Fig. 16-34) is typically the diagnostic test most helpful in defining capsulitis and/or instability of the MP joint. By grasping the involved toe between the fingers and stressing the MP joint in a dorsal plantar direction, exquisite pain can be elicited, likely due to stress on the attenuated plantar capsule or collateral ligaments. (This finding is absent in an isolated interdigital neuroma.)

Not uncommonly, early diagnosis is difficult to make. A patient may be seen on several occasions and isolated injections may be performed with 1% lidocaine into suspected areas of pain (i.e., second IMS, third IMS, second MP joint, third MP joint). A patient is asked to pay close attention to diminution of symptoms with each injection and to help isolate the exact area of pain. The diagnosis of MP instability versus interdigital neuroma formation can be difficult and time-consuming; it should be arrived at by ruling out less likely causes until the examiner and athlete are convinced of the diagnosis.

With time, the diagnosis becomes obvious as the toe deviates[7,8] (Fig. 16-35). Initially the toe deviates medially and with time dorsally, developing into a crossover second toe deformity. This development

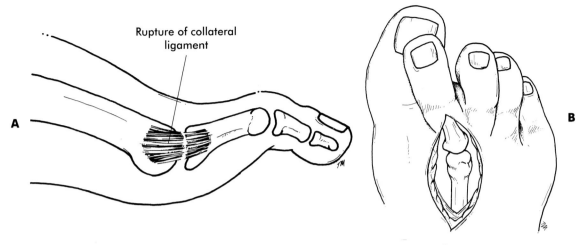

**Fig. 16-35. A,** Instability of the second MP joint with a crossover second toe may occur due to degeneration of the lateral collateral ligament. **B,** Malalignment as demonstrated with a crossover second toe.

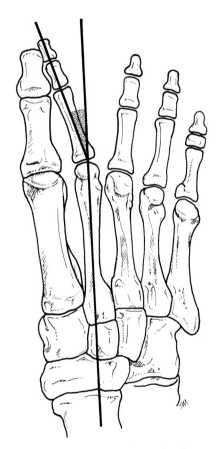

**Fig. 16-36.** Axial malalignment may be demonstrated on radiographic examination.

can be acute, although typically in athletes it occurs insidiously over several months.

Radiographic evaluation involves routine AP and lateral radiographs to determine if there is widening of the joint space (effusion), narrowing (arthritis), or malalignment in relationship to the adjoining MP joints (Fig. 16-36). Occasionally an arthrogram may be obtained, but this is not routinely performed.

### Conservative treatment

Early conservative treatment relies on early diagnosis by the treating physician. Before deformity at the second MP joint, early MP instability is best treated with taping the involved toe, padding, and a change in athletic activity. Taping requires stabilizing the toe to prevent dorsal plantar flexion excursion. Taping to an adjacent toe may be effective. A sling-type taping technique also may be effective (Fig. 16-37). An athlete may need to tape the involved toe for several months, although some athletes find it necessary to tape the toe only during sports activities. A metatarsal pad placed just proximal to the metatarsal head may alleviate pressure and relieve symptoms on the involved MP capsule. Restructuring workouts and modifying athletic activity can be helpful in relieving pain. A runner may find that pain occurs only with greater than 2 miles of jogging and that shorter distances can be accomplished pain-free.

With unsuccessful resolution of discomfort, or insistence on a higher level of athletic activity, surgical intervention may be contemplated. What is presented is a step-by-step approach to MP instability (see Case Study 4).

**Case Study 4.** A 25-year-old female aerobic instructor developed the onset of insidious but increasing pain in the area of her second MP joint over 6 months. No specific injury was noted. She denied neuritic pain. She became unable to tolerate aerobic activity and then noted slight medial deviation of her second toe.

On physical examination, she was noted to have normal sensation and no evidence of a neuroma. She had a negative

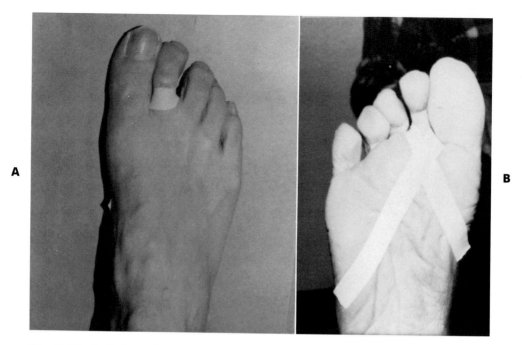

**Fig. 16-37.** Technique of taping toe. (From Coughlin MJ: Cross-over second toe deformity, *Foot Ankle* 8:29, 1987.)

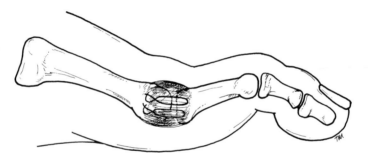

**Fig. 16-38.** Technique of capsular reefing for repair of axial malalignment.

Mulder sign. She had pain on palpation over the second MP joint capsule. She had a positive drawer sign and exquisite pain was elicited. Radiographic examination showed slight medial inclination of the second MP joint.

Initially the patient taped her second toe to the third toe for 3 months and was able to walk without pain. However, her pain resumed with aerobic activity. She requested surgical intervention. A medial MP release, lateral capsular reefing, and flexor tendon transfer were performed. She then taped her toe to stabilize it for 6 weeks postoperatively.

She resumed aggressive walking 6 weeks after surgery, jogging at 3 months, and aerobic instruction at 4 months. She achieved resolution of her pain and is very satisfied with her repair.

### Surgical treatment: metatarsophalangeal instability

1. The foot is cleansed and draped in the routine fashion. The foot is exsanguinated with an Es-

march bandage. The ankle is carefully padded, and the Esmarch is used as an ankle tourniquet.
2. A 2-cm dorsal midline incision is centered over the MP joint. If hyperextension of the toe is present, the extensor digitorum longus tendon is lengthened and later repaired at the conclusion of the procedure.
3. The dorsal MP capsule is released. With medial deviation of the phalanx, the medial capsule is completely released. In this case the lateral capsule is then reefed (Fig. 16-38) with two interrupted 2-0 nonabsorbable sutures to realign the toe in a medial lateral plane. With lateral deviation, the lateral capsule is released and the medial capsule reefed. (This is quite uncommon.)
4. In the presence of remaining hyperextension of the MTP joint, or with remaining dorsal plantar instability, a flexor tendon transfer is then per-

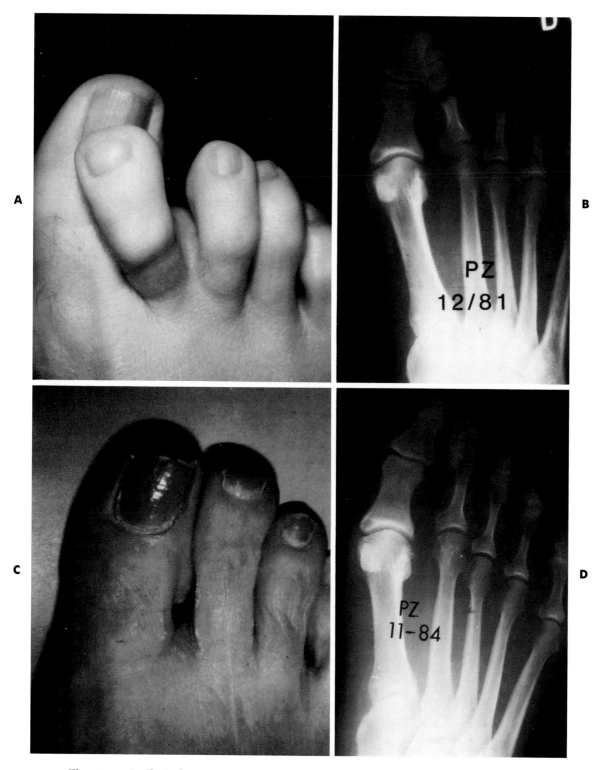

**Fig. 16-39. A,** Clinical appearance of crossover toe deformity. **B,** Radiographic appearance of crossover second toe. **C,** Three-year follow-up demonstrating excellent alignment. **D,** Three-year radiographic follow-up demonstrating excellent alignment. (From Coughlin MJ: Cross-over second toe deformity, *Foot Ankle* 8:29, 1987.)

formed (see section earlier in this chapter).

5. The wound is closed in a routine fashion. A gauze and tape dressing is applied and changed on a weekly basis. The patient is allowed to ambulate in a wooden-soled shoe.

6. Sutures are removed 3 weeks after surgery. If a K-wire has been placed, it is removed at this time (Fig. 16-39). The toe is taped in appropriate position for 6 weeks postoperatively (Fig. 16-37).

The patient is permitted to do aggressive walking 6 weeks following surgery and may increase sporting activity as swelling diminishes and pain permits. Results with this type of approach are gratifying. Significant pain relief can be achieved, although Coughlin[6] reported that several patients had to modify their athletic routine postoperatively.

When possible, the successful conservative treatment of lesser toe problems will allow rapid return to athletic activity with limited downtime. Surgical procedures on the lesser toes take time to heal, are prone to swell, and leave an element of stiffness at the involved joint which may be of some concern to the athlete. Adequate preoperative counseling is important to identify areas of concern, problem areas of recovery, and patient expectations.

**REFERENCES**

1. Betts LO: Morton's metatarsalgia: neuritis of the fourth digital nerve, *Med J Aust* 1:514, 1940.
2. Coughlin MJ: Subluxation and dislocation of the second metatarsophalangeal joint, *Orthop Clin North Am* 20:535, 1989.
3. Coughlin MJ: *Etiology and treatment of the bunionette deformity.* In Greene WB, editor: *American Academy of Orthopaedic Surgeons instructional course lectures,* vol 39, Chicago, 1990, p 37.
4. Coughlin MJ: *Bunionettes.* In Mann RA, Coughlin MJ, editors: *Surgery of the foot and ankle,* ed 6, St Louis, 1992, CV Mosby.
5. Coughlin MJ, Mann RA: *Lesser toe deformities.* In Mann RA, Coughlin MJ, editors: *Surgery of the foot and ankle,* ed 6, St Louis, 1992, CV Mosby.
6. Coughlin MJ: Metatarsophalangeal joint instability in the athlete. *Foot Ankle* 14:309, 1993.
7. Coughlin MJ: Cross-over second toe deformity, *Foot Ankle* 8:29, 1987.
8. Coughlin MJ: When to suspect crossover second toe deformity, *J Musculo Skel Med* 4:39, 1987.
9. Coughlin MJ: *Soft tissue afflictions.* In Chapman M, editor: *Operative orthopaedics,* Philadelphia, 1988, JB Lippincot, p 1819.
10. Coughlin MJ: Mallet toes, hammer toes, claw toes, and corns—causes and treatment of lesser toe deformities, *Postgrad Med* 75:191, 1984.
11. Coughlin MJ: Lesser toe deformities, *Orthopaedics* 10:63, 1987.
12. Coughlin MJ: *Lesser toe abnormalities.* In Chapman M, editor: *Operative orthopaedics,* Philadelphia, 1988, JB Lippincott, p 1765.
13. Coughlin MJ: Treatment of bunionette deformity with longitudinal diaphyseal osteotomy with distal soft tissue repair, *Foot Ankle* 11:195, 1991.
14. Dreeben SM et al: Metatarsal osteotomy for primary metatarsalgia: radiographic and pedobarographic study, *Foot Ankle* 9:214, 1989.
15. Giannestras NJ: Shortening of the metatarsal shaft in the treatment of plantar keratosis, *J Bone Joint Surg* 49A:61, 1958.
16. Mann RA, Coughlin MJ: *Bunionettes.* In *Video textbook of foot and ankle surgery,* St Louis, 1991, Medical Video Productions, p 96.
17. Mann RA, Coughlin MJ: *Lesser toe deformities.* In *American Academy of Orthopaedic Surgeons instructional course lectures,* vol 36, 1987, p 137.
18. Mann RA, Coughlin MJ: *Intractable plantar keratoses.* In *Video textbook of foot and ankle surgery,* St Louis, 1991, Medical Video Productions, p 85.
19. Mann RA, Coughlin MJ: *Lesser-toe deformities.* In Jahss MJ, editor: *Disorders of the foot,* ed 2, Philadelphia, 1991, WB Saunders, p 1205.
20. Mann RA: *Intractable plantar keratosis.* In *American Academy of Orthopaedic Surgeons instructional course lectures,* vol 33, St Louis, 1984, CV Mosby, p 287.
21. Mann RA, Reynolds JC: Interdigital neuroma: a critical clinical analysis, *Foot Ankle* 3:238, 1983.
22. Mann RA, DuVries H: Intractable plantar keratosis, *Orthop Clin North Am* 4:67, 1973.
23. Morton TG: A peculiar painful infection of the fourth metatarsophalangeal articulation, *Am J Med Sci* 71:37, 1876.
24. Mulder JD: The causative mechanism in Morton's metatarsalgia, *J Bone Joint Surg* 33B:94, 1951.
25. Pedowitz WJ: Distal oblique osteotomy for intractable plantar keratosis of the middle three metatarsals, *Foot Ankle* 9:7, 1988.
26. Sponsel KH: Bunionette correction by metatarsal osteotomy, *Orthop Clin North Am* 7:808, 1976.
27. Throckmorton JK, Bradlee N: Transverse V sliding osteotomy: a new surgical procedure for the correction of Tailor's bunion deformity, *J Foot Surg* 18:117, 1978.

# Chapter 17

# Great toe disorders

Roger A. Mann

## HALLUX VALGUS

One normally considers hallux valgus as a problem that affects women who for the most part are not particularly athletically inclined. Although this may be true, the athlete may indeed have a significant hallux valgus deformity, and because of the increased stress placed upon the foot by their athletic endeavors, it may become a significant problem aggravated by athletic activities. Both groups of patients should be treated conservatively if possible; however, the demands placed upon the surgically treated foot by the athlete may result in a less than optimal clinical result, whereas in nonathletic individuals the result would be deemed satisfactory. Thus, when treating athletes, great restraint must be used.

### Etiology

It is generally believed that women's shoes play a predominant role in the development of a hallux valgus deformity. Thus the deformity occurs significantly more frequently in women than in men. When considering the athletic population, however, the increased stress placed along the medial side of the great toe may play a significant role in the development of a hallux valgus deformity. No studies, however, have shown an increased incidence of hallux valgus deformity in athletes, whether they are dancers or football players, than in the normal population. When one considers the stresses placed along the medial side of the great toe by such athletes as high jumpers, pole vaulters, leaping dancers, tennis players serving the ball, and so on, one would almost expect an increased incidence of deformity, but this does not seem to be the case. One can speculate whether these forces result in a greater progression of the deformity once it begins.

Shoe wear for athletes usually is not a significant problem, except for those engaged in ballet dancing, particularly when performing en pointe. Athletic shoe wear, however, certainly can aggravate the problem, particularly if the individual wears a tight, nonyielding shoe that has either seaming or overlapping of materials in the area of the medial eminence. This can result in a chronic neuritis-type picture of the dorsomedial cutaneous nerve or possibly bursal formation.

On rare occasions an acute injury may occur to the medial joint capsule because of an acute valgus stress that could result in an acute acquired valgus deformity, but this is extremely rare.

In athletes as well as the general population, other hereditary predisposing factors must be considered such as anatomic variation of the first metatarsophalangeal joint—for example, a round metatarsal head versus a squared metatarsal head, generalized ligamentous laxity, and overall posture of the foot (e.g., pronated foot).

### Diagnosis

**Clinical evaluation.** The evaluation of the foot begins with a careful history pertaining to the onset of the deformity, area of maximal pain, and activities and shoes that seem to worsen the symptoms. A careful history can provide clues as to whether the individual might have recently changed shoes, training technique, or overall level of activities. The possibility that other joints may be involved, indicating some type of more generalized condition, should also be considered. If possible, the patient's shoe wear should be evaluated as well.

A careful physical examination should be carried out beginning with the patient standing and the physician observing the overall alignment of the foot, specifically the great toe and lesser toes. Following this, the range of motion of the joints of the foot and ankle should be determined. Specifically, the first metatarsophalangeal joint should be evaluated for range of motion of the joint, degree of pronation, size and location of the medial eminence, pain over the dorsal or plantar cutaneous nerves to the great toe, bursal formation, and presence of interphalangeal hallux valgus. At times significant neuritis of the dorsomedial cutaneous nerve is observed, and less frequently, pain over the plantar medial cutaneous nerve (Joplin's neuroma). The plantar aspect of the foot should be examined for evidence of a transfer lesion. The stability of the first metatarsocuneiform joint needs to be carefully observed. The plantar aspect of the metatarsophalangeal joint is carefully palpated to identify possible areas of pain beneath the sesamoids. If one specific activity seems to aggravate the patient's symptoms, he should perform the activity so the examiner can determine whether the pain originates in the hallux valgus deformity or some other problem is occurring, possibly involving weight transfer.

**Radiographic evaluation.** Routine radiographs include weight-bearing anteroposterior (AP), lateral, and oblique views. Occasionally a sesamoid view is added if warranted by the patient's symptoms. The AP radiograph should be used to determine the degree of hallux valgus deformity, intermetatarsal angle, presence of osteophytes or degenerative changes about the metatarsophalangeal joint, size of the medial eminence, location of the sesamoids, distal metatarsal articular angle, and presence of subluxation of the first metatarsophalangeal joint. The AP view also can help indicate the degree of pronation of the great toe (Fig. 17-1).

The lateral radiograph demonstrates evidence of dorsal osteophyte formation on the metatarsal head, the possible presence of sesamoid pathology, and a general assessment of the longitudinal arch of the foot. From the oblique radiograph a better view of the metatarsophalangeal joint can be obtained—again looking for possible osteophytes or evidence of previous trauma to the joint. The sesamoids can be viewed—again looking for possible pathology. The sesamoid view silhouettes the sesamoid bones, allowing one to determine in some cases whether narrowing of the sesamoid metatarsal joint is present and whether possible changes are present in the sesamoids such as avascular necrosis or a stress fracture (Fig. 17-2).

**Differential diagnosis.** Although the bunion deformity may be the most obvious deformity, the differential diagnosis should include hallux rigidus, bursitis over the medial eminence, neuritis of the dorsal or plantar medial cutaneous nerve, sesamoid pathology, or possible metabolic disorder (e.g., gout).

### Treatment

**Conservative management.** As with most bunion deformities, initial management should be conservative. This involves carefully explaining the nature of the problem to the patient, after which shoe modifications should be made for comfort. This may necessitate a wider shoe, a shoe whose seam pattern does not converge over the area of the medial eminence, use of softer shoe material that would better accommodate the deformity, occasionally bowing out of the shoe over the involved area, and in the case of a problem with excessive pronation, a soft orthotic device may be indicated. Some common errors made in the management of this problem include placing layers of moleskin or felt over the prominence, which unfortunately *increases* the pressure over the medial eminence. If padding is used, it should be used around the prominence rather than on it. Occasionally if a large bursa is present, it may require draining; only rarely should cortisone be used. The main factor in conservative management is to precisely identify the problem so it can be adequately treated. For example, if the main problem is pain over the dorsomedial cutaneous nerve, treatment should be directed towards relieving pressure in this area rather than over the medial eminence per se.

In athletes, particularly figure skaters and dancers—who may have highly restricted shoe gear—conservative management at times is difficult but must be undertaken, since the possibility of obtaining results permitting a return to their previous level of activity is somewhat remote.

With any professional athlete who has a bunion problem—unless the bunion problem is interfering with their level of performance—I believe it is probably better to avoid surgery than risk the possibility of failure, which may result in their inability to continue in their career.

**Surgical management.** If the decision to carry out surgery has been made, the selection of the operative procedure becomes highly critical. The decision-making process in the selection of the surgical procedure begins again with a careful physical examination to pinpoint the area of maximal pain. If this area of maximal pain is over a sharp medial eminence, possibly a procedure in which just the eminence is removed and little else is done to correct the toe may be indicated. If the problem involves the enlargement of the entire medial eminence, but there is no subluxation or incongruity of the metatarsophalangeal joint, then a chevron procedure would be

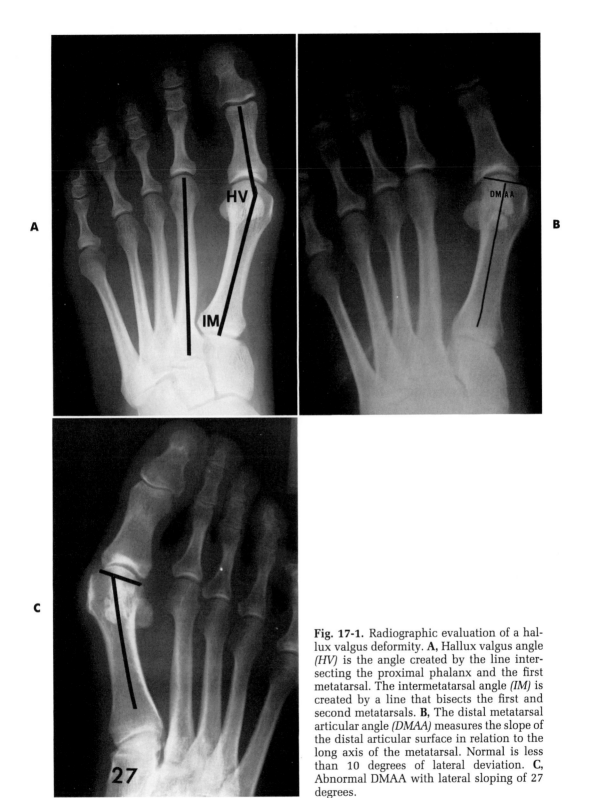

**Fig. 17-1.** Radiographic evaluation of a hallux valgus deformity. **A,** Hallux valgus angle *(HV)* is the angle created by the line intersecting the proximal phalanx and the first metatarsal. The intermetatarsal angle *(IM)* is created by a line that bisects the first and second metatarsals. **B,** The distal metatarsal articular angle *(DMAA)* measures the slope of the distal articular surface in relation to the long axis of the metatarsal. Normal is less than 10 degrees of lateral deviation. **C,** Abnormal DMAA with lateral sloping of 27 degrees.

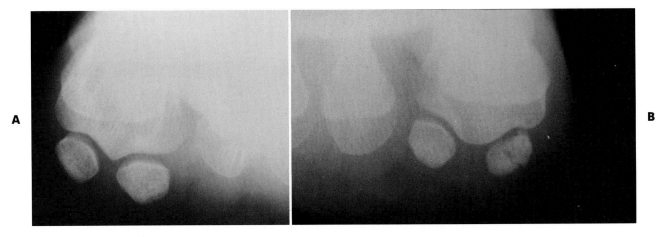

**Fig. 17-2.** Sesamoid view. **A,** Normal sesamoids. **B,** Collapse of the tibial sesamoid secondary to avascular necrosis.

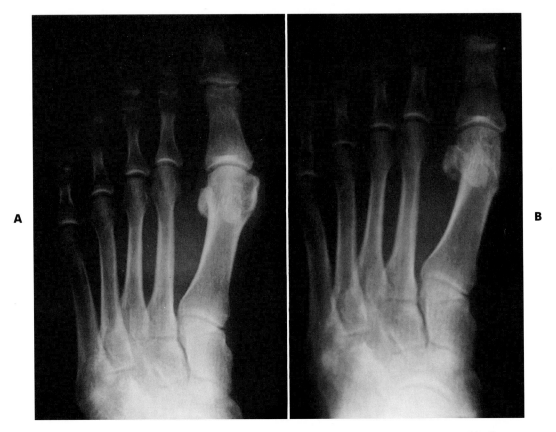

**Fig. 17-3.** Preoperative and postoperative radiographs demonstrate correction of hallux valgus deformity using various procedures. **A,** Preoperative and **B,** postoperative radiographs of a chevron procedure.

indicated (Fig. 17-3). If an interphalangeal hallux valgus is also present and needs to be corrected, an Akin procedure may be performed at the same time as the chevron procedure to produce satisfactory alignment[1] (Fig. 17-4). If the metatarsophalangeal joint is incongruent, the intermetatarsal angle exceeds 13 degrees and the hallux valgus angle 30 degrees, more than likely a distal soft tissue procedure with proximal metatarsal osteotomy is indicated (Fig. 17-5).

In athletic individuals stability of the metatarsophalangeal joint must be maintained. For this reason, one should not consider using a prosthesis or a procedure (e.g., the Keller operation) that would destabilize the first metatarsophalangeal joint.

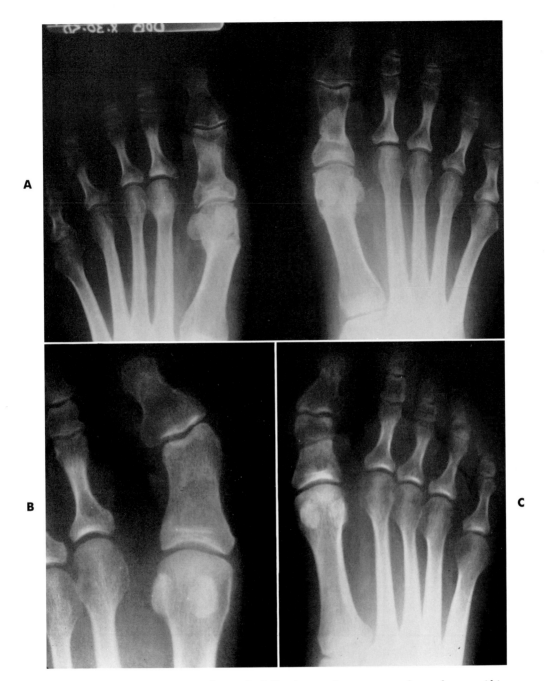

**Fig. 17-4. A,** Postoperative radiograph following a chevron procedure plus an Akin procedure. **B,** Preoperative and **C,** postoperative radiographs following an Akin procedure for interphalangeal hallux valgus.

The postoperative regimen following a hallux valgus repair must ensure adequate immobilization of the first metatarsophalangeal joint and osteotomy for satisfactory healing of the tissues. Usually 6 to 8 weeks of immobilization is required for adequate ligamentous healing about the joint. During this period of immobilization, patients can carry out nonimpact activities such as riding a stationary bicycle and weight lifting, but stress across the operated sites should be avoided. After the dressings have been removed after 6 to 8 weeks, patients should slowly begin a conditioning program probably equal in length to the period of immobilization. To start athletes out too soon on an operated joint is only courting difficulty.

## TURF TOE

A turf toe is most commonly thought of as a sprain of the first metatarsophalangeal joint. The term *turf toe* was coined by Bowers and Martin[4] in 1976. It was

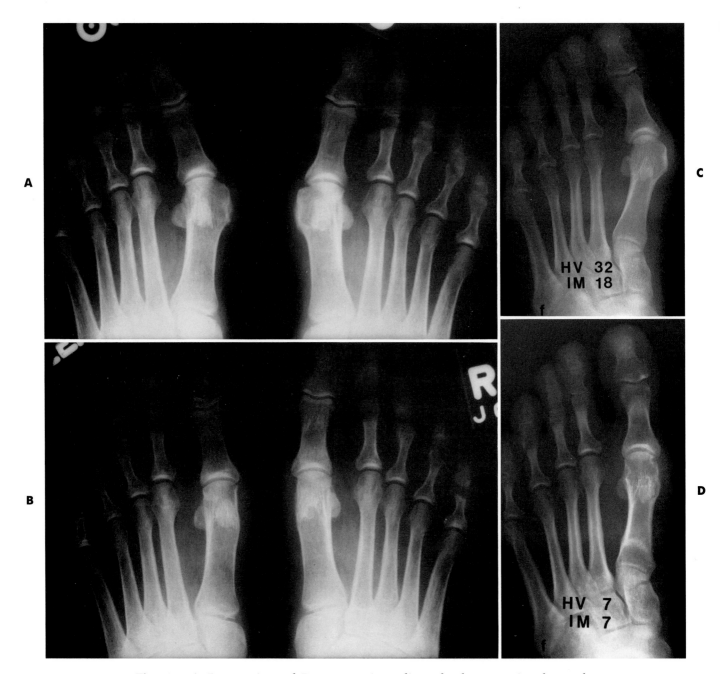

**Fig. 17-5. A,** Preoperative and **B,** postoperative radiographs demonstrating the results following a distal soft tissue procedure for a hallux valgus deformity. **C,** Preoperative and **D,** postoperative radiographs demonstrate a distal soft tissue procedure and proximal metatarsal osteotomy to correct a hallux valgus deformity.

initially believed to be due to a combination of playing on hard artificial surfaces and use of flexible shoe wear. Although it is considered a sprain of the first metatarsophalangeal joint, to a certain extent it is a general term used for any injury around this area—which could include a sprain, osteochondral fracture, sesamoid contusion or fracture, or just "jamming" the joint. An excellent review of the topic has recently been published by Clanton,[5] who noted that the incidence was somewhat variable but approximated 5.4 injuries per season in a population of approximately 500 players at one institution[4] and 4.5 such injuries at his institution.[6] In a series of professional football players, 45% of 80 active players had sustained a turf toe injury.[23]

The problem with turf toe injury is that it carries a significant morbidity, as Cocker et al[9] noted. Although ankle sprains were noted to be four times more common, turf toe accounted for twice the number of missed practices. Clanton's observations were the same.[6]

## Etiology

The metatarsophalangeal joint of the great toe is subjected to significant stress, and being a shallow joint, is supported by a strong capsuloligamentous complex. This complex includes the sesamoid mechanism plantarward, the intrinsic abductor and adductor tendons medially and laterally, respectively, and the weaker extensor hood mechanism dorsally (Fig. 17-6). The most common mechanism of injury is hyperextension of the joint, but injury may also be brought about by a significant varus or valgus stress. Occasionally sharp plantar flexion can be the cause of injury. On rare occasions injury occurs because of direct jamming of the toe against a fixed object, whether it be an opponent's leg, a sprinkler head, or possibly a hard edge surrounding a playing field.

In today's competitive sports world, shoe wear has become lighter and playing surfaces faster in order to increase speed. This combination unfortunately results in less support for the foot and greater stress applied to it. A poll of athletic trainers showed they believed 34% was due to the turf, 21% due to shoes, and 24% due to a combination of both.[9] The remainder had no definite opinions as to the etiology of the problem. Clanton points out in analyzing this injury that the majority occur in football but that turf toe has also been reported in basketball and track. He notes that there has been no mention of turf toe problems in soccer or lacrosse players. Why this happens is difficult to state with assurance, other than the fact that football obviously has the greatest degree of contact involved, as well as the added effects of players piling on one another.

## Diagnosis

**Clinical evaluation.** The clinical evaluation of a suspected turf toe injury starts with a careful history of the injury. Admittedly in sporting events the mechanism may not be recalled by the athlete, but an attempt should be made to define the injury. One would want to know whether the toe was forced into extension, flexion, varus or valgus, or whether it was a jamming type of injury. The area of maximal pain, likewise, needs to be carefully defined, since this will usually greatly aid the clinician in establishing the correct diagnosis.

The physical examination, particularly in the acute injury, is extremely important in making a specific diagnosis. The range of motion of the joint should be carefully observed, the area of maximal tenderness noted, and the medial and lateral collateral ligaments

carefully checked for stability. The sesamoid mechanism needs to be carefully palpated to see whether the injury involved a sesamoid or possibly a tear in the phalangeosesamoid ligament area.

Evaluating athletes with a more chronic problem again includes a careful history as to the mechanism of injury and a detailed physical examination to pinpoint the part of the joint that is injured. At times synovitis is present along with mild crepitation, which would be indicative of a possible chondral lesion. In the more chronic turf toe, a careful evaluation of motor strength may be indicated in defining a problem created by stretching of the phalangeosesamoid ligament. Careful palpation over each sesamoid again provides a good clue as to whether it may be the site of the pathology.

**Radiographic evaluation.** Routine weight-bearing AP, lateral, and oblique radiographs as well as a good sesamoid view should be obtained in the patient with a turf toe injury. Since many times the injury involves the soft tissue, unfortunately no bony abnormality is detected. However, one should look for small avulsion fragments about the joint, a possible sesamoid fracture, and possible preexisting degenerative arthritis. If one suspects injury to the sesamoid mechanism due to hyperextension, comparison AP weight-bearing radiographs may demonstrate that the sesamoids have retracted slightly proximally, indicating that the phalangeosesamoid ligament has been partially or completely disrupted. This is determined by observing the space between the base of the proximal phalanx and the beginning of the sesamoid. If a bipartite sesamoid is present and appears to be painful by the physical examination, one would be justified in obtaining a bone scan using a pinhead collimator to determine if there is increased activity about the involved sesamoid. In my experience the use of magnetic resonance imaging (MRI) has rarely been justified in defining problems about the metatarsophalangeal joint, mainly due to the fact that the resolution of most studies is poor.

**Differential diagnosis.** The differential diagnosis of a turf toe would include injury to the medial or lateral ligamentous structures of the metatarsophalangeal joint, the phalangeosesamoid ligament, a fractured sesamoid, osteochondral or chondral injury to the joint surface, chondral contusion secondary to direct linear stress, dislocation and spontaneous reduction of the metatarsophalangeal joint, and injury to the interphalangeal joint of the great toe.

## Treatment

**Conservative management.** The initial treatment of the acute injury follows the usual concepts: ice, compression, elevation, and rest. A postoperative shoe

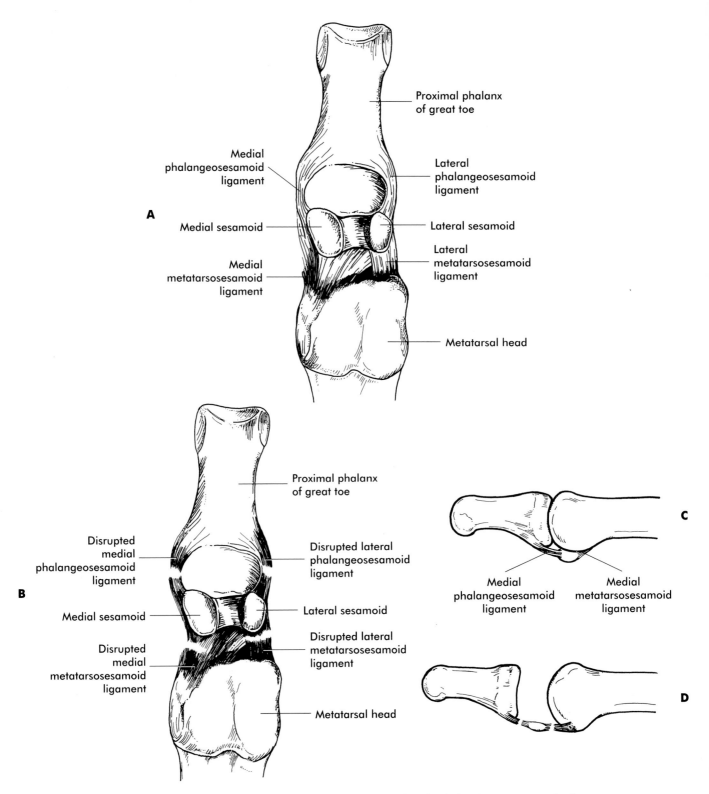

**Fig. 17-6. A,** Anatomic relationships between the head of the first metatarsal, the sesamoids, and the base of the proximal phalanx. **B,** Following a hyperextension injury, at times the metatarsosesamoid ligament and/or the phalangeosesamoid ligament may be partially or totally disrupted. **C,** Normal lateral view. **D,** A hyperextension injury where the metatarsosesamoid ligament and the phalangeosesamoid ligament are totally disrupted.

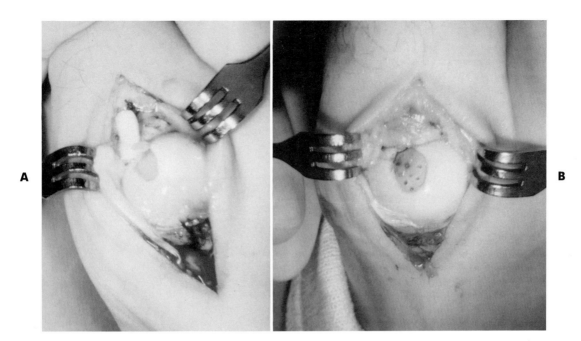

**Fig. 17-7.** Chondral injury to the first metatarsal head. **A,** Preoperative and **B,** postoperative appearance following excision and drilling of the base of the lesion.

with a firm sole is often helpful, particularly if there is a great deal of swelling and pain with motion. If the injury is minor and will resolve rapidly, patients may be progressed with range-of-motion exercises and activities as tolerated. If, however, a more serious injury is present, I favor longer periods of immobilization until the condition has stabilized. If a sesamoid bone has been fractured, the patient should be casted with the toe in about 10 degrees of plantar flexion to keep the stress off of the sesamoid mechanism until healing has occurred, usually in about 8 to 10 weeks. With ligamentous injuries 3 weeks of immobilization is usually adequate. As a rule, if the injury involves the phalangeosesamoid ligaments, 3 weeks of immobilization may be adequate, but vigorous exercise should probably be avoided for several months to allow this structure—which is under maximal stress during athletic endeavors—to adequately reconstitute itself.

If one is dealing with a bipartite sesamoid in which the fibrocartilaginous tissue has been stressed, a longer period of immobilization should probably be carried out to permit adequate healing to occur. If, in the case of a chondral fracture, symptoms persist (e.g., persistent synovitis and pain), an arthrotomy to remove the fragment with drilling of the subchondral bone to enhance the formation of fibrocartilage should be performed (Fig. 17-7).

**Surgical management.** If the problem involves a painful sesamoid due either to a fracture, avascular necrosis, or a painful bipartite sesamoid, a sesamoidectomy may be indicated. The fibular sesamoid

should be removed through a dorsal incision in the first web space, and the tibial sesamoid removed through a medial incision, with care being taken not to disrupt the plantar medial cutaneous nerve or the abductor hallucis tendon. I have obtained satisfactory results in patients following excision of the sesamoid and rarely does a varus or valgus deformity result.[20] Postoperatively the foot should be immobilized for 6 weeks, holding the great toe in a position that allows the abductor hallucis or adductor hallucis tendon to adequately scar down and the joint to re-form adequate capsular tissue before applying stress.

Clanton et al,[6] in their review of this subject, noted a 50% incidence of persistent symptoms in 20 athletes diagnosed with a turf toe injury at greater than 5-year follow-up. This unfortunate sequela may be reduced with early specific diagnosis and treatment of turf toe injury.

## HALLUX RIGIDUS

Hallux rigidus presents a significant problem for the athlete. As a result of this condition, bony proliferation occurs over the dorsal aspect of the metatarsophalangeal joint, resulting in loss of active and passive dorsiflexion. In athletes in particular, dorsiflexion plays an important role in the function of the foot, particularly in activities such as accelerating, jumping, and changing direction. If due to lack of dorsiflexion the athlete is forced to compensate by rolling onto the lateral aspect of the foot, this will frequently result in other areas of the body such as

A 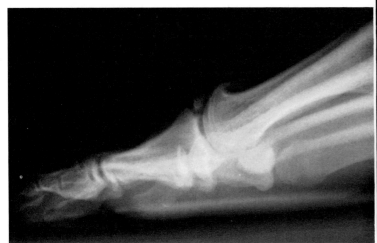 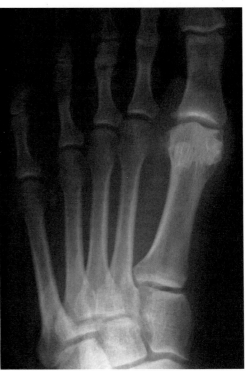 B

**Fig. 17-8.** Radiographs demonstrate hallux rigidus. **A,** The lateral view demonstrates the large dorsal exostosis on the metatarsal head and a fractured fragment on the dorsal aspect of the base of the proximal phalanx. **B,** The anteroposterior radiograph demonstrates some proliferative bone formation along the lateral aspect of the metatarsal head and proximal phalanx.

ankle, knee, hip, or back becoming symptomatic. The added bulk about the joint may result in significant pressure points, which again makes it difficult for the athlete to wear comfortable shoes. This condition also plays a significant role in the so-called "weekend warrior" or the individual just interested in jogging who, because of lack of dorsiflexion, must then compensate by carrying out activity on the lateral border of the foot. In this section only the adult type of hallux rigidus is discussed.

### Etiology

As a general rule hallux rigidus is brought about by degenerative arthritis of the first metatarsophalangeal joint. In the section on turf toe, one certainly could in some cases state that a hallux rigidus type of problem existed; this is why attempting to precisely define turf toe as a specific entity becomes difficult. In the majority of patients with hallux rigidus, there is no specific predisposing factor, although occasionally the individual will recall a specific traumatic episode. Certain predisposing factors have been suggested as possible etiologies of hallux rigidus, including congenital flattening or squaring off of the metatarsal head,[12] metatarsus primus elevatus,[16] osteochondritis

of the metatarsal head,[13,17,25] a long hallux,* pes planus,[8,11,14] pronated foot,[3,15,22] and a long slender foot.[2] It is hypothesized that these conditions tend to place more stress on the first metatarsophalangeal joint, predisposing it to arthrosis. In my experience it is unusual for these conditions to be present in the patient with hallux rigidus.

The pathophysiology in hallux rigidus usually consists of degenerative changes in the articular cartilage, particularly on the metatarsal head, associated with some degree of synovitis. As the condition progresses, there is bony proliferation, particularly over the dorsal, and to a lesser degree, lateral aspect of the metatarsal head. With time these areas enlarge, creating a significant ridge of bone both dorsally and laterally. As the condition progresses, an impingement between the base of the proximal phalanx and metatarsal head occurs which results in lack of dorsiflexion and hence the pain experienced by the patient (Fig. 17-8).

Occasionally a patient sustains an acute injury to the articular cartilage of the metatarsophalangeal joint, which results in loosening or displacement of a

*References 8, 10, 11, 22, 24, 25.

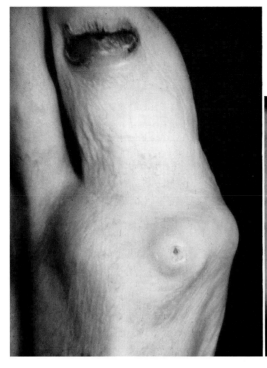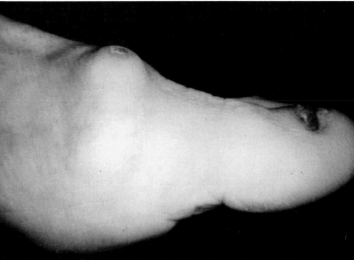

**Fig. 17-9.** Pictures demonstrate the clinical appearance of hallux rigidus. The proliferative bone around the metatarsal head causes increased bulk of the joint and occasionally breakdown of the skin.

fragment. This results in chronic pain and synovitis of the joint, and probably in time, degenerative changes. If the condition is diagnosed early, I believe the possibility of the patient developing degenerative changes probably can be diminished. This is not a true form of hallux rigidus but does show the overlap between this condition and turf toe.

### Diagnosis

**Clinical evaluation.** The physical examination begins by having the patient stand and the physician observing the enlargement due either to bony prominences or synovitis about the first metatarsophalangeal joint (Fig. 17-9). Range of motion of the first metatarsophalangeal joint demonstrates limited dorsiflexion. With forced dorsiflexion one usually will reproduce the patient's pain. Palpation often demonstrates a ridge of bone along the lateral side of the metatarsal head; if the toe is brought into some valgus and motion carried out, this may also reproduce the patient's pain. Palpation about the joint demonstrates the ridge of bone along the dorsal aspect but surprisingly, it is usually absent along the medial aspect. Occasionally synovitis is present. If the bony proliferation is extensive, abrasions over the skin may be observed. Sometimes plantar flexion of the metatarsophalangeal joint will cause the patient discomfort,

probably due to stretching of the extensor tendons and capsule over the bony ridge.

### Radiographic evaluation

The radiographic findings early in the condition may be surprisingly benign, and one must rely more on the clinical evaluation than the radiographs. With time, however, the findings become that of degenerative changes of the joint with narrowing and bony proliferation along the dorsal and lateral aspect of the joint. Occasionally a "kissing spur" is noted along the dorsal aspect of the base of the proximal phalanx. The oblique radiograph is useful in evaluating the extent of the damage to the articular surface. The sesamoids are not usually significantly involved in the degenerative process.

**Differential diagnosis.** Although the diagnosis of hallux rigidus is usually not difficult to make, other conditions such as a turf toe due to chondral damage should be considered. Gout may bring about an acute change in the joint, and occasionally a sesamoid injury or fracture can mimic classic hallux rigidus.

### Treatment

**Conservative management.** Conservative care for hallux rigidus consists of first alleviating pressure against the toe by modifying the shoe wear. Usually a

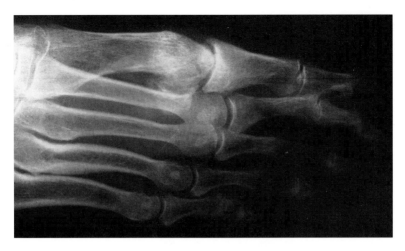

**Fig. 17-10.** Postoperative radiograph following a cheilectomy. Note the way the dorsal ridge of bone has been removed from the first metatarsal, alleviating the dorsal impingement and permitting dorsiflexion of the proximal phalanx on the metatarsal head.

larger toe box, possibly using an athletic shoe with a modified seam pattern to avoid too much pressure over the prominences, or possibly expanding the shoe, may bring about symptomatic relief. At times, if possible, a stiffer shoe or an appliance with a steel shank or rocker-bottom sole can be used. The problem, however, with stiffening the shoe—particularly in athletes involved in ballet, basketball, and other activities that require dorsiflexion and push-off—is that the performance level will probably diminish using a rigid shoe.

The use of nonsteroidal antiinflammatory medications and occasionally even an injection of cortisone into the joint may be of benefit to the patient.

**Surgical management.** Surgical options usually available for patients with hallux rigidus consist of cheilectomy, which has the advantage of restoring some active and passive dorsiflexion; arthrodesis of the joint, which eliminates the pain but sacrifices joint motion; and the Moberg procedure, which is a proximal phalangeal osteotomy that will permit more dorsiflexion in a joint that is rigid or in some plantar flexion. Obviously in athletes arthrodesis is not a viable choice since this would significantly impair athletic performance.

The main advantage of cheilectomy for athletes with limitation of dorsiflexion is that it removes the mechanical obstruction to dorsiflexion, which usually will result in some increased dorsiflexion but usually will eliminate the pain brought about by the impingement of the proximal phalanx against the dorsal ridge of bone. Usually this permits individuals to return to their previous level of activity. One must keep in mind, however, that the joint has undergone and is

undergoing degenerative changes—and this will continue—so the procedure probably does not influence the rate of degeneration but prolongs the athletic life of the individual. As a general rule the dorsal ridge does not recur, although progressive narrowing of the joint will occur. It is important when carrying out this procedure—if there is a ridge of bone laterally—that it be removed at the same time.

**Cheilectomy: surgical technique.** The basic surgical technique for a cheilectomy is to approach the joint through a dorsal incision, sweeping the extensor tendon medially or laterally. The joint capsule is opened and a complete dorsal, medial, and lateral synovectomy is performed. The joint is carefully inspected, and usually the dorsal 20% to 30% of the metatarsal head is removed. At the time of surgery, one attempts to gain 60 to 70 degrees of passive dorsiflexion. If this much motion cannot be attained, possibly enough dorsal bone has not been removed. The object is to permit dorsiflexion to occur without impingement. The lateral side of the metatarsal head is observed, and if there is new bone formation laterally it is removed in line with the lateral side of the metatarsal shaft (Fig. 17-10). If the articular cartilage is damaged, it should be tidied up by sharp dissection. As a general rule, even if hard eburnated bone is present, one does not drill the surface to try to gain formation of fibrocartilage, since this probably results in some fibrosis of the joint. The joint capsule is closed, if possible, under the extensor tendon, and the skin is closed in a routine manner. After using a compression dressing for 18 to 24 hours, a firm dressing is applied and the patient permitted to ambulate in a postoperative shoe. At

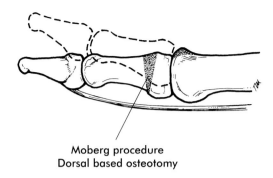

Moberg procedure
Dorsal based osteotomy

Lateral

**Fig. 17-11.** The Moberg procedure is an osteotomy of the base of the proximal phalanx, which permits increased dorsiflexion of the metatarsophalangeal joint.

approximately 8 to 10 days following surgery, the sutures are removed and the patient is encouraged to work on active range-of-motion exercises as frequently as possible throughout the day. These should be both active and passive exercises. Patients also are encouraged at this time to wear a soft shoe that will permit motion of the metatarsophalangeal joint with walking. No significant activities generally are allowed for approximately 10 to 12 weeks following the cheilectomy, giving the joint time to mature following surgery. Athletes may continue to train by bicycling, swimming, running in water, and other activities that avoid significant impact against the metatarsophalangeal joint. It may take many months for the swelling to subside after surgery, but this varies from patient to patient.[7,18]

**Moberg's procedure: surgical technique.** The Moberg procedure[21] is used when there is significant arthrosis of the metatarsophalangeal joint so that a cheilectomy would probably not be of benefit to the patient. In these cases—if dorsiflexion is severely limited but there is some active and passive plantar flexion of 20 to 30 degrees—a Moberg procedure can be successful. What is gained by this procedure is the ability to roll over the first metatarsophalangeal joint because the great toe has been brought out of its slightly plantar-flexed position to one of mild dorsiflexion. From a functional standpoint little or no active motion is gained (Fig. 17-11).

The surgical technique is to approach the proximal phalanx through a dorsal incision, exposing the base of the proximal phalanx. Being certain that one is distal to the metatarsophalangeal joint, a dorsal closing wedge osteotomy is performed. The width of the osteotomy will determine how much dorsiflexion is gained by the procedure. The osteotomy site is fixed, after which the patient is kept in a postoperative shoe with the toe dressed in a dorsiflexed position for approximately 4 weeks. If a large dorsal exostosis is present, it is excised. Following this, gentle range of motion is begun, both actively and passively, until healing has occurred, at which time the postoperative shoe is discontinued.

As stated previously, the use of a fusion in athletes is usually discouraged since they will not be able to perform at their previous level after an arthrodesis has been performed. Any operative procedure that results in destabilization of the joint such as a Keller-type procedure or a prosthesis is contraindicated in the athletic population.

**REFERENCES**

1. Baxter DE, Lillich JS: Bunionectomies and related surgery in the elite female middle distance and marathon runner, *Am J Sports Med* 14:491, 1976.
2. Bingold AC, Collins DH: Hallux rigidus, *J Bone Joint Surg (Br)* 32:214, 1950.
3. Bonney G, McNab I: Hallux valgus and hallux rigidus, *J Bone Joint Surg (Br)* 34:366, 1952.
4. Bowers KD Jr, Martin RB: Turf-toe: a shoe-surface related football injury, *Med Sci Sports Exerc* 8:81, 1976.
5. Clanton TO, Schon LC: Athletic injuries to the soft tissues. In Mann RA, Coughlin MJ, editors: *Surgery of the foot and ankle,* St Louis, 1993, Mosby–Year Book, p 1191.
6. Clanton TO, Butler JE, Eggert A: Injuries to the metatarsophalangeal joints in athletes, *Foot Ankle* 7:162, 1986.
7. Mann RA, Coughlin MJ, DuVries HL: Hallux rigidus. A review of the literature and a method of treatment, *Clin Orthop* 142:57, 1979.
8. Cochrane WA: An operation for hallux rigidus, *Br Med J* 1:1095, 1927.
9. Coker TP, Arnold JA, Weber DL: Traumatic lesions of the metatarsophalangeal joint of the great toe in athletes, *Am J Sports Med* 6:326, 1978.
10. Davies-Colley N: Contraction of the metatarsophalangeal joint of the great toe, *Br Med J* 1:728, 1887.
11. Dickson FD, Diveley RL: *Functional disorders of the foot. Their diagnosis and treatment,* Philadelphia, 1939, JB Lippincott, p 228.
12. DuVries HL: *Surgery of the foot,* St Louis, 1959, Mosby–Year Book, p 392.
13. Goodfellow J: Aetiology of hallux rigidus, *Proc R Soc Med* 59:821, 1966.
14. Jack EA: The aetiology of hallux rigidus, *Br J Surg* 27:492, 1940.
15. Jansen M: Hallux valgus, rigidus, and malleus, *J Orthop Surg* 3:87, 1921.
16. Lambrinudi C: Metatarsus primus elevatus, *Proc R Soc Med* 31:1273, 1938.
17. Lyritis G: Developmental disorders of the proximal epiphysis of the hallux, *Skeletal Radiol* 10:250, 1983.
18. Mann RA, Clanton TO: Hallux rigidus: treatment by cheilectomy, *J Bone Joint Surg (Am)* 70:400, 1988.
19. Mann RA, Rudicel S, Graves SC: Hallux valgus repair utilizing a distal soft tissue procedure and proximal metatarsal osteotomy: a long term followup, *J Bone Joint Surg (Am)* 74:124, 1992.
20. Mann RA et al: Sesamoidectomy of the great toe, American Orthopaedic Foot and Ankle Society, 15th annual meeting, Las Vegas, Jan 24, 1985.

21. Moberg E: A simple operation for hallux rigidus, *Clin Orthop* 142:55, 1979.

22. Nilsonne H: Hallux rigidus and its treatment, *Acta Orthop Scand* 1:295, 1930.

23. Rodeo SA et al: Turf-toe: an analysis of metatarsophalangeal joint sprains in professional football players, *Am J Sports Med* 18:280, 1990.

24. Smith NR: Hallux valgus and hallux rigidus treated by arthrodesis of the metatarsophalangeal joint, *Br Med J* 2:1385, 1952.

25. Vilaseca RR, Ribes ER: The growth of the first metatarsal bone, *Foot Ankle* 1:117, 1980.

# Chapter 18

# Bunion deformity in elite athletes

**Donald E. Baxter**

## THE PROBLEMS

Bunions occur in elite athletes. Often the bunion has a congruous joint that slowly develops over a long period. As long as the athlete wears large enough shoes and accommodates the bunion, he or she will do well. In this type of deformity, there is minimal restriction of motion.

The decompensated bunion usually progresses rapidly. The sesamoids begin to sublux and the joint becomes incongruous. Secondary problems develop such as stress fractures, neuromas, soft corns, and leg pain. The sesamoids and the capsule of the first metatarsophalangeal joint aches. Shoes become less and less comfortable.

What can be done to help? Compensated bunions in athletes are most often treated conservatively. Decompensated bunions need more aggressive, often surgical, treatment.

### The compensated bunion (Fig. 18-1)

The compensated bunion usually develops slowly. There is often a congenitally large metatarsal head. The hallux valgus is usually less than 20 degrees and the intermetatarsal angle less than 11 degrees. Symptoms are periodic with bursitis or neuralgia of the superficial dorsal cutaneous nerve. There is good dorsal motion of the first metatarsophalangeal joint, usually at least 60 to 70 degrees of dorsiflexion.

The articular facet is congruous. The sesamoids are mechanically in a functional position, and the fibular sesamoid is at least 50% covered by the first metatarsal head.

Even though the bunion is compensated, preven-tion of progression or secondary deformities should be considered. These considerations include proper shoes with good arch support and an adequate toe box. It also includes an orthosis when necessary to prevent pronation. In a patient with an inadequate first metatarsal, or "Morton's foot," an orthosis should be considered with a Morton extension (an extension of the orthosis underneath the first metatarsal head). Stretching the Achilles tendon is performed two to three times a day for 10 to 15 seconds if there is tightness of the Achilles tendon. Where the great toe rubs against the second toe, a pad should be inserted in the web space.

As long as the athlete is functional, surgery should be avoided and the athlete observed at 6- to 12-month intervals. If the problem progresses, more aggressive treatment may be necessary.

### The decompensated bunion (Figs. 18-2 and 18-3)

The athlete with a decompensated bunion has a history of a long-standing bunion that suddenly becomes worse. The bunion becomes painful, and the athlete states that the hallux valgus increases, usually showing greater than 25 degrees of hallux valgus. When examining the standing x-rays, the intermetatarsal angle is usually greater than 12 degrees. The joint is incongruous with the proximal phalanx subluxing off of the articular surface of the first metatarsal. The fibular sesamoid is more than 50% uncovered by the first metatarsal head.

Pronation suddenly becomes worse as the first metatarsal no longer supports the medial foot, and the toe rotates laterally.

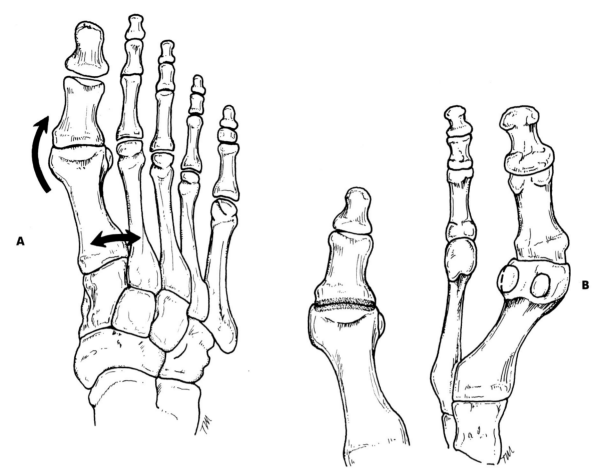

**Fig. 18-1. A,** The compensated bunion has a hallux valgus that is usually less than 20 degrees and an intermetatarsal angle less than 11 degrees. The articular facet is congruous. **B,** With a compensated bunion the articular facet is congruous and the fibular sesamoid is less than 50% uncovered by the first metatarsal head.

The initial treatment is to add an orthosis and, if necessary, a Morton extension underneath the first metatarsal head. Web space padding of the first and second toes is somewhat helpful initially.

As the athlete becomes less and less competitive and misses more and more practice days, surgery becomes more of a necessity.

I feel that a chevron bunionectomy[1,2] gives the best chance of a rapid functional recovery. Other procedures that may be used are the Mann-McBride procedure with or without a proximal osteotomy of the first metatarsal. The chevron-Akin procedure may also be used.[3] Other anatomic repairs may be useful, depending on the surgeon and his experience.

Procedures to avoid are the Silastic implant, fusions, the Lapidus procedure, and Keller arthroplasties. The Silastic implant placement will disintegrate with repetitive use and is usually mechanically unsound. Fusion, even though necessary for salvage situations, should be a last resort. The Lapidus procedure (fusion of the first metatarsal tarsal with a

bunionectomy) is a good procedure in decompensated bunions where the first metatarsal is dorsiflexed and there is a hypermobility of the first metatarsal tarsal joint. However, this procedure is slow-healing and has a long period of recovery. It is better used at the time of retirement of the athlete. The Keller procedure changes the mechanics by eliminating the short flexor tendon, thus affecting push-off. This procedure should also be avoided.

My experience with athletes shows the chevron procedure to be the most beneficial, rapidly healing, and functionally adequate.[2] The chevron-Akin[3] may extend the limits of the chevron procedure. However, the chevron-Akin procedure must create a compensated alignment. Proximal osteotomy of the first metatarsal should be used if the intermetatarsal angle is more than 14 degrees and the fibular sesamoid is completely uncovered by the first metatarsal head (Fig. 18-3).

Problems with the chevron-Akin procedure include some weakening of push-off. However, the

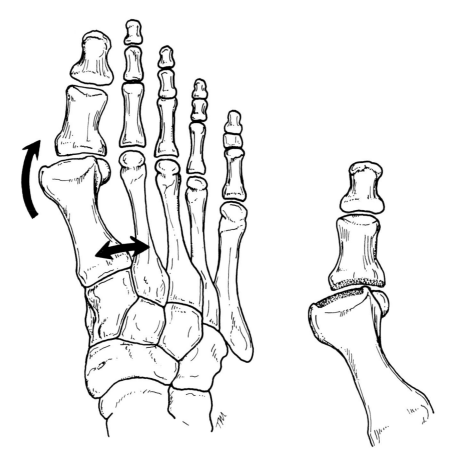

**Fig. 18-2.** The decompensated bunion usually has more than 25 degrees hallux valgus and an intermetatarsal angle more than 12 degrees. The joint is incongruous.

range of motion is actually increased, and the procedure may be used for the athlete with a bunion and early rigidus.

With any procedure it is important to consider a possible dorsal spur of the first metatarsal. Should a dorsal spur be present at the time of surgery, it is removed.

This philosophy of treatment is to change a decompensated bunion into a compensated bunion. By trying to create perfection, function may be affected — that is, by trying to reposition the first metatarsophalangeal joint and the sesamoids anatomically, a stiff painful incongruous joint could be created.

By putting the joint back to a less than perfect but congruous position, function will be improved and the competitive life of the athlete prolonged. Of course, orthosis and appropriate preventive padding should be considered while competing. Should surgery be necessary, proper shoes should be worn postoperatively.

## SECONDARY PROBLEMS

As bunions develop, the complaint is not only the pain at the first metatarsophalangeal joint but often secondary problems — which in many athletes cause the major disability. Some of the many secondary problems are discussed below in the order of their occurrence, with the most prevalent discussed first.

### Stress fractures

Stress fractures occur with biomechanical imbalance. These stress fractures can occur in the second or third metatarsals or the distal fibula. As the athlete with a bunion decompensates and develops more and more pronation, stress is transferred to the second and third metatarsals and to the lateral fibula. Without adequate orthotic foot control, stress fractures may develop to the second and third metatarsals or the fibula. After the initial period of healing, the runner should gradually resume his or her activity with a longitudinal arch support.

### Neuromas

With transfer of forces following bunion development, pressure is increased between the lateral metatarsals, and often neuromas will be seen accompanying bunions. These neuromas are in the second or third interspaces. They are treated with metatarsal

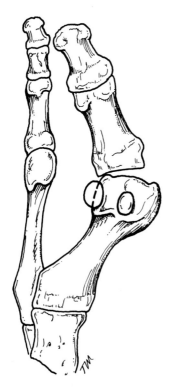

**Fig. 18-3.** With a decompensated bunion the joint is incongruous, and the fibular sesamoid is more than 50% uncovered by the first metatarsal head.

pads and, if necessary, surgery, to excise the neuromas. If the bunion is compensated, a longitudinal arch support can be used and the neuroma removed without performing a bunionectomy. However, if the bunion has decompensated and a neuroma is present, both problems should be treated surgically simultaneously.

**Transfer lesions**

Without adequate orthoses, transfer lesions are very common in runners. These transfer lesions develop under the second, third, or fourth metatarsophalangeal joints. The initial treatment should be flexibility stretching of the toes and use of a metatarsal pad or a Morton extension to rebalance the metatarsals.

**Pronation**

Pronation occurs as a secondary problem and can lead to other problems; therefore a longitudinal arch support should be used once the first metatarsal becomes incompetent. This longitudinal arch support will prevent transfer of pressure to the lesser metatarsals.

**Sesamoid degeneration**

Sesamoid pain is common with the progression of bunions and decompensation of a bunion. As the

sesamoids migrate in a fibular direction, they can develop incongruity and osteochondrosis. U-type pads are placed proximal to the first metatarsal head and underneath the second metatarsal head to eliminate pressure from the sesamoids. Also a more rigid midsole may be placed in the athletic shoe or a rocker on the bottom of the shoe. Rarely an isolated sesamoidectomy is needed.

**Tight Achilles**

With pronation, Achilles tightness can be an associated finding. Stretching of the Achilles tendon is performed two to three times daily for 20 to 30 seconds and, if necessary, a one-half-inch heel lift is placed in both shoes to eliminate some of the pull of the Achilles tendon and to eliminate stress from this area.

**Soft corns**

Soft corns commonly occur with bunions between the first and second toes and even between lesser toes because there is more pressure on the toes from the hallux valgus deformity. Pads may be placed between the toes to eliminate pressure from the corns.

**Flexible or rigid claw toes**

With flexible claw toes, stretching exercises can be performed to stretch the extensor tendons. Metatarsal pads or metatarsal bars are used on the jogging shoe to allow more plantar flexion of the toes. For more rigid deformities surgery may be necessary.

**Posterior tibial tendinitis**

With increased pronation and incompetence of the first metatarsophalangeal joint, posterior tibial tendinitis may result as the foot pronates. This problem is treated with a longitudinal arch support or a medial wedge in the sole and heel of the shoe. By using a three-sixteenth-inch medial sole and heel wedge in the shoe, pressure can be removed from the posterior tibial tendon. The medial sole wedge is more effective in high-level competitive runners than the longitudinal arch support. This medial sole wedge, which is placed in the midsole of the running shoe, keeps the forefoot inverted during push-off and thus does not allow for excessive pressure and pull on the posterior tibial tendon.

**Hallux rigidus**

Hallux rigidus is a common problem that can be associated with a bunion. Hallux rigidus is a dorsal compression of the metatarsophalangeal joint with spur formation. From a conservative point of view a more rigid sole (or an orthotic device) may be used in the athletic shoe. Occasionally a rocker is placed on the outer sole of the shoe to allow better mechanics and to decrease dorsiflexion of the great toe during running.

## Peroneal spasm

As pronation develops, peroneal spasm may result because the peroneus longus tendon—which inserts into the distal aspect of the first metatarsal head—is stretched during running. To compensate for a hypermobile high-riding first metatarsal, the peroneus longus muscle activates and thus causes peroneal spasm. By placing a longitudinal arch support in the shoe with a Morton extension, this pain in the lateral leg can be decreased in long-distance runners.

## Flexor hallucis longus tendinitis

Flexor hallucis longus tendinitis may develop in association with bunions. With pronation and hypermobility of the first metatarsal, the flexor hallucis longus muscle contracts to plantar flex the great toe and balance the great toe joint. With greater use of this tendon, tendinitis may result. Initially, stretching exercises to the great toe will stretch out the flexor hallucis longus tendon and muscle. Following that, a longitudinal arch support with a Morton extension will remove some of the spasm from the flexor hallucis longus tendon.

## Arthritis

Arthritis, even though rare, may develop in the first metatarsal tarsal joint. This develops with long-standing bunion and metatarsus varus. With instability of the first metatarsal and progressive pronation, stress is placed on the first metatarsal tarsal joint. Unless this is corrected with appropriate longitudinal arch support, degenerative or traumatic arthritis may develop in the first metatarsal tarsal joint. For athletes with this problem, a longitudinal arch support should be used in the shoe and, if necessary, a rocker placed on the outer sole to eliminate stress.

## Midfoot stress

As a last result of chronic bunion development and incompetence of the first metatarsophalangeal joint, the midfoot can break down and a Lisfranc type of arthritic change may develop. When there is pain across the midfoot, a longitudinal arch support should be used, and the athlete should be cautioned that the problem may become more progressive, particularly with excessive training and running. With this type of problem the physician should recommend not only shoe modifications and orthosis but a change in activity, using nongravity exercises such as biking or swimming.

## SUMMARY

Bunions and hallux valgus and metatarsus varus should be prevented in athletes with appropriate shoe wear and orthosis and padding.

If bunions develop and are compensated (i.e., no functional loss of performance) and no progression of the deformity occurs, conservative care is the first line of treatment and prevention of progression.

However, if the deformity progresses and the functional capacity of the athlete fails, then a precise, well-planned operation should be performed. The goal of the surgery should be the functional return and restoration of a congruous joint. This often means a less definitive procedure until the athlete retires. For instance, by avoiding a fusion of the first metatarsophalangeal joint or a Lapidus procedure or a Keller procedure (which may ultimately be needed), the athlete may perform on a world-class level for additional years.

In weekend athletes the more definitive procedure is used knowing that some function will be lost. A more supportive shoe, orthosis, or adding rocker-bottom elements to the shoes may be needed postoperatively.

**Case Study 1.** A 25-year-old ballet dancer was seen on several occasions with bursal pain over the first metatarsophalangeal joint. There were hyperkeratotic lesions between the great toe and the second toe; however, the dancer stated that she was able to dance and work out 8 to 12 hours each day, 6 days a week, 50 weeks out of the year. Her range of motion showed that her great toe could dorsiflex 90 degrees and plantar flex 40 degrees. With some change in her shoe wear and stitch pattern of the shoes, she was able to improve and the bursitis subsided. She has never had bunion surgery, a procedure not considered because it would affect the range of motion of her toe and thus her dancing.

**Case Study 2.** A 29-year-old female middle-distance runner presented with pain in her bunion. She stated that the bunion had become worse over the previous 12 months. She had tried using different shoes and a different orthosis; however, she continued to have increasing pain in the area of her bunion and could not wear running shoes or train. At the time of the evaluation, her hallux valgus was 28 degrees. Her intermetatarsal angle was 14 degrees, and her fibular sesamoid was 75% uncovered by the first metatarsal head. The athlete was considered for surgery. She had a chevron procedure, and 8 weeks following surgery she resumed training and ultimately regained world-class form as an athlete 10 months postoperatively.

**Case Study 3.** A 42-year-old world-class master's runner was seen with a progressive bunion that was causing significant pain. She had a bunionectomy with a fusion of the first metatarsal tarsal joint (a Lapidus procedure). She had to be non–weightbearing for 4 weeks; after 3 months it was noted that she had a nonunion of the first metatarsal

tarsal joint. Surgery was again performed and an additional bone graft was carried out. She ultimately recovered after 1 year. However, she never was able to return to world-class form as a master's runner. In my opinion she would have been better served with a chevron procedure or a chevron-Akin procedure; if a Lapidus was indicated, it could have been delayed until her retirement from competitive sports.

**REFERENCES**

1. Johnson K, Cofield R, Morrey B: Chevron osteotomy for hallux valgus, *Clin Orthop* 142:44, 1979.
2. Lillich JS, Baxter DE: Bunionectomies and related surgery in the elite female middle-distance and marathon runner, *Am J Sports Med* 14:491, 1986.
3. Mitchell LA, Baxter DE: A chevron-Akin double osteotomy for correction of hallux valgus, *Foot Ankle* 12:7, 1991.

# Chapter 19

# Chronic leg pain

Lew C. Schon
Thomas O. Clanton

In a typical sports medicine or foot and ankle practice, it is not uncommon for an athlete to present with leg pain. Even though we all know from the popular song "the foot bone is connected to the leg bone, the leg bone is connected to the knee bone etc.", the interrelationships between the foot, ankle, and leg are considerably more complex than a simple skeletal interconnection. The muscles and tendons that provide mobility to the toes, midfoot, hindfoot, and ankle take origin in the leg, and the nerves, arteries, and veins that supply the foot course through the leg. Further, alignment, flexibility, and strength in the foot all have a significant impact on the more cephalad structures in the leg. Our charge is to interpret particular constellations of complaints and physical findings in light of an understanding of the anatomy, biomechanics, and pathomechanics of leg disorders. Although there are certainly sports-specific acute and subacute injuries to the leg, this chapter focuses on injuries caused by repetitive stresses.

Various pathologic entities must be considered in the differential diagnosis of chronic leg pain in athletes: chronic compartment syndrome, medial tibial stress syndrome, stress fractures, gastroc-soleus strain, nerve entrapment syndromes, venous and arterial pathology, fascial herniations, tendinitis, and radiculopathies. Although a multitude of tests are available to assist in the evaluation of these conditions, diagnosis can often be established solely on the basis of a thorough history and physical examination. When analyzing these conditions, it is imperative to recognize their dynamic nature and to alter the standard physical evaluation to include the specific activities that stress the appropriate structures.

## CHRONIC COMPARTMENT SYNDROME

Chronic compartment syndrome is a well-known entity in the sports medicine literature, but it is a relatively uncommon cause of exertional leg pain in the primary-care sports medicine setting.[17] The syndrome is caused by high pressures within the noncompliant fascial boundaries of the leg with resultant ischemia of muscles and nerves (Fig. 19-1). The elevated pressures are felt to arise from increased muscle volume and from increased intracellular and extracellular fluid accumulation with or without muscular microtears and hemorrhage. These increased pressures may cause venous and lymphatic compromise and further compound the situation[43] (Fig. 19-2).

### History

Typically athletes with a chronic compartment syndrome are involved in a running and/or ball or puck sport. The athlete notes the onset of pain after a particular distance, duration, or speed. The pain is progressive and may be described as achy, cramping, deep, or stabbing and is associated with a perceived fullness over the affected compartment. Neurologic symptoms such as numbness, tingling, burning, or electric sensations may occur in the distribution of the involved nerves. If activity is halted shortly after the onset of symptoms, resolution occurs in a relatively short period. If the pain is ignored, resolution may be more prolonged, taking several hours. Involvement of the anterior and deep posterior compartments is most common, and that of the lateral and superficial posterior compartments is less common.[5,17,34,63] In 10 to 17% of patients, a history of previous or concurrent

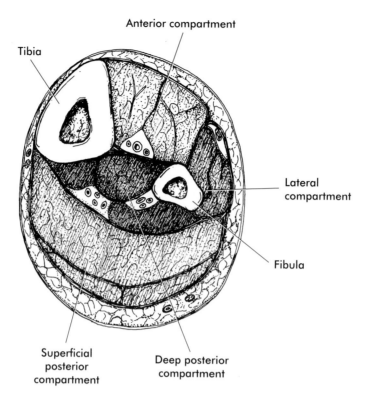

Tibia

Anterior compartment

Lateral compartment

Fibula

Superficial posterior compartment

Deep posterior compartment

**Fig. 19-1.** Compartments of leg in cross-section. (Reprinted with permission from Clanton TO, Schon LC: *Athletic injuries to the soft tissues of the foot and ankle.* In Mann RA, Coughlin MJ, editors: *Surgery of the foot,* ed 6, St Louis, CV Mosby Co, 1993, p. 1113.)

stress fractures may be obtained.[10,17] Medial tibial stress syndrome and stress fractures may also be common and associated with chronic compartment syndromes. Superficial peroneal nerve (SPN) and sural nerve irritations or entrapments can be difficult to distinguish from lateral or superficial posterior chronic compartment syndromes (Fig. 19-3).[40,62]

**Physical examination**

Athletes should be observed during and after running on a treadmill. Typically after the onset of symptoms, there is tenderness over the affected compartment. Decreased sensation or paresthesias may be appreciated along the course of affected nerves. Vascular compromise is rarely encountered. In the physical examination of the athlete at rest (without provocation), the findings may be minimal. Muscle herniations through fascial defects may be noted in 20% to 60% of the athletes[43,54] (Fig. 19-4). Findings of concurrent stress fractures or medial tibial stress syndrome with tenderness over the middle and lower borders of the tibia may also be noted.

Anteroposterior and lateral radiographs of the leg are indicated to appreciate stress fractures and periostitis, as well as to exclude the presence of an occult tumor. A technetium bone scan may demonstrate

focal uptake consistent with a stress fracture or diffuse uptake associated with medial tibial syndrome. There is no specific pattern of uptake associated with the elevated compartment pressures that is useful in establishing the diagnosis of the chronic compartment syndrome.

**PRESSURE MEASUREMENTS**

The diagnosis of chronic compartment syndrome can be made on clinical examination during or after exercise, but confirmation with compartmental pressures is warranted when considering surgical treatment. Although there are many different techniques and criteria for establishing the diagnosis,* the following guidelines are recommended[10]:

1. Preexercise compartment pressures greater than or equal to 15 mm Hg.
2. One minute postexercise compartment pressures greater than or equal to 30 mm Hg.
3. Compartment pressure measured 5 to 10 minutes following cessation of exercise greater than or equal to 15 mm Hg.

*References 1, 4, 43, 49, 53, 58, 59, 63, 66, 67.

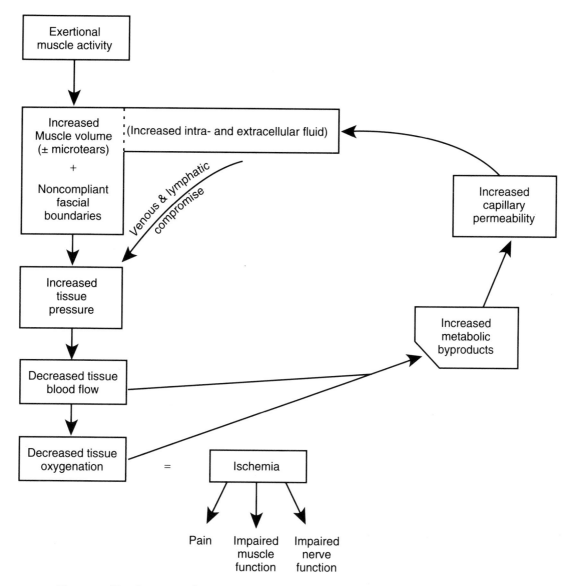

**Fig. 19-2.** Development of a compartment syndrome. (Reprinted with permission from Clanton TO, Schon LC: *Athletic injuries to the soft tissues of the foot and ankle.* In Mann RA, Coughlin MI, editors: *Surgery of the foot,* ed 6, St Louis, CV Mosby Co, 1993, p. 1107.)

Pressures can be reproducibly obtained using the Stryker or other hand-held devices (Fig. 19-5).

**Nonoperative treatment**

Nonoperative treatment of compartment syndrome includes avoidance of the level or intensity of activity responsible for the pain. After a brief period of relative rest, a gradual increase in activity level in association with ice and antiinflammatory medication may be sufficient. Orthotic devices, taping, and therapeutic modalities (ultrasound, massage, etc.) may be tried but usually are not curative. If the athlete is tolerant of the symptoms and is not significantly limited from pursuing their sport, no further aggressive treatment is warranted.

Be aware that an athlete with a history of chronic compartment syndrome may present with an acute compartment syndrome with increasing pain and dysfunction despite the cessation of activity. These cases obviously require more emergent surgical management.

**Operative treatment**
**Operative technique for anterior compartment syndrome release**

1. An anterior longitudinal incision is made 2 to 4 cm lateral to the lateral border of the tibia (Fig. 19-6). The incision extends from just below the level of the tibial tubercle in a distal direction for approximately 8 to 10 cm.

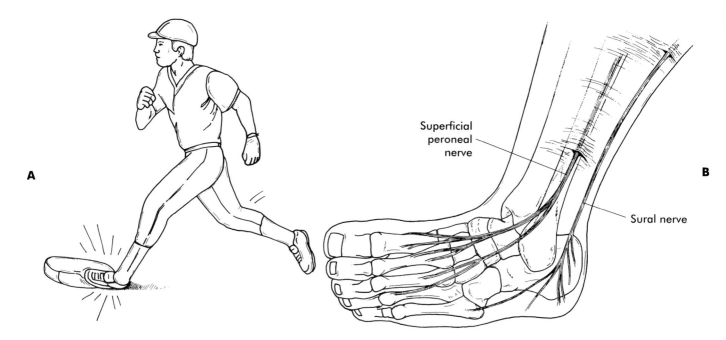

A B

Superficial
peroneal
nerve

Sural nerve

**Fig. 19-3.** Superficial peroneal nerve and sural nerve can be stretched during an ankle sprain and may result in chronic neuritis or entrapment.

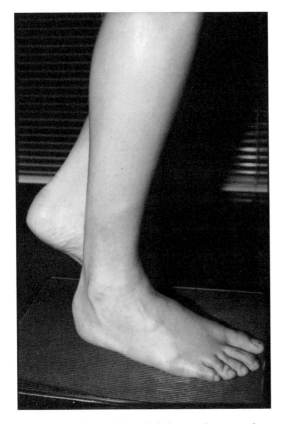

**Fig. 19-4.** Anterolateral fascial defect and peroneal muscle herniation in a runner.

2. The fascia is then released distal and proximal to the skin incision. Care must be taken to avoid the SPN distally.
3. Hemostasis is achieved and the skin is closed.

**Technique for lateral compartment syndrome release**

1. The lateral compartment is released through an anterolateral incision made over the course of the peroneal musculature using an 8- to 10-cm incision (Fig. 19-7).
2. Again in the lower middle and distal aspects of the incision, care must be taken to avoid cutting the superficial peroneal nerve. Identifying the fascial boundary between the anterior and lateral compartment will aid in the identification of the nerve. Typically the nerve runs just posterior to this fascia boundary at this junction. Occasionally the nerve pierces this fascia higher in the leg and runs in the anterior compartment. Although the nerve typically pierces the lateral fascia about 10 cm above the tip of the fibula, it may pierce the anterior fascia in the lower third of the leg.
3. Hemostasis is achieved and the skin is closed.

**Technique for the posterior compartment release**

1. A 10-cm longitudinal incision is made paralleling the posteromedial border of the tibia, beginning at the midtibia level (Fig. 19-8). The saphenous vein and its associated nerve lie subcutaneously and must be preserved.

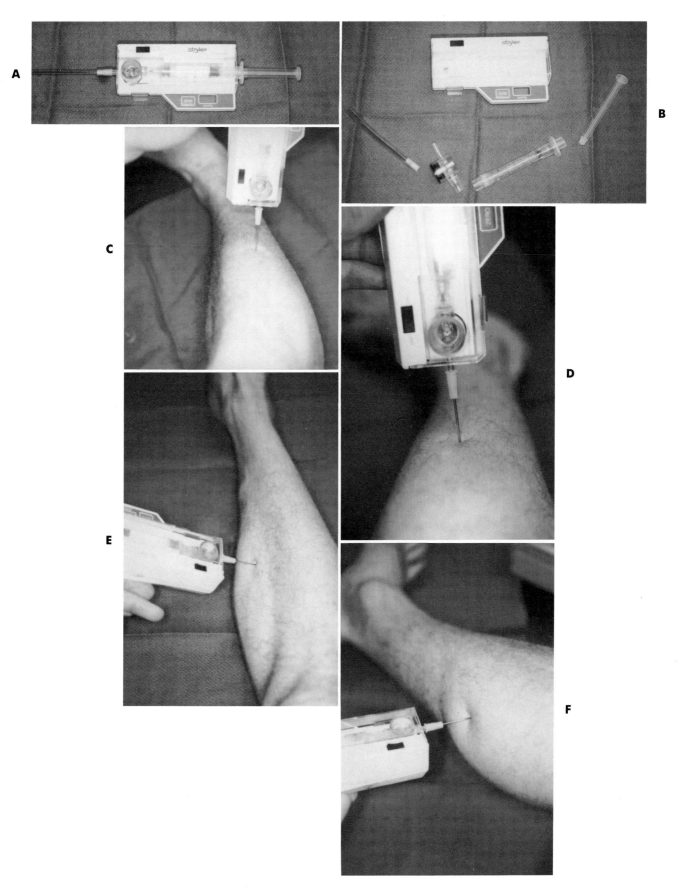

**Fig. 19-5.** Stryker hand-held device for compartment pressure measurement **(A)**, disassembled components **(B)**, measuring anterior **(C)**, lateral **(D)**, deep posterior **(E)**, and superficial posterior compartments **(F)**.

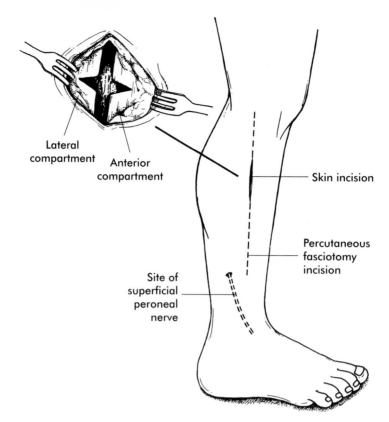

**Fig. 19-6.** Technique for releasing the anterior compartment. (Reprinted with permission from Clanton TO, Schon LC: *Athletic injuries to the soft tissues of the foot and ankle.* In Mann RA, Coughlin MI, editors: *Surgery of the foot,* ed 6, St Louis, CV Mosby Co, 1993, p. 1111.)

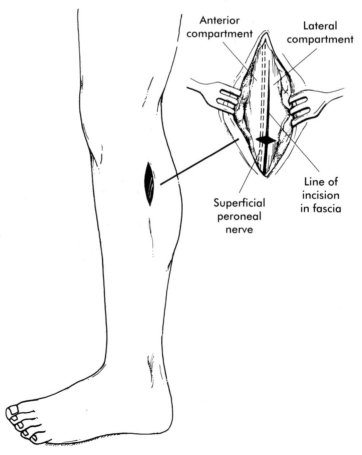

**Fig. 19-7.** Technique for releasing the lateral compartment. (Reprinted with permission from Clanton TO, Schon LC: *Athletic injuries to the soft tissues of the foot and ankle.* In Mann RA, Coughlin MI, editors: *Surgery of the foot,* ed 6, St Louis, CV Mosby Co, 1993, p. 1112.)

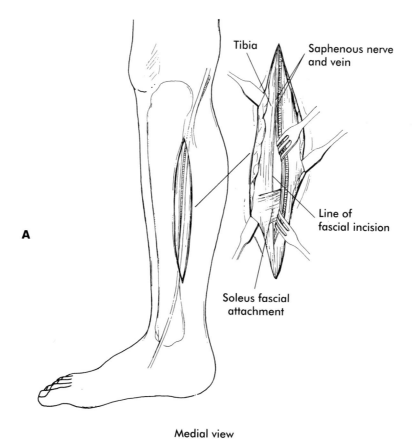

**Medial view**

**Cross section of right leg**

**Fig. 19-8. A,** Technique for releasing the posterior compartment. **B,** Cross-sectional orientation demonstrating posterior compartment release. (Reprinted with permission from Clanton TO, Schon LC: *Athletic injuries to the soft tissues of the foot and ankle.* In Mann RA, Coughlin MI, editors: *Surgery of the foot,* ed 6, St Louis, CV Mosby Co, 1993, p. 1113.)

2. In the middle and distal third of the leg, the fascia of the soleus muscle inserts on the posteromedial border of the tibia. This is released providing exposure to the deep posterior compartment. Based on the surgeon's interpretation of the preoperative findings, a separate release of the tibialis posterior compartment may be performed.

3. The skin is sutured after obtaining hemostasis.

**Postoperative care after compartment release.** Compression bandages are applied in the operating room. Partial progressive weight bearing with crutches may be initiated after surgery. The patient may begin range-of-motion and isometric exercises immediately. By 3 weeks the patient may resume light running. In a posterior compartment release, recovery may be twice as long. The overall success rate of the procedure ranges from 60% to 90% of complete relief of symptoms.[14,34,53,54] Although decreased strength has been demonstrated following fasciotomy, relief of pain and subsequent increased endurance offset this weakness.[24,41] Other potential complications include hematoma, persistent swelling, muscle pain, scar pain, nerve damage, nerve entrapment (especially of the SPN following anterior compartment release), superficial and deep infection, and enlarged fascial defect and muscle herniation.

**Case Study 1.** A 34-year-old female runner has a 2½ year history of right leg pain that intensified with activity. Previously she was able to run 50 miles per week but sustained a metatarsal stress fracture 3 years ago. Once running was resumed, achy dull pain began in both legs. The right leg pain intensified in time and was associated with fullness laterally and anteriorly. Whenever running was increased above 4 miles per day, she would experience shooting pains into the lateral ankle and dorsum of the foot. Occasionally there would be numbness of the foot. This pain would gradually diminish over 30 to 60 minutes.

A static evaluation revealed a small fascial defect and a fatty mass 12.5 cm above the tip of the fibula. The SPN was observed penetrating the fascia at this location (Fig. 19-9). Palpation over the nerve caused discomfort in a similar pattern to her exercise-induced pain. The character of the discomfort was of a different quality. There was no sensory or motion deficit. Vascular status was normal.

In a treadmill stress test, symptoms were induced after about 30 minutes. Examination revealed a positive percussion sign (Tinel's) over the SPN. There was diminished light touch sensation on the dorsum of the right foot. Pulses were normal. There was no tenseness of the compartments, but mild swelling was evident anteriorly and laterally. Pressure measurements anteriorly and laterally were 20 mm Hg at 1 minute and 6 mm Hg at 5 minutes postexercise. Radiographs were normal, and a bone scan was not ordered. A local injection (lidocaine and marcaine) of the SPN at the fascial defect eliminated the pain.

The diagnosis of dynamic SPN entrapment was established on clinical grounds. Since conservative trials were unsuccessful, the patient underwent release of the SPN. She had excellent relief of symptoms with a low level of activity but required 3 months to resume 40 miles a week.

**Case Study 2.** A 36-year-old runner ran 20 to 25 miles per week. He had a 2-year history of lateral leg pain with mild swelling but always the sensation of tightness and fullness. He had no back problems. He used an orthotic without any benefit and managed 20 to 25 miles of running by using ice packs before and after. The patient had compartment pressure studies, which showed elevated pressures in the lateral compartment after exercising. The pressures were 20 mm Hg after 15 minutes.

Static evaluation revealed some mild tenderness over the SPN, but no tenderness over the deep posterior or lateral anterior compartment. There was no tenderness over the bone. Overall alignment of the foot and ankle was good; strength was good. With running on the treadmill, the patient had tightness of the anterior and lateral compartments, but the tenseness in the lateral compartment remained much longer than that in the anterior compartment; pressure studies confirmed the presence of a chronic lateral compartment syndrome.

The patient underwent surgery and had immediate relief postoperatively. At 6 weeks he resumed running 1 to 2 miles per week and then gradually built his way back up to 20 to 25 miles per week. He has no weakness, no swelling, but there is minimal tenderness with deep palpation of the scar.

## MEDIAL TIBIAL STRESS SYNDROME

Medial tibial stress syndrome is a cause of medial leg pain resulting from a stress reaction of fascia, periosteum, and/or bone along the posteromedial aspect of the tibia.[6,16,37,46] The syndrome is a well-established clinical entity that represents a spectrum of associated pathologic conditions. Medial tibial stress syndrome has been subclassified into three types by Detmer.[16] Type I represents posteromedial stress fracture or a bone stress reaction. Type II is a periosteal reaction from overpull of the soleus fascia on the posteromedial border of the tibia. Type III is a deep posterior or posterior tibialis compartment syndrome. The syndrome is quite common in running and in jumping sports.

In Finland medial tibial stress syndrome is thought to occur in 60% of conditions causing leg pain. In the findings of Orava and Puranen this syndrome accounted for 9.5% of all presenting complaints in an athletic population.[48]

### History

Patients with medial tibial stress syndrome complain of recurrent exertional pain along the posterior border of the middle and distal tibia. The pain is usually a dull ache but may increase to intense focal pain and is particularly noticeable during toe-off. Symptoms are also exacerbated by running on banked

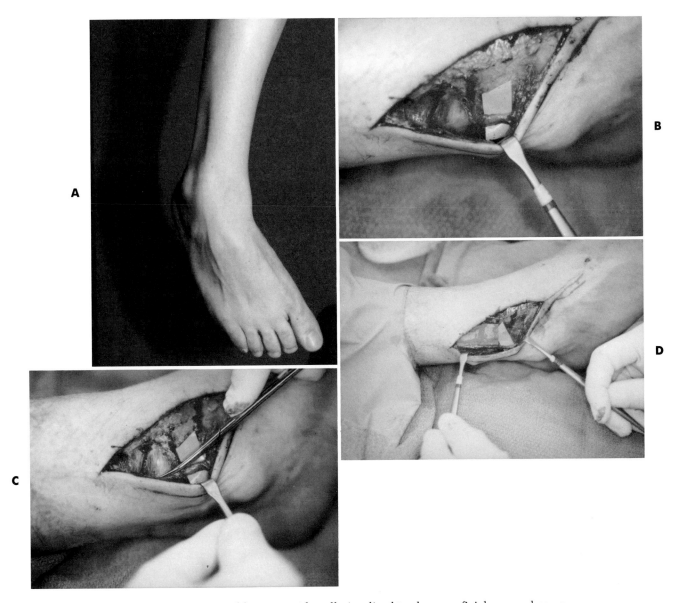

**Fig. 19-9. A,** A 34-year-old runner with well-visualized tender superficial peroneal nerve.
**B** to **D,** Intraoperative photographs demonstrating release of the superficial peroneal nerve.

surfaces. Initially the pain will be present only during the activity but in time pain may occur even during walking or rarely at rest.

### Physical examination

The most characteristic finding of the medial tibial stress syndrome is tenderness along the posteromedial border of the tibia. Local induration may also be appreciated in the region of pain. Neurovascular examination is unremarkable. There is no pain with passive stretching of the involved muscle. Excessive subtalar mobility and/or abnormal pronation with excessive posteromedial muscle or fascial stresses have been noted in this syndrome.[37,50,70]

### Diagnostic studies

Radiographs may demonstrate cortical hypertrophy of the tibia or evidence of healed stress fracture. Typically radiographs are unremarkable. Technetium bone scans may show diffuse linear uptake along the posterior border of the tibia, which may involve as much as one third of the bone length[26] (Fig. 19-10).

Since some authors have maintained that medial tibial stress syndrome results from a superficial posterior, deep posterior, or isolated posterior tibial exertional compartment syndrome, compartmental pressure measurements are frequently obtained.[14,30,52,54,57] The role of these pressure measurements has been debated and some authors have

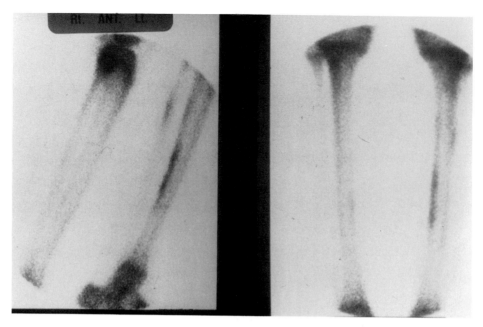

**Fig. 19-10.** Characteristic technetium bone scan in medial tibial stress syndrome demonstrating diffuse linear uptake along the posteromedial border of the tibial cortex. (Scan courtesy of L. Holder, M.D., Department of Radiology, University of Maryland School of Medicine.)

reported normal pressures before, during, and after exercises.[12,44,71,72] The concurrence of a chronic compartment syndrome and medial tibial stress syndrome is 50% according to Allen and Barnes.[1] An injection of a local anesthetic at the posteromedial border of the tibia, which gives relief, supports the diagnosis.

**Nonoperative treatment**

Nonoperative treatment is similar to that for chronic compartment syndrome. In athletes with abnormal subtalar motion and hyperpronation, orthotic devices may be of some benefit.[28] After a period of relative rest, running on grass can be instituted to help recondition the legs. Similarly underwater running may also be of value. Operative treatment is indicated for those athletes who are unresponsive to a supervised program of conservative treatment. Athletes should be symptomatic to the point that they are unable to continue their athletic activity before surgical treatment is considered.

**Operative treatment**

1. A 10-cm longitudinal incision parallel and posterior to the posteromedial border of the tibia is made involving the middle third of the tibia. The saphenous vein and nerve are identified and retracted.
2. The fascia is released from the level of the tibial tuberosity to about 5 cm above the medial malleolus.

3. Hemostasis is achieved and the skin is closed.

Alternatively two incisions can be made, one at the junction of the proximal and middle thirds of the tibia and one at the junction of the distal and middle thirds of the tibia (Fig. 19-11). Puranen believes this permits easier division of the fascia.[51]

**Postoperative care**

In the operating room compression bandages are applied. Partial progressive weight bearing with crutches is initiated after surgery. Isometric and range-of-motion exercises begin immediately. Light running may begin at 2 to 3 weeks, but it may be 4 to 6 weeks before beginning more intense training. Overall success rate is favorable, with 75% to 80% of patients having good-to-excellent results.[10,27]

**Case Study 3.** A 30-year-old male complained of left leg pain for over 1 year. He had been running 4 or 5 times per week for a total of 60 to 70 miles per week. He ran 10-Ks and marathons and in addition was active in racquetball and aerobics. He began having deep pain on the inner side of his leg with slight radiation proximally. He had no back problems. He stated the pain was worse late in the evening for about 3 to 4 hours. Sometimes, he had pain after he stopped exercises. He subsequently modified his workout, changed his shoes, and had some relief of pain. In time, the pain increased and became persistent. The patient had to decrease his activity below a satisfactory level.

The physical examination revealed tenderness along the posteromedial border of the tibia and along the lower third.

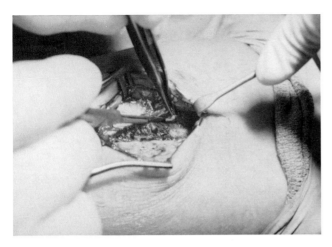

**Fig. 19-11.** Proximal incision for release of medial tibial stress syndrome.

There was normal subtalar motion. The overall alignment was good. Strength of the invertors and plantar flexors were normal. There was no swelling in the compartments and no neurologic findings. The patient was thought to have a medial tibial stress syndrome, which was unresponsive to conservative treatment and indicated the need for a deep posteromedial release. A bone scan was performed, which showed diffuse linear uptake along the medial aspect of the tibia (Fig. 19-10). X-rays and compartment pressures were unremarkable.

A posteromedial release was performed in addition to release of the fascia of the posterior tibialis muscle. The patient had immediate relief of pain but complained postoperatively of some numbness in the foot, which lasted for a few weeks. After 2 weeks the patient began walking without crutches. He had gradual improvement of the pain and swelling over the next 5 months. The patient was able to return to vigorous athletics. He has resumed biking, tennis, and racquetball but runs less than 30 miles per week. He feels he has 100% use of the leg but has had some mild atrophy on the affected side. The patient said he was satisfied with the results of the surgery and was disappointed only that he was not able to return to his previously intense level of running.

## STRESS FRACTURES OF THE TIBIA AND FIBULA

Stress fractures occur when repetitive loads result in an imbalance of the formation and resorption of bone. Both tibia and fibula stress fractures are most common in running and jumping sports. Anterior midtibial stress fractures are seen more commonly in dancers and basketball players. Amenorrheic females and other athletes with diminished bone mineral content appear particularly vulnerable to stress fractures.[29] Stress fractures may also occur in association with other leg overuse syndromes. It is not unusual for athletes to change their activity or technique to alleviate their primary pain and inadvertently overload other structures, causing a secondary problem.

### History

Stress fractures often occur when there are alterations in an athlete's typical routine: changes in shoes, altered terrain, different playing surfaces (i.e., tracks or dance floors), changes in intensity of activity or increased speed. Certainly at the beginning of a season (after a period of relative inactivity), athletes are particularly vulnerable to these fractures. Symptoms begin as a dull ache over the affected bone, which over the course of several weeks may increase to a more persistent deep pain. The pain begins earlier and earlier after the beginning of an activity and typically decreases before it increases as activity persists. Once activity is stopped, pain typically remains. With time the pain will remain for many hours and may even be constant. The pain is often relieved with rest. Jumping and higher-impact activities exacerbate the pain.

### Physical examination

Unlike compartment syndrome, examination at rest often reveals well-localized tenderness over the affected area of the bone. Doughy edema or swelling may be appreciated at the site of the fracture (Fig. 19-12). Increased warmth and erythema may be noted. Stressing the bone by having the patient jump or hop will induce pain. In more chronic stress fractures, local thickening of the bone or periosteum is readily appreciated.

### Diagnostic studies

Radiographs should be obtained in cases of suspected stress fracture but typically are unremarkable within the first several weeks. In time, periosteal reaction may be appreciated with or without hairline cortical lucencies (Fig. 19-13). Radiographs may be persistently normal in some cases. Occasionally a stress fracture will be associated with the presence of a benign bone tumor.

In cases where there is some question of the diagnosis, a technetium bone scan is most sensitive. Focal uptake is considered characteristic of a fracture (Fig. 19-14). More diffuse linear uptake is more consistent with a stress reaction of the bone.

### Nonoperative treatment

Nonoperative treatment consists of avoiding the offending activity coupled with cross-training. In patients with more advanced fractures, partial or non–weight bearing may be instituted until resolution of pain. In patients with preexisting problems and stress fractures due to overcompensation, immobilization may be necessary. During recovery, cycling, pool running, swimming, rowing, and weight training should be emphasized. These lower-impact activities should limit deconditioning while the fracture is

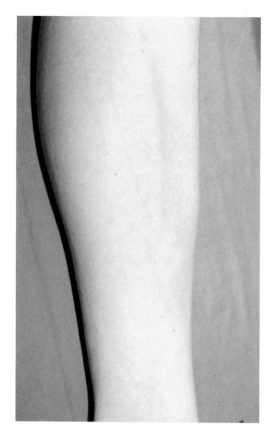

**Fig. 19-12.** Tender bony prominence over tibia with a stress fracture.

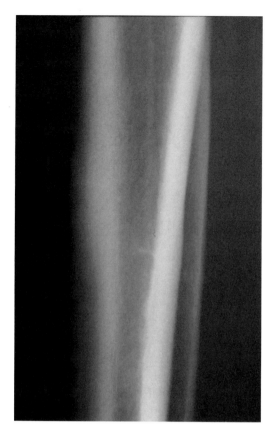

**Fig. 19-13.** Cortical hypertrophy of anterior tibia with a stress fracture.

allowed to heal. A fibula stress fracture usually resolves within 2 to 10 weeks. On the other hand, an anterior tibial stress fracture is usually associated with longer recovery, which may at times be several years (Fig. 19-15).[47] In some of the more ominous stress fractures, especially those with cortical lucency involving the anterior tibia, pulsed electromagnetic fields may be of some benefit.[55] Rettig et al proposed pulsed electromagnetic fields used for 10 to 12 hours for 3 to 6 months with/without immobilization in cases of resistant nonhealing fractures.[55]

### Operative treatment

Operative treatment is reserved for chronic nonhealing stress fractures. Most commonly these are anterior tibial stress fractures.

#### Technique

1. A longitudinal incision is made over the fracture. The periosteum is incised longitudinally and reflected sharply off the bone. The stress fracture is identified by the presence of fibrous tissue or lower-density bone with increased vascular perforations. Fluoroscopic imaging is frequently useful.

2. Fibrous tissue is debrided and/or a small portion of the hypervascular bone is resected in a troughlike manner.
3. Regional cancellous bone graft is harvested and packed in the defect.
4. Using a 2.0 or 2.5 mm drill bit, multiple perforations are created in the surrounding sclerotic bone.
5. Hemostasis is achieved, periosteum is reopposed, and the skin is sutured.

### Postoperative course

A compression dressing is applied in the operating room and partial weight bearing with crutches begins initially and is progressed to full weight bearing to tolerance. Any offending activity is avoided during the recovery. Cross-training may be resumed at 1 to 2 weeks, depending on the condition of the wound.

**Case Study 4.** A 14-year-old baseball player complained of persistent low-grade anterior leg pain for 3 months. Pain was worse with running or jumping and occasionally lasted until the next morning after a game. There was no numbness, tingling, or swelling. The athlete attributed the pain to an injury 3 months earlier when he was struck with a baseball. He presented to the office after experi-

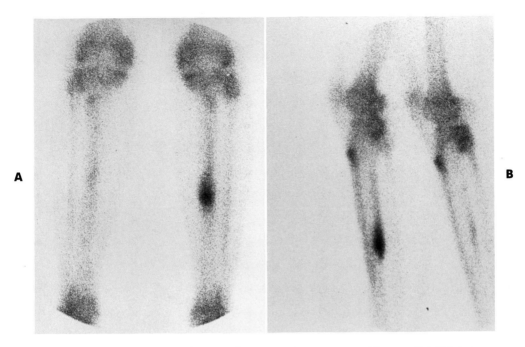

**Fig. 19-14.** Characteristic technetium bone scan in a runner with a medial tibial stress fracture. Notice the intense focal fusiform uptake. (Scan courtesy of L. Holder, M.D., Department of Radiology, University of Maryland School of Medicine.)

encing sudden severe pain and inability to walk. This occurred without trauma while he was walking in the school hallway.

On physical examination, there was marked tenderness over the anterior proximal tibia with procurvatum deformity of the leg. Radiographs revealed an acute fracture through a chronic anterior tibial stress fracture (Fig. 19-16). The fracture was reduced and the leg placed in a long-leg cast in extension. After 6 weeks the cast was removed and a new immobilizer applied for 6 additional weeks. He resumed sports at 3 months with a graduated return to activities and stresses.

## GASTROC-SOLEUS STRAIN

Gastroc-soleus strain or rupture is a common injury in athletes. Although most cases are acute events with relatively rapid recovery, it is not infrequent to encounter cases with chronic symptoms. The injury is common in racket sports, running, basketball, and skiing.

Confusion has existed as to whether this lesion represented a ruptured plantaris. Despite the clinical impression that a plantaris muscle tear had occurred, only one or two plantaris tears identified during surgery have been reported in the literature.[36,64]

### History

Typically acute gastroc-soleus strain occurs when the athlete extends the knee while in the crouched position with the ankles dorsiflexed (Fig. 19-17). The

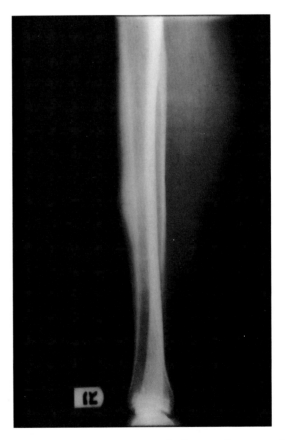

**Fig. 19-15.** Transverse anterior tibial stress fracture with cortical lucency.

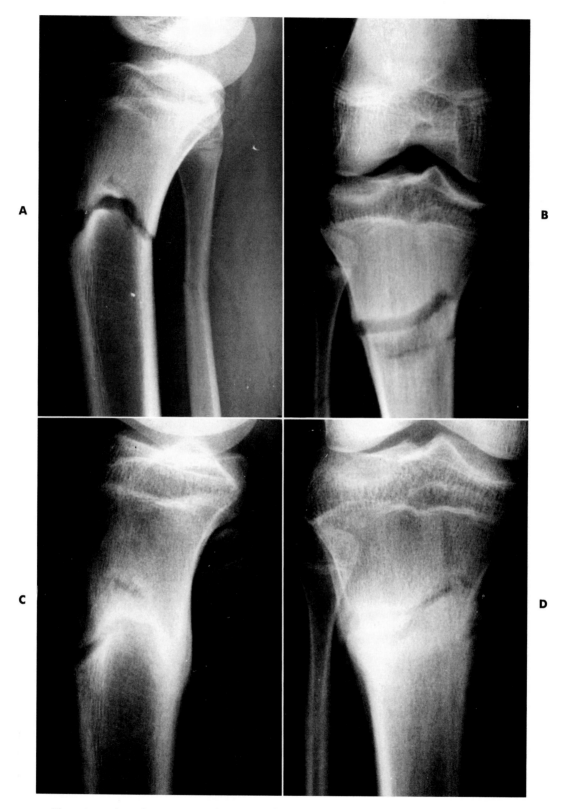

**Fig. 19-16. A** and **B,** Catastrophic tibial fracture with evidence of chronic prefracture sclerosis and hypertrophy. **C** and **D,** Healed fracture following reduction, long-leg casting, and bracing.

push-off leg in the crouched athlete who is lunging forward to meet the ball or another player is particularly vulnerable. Often the athlete experiences sudden intense calf pain, which may or may not be followed by swelling, cramping, and discoloration secondary to local hemorrhage. Depending on the severity of the rupture, athletes may or may not have difficulty walking. Rising up on the toes and the toe-off portion

of the gait are often uncomfortable for the athlete.

Most often the chronic pain is thought to occur as a result of intramuscular scar pain, low-grade venous dysfunction, increased fatigability and/or cramping of the muscle due to alterations in the functional length of the musculotendinous unit. Beware of the unusual case of posterior calf pain, which may represent other pathology (Fig. 19-18).

### Nonoperative treatment

In mild strains the patient begins with a program of rest, ice, compression, and elevation in association with gentle passive stretching. As the pain decreases, standing calf stretches can be instituted.[32] In patients with moderate strains who are unable to stand on their toes, a removable leg brace with the ankle in equinus may be indicated. The use of crutches with weight bearing to tolerance is also effective. Active dorsiflexion and gentle passive stretching should be instituted as soon as tolerated.

### Operative treatment

Operative intervention is rarely indicated. Athletes with painful and tense hematomas may benefit from aspiration or drainage. Some authors have made a case for debridement and repair in selected cases of massive rupture.[39,41]

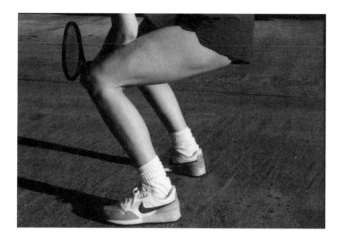

**Fig. 19-17.** Gastrocnemius tear occurs when the athlete extends the knee from the crouched position with the ankles dorsiflexed.

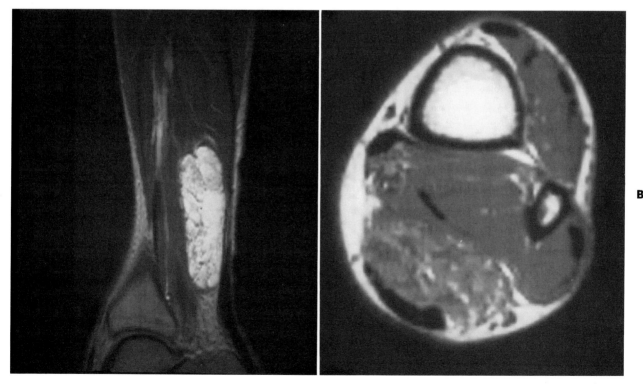

A

B

**Fig. 19-18. A,** Magnetic resonance imaging (MRI) study of a middle-aged runner with what was thought to be a gastroc-soleus tear. Biopsy revealed capillary hemangioma. **B,** MRI study of the calf in an athlete with chronic pain following a gastrocnemius tear reveals local muscle changes consistent with scarring.

## POPLITEAL ARTERY ENTRAPMENT SYNDROME

Popliteal artery entrapment syndrome is a rare cause of calf pain in young athletes. The popliteal artery is compressed as it courses medial to the medial head of the gastrocnemius (Fig. 19-19). Multiple variations of the pathoanatomy have been described.[15,19] The syndrome occurs in athletes and nonathletes participating in football, basketball, soccer, and running sports.* A functional (i.e., dynamic) neurovascular compression by the soleus and plantaris muscles also occurs in athletes. In these cases plantar flexion of the ankle results in lateral displacement of the popliteal artery and tibial nerve.[69]

### History

Patients typically present with cramping, claudication, and calf pain. The pain is associated with exertion and is better with rest. Bilateral symptoms are found in 67% of patients.[7,11]

### Physical examination

As with exertional compartment syndrome, a static evaluation may be completely unremarkable. After an exercise treadmill challenge, pulses may be diminished, particularly with the knee in hyperextension and the foot dorsiflexed.[38,60] The foot may be cool while the knee is warm secondary to collateral circulation.[8]

### Diagnostic studies

Compartment pressure studies should be performed in patients with popliteal artery entrapment syndrome. Additionally, Doppler pressure measurements should be performed before and after exercises.[13,38] Continuous-wave Doppler studies, duplex scanning, and ultrasonography, computed tomography, and MRI may also be of benefit.[18,38,45,69,73] In patients with suspected popliteal artery entrapment, an arteriogram performed after exercise is diagnostic. Medial deviation of the popliteal artery, popliteal artery segmental occlusion, and poststenotic dilation are characteristic. Dynamic stenosis of the artery may occur with hyperextension of the knee and passive dorsiflexion of the ankle.[60] In patients without arterial or muscular abnormalities, the functional lateral compression by the soleus and plantaris can be visualized by MRI with the foot in plantar flexion.[69]

### Nonoperative treatment

In patients with minimal symptoms, nonoperative treatment with relative rest and avoidance of the

*References 7, 13, 19, 21, 33, 64.

offending activity is worthwhile. Physical therapy and antiinflammatory medications are not beneficial.

### Operative treatment

In cases diagnosed early—when there is no damage to the artery—release of the artery is indicated.[19] Turnipseed and Pozniak recommended resection of the plantaris muscle, medial release of the soleus off the tibia, and release of the soleus fascial bands via a medial approach.[69] With more chronic lesions arterial grafting, saphenous vein bypass, endarterectomy, or excision and reanastomosis may be necessary.[8,19,21,35]

## FEMORAL OR EXTERNAL ILIAC ARTERIAL OCCLUSION

Exercise-induced occlusion of the external iliac artery may also cause chronic leg pain. The syndrome has been described in bicycle racers by Chevalier et al.[9]

### History

Cyclists describe severe lower-extremity pain during maximal effort during competition. Painful mus-

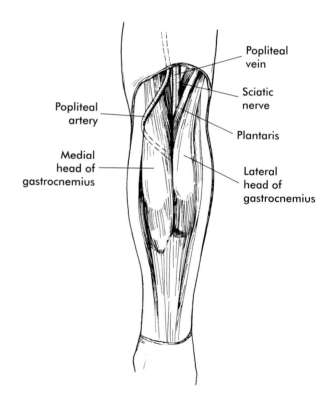

**Fig. 19-19.** Anatomic variation of the popliteal artery where the artery deviates medially around the medial gastrocnemius. (Reprinted with permission from Clanton TO, Schon LC: *Athletic injuries to the soft tissues of the foot and ankle.* In Mann RA, Coughlin MJ, editors: *Surgery of the foot,* ed 6, St Louis, 1993, CV Mosby Co, 1993, p. 1118.)

cular contractions descend in the calf with gradual loss of responsiveness of the extremity. The palsy resolves within a few minutes following cessation of the maximal effort.

### Physical examination

A static evaluation is often unremarkable. Occasionally the affected extremity may have a larger thigh and calf circumference. With the thigh maximally flexed, a systolic bruit may be auscultated. Systolic Doppler pressures performed while the cyclist is stressed on a wind trainer may reveal reduction in flow. In those patients with a suspected lesion, arteriography of the external iliac artery may show stenosis and arterial lengthening.[9]

Avoiding the offending activity may be sufficient for most athletes. For athletes with inability to compete, surgery may be warranted. Chevalier et al performed endarterectomy and shortening of the artery in seven competitive racers. Four of the seven were able to return to competition 2 months following the surgery.[9]

### VENOUS DISEASE

A rare condition known as effort thrombosis has been described in the lower extremities.[24,25,75] Patients present with pain and swelling associated with superficial venous distension and discoloration. The diagnosis is confirmed by venography, and treatment requires anticoagulation with heparin followed by warfarin sodium (Coumadin).

Thrombophlebitis may occur in association with acute and chronic leg injuries. The likelihood of developing phlebitis increases with immobilization after injury, prolonged inactivity (especially sitting during bus or air travel), activity at high altitudes, alcohol or drug abuse, dehydration, oral contraceptives, and hemoglobinopathies. These risk factors are not infrequent in the athletic population.

### SAPHENOUS NERVE ENTRAPMENT

The saphenous nerve, the largest cutaneous branch of the femoral nerve, runs between the vastus medialis and sartorius along the superficial femoral artery in the lower third of the thigh. Approximately 10 cm

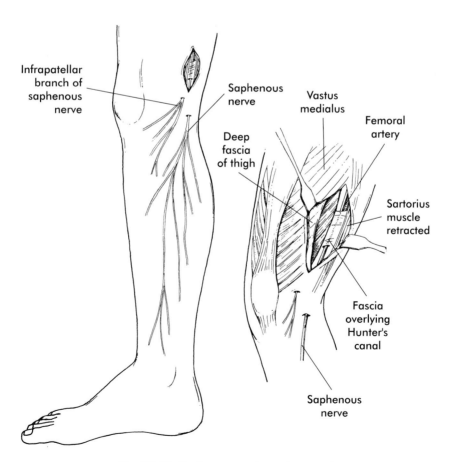

**Fig. 19-20.** Saphenous nerve entrapment.

proximal to the medial femoral condyle, the nerve pierces the subsartorial fascia. The nerve divides into the infrapatellar and sartorial branches. Posterior to the medial femoral condyle, it emerges into the subcutaneous tissue between the sartorius and gracilis. The nerve descends along the medial border of the tibia with the greater saphenous vein (Fig. 19-20). Proximal to the medial malleolus about 15 cm, it branches into one division that provides sensation to the medial aspect of the ankle and another division that provides sensation to the medial side of the foot.[2,3,31,42,61]

Sartorial or saphenous nerve problems may occur following knee surgery or after direct trauma. Patients most commonly complain of medial knee or medial leg pain. Infrequently athletes will complain of medial ankle or foot pain. The pain may be confused with vascular disease. Symptoms of intermittent claudication with fatigue and heaviness of the leg may be elicited.[42] On physical examination, there is point tenderness approximately 10 cm above the medial femoral condyle over the subsartorial canal. There may or may not be sensory changes. No motor changes should be found. In some patients hyperextension of the thigh may cause the pain to radiate distally. Saphenous nerve entrapment has also been seen in athletes with hypertrophied muscles.[20]

Somatosensory-evoked potentials may be helpful in establishing the diagnosis of saphenous nerve entrapment.[20,68] Anesthetic block in the subsartorial canal with a local anesthetic and corticosteroid may be diagnostic as well as therapeutic. The range of success with the injections is from 38%[42] to 80%.[56] Patients with neuromas of the infrapatellar branch may require surgery.[74]

The surgery requires a 10-cm incision along the anterior border of the sartorius muscle in the lower third of the thigh. The fibrous roof of Hunter's canal is released, and the perforating nerves are dissected from the surrounding fascia.[31,42] For patients with a infrapatellar neuroma, Worth et al recommended a nerve transection.[74]

## EXERCISE-INDUCED MUSCLE PAIN

Muscle pain may follow athletic activity, especially when associated with eccentric contractions. The athlete may complain of muscle pain as well as fatigue, stiffness, and loss of performance 24 to 48 hours following exercises. This may require 5 to 7 days for resolution.[22] Treatment involves rest, ice, and conservative modalities.

## SUMMARY

Exercise-induced leg pain is common in athletes. Although some cases are easy to analyze, others are more complex requiring a dynamic evaluation. In the more challenging problems, additional tests such as compartment pressure studies, static and dynamic arterial or venous Doppler examinations, and bone scans may be necessary. Treatment involves relative rest, common sense, and cross-training to avoid deconditioning while the body heals itself.

Certain conditions such as acute compartment syndrome, thrombophlebitis, and arterial disorders that require more aggressive intervention should be excluded. Athletes who fail a conservative trial and are limited in their activities may benefit from surgery.

## REFERENCES

1. Allen JM, Barnes MR: Exercise pain in the lower leg, *J Bone Joint Surg* 68B:818, 1986.
2. Arthornthurasook A, Gaem-Im K: Study of the infrapatellar nerve, *Am J Sports Med* 16:57, 1988.
3. Arthornthurasook A, Gaem-Im K: The sartorial nerve: its relationship to the medial aspect of the knee, *Am J Sports Med* 18:41, 1990.
4. Awbrey BJ, Sienkiewicz PS, Mankin HJ: Chronic exercise-induced compartment pressure evaluation measured with a miniaturized fluid pressure monitor. A laboratory and clinical study, *Am J Sports Med* 16:610, 1988.
5. Bourne RB, Rorabeck CH: Compartment syndromes of the lower leg, *Clin Orthop* 240:97, 1989.
6. Brody DM: Running injuries, *CIBA Clin Symp* 32:1, 1980.
7. Carter AE, Eban R: A case of bilateral developmental abnormality of the popliteal arteries and gastrocnemius muscles, *Br J Surg* 51:518, 1964.
8. Casscells SW, Fellows B, Axe MJ: Another young athlete with intermittent claudication. A case report, *Am J Sports Med* 11:180, 1983.
9. Chevalier J et al: Endofibrosis of the external iliac artery in bicycle racers: an unrecognized pathological state, *Ann Vasc Surg* 1:297, 1986.
10. Clanton TO, Schon LC: *Athletic injuries to the soft tissues of the foot and ankle.* In Mann RA, Coughlin MJ, editors: *Surgery of the foot,* ed 6, St Louis, 1993, CV Mosby Co, 1993, p. 1095-1224.
11. Collins PS, McDonald PT, Lim RC: Popliteal artery entrapment: an evolving syndrome, *J Vasc Surg* 10:484, 1989.
12. D'Ambrosia RD et al: Interstitial pressure measurements in the anterior and posterior compartments in athletes with shin splints, *Am J Sports Med* 5:127, 1977.
13. Darling RS et al: Intermittent claudication in young athletes: popliteal artery entrapment syndrome, *J Trauma* 14:543, 1974.
14. Davey JR, Rorabeck CH, Fowler PJ: The tibialis posterior muscle compartment. An unrecognized cause of exertional compartment syndrome, *Am J Sports Med* 12:391, 1984.
15. Delaney TA, Gonzalez LL: Occlusion of popliteal artery due to muscular entrapment, *Surgery* 69:97, 1971.
16. Detmer DE: Chronic shin splints: classification and management of medial tibial stress syndrome, *Sports Med* 3:436, 1986.
17. Detmer DE et al: Chronic compartment syndrome: diagnosis, management and outcomes, *Am J Sports Med* 13:162, 1985.
18. di Marzo L et al: Diagnosis of popliteal artery entrapment syndrome: the role of duplex scanning, *J Vasc Surg* 13:434, 1991.
19. di Marzo L et al: Surgical treatment of popliteal artery entrapment syndrome: a ten year experience, *Eur J Vasc Surg* 5:59, 1991.
20. Dumitru D, Windsor RE: Subsartorial entrapment of the saphenous nerve of a competitive female bodybuilder, *Phys Sports Med* 17:116, 1989.

21. Duwelius PJ et al: Popliteal artery entrapment in a high school athlete. A case report, *Am J Sports Med* 15:371, 1987.

22. Ebbeling CB, Clarkson PM: Exercise-induced muscle damage and adaptation, *Sports Med* 7:207, 1989.

23. Garfin SR et al: The role of fascia in the maintenance of muscle tension and pressure, *J Appl Physiol* 51:317, 1981.

24. Gorard DA: Effort thrombosis in an American football player, *Br J Sports Med* 24:15, 1990.

25. Harvey JS Jr: Effort thrombosis in the lower extremity of a runner, *Am J Sports Med* 6:400, 1978.

26. Holder LE, Michael RH: The specific scintigraphic pattern of "shin splints in the lower leg," *J Nucl Med* 25:865, 1984.

27. Jarvinen M, Aho H, Niittymaki S: Results of the surgical treatment of the medial tibial syndrome in athletes, *Int J Sports Med* 10:55, 1989.

28. Jones DC, James SL: Overuse injuries of the lower extremity: shin splints, iliotibial band friction syndrome and exertional compartment syndromes, *Clin Sports Med* 6:273, 1987.

29. Kadel NJ, Teitz CC, Kronmal RA: Stress fractures in ballet dancers, *M J Sports Med* 20:445, 1992.

30. Kirby NG: Exercise ischemia in the fascial compartment of the soleus, *J Bone Joint Surg* 52B:738, 1970.

31. Kopell HP, Thompson WAL: *Peripheral entrapment neuropathies*, Malabar, Fla, 1976, RE Krieger.

32. Leach RE: Editorial comment, *Am J Sports Med* 5:193, 1972.

33. Lysens RJ et al: Intermittent claudications in young athletes: popliteal artery entrapment syndrome, *Am J Sports Med* 11:177, 1983.

34. Martens MA, Moeyersoons JP: Acute and recurrent effort-related compartment syndrome in sports, *Sports Med* 9:62, 1990.

35. McDonald PT et al: Popliteal artery entrapment syndrome. Clinical, noninvasive and angiographic diagnosis, *Am J Surg* 139:318, 1980.

36. Mennen U: Letter to the editor, *J Bone Joint Surg* 65A:1030, 1983.

37. Michael RH, Holder LE: The soleus syndrome. A cause of medial tibial stress (shin splints), *Am J Sports Med* 13:87, 1985.

38. Miles S et al: Doppler ultrasound in the diagnosis of the popliteal artery entrapment syndrome, *Br J Surg* 64:883, 1977.

39. Miller WA: Rupture of the musculotendinous juncture of the medial head of the gastrocnemius muscle, *Am J Sports Med* 5:191, 1977.

40. Moller BN, Kadin S: Entrapment of the common peroneal nerve, *Am J Sports Med* 15:90, 1987.

41. Mozan LC, Keagy RD: Muscle relationship in function fascia, *Clin Orthrop* 67:225, 1969.

42. Mozes MM, Ouaknine G, Nathan H: Saphenous nervous entrapment simulating vascular disorder, *Surgery* 77:299, 1975.

43. Mubarak SJ: *Exertional compartment syndromes*. In Mubarak SJ, Hargens AR, editors: *Compartment syndromes and Volkmann's contracture*, Philadelphia, 1981, WB Saunders, p 209.

44. Muburak SJ et al: The medial tibial stress syndrome. A cause of shin splints, *Am J Sports Med* 10:201, 1982.

45. Muller N, Morris DC, Nichols DM: Popliteal artery entrapment demonstrated by CT, *Radiology* 151:157, 1984.

46. O'Donoghue DH: *Injuries of the leg*. In *Treatment of injuries to athletes*, ed 4, Philadelphia, 1984, WB Saunders, p 586.

47. Orava S et al: Diagnosis and treatment of stress fractures located at the mid-tibial shaft in athletes, *Int J Sports Med* 1991.

48. Orava S, Puranen J: Athletes' leg pain, *Br J Sports Med* 13:92, 1979.

49. Pedowitz RA et al: Modified criteria for the objective diagnosis of chronic compartment syndrome of the leg, *Am J Sports Med* 18:35, 1990.

50. Prost WJ: Biomechanics of the foot, *Can Family Phys* 25:827, 1979.

51. Puranen J: The medial tibial syndrome, *Ann Chir Gynaecol* 80:215, 1991.

52. Puranen J: The medial tibial syndrome. Exercise, ischemia in the medial fascial compartment of the leg, *J Bone Joint Surg* 56B:712, 1974.

53. Puranen J, Alavaikko A: Intracompartmental pressure increase on exertion in patients with chronic compartment syndrome in the leg, *J Bone Joint Surg* 63A:1304, 1981.

54. Reneman RS: The anterior and the lateral compartmental syndrome of the leg due to intensive use of muscles, *Clin Orthop* 113:69, 1975.

55. Rettig AC et al: The natural history and treatment of delayed union stress fractures of the anterior cortex of the tibia, *Am J Sports Med* 16:250, 1988.

56. Romanoff ME et al: Saphenous nerve entrapment of the adductor canal, *Am J Sports Med* 17:478, 1989.

57. Rorabeck CH: Exertional tibialis posterior compartment syndrome in athletes, *Clin Orthop* 208:61, 1986.

58. Rorabeck CH, Bourne RB, Fowler PJ: The surgical treatment of exertional compartment syndrome in athletes, *J Bone Joint Surg* 65A:1245, 1983.

59. Rorabeck CH, Fowler PJ, Nott L: The results of fasciotomy in the management of chronic exertional compartment syndrome, *Am J Sports Med* 16:224, 1988.

60. Rudo ND et al: Popliteal artery entrapment syndrome in athletes, *Phys Sports Med* 10:105, 1982.

61. Sarrafian SK: *Anatomy of the foot and ankle: descriptive, topographic, functional*, Philadelphia, 1983, JB Lippincott.

62. Schon LC: Nerve entrapment, neuropathy and nerve dysfunction in athletes, *Orthop Clin North Am* 25:47-59, 1994.

63. Sejersted OM et al: Intramuscular fluid pressure during isometric contraction of human skeletal muscle, *J Appl Physiol* 65:287, 1984.

64. Severance HW, Bassett FH: Rupture of the plantaris—does it exist? *J Bone Joint Surg* 64A:1387, 1982.

65. Snook GA: Intermittent claudication in athletes, *J Sports Med* 3:71, 1975.

66. Styf J, Korner L: Chronic anterior compartment syndrome of the lower leg: results of treatment with fasciotomy, *J Bone Joint Surg* 69A:1338, 1986.

67. Styf JR, Korner LM: Diagnosis of chronic anterior compartment syndrome in the lower leg, *Acta Orthop Scand* 58:139, 1987.

68. Tranier S et al: Value of somatosensory evoked potentials in saphenous entrapment neuropathy, *J Neurol Neurosurg Psychiatry* 55:461, 1992.

69. Turnipseed WD, Pozniak M: Popliteal entrapment as a result of neurovascular compression by the soleus and plantaris muscles, *J Vasc Surg* 15:284, 1992.

70. Viitasalo JT, Kvist M: Some biomechanical aspects of the foot and ankle in athletes with and without shin splints, *Am J Sports Med* 11:125, 1983.

71. Wallensten R: Results of fasciotomy in patients with medial tibial syndrome or chronic anterior compartment syndrome, *J Bone Joint Surg* 65A:1252, 1983.

72. Wallensten R, Eriksson E: Intramuscular pressures in exercise-induced lower leg pain, *Int J Sports Med* 5:31, 1984.

73. Williams LR et al: Popliteal artery entrapment: diagnosis by computed tomography, *J Vasc Surg* 3:360, 1986.

74. Worth RM et al: Saphenous nerve entrapment, *Am J Sports Med* 12:80, 1984.

75. Zigun JR, Schneider SM: "Effort" thrombosis (Paget-Schroetter's syndrome) secondary to martial arts training, *Am J Sports Med* 16:189, 1988.

# Unique Problems in Sports and Dance

# Chapter 20

# Ballet injuries

**Ronald Quirk**

Ballet injuries have much in common with sporting injuries, but they are not identical. The difference is due to the different physical demands placed on dancers and on athletes.

The majority of young dancers are girls, and they begin ballet classes at a young age, typically 5 years. There is much greater emphasis on flexibility in dance than in any sport except perhaps gymnastics. By a process of natural selection, only those who are naturally flexible survive to become professional dancers. Daily exercises increase this natural flexibility, and a dancer who has limited motion in, say, the arch of the foot, may suffer an injury as a result.

Professional dancers and advanced students normally spend 6 or more hours each day in the studio, and their exercises are both forceful and repetitious. This leads to a high incidence of overuse injuries such as tendinitis.

Dance is characterized by outbursts of explosive energy in which the dancer, particularly the male dancer, performs large leaps. There is a technique for taking off and a technique for landing, and poor technique will cause traumatic injuries such as stress fractures, and at the same time may aggravate overuse injuries.

Two particular aspects of ballet deserve mention because they are absolutely fundamental to ballet technique, and they are a potent source of injury.

The first is the practice of rising onto the front part of the foot. Both boys and girls rise onto the ball of the foot (Fig. 20-1); this is called the *demipointe* position (ballet terms are universally in French). Girls also use a special shoe to allow them to rise onto the tips of their toes, a position colloquially called *en pointe* but correctly called *sur les pointes* (Fig. 20-2).

Dancing on the tips of the toes was popularized in the early 1830s by Marie Taglione, the most famous dancer of her day. She has bequeathed to her followers a legacy of beauty, but also of nail problems, bunions, corns, calluses, tendinitis, and stress fractures.

The other aspect of ballet technique that deserves a mention is the turned-out position of the feet (Fig. 20-3). It is impossible to abduct the leg far at the hip with the foot pointing forward, because the greater trochanter of the femur soon comes up against the side of the pelvis and limits movement. External rotation of the femur gets the trochanter out of the way, and allows the high positions so often seen in classical ballet.

Turnout should take place at the hip, and it requires progressive stretching of the hip ligaments over years. Young dancers like to show that they have a good turnout, and in doing this mistakenly they often turn the feet out rather than the hips. This imposes a rotary strain on the lower limb, which leads to "rolling" of the foot into an everted position (Fig. 20-4). This puts a strain on the structures on the medial side of the foot, leading to pain in this area. It also increases the risk of tendinitis, especially of the flexor hallucis longus tendon.

The balance of this chapter deals with some of the more common foot and ankle injuries seen in ballet.

## THE HALLUX
### Nail problems

When standing en pointe, the dancer's weight is largely on the tip of the big toe. Pressure on the nail is transmitted back to the nail bed and as a result the nail may become deformed, thickened, and discolored. Bleeding around the nail, or the occasional loss of the

287

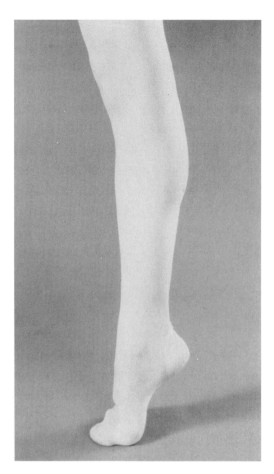

**Fig. 20-1.** Demipointe position, with the weight on the ball of the foot. This position is used by both boys and girls.

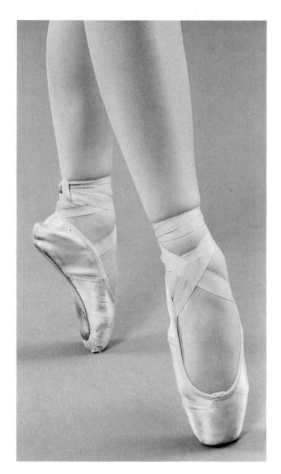

**Fig. 20-2.** A dancer "en pointe" wearing traditional pointe shoes. This technique is usually confined to girls.

nail, is regarded by dancers as part of the day's work. None of these conditions requires any specific treatment.

An ingrown big toenail is another matter, and forcing such a nail into the toe of a pointe shoe produces a level of pain that even dancers are not prepared to tolerate. A wedge resection gives excellent relief.

**Bunions**

The forces on the hallux in ballet are up the axis of the big toe, and in a pointe shoe the toe is supported by the tight toe cap and by the neighboring toes. I do not believe that a normal foot will develop hallux valgus solely as a result of doing ballet.

Dancers who have a natural tendency to hallux valgus, however, seem to deteriorate more rapidly than usual as a result of dancing en pointe, and surgery should not be delayed until a major reconstructive procedure is needed.

When choosing an operation for a dancer with hallux valgus, the usual criteria apply, with the exception that the surgeon must preserve both power

and movement in the big toe. Dancers need a full range of dorsiflexion to allow them to stand in the demipointe position.

The best operation is one that does not directly involve the first metatarsophalangeal joint. The various types of distal metatarsal osteotomy are suitable, and a number of dancers have continued their career following a Mitchell or a chevron operation. Soft tissue procedures should be used with caution because of the risk of joint stiffness. Arthrodesis of the first metatarsophalangeal joint is obviously unsuitable for a dancer, and destructive procedures such as a Keller arthroplasty produce so much weakness and instability of the toe that dancing at a high level becomes impossible.

**Hallux rigidus**

Hallux rigidus is a highly disabling condition for dancers. As stiffness increases, the toe is traumatized by the dancer's efforts to get into the demipointe position; this leads to increasing stiffness. The dancer tries to compensate by "sickling" (adducting) the forefoot; this leads to further problems (Fig. 20-5).

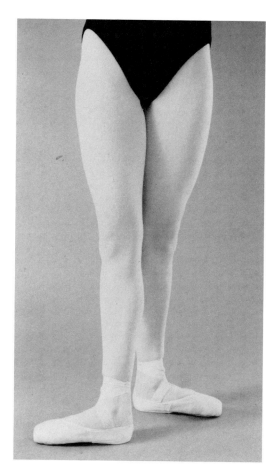

**Fig. 20-3.** Turned-out position of the feet, which is a basic part of ballet technique.

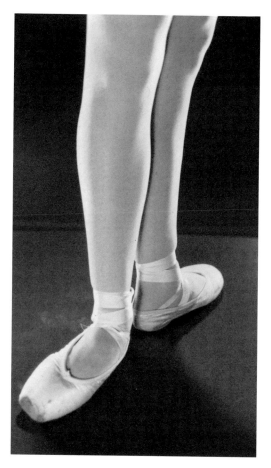

**Fig. 20-4.** Rolling of the foot, which occurs when a dancer with limited turnout at the hips strains to turn the feet out further. This creates a rotary force down the leg and encourages "rolling" into eversion, which can lead to injury.

A cheilectomy (radical excision of osteophytes) has proved to be the best operation for dancers with hallux rigidus and in most cases will give an acceptable result (Fig. 20-6).

Unfortunately the range of movement required in ballet is great, and some patients fail to achieve this range even after a technically successful cheilectomy. In these cases a dorsally based wedge osteotomy of the proximal phalanx may provide just enough additional movement (Fig. 20-7).

Those who are still left with inadequate movement will usually have to give up, because the demipointe position is such a fundamental part of ballet technique and cannot be "faked."

## SESAMOIDITIS
### Anatomy

The sesamoids are two small bones that lie beneath the head of the first metatarsal. Their general structure is similar to that of the patella. The upper surface of each sesamoid is covered with articular cartilage, and the two bones, which appear isolated on x-ray, actually lie within the tendons of the flexor hallucis

brevis and have complex soft tissue attachments (Fig. 20-8).

### Diagnosis

**History.** Dancers who develop pain in the sesamoids often have a poor technique of landing from jumps. Instead of a springy landing with a small plié (knees bent) to decelerate slowly, they come down with an audible thump on the ball of the foot. The pain is felt under one of the sesamoids, usually the medial one.

**Examination.** There is tenderness directly under and around the margins of the sesamoid. When the big toe is dorsiflexed, the sesamoid moves forward because of its soft tissue attachments, and the tenderness moves with it.

**Diagnostic tests.** Fractures of the sesamoids are rare, but recent fractures can be recognized on plain x-ray because of the sharply defined edges of the fragments.

Often a sesamoid (usually the medial one) is

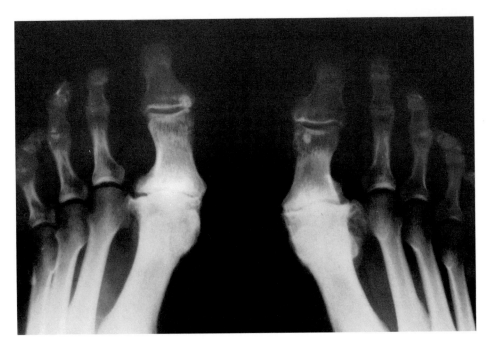

**Fig. 20-5.** X-ray of a male dancer with advanced hallux rigidus.

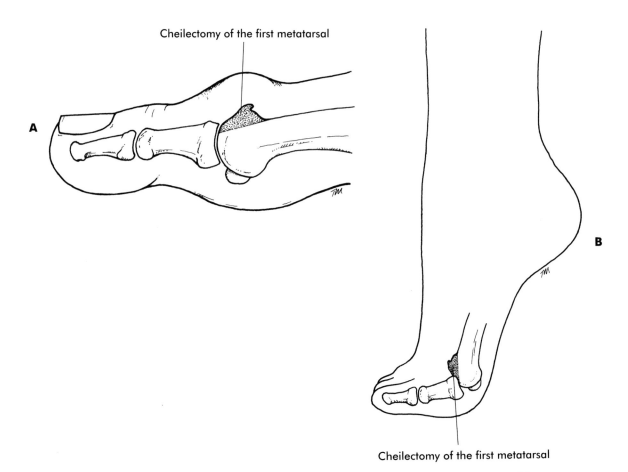

Cheilectomy of the first metatarsal

A

B

Cheilectomy of the first metatarsal

**Fig. 20-6. A,** Cheilectomy operation. The dark area shows the amount of bone excised from the metatarsal head. **B,** Demipointe position.

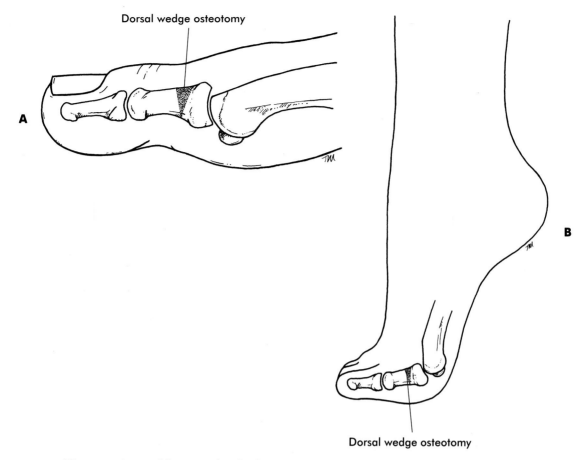

Fig. 20-7. **A,** In addition to the cheilectomy, a dorsal wedge osteotomy of the proximal phalanx may be necessary. The dark area shows the bone to be removed. **B,** Demipointe position.

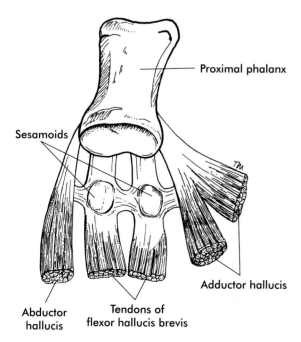

Fig. 20-8. A view of the sesamoids, showing their soft tissue connections.

bipartite, but the rounded bone edges distinguish this from a fresh fracture. A special tangential view of the sesamoids (Fig. 20-9) will demonstrate loss of joint space and marginal osteophytes. Stress fractures of the sesamoids are occasionally seen, and a nuclear bone scan may be necessary to confirm the diagnosis.

### Treatment

**Conservative.** The main treatment is rest. The usual pathology is chondromalacia affecting the articular cartilage of the sesamoid, and this will usually settle when trauma to the bone ceases. Discussion with the dance teacher about correction of technique should help to prevent recurrence. An orthosis can be fitted to the patient's street shoes, but it is not practical to wear an orthosis in a ballet shoe.

**Surgical.** In resistant cases excision of the sesamoid or part of it may be the only way to relieve the pain.

To excise the medial sesamoid:

1. Make a medial incision to avoid the weight-bearing skin. For a lateral sesamoid a plantar incision cannot be avoided.

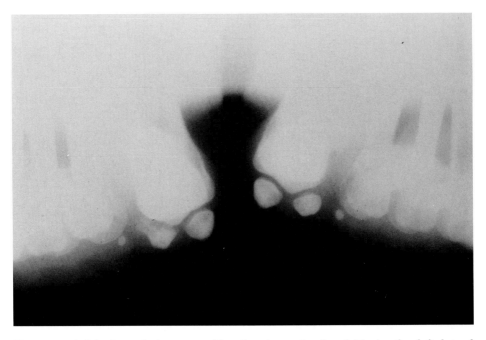

**Fig. 20-9.** Axial view of the sesamoids, showing osteochondritis in the left lateral sesamoid.

2. Deepen the incision and expose the sesamoid without damaging its ligamentous attachments.
3. Partial sesamoidectomy (Fig. 20-10) seems to give as good relief as total sesamoidectomy. Using a power saw, cut horizontally slightly above the middle of the bone, and discard the lower piece. Smooth the remaining bone using nibblers or a powered burr.
4. If circumstances make complete excision desirable (e.g., a symptomatic multipartite patella), cut close to the sesamoid, with care being taken to repair the ligamentous defect left by removal of the bone.

## STRESS FRACTURES
### Pathology

By far the most common stress fracture in dancers occurs in the neck of the second metatarsal (Fig. 20-11). This is because the second metatarsal is always the longest, and in the demipointe position the whole body weight centers on the second metatarsal head. Even dancers who do not have a stress fracture often show marked hypertrophy of the second metatarsal, which can confuse even experienced radiologists (Fig. 20-12).

Stress fractures are also found, in order of frequency, at the base of the second metatarsal; in the other metatarsals, in the lower fibula (Fig. 20-13); and occasionally in the tarsal bones, especially the talus, calcaneum, and navicular.

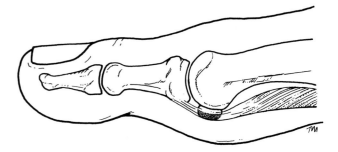

**Fig. 20-10.** Partial excision of a painful sesamoid usually gives adequate relief and does not disturb the soft tissue attachments. The dark area shows the amount of bone to be excised.

### Diagnosis

**History.** Stress fractures typically present as a dull pain that at first comes on toward the end of a period of activity. The pain tends to begin earlier and earlier in the active period and soon is felt in the periods between activity. Finally the pain prevents dancing altogether.

**Examination.** Apart from some localized tenderness, there may be little to see on physical examination. In very late cases a swelling may be felt due to callus at the fracture site, but this is rare in dancers, who tend to present well before this stage is reached.

**Diagnostic tests.** Plain x-rays are often normal and cannot be relied on. A nuclear bone scan is the most useful investigation; if the typical area of increased

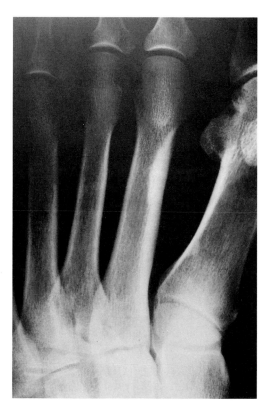

**Fig. 20-11.** Cortical thickening in a stress fracture of the neck of the second metatarsal. Most stress fractures in dancers are diagnosed before anything is seen on plain x-ray.

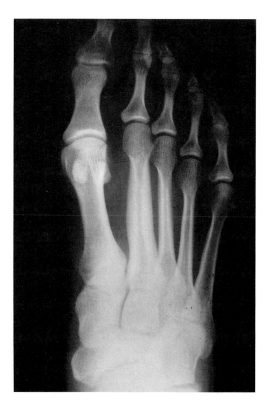

**Fig. 20-12.** Hypertrophy of the second metatarsal in a professional female dancer. This is the normal response to overuse and is not pathological.

uptake is seen, the diagnosis may be made with confidence (Fig. 20-14).

In the case of the navicular, a CT scan is a useful additional test, because it shows the exact appearance of the fracture line.

### Treatment

**Conservative.** Most stress fractures are treated conservatively. In many cases the fracture would heal if the dancer was to simply stop dancing for a few months. Most dancers, however, want the fracture healed in minimal time, and are happy to invest 6 weeks of non–weight bearing on crutches to achieve this. I normally do not put dancers in a cast, because it does not seem to help union and it causes muscle wasting and joint stiffness that must then be corrected when the cast is removed.

Recovery from a stress fracture must be judged on clinical grounds as the bone scan remains "hot" for some time after the fracture heals. Activity must be resumed gradually to prevent recurrence.

**Surgical.** Stress fractures of the navicular, which fortunately are rare in dancers, are unusual in having a strong tendency to nonunion. In cases where conservative treatment fails, bone grafting and the

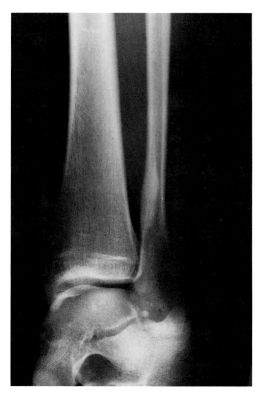

**Fig. 20-13.** Cortical thickening showing the usual site of a stress fracture in the fibula.

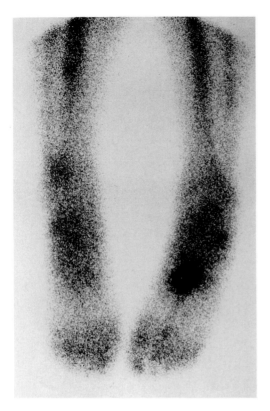

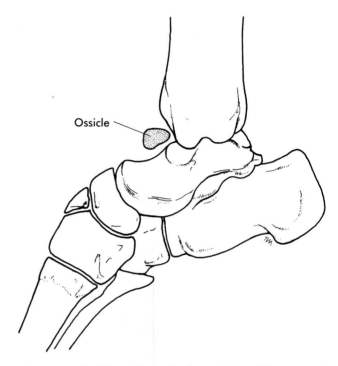

**Fig. 20-15.** Small ossicles at the front of the ankle represent pieces broken off from anterior tibial osteophytes.

**Fig. 20-14.** Typical appearance on nuclear bone scan of a stress fracture of the fibula.

insertion of a compression screw across the fracture line generally causes the fracture to unite.

## ANTERIOR ANKLE OSTEOPHYTES

It is not uncommon in dancers to find a traction osteophyte on the front of the lower tibia, just above the ankle joint, where the capsule attaches to the tibia.

This results from forcible plantar flexion of the foot, which is a part of many ballet movements. The resulting exostosis may then limit dorsiflexion of the ankle and cause it to be painful.

Sometimes the osteophyte may break off, eventually becoming a rounded ossicle lying in front of the ankle joint (Fig. 20-15).

### Diagnosis

The diagnosis should be suggested by pain in the front of the ankle joint on dorsiflexion of the foot. It can be confirmed by plain x-rays.

### Treatment

**Conservative.** Once the condition becomes symptomatic, and fails to improve with rest, conservative treatment is unlikely to help.

**Surgical.** The front of the ankle joint can be evaluated by arthroscopy, and the excess bone removed, together with any inflamed synovial mem-

brane, using arthroscopic instruments. This should produce complete resolution of symptoms.

If the surgeon is not experienced in ankle arthroscopy, it is much better to make a small anterior arthrotomy of the ankle and ensure that the abnormal tissue is completely excised.

## SPRAINED ANKLE

Sprained ankles are probably the most common single injury in ballet. Dancers frequently work at the limits of their strength and adhesion to the floor. A momentary lapse in concentration or a slight loss of balance can lead to an inversion injury, with tearing of the lateral ligament.

### Anatomy

The lateral ligament of the ankle is in three parts: the anterior and posterior talofibular ligaments and the calcaneofibular ligament. The posterior talofibular ligament is relatively unimportant, but complete rupture of either or both of the other ligaments will lead to ankle instability.

### Diagnosis

**History.** Usually there is a clear history of an inversion injury, most often sustained in a turn, a jump, or when overbalancing from the pointe position. The dancer will complain of pain and swelling.

**Examination.** It is difficult to examine a painful swollen ankle adequately. It is, however, important to

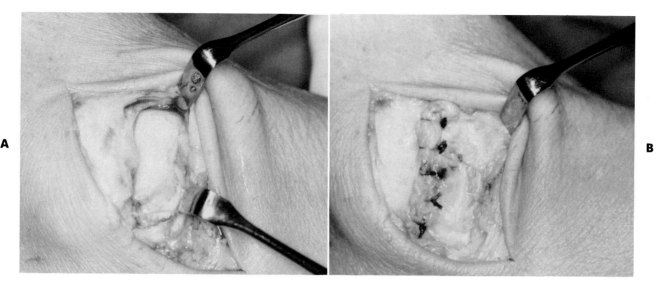

**Fig. 20-16. A,** Complete rupture of the lateral ligament. **B,** Same ankle as shown in **A,** following repair of the lateral ligament.

exclude a complete ligament rupture, because immediate repair of such an injury gives much better results than a late tenodesis following delayed diagnosis.

When examining the ankle, look for an excessive range of inversion, indicating tearing of the calcaneofibular ligament. Observe also for abnormal forward movement of the talus within the ankle mortice (anterior drawer sign). Bear in mind that a completely torn ligament causes less pain when it is stressed than an incompletely torn ligament.

**Diagnostic tests.** If there is any doubt about the integrity of the lateral ligament, an x-ray should be taken with stress views. These should include an anteroposterior view with forced inversion to see if there is tilting of the talus in the ankle mortise. There is usually slight tilting (10 to 15 degrees); if one is unsure whether the degree of tilting is significant, one should perform the same test on the uninjured ankle.

The other important x-ray is a lateral view, in which one hand presses back against the tibia, while the other draws the heel forward. If the talus subluxes forward, there is significant damage to the anterior talofibular ligament.

X-rays must be taken with sufficient force applied to demonstrate the instability. If pain makes this difficult, some surgeons advocate infiltrating the lateral ligament with a local anesthetic before obtaining the x-ray.

An alternative to stress x-rays is an arthrogram of the ankle, with the radiopaque fluid injected under pressure. If there is a complete ligament tear, the contrast medium escapes to give a characteristic appearance.

**Treatment**

**Conservative.** The vast majority of sprained ankles are treated, depending on their severity, with one or more of rest, crutches, a cast, strapping, physiotherapy, antiinflammatory tablets, and steroid injections. Recovery time depends on the severity of the sprain, but it is usually several weeks before the dancer is fit for full activity.

**Surgical.** In cases where there is a complete tear, the choice of surgical treatment depends on how long ago the accident occurred.

If surgery can be performed within several days of the injury, a straightforward repair of the torn ligament is possible using interrupted absorbable sutures (Fig. 20-16). A below-the-knee plaster is applied for 6 weeks and following its removal, intensive rehabilitation is commenced.

If a serious tear is discovered weeks or months after the injury and the patient has instability, then repairing the remains of the ligament is not practical, and a substitute for the ligament must be provided.

The most common operation is a tenodesis, and commonly the peroneus brevis tendon is passed through drill holes in the bones around the ankle to compensate for the torn ligament and to provide stability.

Many methods of tenodesis have been described. One that has been popular for many years is the Watson-Jones tenodesis (Fig. 20-17) in which the tendon of peroneus brevis is detached from its muscle belly and is then passed through drill holes in the lower fibula and the neck of the talus. Finally, it is sutured back onto itself. This replaces the anterior

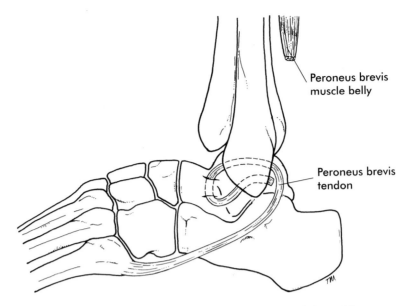

**Fig. 20-17.** Watson-Jones method of tenodesis of the ankle.

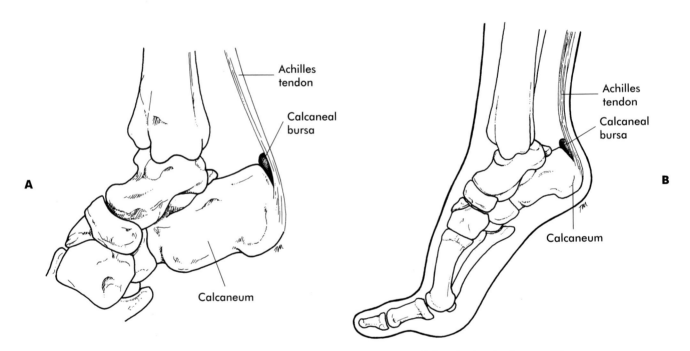

**Fig. 20-18. A,** Anatomy of calcaneal bursa. **B,** Anatomy with foot in demipointe position.

talofibular and calcaneofibular ligaments, although the direction taken by the tendon differs considerably from that of the ligaments it is replacing. Nevertheless, this operation has produced many excellent results, and one of the most famous dancers of the century danced for years following a Watson-Jones tenodesis.

Later modifications of the operation use half of a split peroneus brevis tendon to avoid completely sacrificing the tendon, and the tenodesis is performed so as to more nearly reproduce the direction of the original ligaments.

Following this type of surgery the patient is kept non–weight bearing in a below-the-knee cast for 6 weeks and is then given intensive rehabilitation.

## CALCANEAL BURSITIS

The Achilles tendon is attached to the lower part of the back of the calcaneum. This arrangement gives the tendon maximal leverage when rising onto the ball of the foot or when running. There is thus a small area in which the tendon is intermittently in contact with the bone but is not attached to it. To minimize friction

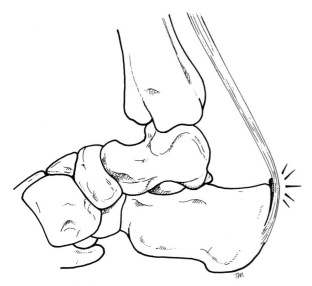

**Fig. 20-19.** Haglund deformity of the posterior part of the calcaneum: plié position.

on the tendon, there is a bursa called a *calcaneal bursa* between the tendon and the bone (Fig. 20-18).

With overuse the bursa may become inflamed, distended, and painful. This is more likely to occur if the posterosuperior angle of the calcaneum is sharp or prominent (Fig. 20-19).

### Diagnosis

**History.** Dancers will often admit to overuse of the ankle in preparation for an audition, examination, or special performance. The main complaint is of pain in the lower part of the Achilles tendon, often with localized swelling.

**Examination.** In severe cases the localized swelling is obvious, and the bursa can easily be felt where it bulges on either side of the Achilles tendon. In less severe cases the upper part of the heel still has a spongy feeling on palpation, in contrast to the firm texture of the unaffected heel.

**Diagnostic tests.** By far the most useful test is ultrasound, which clearly shows the size of the bursa and whether it contains fluid. Plain x-rays are usually not helpful, and arthrography is a painful and invasive procedure that gives no more information than ultrasound.

### Treatment

**Conservative.** Most cases of calcaneal bursitis settle with rest, physical therapy, and antiinflammatory medication. The usual reason for chronic bursitis to develop is that the dancer ignores the pain and continues dancing.

**Surgical.** When conservative treatment fails, excision of the bursa gives reliable relief (Fig. 20-20). I prefer a medial approach with the patient supine and

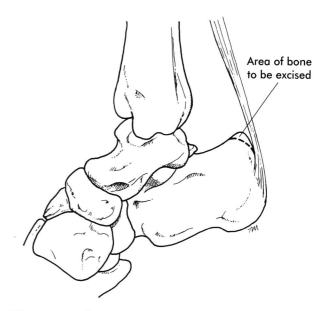

**Fig. 20-20.** Following excision of the bursa, a small amount of bone *(dotted line)* should be excised from the calcaneum.

a large sandbag under the opposite buttock, although many surgeons use a lateral approach with the patient placed in the lateral position.

1. Through a short vertical incision, identify the calcaneum and the Achilles tendon.
2. Find the bursa in the interval between the tendon and bone and excise it completely.
3. Check the lower Achilles tendon, which may be chronically inflamed. It may be necessary to extend the incision upward to deal with adhesions between the paratenon and the tendon.
4. Using bone nibblers or an osteotome, round off the posterosuperior angle of the calcaneum. The large-scale removal of bone described in some older textbooks is not necessary.
5. The patient should be kept non–weight bearing on crutches for 10 days and should be able to return to limited ballet activity in about 4 weeks.

### POSTERIOR IMPINGEMENT SYNDROME OF THE ANKLE

Posterior impingement syndrome of the ankle was first recognized in dancers but has since been found commonly in athletes, especially those who jump or who play football.

The pain is felt at the back of the ankle when the toe is pointed. It is due to a piece of bone that occupies space behind the ankle, leading to compression of the soft tissues.

The posterior tubercle of the talus varies greatly in size. It arises from a separate ossific center, and in about 10% of cases it fails to fuse with the main bone. It is then called an *os trigonum* (Fig. 20-21). The fact

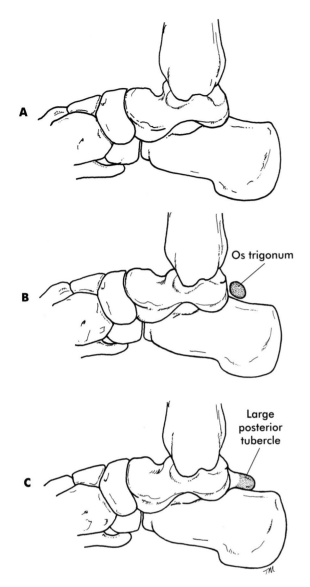

A, Some ankles show no bony protrusion at the back of the talus.

Os trigonum

B

Large posterior tubercle

C

**Fig. 20-21. A,** Some ankles show no bony protrusion at the back of the talus. **B,** Some ankles (between 7% and 11%) show an os trigonum. **C,** Some ankles show a large posterior tubercle.

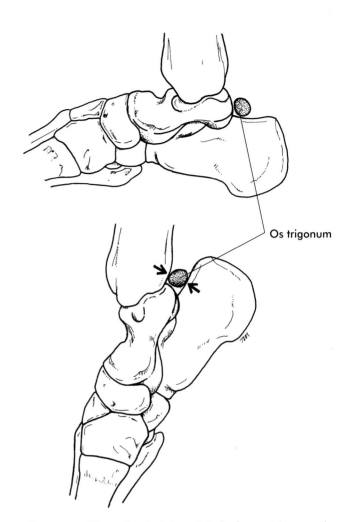

Os trigonum

Os trigonum

**Fig. 20-22.** When the foot is pointed, the os trigonum is jammed between the lower tibia and the upper calcaneum.

that it is unfused is not the source of the pain, however. It is the crowding of the soft tissues that causes the problem.

When the foot is pointed, the lower tibia and the upper calcaneum come together, so that a large posterior tubercle or an os trigonum is caught like a nut in a nutcracker and the surrounding tissues may be severely traumatized (Fig. 20-22).

## Diagnosis

**History.** The dancer will usually complain of heel pain during activity. She may have noticed that the pain is related to pointing the foot.

**Examination.** There may be tenderness deep behind the ankle joint, but the main diagnostic test is for the doctor to *passively* plantar flex the dancer's foot. If this produces pain, an impingement syndrome is probable. If the injection of a little local anesthetic into the back of the ankle joint abolishes the pain, the diagnosis is confirmed.

**Diagnostic tests.** A lateral x-ray with the foot in full plantar flexion is often performed (Fig. 20-23 and 20-24); it shows the size and position of the bone but cannot add much to the clinical findings. A nuclear bone scan usually shows an area of increased uptake just behind the talus.

## Treatment

**Conservative.** In many cases rest, physical therapy, and antiinflammatory medications are effective. Local steroid injections are also sometimes indicated.

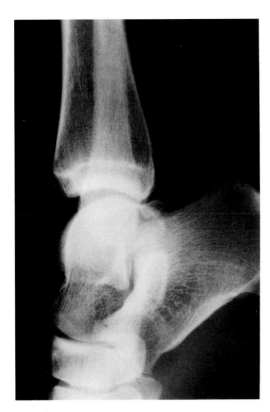

**Fig. 20-23.** X-ray of a patient with a symptomatic os trigonum, which required surgical removal.

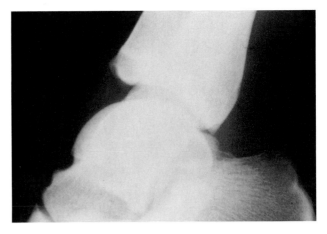

**Fig. 20-24.** X-ray of a patient with a large symptomatic posterior process, which required surgical removal.

**Surgical.** In those cases where the pain does not settle despite conservative treatment, the bony prominence must be removed. I prefer to use a medial approach, because I can visualize and protect the neurovascular bundle and can also inspect the flexor hallucis longus tendon.

1. The patient should be supine with a large sandbag under the opposite hip.
2. Make a curved vertical incision midway between the medial malleolus and the Achilles tendon.
3. Divide the deep fascia and dissect out the neurovascular bundle. Protect the nerve, which is posterior to the vessels, and is similar in color to the surrounding fat. Retract the nerve and vessels forward.
4. Find the flexor hallucis longus just deep to the neurovascular bundle. Divide its sheath and inspect the tendon. If it is inflamed or partly torn, extend the division of the sheath as far as practical. Retract the tendon forward with the nerve and vessels.
5. Open the capsule of the ankle joint. The posterior tubercle or os trigonum can now be easily seen and excised (Fig. 20-25).

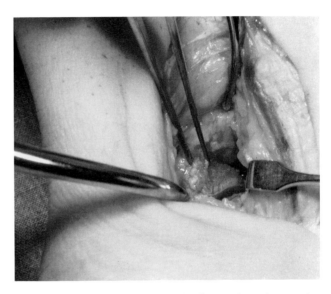

**Fig. 20-25.** Stage in the removal of an enlarged posterior tubercle.

6. Close the wound in layers and apply a compression dressing.
7. Have the patient non–weight bearing on crutches for 10 days and then mobilize the ankle with the help of a physical therapist.

Classes can be resumed 4 to 6 weeks postoperatively.

## TENDINITIS

Because of the repetitive nature of ballet, inflammation of the tendons and tendon sheaths is common especially around the ankle. Ask any professional dancer to circumduct the foot, and you will probably hear a good deal of crepitus due to tendinitis.

Any of the tendons around the ankle can be

affected, but the flexor hallucis longus tendon gives the greatest trouble in dancers. This contrasts with athletes, where the Achilles tendon causes most of the problems.

## FLEXOR HALLUCIS LONGUS TENDON

The flexor hallucis longus tendon is on the medial side of the ankle. It has a long powerful muscle belly, and the tendon passes through a fibrous sheath at the point where it changes direction behind and below the medial malleolus.

Quite commonly, following prolonged overuse, a nodule develops on the tendon, and this may then cause clicking as it enters and leaves the fibrous tunnel, in much the same way as a trigger finger. Ultimately the nodule may reach a size where the big toe begins to trigger, and the dancer may find that the toe sticks in the plantar-flexed position, so that she has to push it back with her fingers.

### Diagnosis

**History.** The dancer complains of pain and sometimes clicking or crepitus on the medial side of the ankle. This is felt particularly when rising en pointe. There may be triggering of the toe.

**Examination.** Hold the dancer's foot firmly so that the ankle is immobilized and then ask her to move the big toe. Feel behind the medial malleolus for crepitus and for a nodule that moves with the tendon (Fig. 20-26).

**Diagnostic tests.** The diagnosis is mainly a clinical one, but ultrasound may show the presence of a nodule.

### Treatment

**Conservative.** Physical therapy and antiinflammatory medication may help. It is difficult to ask the dancer to rest the tendon, because it is involved in some of the most basic movements in ballet. This is why a number of these patients come to operation.

**Surgical.** The approach to the tendon and its sheath is exactly as described in the section, Posterior Impingement Syndrome of the Ankle (Fig. 20-27).

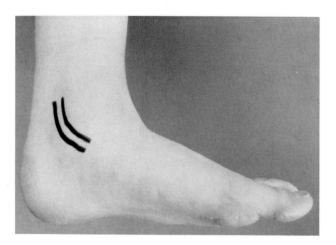

**Fig. 20-26.** Lines show where a nodule on the flexor hallucis longus tendon is felt.

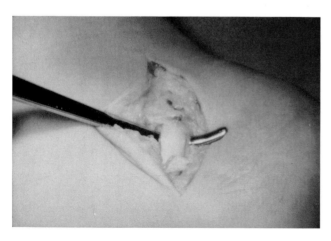

**Fig. 20-27.** This girl had a fusiform swelling on the flexor hallucis longus tendon and as a result experienced triggering of the big toe.

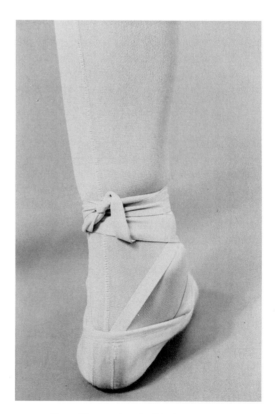

**Fig. 20-28.** The ribbons that hold the pointe shoe on can aggravate an Achilles tendon problem if they are tied too tightly.

Divide the sheath as far distally as possible to ensure free movement of the damaged tendon.

## THE ACHILLES TENDON

The Achilles tendon becomes inflamed in the same way and for the same reasons in dancers as it does in athletes.

An additional problem in dancers is that the ballet shoe is held on by ribbons that tie at the back of the ankle directly over the Achilles tendon. Some dancers, to ensure that their shoes will not fall off, tie their ribbons too tightly, and thus aggravate the damage that has resulted from overuse (Fig. 20-28).

### Diagnosis

**History.** The dancer will complain of pain over the Achilles tendon following activity. There may also be crepitus.

**Examination.** The tendons should be examined with the patient prone. Often the tissues surrounding the tendon are thickened and irregular. There may be crepitus on movement. Sometimes a tender nodule can be felt which moves with the tendon.

**Diagnostic tests.** Ultrasound is helpful in demonstrating the swelling of the tendon, inflammation of surrounding structures, and partial or complete tearing of the tendon.

### Treatment

**Conservative.** This is exactly the same as described for the flexor hallucis longus tendon.

**Surgical.** I prefer a posteromedial approach, with the patient supine and a large sandbag under the opposite hip.

1. Make a vertical 4-in. incision, extending upward from the upper border of the calcaneum.
2. Split the paratenon vertically and peel it off the tendon, dividing adhesions as you go. Be sure to take the division of the paratenon to the upper limit of the tendon.
3. Remove any obviously inflamed tissue and clean up the tendon. Check the calcaneal bursa, and if it is obviously inflamed, remove it.
4. Close the wound in layers and apply a compression dressing.
5. Keep the patient non–weight bearing on crutches for 10 days. Then allow mobilization of the ankle with the help of a physical therapist. Classes can be resumed 4 to 6 weeks postoperatively.

## SHINSPLINTS

Although shinsplints is strictly a condition involving the lower leg, its effects are felt as far down as the ankle, and it will often come to the attention of the foot and ankle surgeon.

*Shinsplints* is a lay term that covers any pain in the shin. The most common cause is fasciitis in the region of the tibia. Two less common but important conditions that cause similar pain are anterior compartment syndrome and stress fracture of the tibia.

Compartment syndromes arise because certain muscle groups (Fig. 20-29) are enclosed in a fascial envelope that cannot stretch. The anterior tibial muscles are a good example. With exercise, the increased blood flow causes the muscle to swell. In a few individuals the confined muscle cannot swell sufficiently and ischemic pain results.

### Diagnosis

**History.** Painful shins are common in ballet. The usual complaint is of pain and tenderness in the tissues adjacent to the subcutaneous surface of the tibia, especially near its anterior border. The pain is felt mainly on activity, but in severe cases it is felt between classes also.

**Examination.** The leg usually looks normal, and swelling is not a feature. The only physical sign in most cases is tenderness down one or other border of the subcutaneous surface of the tibia.

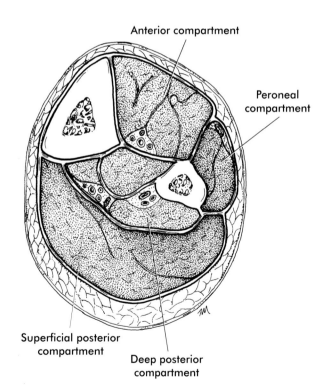

Anterior compartment

Peroneal compartment

Superficial posterior compartment

Deep posterior compartment

**Fig. 20-29.** The four compartments of the lower leg: (1) anterior compartment, (2) peroneal compartment, (3) superficial posterior compartment, and (4) deep posterior compartment.

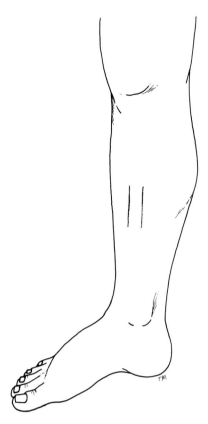

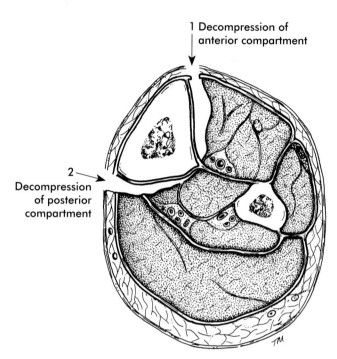

**Fig. 20-31.** Illustration of how (1) the anterior compartment and (2) the posterior compartment are decompressed. Note that the deep posterior compartment has also been decompressed.

**Fig. 20-30.** Decompression of the anterior compartment is done through a short incision parallel to the anterior border of the tibia. The posterior compartment is reached through an incision parallel to the medial border of the tibia.

**Diagnostic tests.** In severe cases where conservative treatment is not helping, it is advisable to order a nuclear bone scan and to perform compartment pressure studies.

A nuclear bone scan will show a stress fracture of the tibia as a localized area of intense uptake. The more common fasciitis often shows on a bone scan as a faint line of increased uptake close to the anterior border of the tibia.

Compartment pressure studies are performed by inserting a needle into the anterior tibial muscles and connecting this to a water manometer. The leg is then exercised. Normally there is a moderate rise in compartment pressure followed by a fairly rapid fall when exercise ceases. In a compartment syndrome the pressure rises several times higher and takes much longer to fall.

**Treatment**

**Conservative.** Dancers with fasciitis often recover spontaneously and need no special treatment. In more resistant cases, rest, physical therapy, and antiinflammatory medication may help.

Stress fractures must be treated by rest, as described in the section, Stress Fractures.

Compartment syndrome responds to rest and the other previously mentioned measures but may recur when other activity is resumed.

**Surgical.** Patients with fasciitis seldom need surgery. In those rare cases who do, the operation is exactly as described for compartment syndrome.

Patients with a stress fracture of the tibia might occasionally progress to a complete fracture and then need some form of internal fixation. Apart from this, stress fractures of the tibia are always treated conservatively.

To decompress the anterior compartment of the leg, the steps are as follows:

1. Make a 2-in. vertical skin incision parallel with the anterior border of the tibia, halfway between the knee and ankle (Fig. 20-30).
2. Incise the deep fascia of the muscle vertically a few millimeters from the bone.
3. Using a long fine scissors, make a blind cut in the fascia extending up almost to the knee and down almost to the ankle (Fig. 20-31).
4. Close the wound and apply a pressure dressing.
5. Restrict walking for 10 to 14 days and then allow increasing activity. Recovery is usually rapid following this type of surgery.

6. The superficial and deep posterior compartments and the peroneal compartments can be decompressed in a similar way.

**Case Study 1.** A well-known ballerina, at the height of her career, developed a click in the medial side of her ankle. This persisted and became painful. Finally she developed "triggering" of the big toe. She could point the toe but had to straighten it by pushing it up with her fingers.

She was found to have a nodule on her flexor hallucis longus tendon, and this was jamming in the fibrous flexor sheath behind the medial malleolus.

Following surgical division of the tendon sheath, the click disappeared, and she was able to dance normally.

**Case Study 2.** A young student was allowed to start dancing en pointe regularly at the age of 8 years, instead of at the usual age of 11 to 12 years.

This resulted in premature fusion of the epiphysis of the proximal phalanx of one of her big toes, leading to marked shortening.

As a result she was unable to dance properly in a pointe shoe. She continued to dance in a limited way but was unable to fulfill her ambition to be a professional classical ballet dancer.

Ballet teachers currently are better informed, and cases like this are becoming rare.

**Case Study 3.** A professional company with a good injury record suddenly found a number of their dancers experiencing stress fractures of the feet. The only recent change in the company's routine had been the use of a different practice studio. It was found that the wooden floor of the new studio had been laid directly on a concrete slab and lacked resilience. A properly sprung modular floor was laid on top of the existing floor, and the rate of occurrence of stress fractures immediately fell to normal.

The company now takes the modular floor with it when touring to centers where the dancers will have to use a floor not designed for ballet. The overall rate of injury has dropped considerably as a result.

**Case Study 4.** A male dancer who was practicing hard for an important performance developed severe pain under the sesamoids of both feet. This made it almost impossible for him to rehearse.

He was sent for a medical opinion and fortunately the doctor called the boy's teacher. Apparently the pain was due to his method of landing from jumps, in which he took most of the shock of impact on the forefoot. He should have been using the forefoot, then the heel, and then the knees to slow his descent progressively.

Under strict supervision by his teacher, he continued rehearsals but at first omitted jumping altogether. When the pain had settled, he reintroduced jumps but with strict attention to correct technique.

He got through the performance almost without pain. He needed no medical treatment at all, because the doctor had been enterprising enough to contact his teacher.

## SUGGESTED READING

Fricker PA, Williams JGP: Surgical management of os trigonum and talar spur in sportsmen. *Br J Sports Med* 13:55-57, 1979.

Howse AJG, Hancock S: *Dance technique and injury prevention*, London, 1988, A & C Black.

Quirk R: Talar compression syndrome in dancers. *Foot Ankle* 3:65-68, 1982.

Ryan AJ, Stephens RE, eds: *Dance medicine*, Chicago, 1987, Pluribus.

Sammarco J: In Jahss M, ed. *Disorders of the foot*, Philadelphia, 1982:1626-1659, WB Saunders.

Sarraffian SK: *Anatomy of the foot and ankle*, Philadelphia, 1983, JB Lippincott.

# Chapter 21

# Overuse syndromes of the running athlete

**Roy S. Benedetti**

## EVALUATION

Evaluation of the running athlete can require a significant amount of time and effort. The patient typically has a variety of complaints with numerous concerns and theories as to their etiology. This group of patients is extremely concerned about their condition and often intolerant of treatments that will impair their ability to compete or exercise. For these reasons, the treating physician must have a preplanned systematic approach for these patients. The following provides a guideline for acquiring the necessary information required to make a diagnosis and for subsequent treatment planning.

### History

Many physicians who treat runners routinely provide a well-organized and thorough questionnaire from which a majority of the pertinent history can be obtained in a time-efficient manner. The questionnaire also allows patients to organize their thoughts before being examined. Since patients commonly have a variety of complaints, it is helpful to have them list their symptoms in order of severity. A description of each symptom is then obtained and should include whether it occurs before, after, or during activity. Other important information includes associated symptoms such as swelling, popping, or radiating pain and whether any factors, such as running up or down hills, that affect their symptoms.

All prior treatments should be elicited including all medications used, the number and location of injections, as well as previous surgical procedures. Any changes in symptoms as a result of these treatment modalities should be documented.

With over 60% of injuries in the running athlete occurring secondary to errors in training, it is imperative that the patient's training history be carefully evaluated.[7] This should include the type of stretching performed, if any, before and after exercise, as well as the amount and type of exercise performed including the number of miles run per week. The type of surface, as well as the geography of the patient's running courses, is important information. Any recent changes in the type or amount of training should be documented. Runners—especially the amateur athlete—commonly attempt to increase running mileage too rapidly in preparation for an upcoming event. This can lead to a sudden onset of symptoms.

The type of shoe wear used can be helpful since each shoe has different characteristics with respect to hindfoot alignment, the amount of cushioning, sole rigidity, forefoot space, etc. It is helpful to be able to inspect the patient's running shoes and orthoses so that any evidence of abnormal wear can be noted. Patients should be asked whether they rotate their shoes as well as the amount of mileage allowed before obtaining new shoes. The type of orthotic devices used should be examined and the effect of their use determined.

Information with respect to the runner's diet should be obtained. Particular references are made to adequate caloric, mineral, and vitamin intake as well as adequate hydration during exercise. Dehydration may lead to a variety of symptoms such as muscle cramps and fatigue secondary to electrolyte disorders and hypovolemia.

## Physical examination

Since many abnormalities may be subtle, a thorough physical examination of the spine and lower extremities should be performed with the patient sitting, standing, supine, and prone. Particular attention is given to the presence of any asymmetries in the examination, since these differences can often aid in the determination of the underlying causative factors.

In the standing position the spinal alignment can be assessed. This includes any evidence of scoliosis or increased lumbar lordosis. Leg lengths can be assessed by evaluating relative iliac wing height. It is important to have the patient bend forward and touch the floor to test for hamstring or Achilles tightness. Lower-extremity alignment is assessed by observing the direction of the patellae and the feet. Inward rotation of the patellae may suggest increased femoral anteversion. Evidence of intoeing with a neutral patella suggests internal tibial torsion. Angular alignment (varus/valgus) of the knee should also be observed. The hindfoot position (varus/valgus) while standing should be carefully examined, and the function of the subtalar joint assessed by observing its motion during toe standing. The hindfoot should move into varus as the patient stands up on the toes. The midfoot and forefoot alignment is examined by assessing the longitudinal arch. The presence of hammertoes and claw toes is also noted. Sometimes it is helpful to observe the patient walking or, if necessary, running to better appreciate the dynamics involved in that patient's running style.

In a sitting position, hamstring tightness and evidence of sciatica can be appreciated. The rotational range of motion of the hip can be measured. A thorough examination of patellar tracking can be performed by actively extending the knee. Tibial torsion can be more accurately assessed by measuring the malleolar axis in the sitting position with the patella facing forward. Ankle and subtalar joint motion is documented. The alignment of the forefoot is noted with the hindfoot held in the neutral position. The amount of midfoot mobility is assessed with particular attention given to the first metatarsocuneiform joint. The range of motion of the metatarsophalangeal joints, particularly the first metatarsophalangeal joint, is documented as is the presence and location of callosities and areas of tenderness and swelling. Toe deformities are observed and attention given to whether the deformity is static or dynamic.

The supine position allows additional examination for signs of sciatica and allows completion of the measurement of hip range of motion. A thorough examination of the knee is best performed in this position. Ankle and subtalar motion is assessed again with the knee extended.

In the prone position with the knee flexed at 90 degrees, an accurate assessment of subtalar motion can be obtained. Normal subtalar motion is 25 to 30 degrees of inversion and 10 degrees of eversion with the hindfoot in neutral position.[16] The hip rotational range of motion can be compared with that previously obtained in the sitting opposition.

## Diagnostic studies

Once a complete history and physical examination have been obtained, one or several diagnostic studies may be indicated to provide additional information necessary to determine a diagnosis.

Initial studies should be routine x-rays of the involved area. They generally will rule out disorders such as osteoarthritis, infection, tumors, fractures, and bony avulsions. The presence of extra ossicles such as an accessory navicular or an os trigonum will be evident with routine x-rays and may explain the patient's symptoms. Stress fractures, if over 3 to 4 weeks old, may be seen with routine x-rays by visualizing periosteal reaction or callus formation. Weight-bearing views of the foot add additional information about the alignment of the foot under a static load.

Stress views may be indicated if the patient has evidence of ligamentous instability. The two most common indications for stress views are suspected instability of the lateral ankle or Lisfranc joint. The competency of the lateral ligaments of the ankle can be objectively evaluated by obtaining two views: an anteroposterior view of the ankle with varus stress and a lateral view with anterior stress. In the patient with suspected Lisfranc joint strain or instability, stress views may reveal instability not appreciated with routine or weight-bearing x-rays. Obtaining an anteroposterior and an oblique view of the foot while applying abduction stress at Lisfranc's joint may reveal instability at one or more of the metatarsal tarsal joints. These injuries can be difficult to treat, but with early diagnosis and early treatment, chronic symptoms and the necessity for surgical arthrodesis may be avoided. Stress views to assess subtalar instability have been less informative, and the diagnosis of this entity may have to be obtained by the exclusion of other disorders.

In those cases where difficulty is encountered in obtaining a diagnosis, a bone scan can sometimes provide additional information. The bone scan is highly sensitive for stress fractures and is helpful in their early diagnosis before x-ray changes. Since a bone scan is sensitive but nonspecific, a normal bone

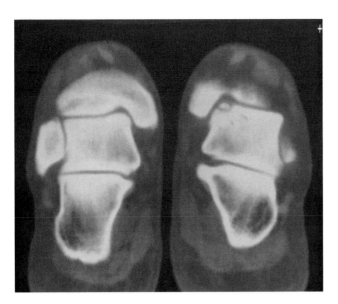

**Fig. 21-1.** CT scan illustrating an osteochondral lesion of the medial talar dome. The subtalar joint is also well visualized.

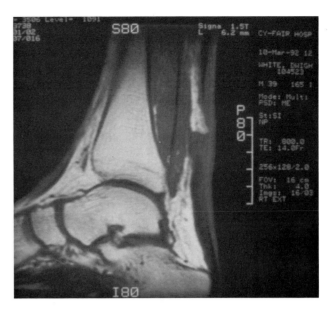

**Fig. 21-2.** Sagittal MRI scan of the ankle revealing a complete Achilles tendon rupture. The Achilles tendon is the black structure at the posterior aspect of this section. The disrupted section of tendon is interposed with fat that appears white on this T1-weighted image.

scan can rule out numerous entities such as stress fractures, infections, tumors, and significant inflammatory processes.

The CT scan provides useful information in the assessment of the ankle, subtalar joint, and small joints of the midfoot and forefoot. Degenerative changes are easily visualized by the presence of osteophytes and/or intraosseous cysts involving these joints. Osteochondral lesions of the talus are well visualized and the CT scan can be used to determine the precise location and size of the lesion, which can be useful in preoperative planning (Fig. 21-1).

Magnetic resonance imaging (MRI) has become a highly useful diagnostic tool in the assessment of disorders within bone, cartilage, tendons, ligaments, muscles, and fat.[9] By careful analysis of T1- and T2-weighted images, a great deal of information can be obtained. The T1-weighted images enhance the tissues with high fat content, such as bone marrow, and can aid in the diagnosis of occult fractures and avascular necrosis. The T2-weighted images enhance tissues with high water content, such as joint effusions and fluid within tendon sheaths. MRI allows assessment of articular cartilage and identifies the presence of soft tissue masses. Tendons are well visualized, and by using T1- and T2-weighted images, intrasubstance degenerative tears as well as complete ruptures can be visualized (Fig. 21-2). Unfortunately MRI is a costly diagnostic tool and should be used only if it will provide information necessary to establish a specific treatment regimen. Often in treating the running athlete, a specific diagnosis will not alter the early treatment. In this situation, it may

be prudent to obtain the MRI scan only if the patient's symptoms persist and a precise diagnosis becomes necessary.

### Primary versus secondary disorders

Once all the necessary information has been obtained, a determination of primary versus secondary disorders must be made. A secondary disorder results as a consequence of a primary disorder. Therefore by correcting a primary disorder, one would expect concomitant resolution of the secondary disorder (see Case Study 1). One example is a runner with hyperpronation of the hindfoot who develops medial knee pain secondary to repetitive strain of the medial collateral ligament of the knee from the hyperpronation placing increased valgus stress on the knee during impact. Hyperpronators also may develop some symptoms of lateral patellar subluxation secondary to the valgus stress placed on the knee.[7] In these situations correction of the hindfoot pronation with longitudinal arch supports or medial sole and heel wedges will resolve the secondary knee symptoms. Another example is a runner who presents with recurrent second metatarsal pain and is diagnosed with a stress fracture of the metatarsal. During the physical examination, it is noted that the patient has only 10 degrees of dorsiflexion at the ankle on the injured side as compared with 30 degrees on the unaffected side. An x-ray reveals a large anterior tibial osteophyte which is limiting dorsiflexion. Upon removing this osteophyte, the involved ankle achieves

30 degrees of dorsiflexion and the patient returns to full activities without a recurrence of the second metatarsal symptoms. In this situation the limitation of ankle dorsiflexion was a primary disorder and led to increased stress at the second metatarsal, with a resultant stress fracture.

These are only two examples of how the determination of primary and secondary disorders is imperative to the treatment of the running athlete. Throughout this chapter an emphasis is placed on the determination of primary disorders and developing an understanding of the secondary disorders that may result.

**Case Study 1.** A 25-year-old male presented with insidious onset of right leg pain. He stated that the pain had increased over the past 2 to 3 months such that he now had symptoms even with walking. He ran competitively in high school until he fractured his right tibia in a motorcycle accident. Since that time he ran approximately 20 to 30 miles per week on the streets surrounding his neighborhood. He had one episode of right leg pain several years ago, but this resolved with a decrease in his weekly mileage.

On physical examination the patient had a leg length discrepancy, with the right lower extremity being 2 cm shorter than the left. The patient also had a noticeable varus deformity of the right tibia and point tenderness at the middle third of the tibia. The x-rays of his right tibia (Fig. 21-3) revealed a healed proximal third tibia/fibula fracture that united in a shortened varus position. The middle third of the tibia has abundant callus at the lateral tibia, which suggested a long-standing stress fracture and corresponded to his area of tenderness.

The primary disorder, in this case, was a tibial malunion that caused increased stresses to be placed on the tibia from the varus angulation as well as the anatomic short-leg syndrome. The secondary disorder was the tibial stress fracture.

This patient was advised to decrease his activities to nonimpact activities until all symptoms resolved. At that time he was allowed to run using a 1-cm lift in his right shoe. His symptoms improved, and he has been able to run 30 miles per week without recurrence of leg symptoms.

## TORSIONAL JOINT INJURIES

Running involves a complex series of linear and rotational movements of the spine and lower extremities. A limitation in the range of motion at one segment will thereby cause increased demands on the adjacent structures. Runners commonly have stretching routines that include linear stretching of the hamstrings, quadriceps, and gastrocnemius muscles while neglecting rotational stretching of the spine and hips. Runners should perform both linear and rotational stretching to maintain full range of motion and to prevent torsional joint injuries.

A 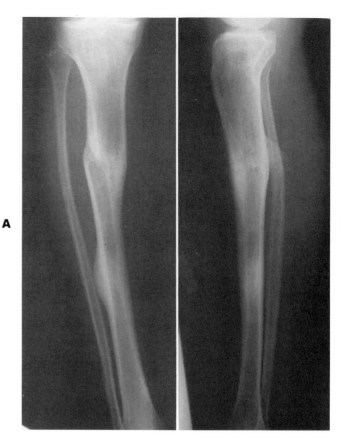 B

**Fig. 21-3.** AP and lateral radiographs of the tibia and fibula. A previous tibia/fibula fracture has healed with some shortening and varus angulation. More distally, lateral callus of the tibia indicates healing of a tibial stress fracture that has resulted from the abnormal stresses placed on the tibia secondary to the more proximal tibial malunion.

During the stance phase of running, the ipsilateral hip internally rotates, allowing the contralateral leg to advance. A limitation of internal rotation of the hip, whether secondary to external rotation contracture or femoral retroversion, will cause increased torque at the ipsilateral knee and ankle, which may lead to secondary disorders at these adjacent sites.

Treatment should consist of the patient running with the involved leg more externally rotated. This will lessen the amount of internal rotation required at the hip and lessen the torque demands on the adjacent knee and ankle. If the limitation of motion is secondary to an external rotation contracture of the hip, an aggressive regimen of internal rotation stretching exercises should be initiated. As the internal rotation of the hip increases with stretching, the runner can resume running with a normal stride. Patients with limited external rotation of the lower extremities secondary to internal rotation contracture of the hip, increased femoral anteversion, or internal tibial torsion rarely develop problems.

## SURFACE INJURIES

Surface injuries occur secondary to two factors: increased traction and/or decreased shock absorption. Recreational runners commonly run on cement or gravel surfaces, which have decreased shock absorption and increased traction as compared with surfaces such as grass or cinder. Competitive runners commonly train and compete on synthetic surfaces that allow more efficient transmission of forces between the foot and the running surface by eliminating the skid phase of gait. Certainly the use of these surfaces has led to Olympic records that would be unachievable on "less efficient" surfaces. Unfortunately the tremendous traction achieved, as well as the increase in impact loads from decreased shock absorption, has led to a multitude of injuries for the running athlete.

Increased traction causes increased shear and torsional stresses on the lower extremities since the foot has limited ability to "slide" during the stance phase. Minimal limitations of motion, which may not have been significant on a cinder surface, may lead to increased demands on adjacent joints with resultant symptoms. Increased traction may also lead to increased risk of blister formation secondary to high shear forces at the skin surface.

Increased impact forces that occur secondary to less shock absorption can lead to disorders of the spine, hips, knees, ankles, and feet. Repetitive impact forces can lead to stress fractures as well as intraarticular pathology.

Treatment for these disorders consists of training and shoe modifications. The runner should make an effort to train on a more "friendly" surface such as grass or dirt whenever possible and to limit running on synthetic or cement surfaces to periodic training sessions and competitions. The athlete also can use a more cushioned shoe during training to lessen the impact loads further.

## SHORT-LEG SYNDROME

A short-leg syndrome may result from either an anatomic or functional disorder. An anatomic short-leg syndrome results from an actual leg length discrepancy secondary to a short femur or tibia or from pelvic obliquity. This entity should be evident during the physical examination. A functional short-leg syndrome results from increased stresses placed on one extremity during training. This occurs when a runner runs in one direction on a circular track or on an incline with the same leg downhill. In both instances one leg is subjected to constant increased stresses. The outer leg on a circular track and the down leg on a lateral incline will experience higher stresses than the opposite leg.

The short-leg syndrome may present with one of many disorders. The shorter leg may present with stress fractures from the increased loads. The knee of the shorter leg experiences valgus stresses and may develop either medial knee pain from the strain of the medial structures or lateral knee pain from increased impact loads on the lateral aspect of the knee. The foot of the shorter leg commonly undergoes increased pronation during stance, which may lead to iliotibial band tendinitis at the lateral knee, medial tibial stress syndrome, tarsal tunnel syndrome, or plantar fasciitis. The longer leg, on the other hand, may present with iliotibial band tendinitis at the hip or knee from repetitive adduction of the hip and varus strain of the knee. Back pain may also occur as part of a short-leg syndrome.

Treatment of the anatomic short-leg syndrome is to add a shoe lift to the shorter extremity. Shoe lifts should be added in small increments such as 0.5 cm until symptoms resolve. Often it is unnecessary to fully correct the leg length discrepancy. If more than 1 to 1.5 cm of lift is required, the lift often must be incorporated into the midsole of the shoe to prevent significant alteration in the fit of the shoe.

The functional short-leg syndrome is treated by alteration of running habits. If using a circular course, the runner should alternate directions so that one leg is no longer constantly receiving increased stresses. If the runner runs on a lateral incline, as is often the case when running along the side of the road, the runner should run equal time against and with traffic. This will prevent one extremity from constantly being downhill and subjected to higher stresses.

## STRESS FRACTURES

Repetitive impact loads experienced during running cause ongoing microdamage of bone. If the body's normal reparative mechanisms cannot keep pace with the microdamage, a stress fracture may occur. Therefore conditions that increase the rate of microdamage or impair physiological remodeling will increase the risk of developing a stress fracture. In the running athlete stress fractures usually are the result of either a sudden increase in load conditions or are secondary to biomechanical imbalances.

A sudden increase in load conditions may occur secondary to a rapid increase in training such as occurs when recreational runners do not allow enough time to prepare for an upcoming event (e.g., 10-K run or ½ marathon). In this situation runners suddenly increase their mileage and running frequency. The rate of bone microdamage suddenly increases and before the rate of remodeling can adapt, an area of weakness develops and a stress fracture results. Another situation that causes a sudden increase in loading conditions is an injury to the opposite limb. This causes a sudden increase in loads and subsequent risk of stress fracture to be placed on the noninjured side. Muscle fatigue may also contribute to sudden increases in load conditions. Normal functioning muscle has a stress-distributing effect on bone at its site of insertion.[5] This protective effect is lost with muscle fatigue. Also, with muscle fatigue, a runner's gait becomes affected and results in a less fluid rhythm with increased impact forces. The combination of decreased stress distribution and increased impact forces may lead to a stress fracture.

Stress fractures may also occur secondary to biomechanical imbalances. These often are subtle abnormalities that may cause no difficulties until the runner reaches a specific level of training. Runners who run on hard surfaces with a heavy heel strike and in poorly cushioned shoes may develop tremendous impact forces throughout their lower extremities and spine. They may reach a level of training in which the balance of microdamage to repair is exceeded, leading to a stress fracture. A runner with a rigid cavus foot will have less shock absorption at the midfoot during the loading response phase of gait and therefore will develop higher resultant impact loads. Runners who hyperpronate may transfer increased stresses along the medial aspect of the tibia, or if the degree of hindfoot pronation is severe enough, may actually transmit stresses through the distal fibula. Runners with a short first metatarsal, long second metatarsal, or a hypermobile first metatarsal cuneiform joint will transfer increased loads at the metatarsals, placing them at risk for developing stress fractures.

Symptoms of a stress fracture may be vague and insidious in onset. This can sometimes lead to a delay in diagnosis. Careful physical examination, however, can usually elicit a focal area of tenderness over the involved site as well as associated swelling and warmth. Radiographic changes are rarely evident on routine x-rays in the first 3 to 4 weeks after a stress fracture. If a definitive diagnosis is required, a bone scan can be helpful and is highly sensitive in the diagnosis of a stress fracture. Common locations for stress fractures in the running athlete include the metatarsals, tibial diaphysis, distal third of the fibula, tarsal navicular, hallucal sesamoids, and rarely the medial malleolus.[30,35]

Treatment of a stress fracture in the running athlete consists of treatment of the fracture as well as correction, if possible, of underlying etiological factors. Initial treatment, if symptoms are mild, can be a limitation in running mileage to a level below which the symptoms occur. If the patient's symptoms are severe or if a limitation of running does not alleviate the symptoms, running should be avoided and replaced with cross-training activities until symptoms resolve. Stress fractures may require anywhere from 4 to 15 weeks to resolve. In general, the running athlete will not accept a recommendation to stop all running activities unless an alternative source of conditioning is offered. Recommended low-impact cross-training activities include swimming, bicycling, cross-country skiing, and skating. Casting should be used as a last resort since the resultant joint stiffness and muscle atrophy can be extremely disabling to the running athlete. An exception to this treatment regimen is when displacement of the stress fracture would lead to significant morbidity. This occurs with stress fractures involving a joint such as the hip or tarsal navicular or with stress fractures of the spine or femur. In these situations cessation of all activities is recommended until symptoms resolve and there is radiographic evidence of healing.

Concurrent with treating the stress fracture, correction of the underlying primary disorder should be addressed. In cases resulting from training errors or injury, simple education of the patient in proper training techniques may be all that is required. If underlying biomechanical imbalances exist, however, the physician must be prepared to prescribe appropriate shoe modifications. For patients who run on hard surfaces with a heavy heel strike, a recommendation for a more cushioned shoe and a change to a softer running surface should be emphasized. Runners with a rigid cavus foot will benefit from placement of a flexible arch support within a highly cushioned shoe. Patients with a tibial or fibular stress fracture secondary to hyperpronation will benefit from a soft medial arch support. If a metatarsal stress fracture is secondary to a hypermobile first metatarsal cuneiform joint or a short first metatarsal, a soft medial arch support may also be indicated. A stress fracture of a long second metatarsal is best treated with a pad placed just proximal to the second metatarsal head to more evenly distribute stresses.

As mentioned earlier, stress fractures can occur from increased microdamage or decreased reparative capability. In a runner with recurrent stress fractures and no underlying biomechanical imbalances, and who does not respond to normal treatment modalities, consideration of an underlying metabolic disorder should be made. Impaired bone reparative processes may occur with hormonal, nutritional, hematologic, or oncologic disorders. Routine laboratory studies such as a complete blood cell count and calcium and phosphate levels should be obtained as an initial screen, and additional consultations obtained as is deemed appropriate.

## LEG PAIN

Leg pain is a common complaint of the running athlete and may be caused by one of several disorders. *Shinsplints* is a general term to describe leg pain from a variety of disorders including stress fractures, periostitis, soft tissue injuries, and compartment syndromes.[8,31] A physician should be familiar with this term as it is used commonly in describing leg pain; however, for the purposes of diagnosis and treatment, more definitive terms should be used.

### Stress fractures of the tibia and fibula

Stress fractures of the tibia and fibula may be a source of leg pain. The tibia is most commonly affected at the middle third, and the fibula is most commonly affected at the distal third. As mentioned previously, stress fractures may result from a rapid increase in loading conditions or from biomechanical imbalances. Diagnosis is based on suspicion and localized tenderness. If the injury is in the acute stages before radiographic changes and a definitive diagnosis is desired, a bone scan is the study of choice. Treatment consists of a limitation or modification of activities until symptoms resolve, as well as the correction of underlying biomechanical imbalances.

### Medial tibial stress syndrome

Medial tibial stress syndrome is characterized by pain at the posterior medial aspect of the distal third of the tibia.[4,23] The pain occurs with exercise and is not associated with an elevation in compartment pressure.[3] The cause of the syndrome is most likely a soleus insertional fasciitis or local periostitis. The diagnosis is based on the presence of localized tenderness at the posteromedial border of the distal third of the tibia which is relieved with a local injection of lidocaine. A bone scan, if deemed necessary for a definitive diagnosis, will demonstrate a characteristic increased longitudinal uptake at the posterior border of the tibia involving one third or more of the length of the tibia with varying intensity.[19] Treatment consists of decreased activity, isometric exercises, and well-cushioned shoes. A return to full activities may resume when symptoms resolve. This entity occurs more commonly in runners with increased subtalar mobility and increased pronation during the loading response phase of gait.[37] Therefore, in patients with these characteristics, a soft medial arch support should be used. If conservative treatment is ineffective, a fasciotomy of the posteromedial insertion of the soleus may be considered.[20]

### Compartment syndromes

A *compartment syndrome* is defined as a condition in which the circulation and function of tissue within a closed space is compromised by increased pressure. With exercise, muscle volume can increase 20% from increased capillary infiltration and blood content.[8] Since the fascial constraints of the leg can be unyielding, there may not be enough space to compensate for this 20% increase in volume. Therefore it is not surprising that exercise can sometimes lead to compartment syndromes. Of the four compartments of the leg, the anterior compartment is the most commonly involved followed by the deep posterior compartment.

Fortunately acute compartment syndromes rarely occur in runners. Fewer than 100 cases of acute exertional compartment syndrome have been reported; in one study of 100 acute compartment syndromes, only 2 were secondary to exercise.[8,21] The symptoms consist of pain and a feeling of unyielding pressure that occurs during exercise or soon thereafter. There is tenderness over the affected compartment and a palpable fullness. An early sign of acute compartment syndrome is increased pain with passive stretching of the muscles within the compartment. Paresthesias involving the nerves that travel within the compartment are also a relatively early finding. An acute anterior compartment syndrome would cause pain with passive ankle plantar flexion and paresthesias in the deep peroneal nerve distribution between the first and second toes. A deep posterior compartment syndrome would cause pain with passive ankle dorsiflexion and dysfunction of the posterior tibial nerve. Late findings include anesthesia and motor weakness followed by paralysis. If an acute compartment syndrome is suspected, compartment pressures should be obtained, and, if consistent with the findings, a fasciotomy should be performed immediately.

More commonly, runners develop a chronic exertional compartment syndrome. Symptoms initially are mild and occur after running several miles. Over the course of time, the pain becomes more consistent and limits the patient's exercise routine. It is at this time that the physician is consulted. Athletes usually are asymptomatic when examined but can describe the temporal characteristics as well as the location of the symptoms. If the symptoms are in the anterior compartment, it is common for paresthesias to occur along the superficial peroneal nerve distribution (i.e., the dorsum of the foot). Several authors have found an increased incidence of fascial defects in these patients ranging from 30% to 60%.[21,25] Closure of these fascial defects can cause acute compartment syndromes and is contraindicated. Diagnosis of this disorder is confirmed by tissue pressure measurements. Numerous studies have been written on resting, exercise, and postexercise intracompartmental pressure measurements with respect to diagnosis of this disorder. Normal resting intracompartment pressure is 0 to 8 mm Hg and can rise to over 50 mm Hg during exercise. Postexercise the pressure will immediately drop to below 30 mm Hg and, after 15 minutes, should return to resting values. In patients with chronic exertional compartment syndrome, some have shown that the resting tissue pressure is higher in the affected compartment, and others have not been able to show significant differences.[24,32] In one study of 55 athletes, 24 of which had symptoms consistent with chronic compartment syndrome, the most reliable finding was whether the compartment pressure fell below 15 mm Hg within 15 minutes of cessation of exercise.[26]

Treatment of chronic exertional compartment syndrome should initially consist of decreased activity, change in shoe wear, and antiinflammatory medications. If this is not successful, a fasciotomy may be indicated to relieve the symptoms. Surgical treatment has been highly successful for anterior compartment syndromes, with anterior compartment fasciotomy allowing a return to full activities in 92% to 100% of cases.[6,27,28] The majority of reported failures with fasciotomy have occurred in cases involving the deep posterior compartment.[27,28] This has led to the recommendation that when a deep posterior compartment fasciotomy is performed, a formal release of the tibialis posterior muscle should also be included.[28]

## HEEL PAIN

It is not uncommon for the running athlete to develop pain about the heel, which may become quite bothersome. Heel pain may be secondary to a number of causes including Achilles tendinitis, plantar fasciitis, compressive neuropathy, calcaneal stress fracture, or calcaneal fat pad trauma.

### Achilles tendinitis

Achilles tendinitis has an incidence ranging from 6.5% to 18% in the running athlete and, in one study of competitive track athletes, caused 16% of those affected to give up competitive running.[2,10,38] As such, not only is this a common disorder, it also is disabling (see Case Study 2). Achilles tendinitis involves a continuum of pathology that initially involves inflammation of the peritendinous structures such as bursae and the tendon sheath. As the severity of inflammation progresses, the tendon itself becomes involved in the process. The condition in which damage to the tendon occurs is termed *tendinosis.*[29] Tendinosis can be in the form of tendon necrosis, attritional longitudinal tears of the tendon, intratendinous calcification, or complete tendon rupture. It is

the physician's and trainer's goal to prevent the tendinitis process from progressing to tendinosis. In general, this can be achieved by effective stretching and early treatment of tendinitis.

**Case Study 2.** A 28-year-old female Olympic middle-distance runner had recurrent posterior heel pain for several years. She was currently training for the Olympic trials and was in significant pain. She had tried heel lifts and routinely performed Achilles stretching exercises. Previous radiographs revealed no evidence of Achilles tendon calcification or a Haglund deformity.

Physical examination revealed tenderness at the medial aspect of the Achilles tendon insertion. She had no palpable prominences at the site of tenderness and no limitation of ankle or subtalar motion. While walking and running, she exhibited significant hindfoot pronation; with the hindfoot held in neutral position, her forefoot had limited motion and assumed a supinated position.

The secondary disorder and cause of her symptoms was insertional Achilles tendinitis. The primary disorder was hindfoot pronation and the supinated posture of her forefoot, which placed increased stress on the medial fibers of the Achilles tendon.

She was given an orthosis that incorporated a mediolongitudinal arch support and a lift under her first metatarsal head to compensate for the forefoot supination. After a week of limiting her running and substituting bicycling, she was allowed to resume her training with a gradual increase in running. She did well and qualified for the Olympic team without heel pain.

Achilles tendinitis occurs in two distinct forms: insertional and noninsertional. Insertional Achilles tendinitis occurs near the insertion of the Achilles tendon at the posterior aspect of the calcaneal tuberosity and presents as posterior heel pain. In this entity the inflammatory process initially involves the retrocalcaneal and superficial Achilles bursae as well as the peritenon of the Achilles tendon. Initial symptoms include local pain and increased discomfort running uphill. The runner often describes heel pain that improves as he or she stretches and warms up. On physical examination there is tenderness at the Achilles insertion and there may be associated crepitance with plantar flexion and dorsiflexion of the ankle. Commonly the patient will have limited dorsiflexion of the ankle secondary to a "tight" Achilles tendon. As the process of insertional tendinitis and tendinosis progresses and becomes chronic, intratendinous calcification may be visualized on x-ray. On physical examination it is not uncommon for the intratendinous calcification to be palpable as a bony prominence posteriorly.

Insertional Achilles tendinitis may be associated with a Haglund deformity, which refers to the presence of a posterosuperior prominence of the calcaneal

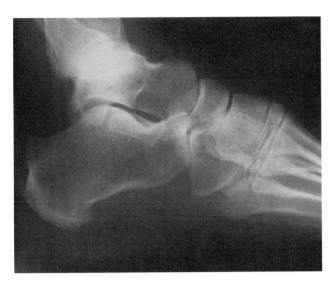

**Fig. 21-4.** Lateral radiograph of the calcaneus illustrating a Haglund deformity and a small amount of calcification at the Achilles insertion.

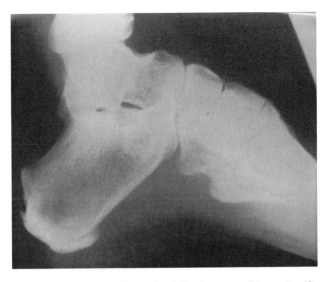

**Fig. 21-5.** Lateral radiograph of the foot revealing a significant cavus deformity as well as a Haglund deformity with calcification at the Achilles tendon insertion.

tuberosity (Fig. 21-4). This prominence predisposes to mechanical irritation at the anterior aspect of the Achilles tendon near its insertion. In a cavus foot this posterosuperior prominence becomes positioned even closer to the anterior aspect of the Achilles tendon and can increase the risk of developing insertional tendinitis (Fig. 21-5).

Initial treatment of insertional Achilles tendinitis consists of rest, intermittent ice massage, Achilles stretching, and antiinflammatory medication. A heel lift should be used in all shoes, especially those used for running. Runners who hyperpronate will often have a majority of their pain at the medial aspect of the heel, whereas supinators will have more discomfort laterally. If this is the case, a heel lift that incorporates a medial sole and heel wedge should be used for hyperpronators and one with a lateral sole and heel wedge for supinators to improve hindfoot alignment throughout the stance phase of gait. In a patient with a Haglund deformity with or without a cavus foot, the heel lift serves not only to decrease the chronic stretch placed upon the Achilles tendon but also rotates the posterosuperior calcaneal prominence away from the Achilles tendon.

If conservative treatment is not effective after an adequate period (approximately 1 year), surgery may be considered. The recommended procedure is a debridement of the Achilles tendon and removal of the Haglund deformity if present. If the tendinous involvement is localized to the medial or lateral aspect, a longitudinal incision is made over the involved area. This simplifies the removal of all of the necrotic and calcified tendon while minimizing disruption of the Achilles insertion. If the pathology is not localized, placing the patient prone and using a midline, longitudinal, tendon-splitting approach is recommended. Regardless of the approach, all necrotic debris and calcification must be removed from the Achilles tendon. If a significant portion of the Achilles tendon is disrupted, a tendon transfer may be indicated. Tendons appropriate for use in the tendon transfer include the peroneus brevis, flexor digitorum longus, or flexor hallucis longus.[15,34,36] Postoperatively a period of casting ranging from 6 to 10 weeks may be required, depending on the amount of tendon disruption and whether a tendon transfer was performed. After the period of casting is completed, the runner will require aggressive rehabilitation to regain range of motion and lower-extremity strength before returning to running activities. This process may require up to 6 months before full activity is achieved.

The noninsertional form of Achilles tendinitis presents with pain in the tendon 2 to 6 cm above the insertion. This region of involvement corresponds to an area of tenuous blood supply within the tendon.[11] With the exception of the location of the pain, the patient's symptoms are similar to those of insertional Achilles tendinitis. Conservative treatment is also similar with rest, ice massage, Achilles stretching, and antiinflammatory medication being the initial treatment regimen. An injection of local anesthetic (e.g., lidocaine or Marcaine) into the tendon sheath to disrupt adhesions may be attempted; however, because of the risk of Achilles tendon rupture, the use of steroid injection near the Achilles tendon is contraindicated.

If conservative treatment fails to provide relief, surgical intervention may be required. The recommended surgical treatment includes debridement of the involved peritendinous sheath as well as debridement of the tendon itself. If significant Achilles tendon disruption is evident, a tendon transfer or tendon augmentation with the plantaris tendon may be indicated. A longitudinal incision just medial to the Achilles tendon is recommended, since it avoids involvement of the sural nerve as well as provides easy access to the plantaris tendon for augmentation or to the FDL tendon if a tendon transfer becomes necessary.

### Plantar fasciitis

Plantar fasciitis may also be a source of heel pain in the running athlete. This entity is a result of microtears that develop within the plantar fascia near its attachment to the medial calcaneal tuberosity secondary to the repetitive loads placed on the foot during running. The microtears, as well as the subsequent inflammation, can result in significant plantar heel pain. A history of severe pain upon arising in the morning or after sitting a prolonged time is typical. The pain usually subsides after warming-up, only to return upon resting. Physical examination reveals tenderness at the medial calcaneal tuberosity and occasionally along the plantar fascia itself. Dorsiflexing the toes may increase the heel pain. Initial treatment consists of decreased activity, Achilles tendon stretching, heel pads, and antiinflammatory medications. A large majority of patients will improve with conservative treatment. A local steroid injection into the maximal area of tenderness may be indicated in patients with significant discomfort or to initiate treatment. If symptoms persist for 1 year despite conservative treatment, surgical intervention may be considered.

The recommended surgical treatment for plantar fasciitis is a partial plantar fascial release with resection of the calcaneal spur if present. All the inflamed and necrotic tissue must be removed to provide an environment that will allow healing of the plantar fascia. Postoperatively the patient is allowed to fully weight bear immediately in a postoperative shoe and is encouraged to perform Achilles stretching exercises. At 12 to 14 days postoperatively, the sutures are discontinued and nonimpact activities such as swimming, bicycling, and skating are allowed. Running is initiated at 4 weeks after surgery. Results following surgical treatment of plantar fasciitis in running athletes is favorable, with 12 of

13 runners returning to full activity in one recent study.[12]

### Compressive neuropathies

A compressive neuropathy may also lead to heel pain. Tarsal tunnel syndrome and compression of the first branch of the lateral plantar nerve (FBLPN) are two such compressive neuropathies that must be considered when evaluating heel pain. In general, neurogenic sources of pain are typically described as burning in nature. In tarsal tunnel syndrome the patient may describe the pain as involving not only the heel but also the plantar aspect of the foot and toes. The pain may be described as radiating up the leg and down into the foot. Tenderness will not only be located at the medial plantar heel but also along the course of the posterior tibial nerve as it courses posterior to the medial malleolus under the flexor retinaculum. Manual compression of the nerve at this location may reproduce the heel and plantar foot complaints. Initial treatment of tarsal tunnel syndrome includes rest, ice massage, and antiinflammatory medications. This entity is more common in hyperpronators; therefore Achilles stretching exercises and longitudinal arch supports may be indicated as well. If symptoms persist, nerve conduction studies and an electromyogram may be desired to confirm the diagnosis before performing surgical decompression of the tarsal tunnel.

Compression of the FBLPN may also contribute to heel pain in the running athlete. A thorough discussion of the anatomy and location of compression of this nerve is offered in Chapter 2, Functional Nerve Disorders, and should be reviewed. The FBLPN can become compressed in the running athlete secondary to abductor hallucis hypertrophy or plantar fascia thickening. Heel pain can sometimes be distinguished from simple plantar fasciitis pain by its burning nature and radiation up the leg or to the lateral plantar foot. The key to the diagnosis, however, is tenderness along its course as it passes deep to the abductor hallucis muscle along the medial heel. Patients often have paresthesias along the course of the nerve with manual compression at the site of maximal tenderness. Conservative treatment consists of rest, contrast baths, Achilles stretching, and antiinflammatory medications. Runners with hyperpronation should also be given longitudinal arch supports. Steroid injections at the area of maximal tenderness may be indicated. Surgical intervention is offered if symptoms persist for over 1 year.

The recommended surgical treatment for compression of the first branch of the lateral plantar nerve is performed through an oblique medial incision. Of importance is to release the entire deep fascia of the abductor hallucis muscle over the FBLPN and to remove enough of the plantar fascia to fully decompress the nerve as it passes transversely plantar to the quadratus plantae muscle. Postoperatively management is the same as for partial plantar fascia release previously described.

### Calcaneal stress fractures

With the repetitive impact and shear forces experienced during heel strike, stress fractures of the calcaneus as well as injury to the calcaneal fat pad may develop. Calcaneal stress fractures may present with a variety of complaints; on physical examination it is often difficult to localize the tenderness to the calcaneus while excluding other disorders. A bone scan is helpful in this situation and may be the only test that can definitively rule out a calcaneal stress fracture.

### Calcaneal fat pad trauma

Calcaneal fat pad trauma refers to injury to the plantar fat pad under the calcaneal tuberosity. The patient's complaints consist of pain at the plantar heel that are exacerbated with weight bearing and especially with impact on the heel. Examination reveals diffuse tenderness limited to the fat pad. The treatment for both a calcaneal stress fracture and calcaneal fat pad trauma is decreased activity, heel cushioning, and running on low-impact surfaces.

## FOREFOOT PAIN

The treatment of forefoot pain in the running athlete can be challenging. Numerous disorders may lead to forefoot pain and a careful physical examination, as well as a complete understanding of gait biomechanics, is helpful. Subtle and seemingly insignificant abnormalities may result in forefoot complaints.

### Metatarsalgia

Metatarsalgia is the most common forefoot complaint and can have numerous etiologies. A limitation of ankle dorsiflexion secondary to a tight Achilles tendon or intrinsic ankle pathology will increase the stresses placed on the forefoot and may lead to symptoms. Metatarsal stress fractures may occur from the increased chronic forefoot impact forces. Initial treatment should consist of decreased activity, metatarsal padding as necessary, and Achilles stretching exercises. If an anterior distal tibial osteophyte or a dorsal talar osteophyte is causing anterior ankle impingement and limitation of ankle dorsiflexion, it may be necessary to surgically remove the offending osteophytes to improve the ankle range of motion.

Claw toes, if present, may lead to metatarsalgia secondary to distal displacement of the forefoot plantar fat pad and increased plantar flexion of the metatarsals resulting from the foot's windlass mechanism. Initial treatment consists of placing a plantar metatarsal pad proximal to the metatarsal head to unload the metatarsal head and also to correct the "dynamic" component of the claw toe. The patient may have to wear running shoes with an increased toe box depth to avoid contact of the dorsum of the toes against the shoe with the metatarsal pad in place. If metatarsal padding is not effective, surgical correction of the claw toes may be indicated.

Metatarsophalangeal joint capsulitis is another source of metatarsalgia in the running athlete. The pain may be sudden or gradual in onset and is characterized as a local area of pain and tenderness at the plantar metatarsal head area (see Case Study 3). It is important during the physical examination to exclude a neuroma as the source of pain. A capsulitis is tender at the plantar aspect of the involved metatarsophalangeal joint and pain may sometimes be evoked with a range of motion of the metatarsophalangeal joint. A neuroma is tender in the interspace between the metatarsal heads plantarly and may be associated with pain that radiates to the toes. Capsulitis may be associated with an irritation of the adjacent interdigital nerve; therefore it is not uncommon to have findings of capsulitis with interdigital nerve tenderness. Metatarsophalangeal joint capsulitis occurs most commonly at the second metatarsophalangeal joint and is often associated with a long second metatarsal. Some patients will develop subluxation of the metatarsophalangeal joint which can be appreciated by performing a Lachman-type test at the metatarsophalangeal joint. If subluxation is evident, this indicates a more chronic process with significant involvement of the plantar plate of the metatarsophalangeal joint. Initial treatment should be the same whether or not there is subluxation and consists of decreased activity, antiinflammatory medications, and a metatarsal pad just proximal to the metatarsal head. In some instances a metatarsal bar may be added to the outside of the running shoe to create a type of rocker-bottom sole.

**Case Study 3.** A 52-year-old male who ran 20 miles per week had gradual onset of severe pain at the plantar aspect of his left foot. It became so painful that he was unable to walk barefoot on hard surfaces. He was no longer able to run at all secondary to the pain.

On physical examination he had normal hindfoot and forefoot alignment without any appreciable deformities. He was exquisitely tender at the plantar aspect of his foot directly over the second metatarsal head. He also was mildly tender at the interspace between the second and third

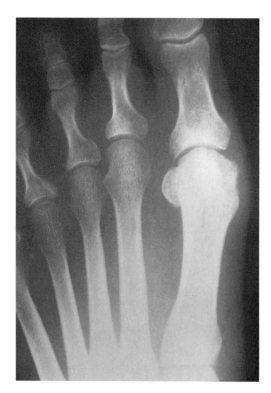

**Fig. 21-6.** Radiograph showing a patient with a long second metatarsal who developed capsulitis of the second metatarsophalangeal joint.

metatarsal heads. Increased pain was elicited with range of motion of the second metatarsophalangeal joint. There was no evidence of subluxation at the joint. The x-ray of his left foot (Fig. 21-6) revealed the presence of a long second metatarsal without evidence of degenerative changes within the joint.

In this case a diagnosis of second metatarsophalangeal joint capsulitis was made secondary to the long second metatarsal. The patient was advised to avoid running for 2 weeks and was given antiinflammatory medications. He also was prescribed a metatarsal pad to be placed just proximal to the second metatarsal head. This regimen led to a total resolution of his symptoms by 6 weeks.

Most cases of metatarsophalangeal joint capsulitis will resolve with conservative measures; however, if the second metatarsal is long or if subluxation is evident, conservative measures may not be successful and surgery may be required. Shortening of the long second metatarsal can be performed either by a proximal metatarsal osteotomy or by a metatarsophalangeal joint arthrotomy and partial metatarsal head resection. Proximal metatarsal osteotomy has the advantage of preserving articular congruity and causing minimal stiffness at the metatarsophalangeal joint. A significant disadvantage is the greater time required to unite a metatarsal osteotomy and the greater risk of causing a transfer metatarsalgia if sagittal alignment is not maintained during the

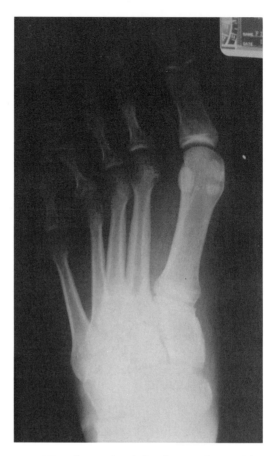

**Fig. 21-7.** AP radiograph of the foot with a mild hallux valgus deformity and a painful tibial sesamoid fracture.

healing process of the osteotomy. With a metatarsophalangeal joint arthrotomy, a partial head resection is performed through a longitudinal dorsal capsulotomy of the metatarsophalangeal joint, with removal of several millimeters of the distal metatarsal head, thereby making the second metatarsal shorter. A plantar condylectomy is performed only if evidence of plantar keratosis exists. Although the intraarticular procedure results in a disruption of articular congruity with subsequent stiffness, this procedure is preferred since it has a more predictable result and allows a more rapid return to full activities. If a subluxatable joint exists, it may be necessary to perform a flexor-to-extensor tendon transfer to achieve stability of the metatarsophalangeal joint.[1,33]

Metatarsalgia may be a result of a metatarsal imbalance, such as a prominent metatarsal plantar condyle or result from hypermobility of the first metatarsal cuneiform joint. The presence of one or several prominent metatarsal plantar condyles can initially be treated with metatarsal padding. If symptoms persist, a plantar condylectomy may be considered. A runner with a hypermobile first metatarsal

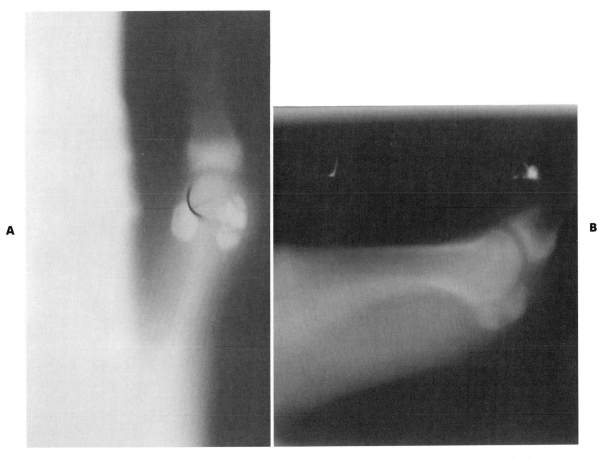

**Fig. 21-8.** AP **(A)** and lateral **(B)** tomograms illustrating fragmentation of the tibial sesamoid of the hallux.

cuneiform joint should be given a medial longitudinal arch support with a Morton extension to increase the weight-bearing contribution of the first metatarsal head and to unload the symptomatic lesser metatarsal heads.

### Sesamoid disorders

Disorders of the hallucal sesamoids may lead to metatarsalgia of the first metatarsal. Predisposing factors include a cavus foot with a plantar-flexed first metatarsal or hyperpronation of the foot. Both situations lead to increased stresses on the sesamoids, which may result in sesamoiditis, osteochondritis, or sesamoid fracture (see Case Study 4). A thorough explanation of sesamoid disorders is offered in a previous chapter and should be reviewed. A runner typically presents with a history of significant pain at the plantar aspect of the first metatarsal head that increases with impact as well as pushing off. On examination there is tenderness at the plantar aspect of the involved sesamoid (usually the tibial sesamoid) and discomfort with dorsiflexion at the first metatarsophalangeal joint. Appropriate x-rays and, if

necessary, a bone scan may be obtained to make a diagnosis, although the initial treatment will not significantly be affected by the specific diagnosis. Initial treatment consists of a decrease in activity, antiinflammatory medications, and an orthosis that incorporates a Morton extension and a U-shaped pad to unload the symptomatic sesamoid. If the patient hyperpronates, a soft medial longitudinal arch is added to the orthosis. As symptoms improve, activity may increase. The orthosis should be continued for a minimum of 6 months and indefinitely if symptoms return. If conservative treatment is ineffective, surgical intervention may be required. Numerous surgical procedures are available for treatment of sesamoid disorders. These include partial or complete sesamoidectomy, plantar sesamoid shaving, as well as bone grafting.[17,18] A runner with a plantar-flexed first metatarsal may benefit from a proximal dorsal wedge osteotomy, which will unload the sesamoids. Sesamoidectomies should be performed with caution as they may result in development of an angular deformity of the hallux as well as decreased push-off strength.[14]

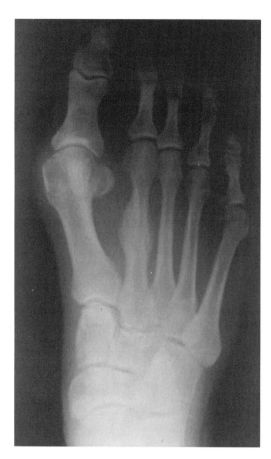

**Fig. 21-9.** Radiograph illustrating a foot with significant hallux valgus and abundant callus at the second metatarsal from a healed stress fracture. The hallux valgus decreases the weight distribution of the hallux, placing increased loads on the lesser metatarsals.

**Case Study 4.** A 28-year-old college track athlete developed gradual onset of pain at the plantar aspect of his left first metatarsal head that was exacerbated when he tried to increase his speed. The pain progressed such that he was no longer competitive.

Physical examination was significant for mild hallux valgus deformity, mild hindfoot pronation while running, and point tenderness at the plantar aspect of the tibial hallucal sesamoid. He had normal range of motion at the first metatarsophalangeal joint, and there was no tenderness at the medial aspect of the first metatarsal head or the lesser metatarsal head. An x-ray (Fig. 21-7) of the left foot revealed a fracture of the tibial sesamoid. Tomograms were subsequently obtained (Fig. 21-8) and clearly showed that the tibial sesamoid had been fragmented into three main pieces.

Initial treatment consisted of a decrease in running activities, fitting of an orthosis incorporating a soft medial longitudinal arch support to limit hindfoot pronation, and a U-shaped pad to unload the tibial sesamoid. This improved his symptoms; however, whenever he attempted to train at a competitive level, his symptoms recurred. When his symptoms returned the following track season, surgical intervention was offered. A decision was made to remove

the distal fragmented portion of the tibial sesamoid while retaining the proximal fragment. In this patient with mild hallux valgus, a total tibial sesamoidectomy would increase his risk of developing a progressive hallux valgus deformity. A partial tibial sesamoidectomy was performed through a medial longitudinal incision, and the distal pole of the sesamoid was approached intraarticularly. He used a postoperative shoe with wooden soles for 1 month, after which he was allowed to ambulate in a regular shoe with his previously prescribed orthosis. Activities such as swimming and bicycling were also begun at this time. Two months postoperatively he was started on a gradual increase in running activities; by 3 months he was able to run without restrictions and without discomfort.

### Interdigital neuromas

An interdigital neuroma may cause significant disability for the running athlete. Presenting complaints include a sharp pain at the plantar metatarsal head area that often radiates to the adjacent toes. On examination significant tenderness is present at the involved interspace, and there may be an associated "Mulder's click" with lateral forefoot compression.[22] Initial treatment consists of a metatarsal pad placed proximal to the metatarsal head to decrease the traction placed on the nerve. A steroid injection into the involved interspace may also be performed. If symptoms persist, resection of the neuroma through a dorsal longitudinal incision with release of the distal half of the intermetatarsal ligament may be considered.

### Hallux valgus

Numerous sources of forefoot pain may result from a hallux valgus deformity. The runner may have pain at the medial eminence of the first metatarsophalangeal joint or may have pain secondary to metatarsalgia, claw toes, or neuromas that result from the angular deformity of the hallux. As the hallux drifts into more valgus, increased weight is transferred to the lesser metatarsals, which may lead to metatarsalgia and metatarsal stress fractures (Fig. 21-9). Claw toes and second metatarsophalangeal joint subluxation may develop from the decreased space available with increasing hallux valgus. Neuromas occur secondary to the increased traction placed on the interdigital nerves as claw-toeing develops. Initial treatment consists of a decrease in activity, antiinflammatory medications, and shoe modifications. The runner should use a shoe with a wide well-cushioned toe box. If metatarsalgia, claw toes, or neuromas are present, metatarsal padding must also be used. If hyperpronation exists, the orthosis should incorporate a soft medial longitudinal arch support to minimize the valgus stresses placed on the hallux during running. If symptoms persist and surgery is considered, the goal should be to achieve a stable

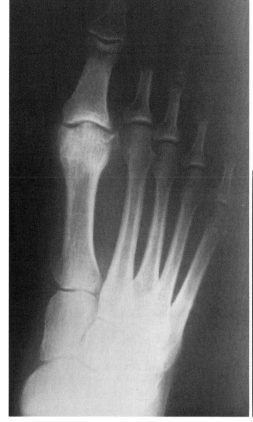
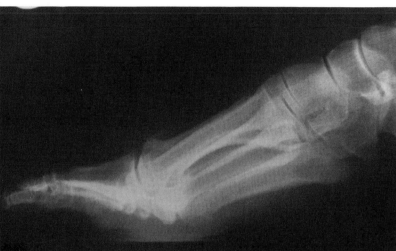

**Fig. 21-10.** AP and lateral radiographs of the foot illustrating the medial, lateral, and dorsal osteophytes seen with hallux rigidus. The joint space of the first metatarsophalangeal joint also is diminished.

realignment of the hallux as well as maintain adequate first metatarsophalangeal joint range of motion. The recommended procedure is a bunionectomy using a distal chevron osteotomy of the first metatarsal, which has proven to be highly successful in middle-distance and marathon runners.[13] The postoperative regimen allows a return to running activities by 8 weeks after surgery.

## Hallux rigidus

Hallux rigidus may result in limited range of motion at the first metatarsophalangeal joint and subsequent pain in the running athlete. The runner's pain is exacerbated with starting from a stance, squatting, or when trying to increase speed. Radiographs reveal degenerative changes within the first metatarsophalangeal joint and the presence of medial, lateral, and dorsal osteophytes (Fig. 21-10). Initial treatment consists of decreased activity, antiinflammatory medication, and a metatarsal bar that adds a rocker bottom to the running shoe. A shoe with a rigid sole and the use of an orthosis with a rigid Morton extension may be tried as well to limit the dorsiflexion

required by the first metatarsophalangeal joint during running. If these conservative measures are not successful, a cheilectomy of the first metatarsophalangeal joint can be performed, at which time the medial, lateral, and dorsal osteophytes are removed. If 60 degrees of dorsiflexion of the first metatarsophalangeal joint is not achieved after sufficient removal of osteophytes, a closing dorsal wedge osteotomy at the base of the proximal phalanx of the great toe should also be performed. A dorsal longitudinal incision just lateral to the extensor hallucis longus is recommended, which allows adequate exposure and minimizes adhesions involving the extensor hallucis longus tendon. If additional exposure is required, a medial longitudinal incision may be added. Postoperatively, aggressive range-of-motion exercises are initiated to regain as much motion as possible at the first metatarsophalangeal joint.

## Blisters

Blisters may develop as the amount of activity increases. Blisters occur secondary to excessive shear forces at the skin surface. Conditions that increase shear forces include high-traction artificial surfaces and the use of spiked running shoes. Initial treatment consists of draining the blister with a sterile needle and covering the area with an adhesive pad such as moleskin. To prevent recurrences, shear reduction in the form of double socks, skin lubrication, and avoidance of high-traction surfaces and spiked shoes should be recommended.

### Toenail disorders

Toenail disorders may also become problematic and lead to significant discomfort. The etiology of toenail disorders in the running athlete is usually direct trauma of the nail against the toe box of the shoe. This may occur secondary to several possible conditions. A poor-fitting shoe with inadequate toe box length or depth will cause the toenail to come in contact with the shoe while running. A shoe that is too wide in the midfoot will allow the foot to slide forward, allowing the toes to strike the distal end of the toe box during the stance phase of gait. Both of these conditions can be alleviated by a shoe with adequate toe box depth and length while being snug at the midfoot. Some runners have hyperextension of the toes, which causes the distal end of the toenails to be more prominent dorsally. In this situation there should be sufficient toe box depth to prevent the toenail from striking the shoe while running. A metatarsal pad may be used in a patient with hyperextension to decrease hyperextension deformity. The result of repetitive toenail trauma is usually a thickening of the nail. Acutely, however, there may be an associated subungual hematoma or ingrowing of the toenail, which may require treatment.

### REFERENCES

1. Barbari SG, Brevig K: Correction of clawtoes by the Girdlestone-Taylor flexor-extensor transfer, *Foot Ankle* 5:67, 1984.
2. Clement DB, Tauton JE, Smart GW: A survey of overuse running injuries, *Phys Sports Med* 9:47, 1981.
3. D'Ambrosia RD et al: Interstitial pressure measurements in the anterior and posterior compartments in athletes with shin splints, *Am J Sports Med* 5:127, 1977.
4. Detmer DE: Chronic shin splints: classification and management of medial tibial stress syndrome, *Sports Med* 3:436, 1986.
5. Frankel VH: Fatigue fractures: biomechanical considerations, *J Bone Joint Surg* 54A:1345, 1987.
6. Fronek J et al: Management of chronic exertional anterior compartment syndrome of the lower extremity, *Clin Orthop* 220:217, 1987.
7. James SL, Bates BT, Ostering LR: Injuries to runners, *Am J Sports Med* 6:40, 1978.
8. Jones DC, James SL: Overuse injuries of the lower extremity: shin splints, iliotibial band friction syndrome, and exertional compartment syndromes, *Clin Sports Med* 6:273, 1987.
9. Kingston S: Magnetic resonance imaging of the foot and ankle, *Clin Sports Med* 7:15, 1988.
10. Krissoff WB, Ferris WD: Running injuries, *Phys Sports Med* 7:64, 1978.
11. Lagergren C, Lindholm A: Vascular distribution in the Achilles tendon, *ACTA Chir Scand* 116:491, 1958.
12. Leach RE, Seavey MS, Salter DK: Results of surgery in athletes with plantar fasciitis, *Foot Ankle* 7:156, 1986.
13. Lillich JS, Baxter DE: Bunionectomies and related surgery in the elite female middle-distance and marathon runner, *Am J Sports Med* 14:491, 1986.
14. Lillich JS, Baxter DE: Common forefoot problems in runners, *Foot Ankle* 7:145, 1986.
15. Mann RA et al: Chronic rupture of the Achilles tendon: a new technique of repair, *J Bone Joint Surg* 73A:214, 1991.
16. Mann RA, Baxter DE, Lutter LD: Running symposium, *Foot Ankle* 1:190, 1981.
17. Mann RA, Wapner KL: Tibial sesamoid shaving for treatment of intractable plantar keratosis, *Foot Ankle* 13:196, 1992.
18. McBryde Jr AM, Anderson RB: Sesamoid foot problems in the athlete, *Clin Sports Med* 7:51, 1988.
19. Michael RH, Holder LE: The soleus syndrome: a cause of medial tibial stress (shin splints), *Am J Sports Med* 13:87, 1985.
20. Mubarek SJ et al: The medial tibial stress syndrome. A cause of shin splints, *Am J Sports Med* 10:201, 1982.
21. Mubarek SJ, Hargens AR: *Exertional compartment syndromes.* In *Symposium on the foot and leg in running sports*, St Louis, 1982, CV Mosby.
22. Mulder JD: The causative mechanism in Morton's metatarsalgia, *J Bone Joint Surg* 33B:94, 1951.
23. Puranen J: The medial tibial syndrome, *J Bone Joint Surg* 56B:712, 1974.
24. Reneman RS: *The anterior and lateral compartment syndrome of the leg*, The Hague, 1968, Mouton.
25. Reneman RS: The anterior and lateral compartment syndromes of the leg due to intensive use of muscles, *Clin Orthop* 113:69, 1975.
26. Rorabeck CH et al: The role of tissue pressure measurements in diagnosing chronic anterior compartment syndrome, *Am J Sports Med* 16:143, 1988.
27. Rorabeck CH, Bourne RB, Fowler PJ: The surgical treatment of exertional compartment syndrome in athletes, *J Bone Joint Surg* 65A:1245, 1983.
28. Rorabeck CH, Fowler PJ, Nott L: The results of fasciotomy in management of chronic exertional compartment syndrome, *Am J Sports Med* 16:224, 1988.
29. Shepsis AA, Leach RE: Surgical management of Achilles tendinitis, *Am J Sports Med* 15:308, 1987.
30. Shelbourne KD et al: Stress fractures of the medial malleolus, *Am J Sports Med* 16:60, 1988.
31. Slocum DB: The shin splint syndrome: medical aspects and differential diagnosis, *Am J Surg* 114:875, 1967.
32. Styf J, Korner L: Intramuscular pressure and muscle blood flow during exercise in chronic compartment syndrome, *J Bone Joint Surg* 69B:301, 1987.
33. Taylor RG: The treatment of clawtoes by multiple transfers of flexor to extensor tendons, *J Bone Joint Surg* 33B:539, 1951.
34. Teuffer AP: Traumatic rupture of the Achilles tendon: reconstruction by transplant and graft using the lateral peroneus brevis, *Orthop Clin North Am* 5:89, 1974.
35. Ting A et al: Stress fractures of the tarsal navicular in long-distance runners, *Clin Sports Med* 7:89, 1988.
36. Turco VJ, Spinella AJ: Achilles tendon-peroneus brevis transfer, *Foot Ankle* 7:253, 1987.
37. Viitasalo JT, Kvist M: Some biomechanical aspects of the foot and ankle in athletes with and without shin splints, *Am J Sports Med* 11:125, 1983.
38. Welsh RP, Clodman J: Clinical survey of Achilles tendinitis in athletes, *Can Med Assoc J* 122:193, 1980.

# Chapter 22

# Foot and ankle injuries in the professional athlete

**J. Bruce Moseley, Jr.**
**Brian T. Chimenti**

Athletic participation involves an inherent risk of injury. Even professional athletes, who possess superior ability and training, cannot escape injuries. These professionals are also under added pressure to recover more quickly and to perform while recovering.

Injuries of the foot and ankle in professional athletes have received little attention in the literature. Rodeo et al found "turf toe" injuries were common and disabling in professional football players.[2] Henry et al studied all injuries in professional basketball over seven years; they found that the ankle was the most frequently injured joint.[1] Zelisko et al also reported that the ankle was the most frequently injured body part in both men's and women's professional basketball.[3] There is little else on the subject.

This chapter discusses foot and ankle injuries in professional football, baseball, and basketball. The information was obtained from the physicians and trainers who care for the athletes on the professional teams.

## METHODS

A survey was mailed to 42 physicians and trainers who cared for 21 professional football, baseball, and basketball teams. In cases where several physicians worked with the team, the physician who most frequently treated foot and ankle injuries was asked to participate. The participants were chosen in order to have equal input from all three sports and from a variety of geographic areas. Of the 42 questionnaires, 32 were returned. Physicians and trainers were equally represented with 16 of each responding. All

three sports were similarly represented, with 11 physicians and trainers from football, 11 from basketball, and 10 from baseball responding. The following team physicians and trainers participated:

- California Angels — Trainer — Ned Bergert
- Chicago Bears — Physician — Michael Shafer, M.D.
  — Physician — Gordon Nuber, M.D.
- Chicago Bulls — Physician — John Hefferon, M.D.
  — Trainer — Chip Schafer
- Chicago Cubs — Physician — Gordon Nuber, M.D.
  — Physician — Michael Shafer, M.D.
  — Trainer — John Fiero
- Dallas Mavericks — Physician — James Evans, M.D.
  — Trainer — Doug Atkinson
- Dallas Cowboys — Trainer — Kevin O'Neal
- Houston Rockets — Physician — Charles Baker, M.D.
  — Trainer — Ray Melchiorre
- Houston Oilers — Physician — Thomas Cain, M.D.
  — Trainer — Brad Brown
- Houston Astros — Physician — William Bryan, M.D.
  — Trainer — David Labossiere
- Indianapolis Colts — Physician — K. Donald Shelbourne, M.D.
  — Trainer — Hunter Smith
- Los Angeles Lakers — Physician — Stephen Lombardo, M.D.
  — Trainer — Gary Vitti
- Los Angeles Dodgers — Physician — Ralph Gambardella, M.D.
- Los Angeles Rams — Physician — Clarence Shields, M.D.
  — Trainer — Jim Anderson
- New York Giants — Trainer — Ronnie Barnes
- New York Mets — Physician — David Altchek, M.D.
- New York Knicks — Trainer — Mike Saunders

- Pittsburgh          Physician     Jim Bradley, M.D.
  Steelers           Trainer       John Norwig
- San Antonio        Trainer       John Anderson
  Spurs
- St. Louis          Physician     Glen Johnson, M.D.
  Cardinals
- Texas Rangers      Physician     Michael Mycoskie, M.D.
                     Trainer       Daniel Wheat
- Utah Jazz          Physician     Gordon Affleck, M.D.

The following four questions were asked of survey participants:

1. What are the *five most common* foot and ankle injuries that you see in the professional athlete?
2. What is the *most difficult* foot and ankle injury in the professional athlete that you have to treat? Why?
3. *Lateral ankle sprains*
   A. How are severely sprained ankles generally treated in the professional athletes on your team? (Early rehabilitation, Cast, Surgery, Other)
   B. Do you try to distinguish between grades of lateral ankle sprain severity? (Yes or No)
   C. If so, how do you distinguish the more severe injuries from the least severe? (Clinical exam, X-rays, or Other)
   D. Are lateral ankle sprains ever immobilized or casted in the professional athletes on your team? (Yes or No)
   E. Do you ever operate on lateral ankle sprains in the professional athlete? (Physicians only) (Yes or No)
4. What is your *most memorable* injury of the foot or ankle in a professional athlete? What made it so memorable? Was it career ending?

## RESULTS
### Most common injuries

Participants were asked to list the five most common foot and ankle injuries they saw in professional athletes. Equal weight was given to all responses, regardless of whether they were listed first or fifth. Participants occasionally listed fewer than five responses.

By far the most common foot and ankle injury reported by both physicians and trainers was the ankle sprain (Fig. 22-1). This injury was reported by all physicians and trainers in every sport, and it was the first or second most common injury seen by 29 of the 32 respondents. The second most common injury was "turf toe", or a sprain of the capsule of the first metatarsophalangeal joint. This injury occurred frequently in all three sports but particularly in football. Two overuse injuries—plantar fasciitis and Achilles tendinitis—were the next most frequently mentioned

problems. Fractures and stress reactions of one of the metatarsals, especially of the fifth metatarsal (Jones fracture), were the fifth most common injury. These were the only fractures reported among the 10 most common injuries, and they were most commonly noted in basketball players. Midfoot (Lisfranc) sprains, syndesmosis/interosseus membrane sprains, and medial (deltoid) ankle sprains were the next three most frequently listed injuries. The Lisfranc and syndesmosis sprains were particularly common in football players. Contusions and arch sprains were the ninth and tenth most common injuries.

All the other injuries listed by respondents as being most common were reported only once or twice. These included Lisfranc's fractures, navicular fractures, sesamoid fractures, subungual hematomas, ingrown toenails, fibula/ankle fractures, foot fractures (unspecified), toe fractures, shin splints, metatarsalgia, corns and calluses, and other injuries.

Physicians and trainers tended to report similar injuries most commonly (Fig. 22-2). The top five most common injuries for both groups were lateral ankle sprains, turf toe, plantar fasciitis, Achilles tendinitis, and fractures and stress reactions of the metatarsals (especially the fifth metatarsal). Physicians listed Achilles tendinitis, metatarsal fractures, and midfoot sprains more frequently than did trainers, and trainers reported medial ankle sprains, contusions, and arch sprains more commonly than did physicians.

There were some differences in the most frequently noted injuries when analyzed by sport (Fig. 22-3). Although ankle sprains were the most common injury listed by physicians and trainers in all three sports, other injuries varied in frequency by sport. Fractures and stress reactions of the metatarsals were the second most common injury in basketball, but these injuries were infrequent in football and baseball. Basketball was also the only sport listing Lisfranc's fractures and navicular fractures among its most common injuries. Physicians and trainers for football players reported that syndesmosis/interosseus membrane sprains, Lisfranc/midfoot sprains, and medial ankle sprains were all among the most common injuries, but their colleagues in basketball and baseball did not frequently list these among the most common injuries. Baseball was the only sport in which contusions were among the most common injuries. All of the contusions were from foul balls, most frequently off of the front leg or foot of the batter.

### Most difficult injuries

Participants were asked what injury was most difficult to treat and to describe why it was so difficult. Thirty of the 32 participants responded to this

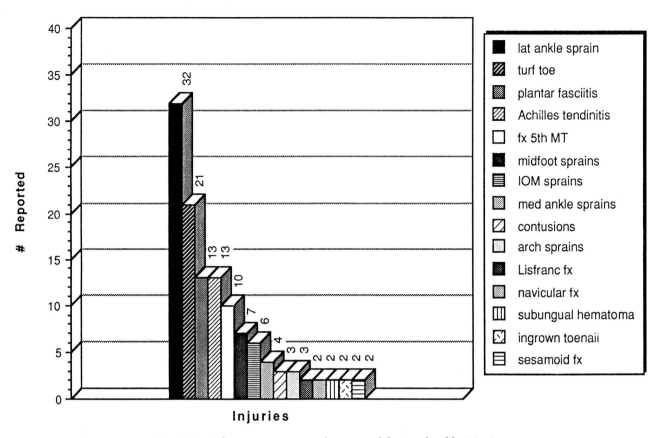

**Fig. 22-1.** Fifteen most commonly reported foot and ankle injuries.

question, and some participants listed more than one injury.

The injury most frequently cited and most difficult to treat was to the interosseous membrane or syndesmosis of the ankle (Fig. 22-4). It was mentioned in responses from physicians and trainers from all three sports, particularly football. The reasons given for why it was such a difficult problem were the prolonged healing time (longer than most athletes expect) and the lack of an effective treatment. The second most frequently cited most difficult injury was a Lisfranc or midfoot sprain, but it was mentioned exclusively by football physicians and trainers. It presented a problem because it was difficult to diagnose and also because it took a long time to heal. Stress fractures and stress reactions were the third most common most difficult injury, and they were mentioned exclusively by basketball team physicians and trainers. They presented problems because of prolonged healing time, limitation of conditioning activities allowable during the healing period, difficulty in knowing when it was safe for the athlete to return to their sport without refracturing, and difficulty selecting the best treatment option for a stress fracture of the fifth metatarsal. Navicular and fifth

metatarsal stress fractures were specifically mentioned as being difficult to treat. Achilles tendinitis and turf toe were tied for the fourth most frequently mentioned most difficult injury. Achilles tendinitis was a particular problem for baseball, and turf toe was mentioned in all three sports. Achilles tendinitis presented problems because it had a prolonged healing time, high recurrence rate, was difficult to treat, and ran the risk of Achilles tendon rupture if athletes returned to their sport too soon. Turf toe presented problems because it was difficult to play with, it was difficult to predict when an athlete would be ready to play, it could linger all season, and it could result in degeneration of the joint.

Ankle sprains, plantar fasciitis, severe plantar/dorsiflexion injuries of the ankle, Achilles tendon rupture, foul balls causing a contusion of the shin, and chronic heel pain were all mentioned once or twice as the most difficult injury to treat. Reasons for their difficult nature were difficulty in treatment or a lack of effective treatment, prolonged rehabilitation, recurrence or persistence of the problem (especially with overuse injuries), and an unwillingness on the part of athletes to take time off from their sport to let overuse problems resolve.

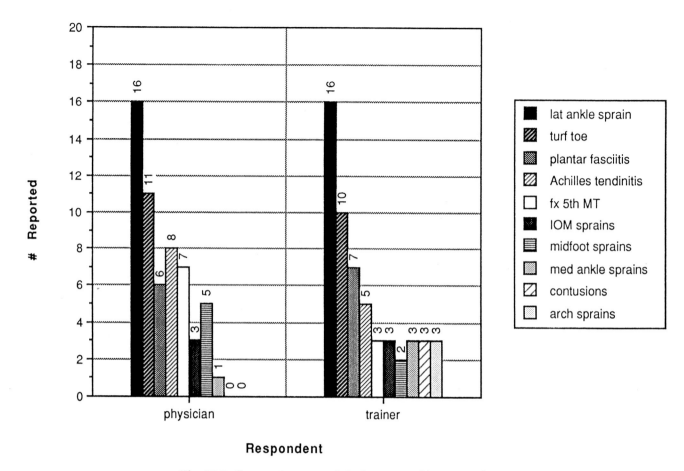

**Fig. 22-2.** Ten most common injuries reported by respondents.

### Lateral ankle sprains

Participants were asked five questions (four questions for trainers) specifically regarding lateral ankle sprains (see the section, Methods). All physicians and trainers responded.

The first question asked about lateral ankle sprains was how the participants generally treated *severe* (grade III) sprains. Participants were given choices of early rehabilitation, cast, surgery, or "other". Of the 32 participants, 29 responded with "immediate rehab", although many participants used an Aircast splint, Unna boot, Cryocuff compression wrap, or removable splint/walker during the "immediate rehab". Two physicians responded with "cast then rehab". One physician mentioned "cast then rehab" and also surgery for severe grade III lateral ankle sprains. Although not specifically asked, many participants volunteered different treatment modalities that they used during immediate rehabilitation. These modalities included transcutaneous electrical nerve stimulation (TENS) units, compression (with and without ice), active exercise with heel cord stretching, static stretching on a slant board, and contrast baths.

The second question asked about lateral ankle sprains was whether participants tried to distinguish between grades of severity (i.e., a grade I, II, or III sprain). Eighty-one percent of respondents said that they try to distinguish between grades of severity, and several volunteered that this was done for prognosis and not treatment. Nineteen percent of respondents, equally distributed among the three sports, did not try to distinguish between grades of severity.

The next question asked those participants who did grade severity of ankle sprains whether they used clinical examination, x-ray films, or other means to assess the severity of sprain. Every participant (100%) used the clinical examination to assess severity of ankle sprains, although 14 participants (44%) also used x-ray for stress views to rule out a fracture or to assess the syndesmosis. Two respondents also mentioned using magnetic resonance imaging (MRI) on occasion to evaluate severe injuries. The responses were similar for all three sports.

Physicians and trainers were next asked if they ever immobilized or casted lateral ankle sprains in professional athletes, and if so, what percentage of ankle

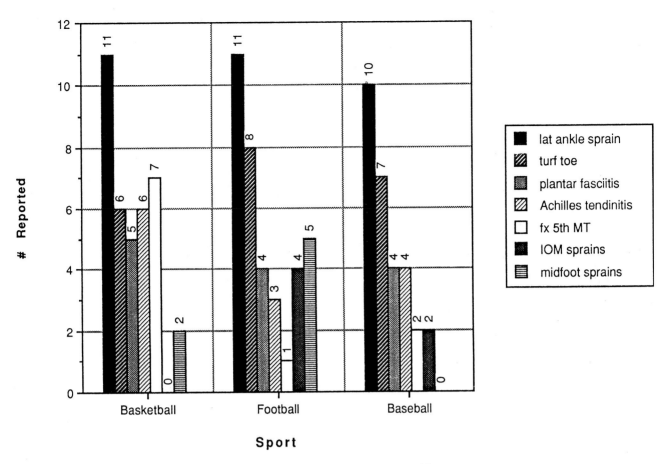

**Fig. 22-3.** Most common injuries, reported by sport.

sprains were casted. Twenty-one of the thirty-two participants (66%) said that they did on occasion cast ankle sprains. However the majority (19 of 21) said that they casted 10% or less of ankle sprains. Although not specifically asked, several participants mentioned that immobilization was temporary until symptoms decreased and athletes could begin rehabilitation. Eleven of the thirty-two respondents (33%) never casted ankle sprains. The responses were similar for all three sports.

The last question regarding ankle sprains asked physicians whether they ever operated on ankle sprains in professional athletes and, if so, what percentage was operated on. Thirteen of the sixteen physicians (81%) never operated on lateral ankle sprains. Three of sixteen physicians (19%) rarely operated on lateral ankle sprains; these three physicians operated on less than 5% of ankle sprains. One of the three physicians mentioned that he only operated on chronic recurrent sprains with peroneal tendon subluxation.

**Most memorable injuries**

The last question asked participants to describe their most memorable foot and ankle injury in the

professional athlete, to discuss what made the injury so memorable, and to note whether the injury in question was career ending. Twenty-seven of the thirty-two participants responded to the question.

Responses varied widely, and reasons the injuries were memorable included the fame of the athlete, the severe nature of the injury, and the persistence of the problem. Many of the "most memorable" injuries were not injuries per se but rather chronic problems that persisted despite treatment. Because it was difficult to characterize the responses, they are (by default) reported by sport.

Baseball physicians and trainers listed a wide variety of most memorable problems, none of which were career ending. One physician reported that the worst fracture-dislocation of an ankle that he had ever seen occurred in a baseball player, but it was successfully treated and the player returned to his sport. Another physician reported a plantar fascia rupture that resulted in severe scarring and swelling in the proximal arch/heel pad region; this injury, however, did not prevent the athlete from resuming his career. One trainer reported a severe contusion of the shin in a prominent player, which was so debilitating that the player missed four games as a result. One reason this

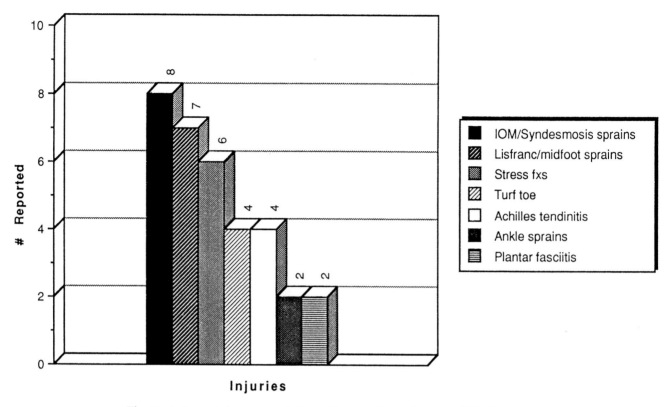

**Fig. 22-4.** Seven injuries reported most frequently as the most difficult to treat.

injury was so memorable was that it led the team to seek increased use of and better manufacturing of shin guards. They also standardized their treatment of these injuries to include sequential compression ice pumps and Russian-frequency muscle stimulation. This eliminated the problems of the "chronic shin abuser" on the team. One physician described a 20-game winner with chronic grade III instability of the ankle who functioned well despite his problem. One trainer was impressed with a severe ankle sprain that tore all of the ankle ligaments; another trainer mentioned a chronic Achilles tendinitis that required special shoes and attention for many years. One physician recalled a dislocated ankle without a fracture that was unusual but not career ending.

Football physicians and trainers most memorable injuries were usually severe injuries or ones that required prolonged recovery, and none were career ending. Two physicians and two trainers recalled Lisfranc/midfoot injuries that were particularly memorable. Two of the four respondents felt that the Lisfranc sprains were memorable because of the long recovery time (one because of an initial misdiagnosis). The other two respondents felt that the Lisfranc injuries (one a ligament injury and the other a fracture) were memorable because they were so severe that they required surgery. One physician and two

trainers recalled injuries to the great toe, two of which were dislocated. They were memorable because they took a long time (>8 weeks) to recover, and in one case (which was not dislocated) it continued to bother the athlete 4 years later. Two trainers remembered severe fracture-dislocations of the ankle that were challenging because of the rehabilitation but they were not career ending. One trainer remembered three ankle fractures requiring surgery in one season, two of which required removal of a syndesmosis screw 8 weeks later. All three players returned to play the next year. One physician was impressed with a complete plantar fascia rupture that responded well to rehabilitation and did not threaten the player's career. One physician had been treating a starting tight end with chronic plantar fasciitis for 2 years; one thing that made it particularly memorable was dealing with the team podiatrist and the head coach. One physician remembered several syndesmosis ankle injuries that looked relatively benign but which caused pain the athletes referred to as "Achilles tendon" pain when running. These athletes required a prolonged recovery.

Most of the basketball team physicians and trainers recalled fractures as their most memorable foot and ankle injury in professional athletes. Many were remarkable because they involved all-star athletes.

Three respondents recalled tarsonavicular stress fractures, two in all-stars, and one that required a full year to recover. One physician remembered a fracture of the fifth metatarsal that required surgery, and the athlete returned to his all-star status. Two trainers were impressed with complete Achilles tendon ruptures, but neither injury was career threatening. One trainer recalled a grade II ankle sprain in a premier center during the NBA playoffs, but with rehabilitation the player returned for the next game and performed well. One physician who cares for an NBA team was most impressed with an injury to a professional rodeo bull rider. The rider fractured all of his metatarsals, and this required open reduction with internal fixation (ORIF). However, the rider had a spur attached to the cast and rode bulls less than 4 weeks after surgery; he recovered to ride another 8 or 9 years.

## DISCUSSION

This study asked participants to recall and estimate frequencies and occurrences of injuries. Studies such as this are prone to inaccuracies, which should be taken into account when reviewing the results. Nonetheless we believe that the information in this study accurately reflects the experience of the respondents as they recall it.

Lateral ligament sprains were the most frequently occurring injury, but they were not considered particularly difficult to treat by most respondents. The majority of respondents favored early rehabilitation of severe lateral ankle sprains, and they used a cast or immobilization less than 10% of the time. The majority of physicians never operated on lateral ankle sprains.

There was surprising similarity in all three sports in regard to the most commonly seen injuries of the foot and ankle. Lateral ligament sprains of the ankle were the most frequently reported injury in all three sports. Turf toe—an injury commonly associated with football players who play on artificial turf—was reported in all three sports including basketball. However, some of the more common and more difficult injuries varied according to sport. Interosseous membrane/syndesmosis injuries and Lisfranc/midfoot sprains were considered the most difficult to treat only in football. Stress fractures and stress reactions were considered the most difficult to treat only in basketball. Contusions (from foul balls) were considered among the most difficult to treat in baseball. Although there were similarities among the three sports surveyed, there were obvious differences for the physicians and trainers in each sport as well.

Physicians and trainers tended to respond similarly to all of the questions. The only trend seemed to be for trainers to see and treat contusions and minor sprains before they were brought to the attention of the physician.

Terminology was not uniform among the respondents, and certain assumptions were made by the authors that allowed grouping seemingly similar injuries. Lateral ligament sprains and inversion ankle sprains were considered the same injury. Interosseous membrane, syndesmosis, and anterior tibiofibular ligament ankle sprains were considered the same entity. Lisfranc sprains and midfoot sprains were considered the same injury. Fractures of the metatarsals, stress fractures of the metatarsals, and stress reactions were grouped as one entity. By grouping seemingly similar injuries, some of the responses may have been analyzed in a way different than the respondent had intended. However, these associations seemed appropriate based on similarities in the way the questionnaires were completed. Perhaps the professionals who treat the athletes should adopt standardized terminology for reporting these injuries.

This study primarily reported the incidence of certain types of injuries in professional athletes. Treatment was not a major part of the questionnaire except in regard to ankle sprains. Drawing major conclusions about treatment results of any injury would be inappropriate based on this study alone.

Physicians and trainers in the high-stress, high-profile world of professional sports mentioned overuse injuries frequently among their most difficult and most memorable problems treated. Plantar fasciitis, Achilles tendinitis, and stress fractures and reactions were all frequently mentioned as being difficult and memorable. Much of the frustration was centered on the struggle to return athletes to the court or field, playing at top performance levels, without aggravating or worsening the condition. Physicians and trainers who struggled with these problems seemed to perform well despite the added stress, because none of the memorable problems developed into a career-threatening injury. Nonetheless, the stress associated with treating professional athletes was indicated in the frustration associated with treating overuse injuries.

## SUMMARY

Lateral ankle sprains were the most common injury reported in professional football, baseball, and basketball. Despite their frequent occurrence, lateral ankle sprains were infrequently noted to be the most difficult injury to treat, and the majority of participants favored immediate rehabilitation for even the most severe ankle sprains. Injuries considered most difficult and most memorable varied by sport, and the reasons cited usually centered on prolonged healing time, recurrence of the problem if athletes returned to their sport too soon, and frustration associated with returning an athlete to their sport as soon as possible and at peak performance level.

## REFERENCES

1. Henry JH, Lareau B, Neigut D: The injury rate in professional basketball, *Am J Sports Med* 10:16, 1982.
2. Rodeo SA et al: Turf-toe: an analysis of metatarsophalangeal joint sprains in professional football players, *Am J Sports Med* 18:280, 1990.
3. Zelisko JA, Noble HB, Porter M: A comparison of men's and women's professional basketball injuries, *Am J Sports Med* 10:297, 1982.

# Chapter 23

# Pediatric problems

**Lowell D. Lutter**

Children have open epiphyses and greater flexibility than adults, which gives a different frequency to injuries with a similar etiology. Children respond to injury with quicker recovery and less residual effects than do older groups. The growing skeletal system reacts differently from the mature frame. Torus or greenstick fractures, apophyseal injuries, and epiphyseal fractures occur in children and not in adults.[33]

Through involvement in football and ice hockey, boys experience a higher injury rate, whereas girls experience a higher risk of injury with involvement in gymnastics and volleyball. Injury rates are equal for sports requiring comparable training and physical skills such as track and cross-country skiing.

Injuries of the leg, foot, and ankle account for 21% of athletic problems in children and adolescents.[5] The distribution of sports-related injuries in the pediatric age group mirrors the types and frequencies seen in adults, with the exception of higher soft tissue and apophysis involvement in children and adolescents.

## OVERUSE INJURIES

In the past, weekend athletes or those on high-level training programs were the only ones to develop overuse injuries. With the advent of increased training as the avenue to better performances, children are increasingly developing overuse injuries.

Risk fractures, which predispose children to stress or overuse injuries, are well known. These result from anatomic problems, training problems, surface changes, and poor footwear.[24]

## Anatomic problems

Anatomic patterns at the extremes of normal have a greater problem accommodating stresses applied during sports activities. For example, those with severe pronation will more frequently have midfoot pain and long arch pain. They may be more susceptible to stress fractures of the metatarsal.

The high-arch foot is disadvantaged in that its shock-absorbing abilities are decreased compared with a more flexible foot. Affected young athletes are more prone to injuries on the lateral side of the foot and the heel area.

## Training problems

Injuries are produced when athletes embark on a training program without supervision. The child/adolescent athlete is susceptible to the same "breakdown" problems that older athletes experience if excess stress is applied to the foot and ankle. The key with this age group is to allow a gradual increase in training stresses. Children and adolescents are likely to overtrain if not provided clear guidelines.

## Surface changes

When a running athlete changes from a soft surface to the firmness of a track or court, overuse injuries can occur. This often happens in individuals who play multiple sports and change too rapidly from one seasonal sport to another without allowing transition time for acclimation of the different stresses.

## Poor footwear

Proper attention must be paid to the condition of training and competing shoes. Usually the counter of a shoe will break down before wear on the outer sole. Once the outer surface has worn into the midsole of any sport shoe, it is time for a replacement. Unfortunately resoling of a training shoe does not work unless the new midsole is similar to the preexisting material (Fig. 23-1).

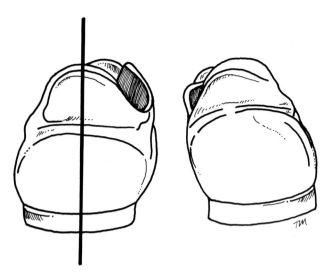

**Fig. 23-1.** Shoe wear pattern illustrates medial breakdown associated with significant foot pronation.

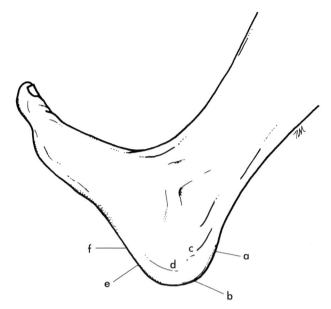

**Fig. 23-2.** Foot shows various areas of abnormality in terms of pain: *(a)* Achilles tendinitis, *(b)* pre-Achilles tendinitis, *(c)* retrocalcaneal bursitis, *(d)* stress fracture, *(e)* calcaneal bursal pain, and *(f)* plantar fasciitis.

Children are susceptible to the same injuries as adults (stress fractures, muscle and tendon injury, ligament strains).[28] The theoretical possibility is that children involved in endurance activities could damage their epiphyses. In our series of over 300 young runners with injuries and the series from two other major running clinics,[4,22] there has not been a documented case of epiphysis damage, ankle angular abnormalities, or growth disturbance from long-distance running.

### HEEL PAIN

Multiple possibilities exist in the diagnosis of heel pain (Fig. 23-2) including overuse or trauma, developmental problems, inflammations, infections, rheumatoid processes, tumor, and neurologic disorders.[23] Many of these can be placed far down on the list in young athletes because they are not associated with the characteristic repetitive stress.

The most prevalent heel injuries include:

- Calcaneal apophysitis (Sever's disease)
- Achilles tendinitis
- Retrocalcaneal bursitis and Achilles bursitis
- Calcaneal stress fracture
- Plantar fasciitis/calcaneal bursitis
- Fat-pad shear syndrome

### Calcaneal apophysitis

Calcaneal apophysitis is the most common etiology of the athlete's heel pain before epiphyseal closure.[23] This entity affects preadolescent athletes, and in our series was rare in children with near apophyseal closure. The average age was 11½ years, with boys affected twice as frequently as girls.

J. W. Sever described a child's inflammatory disorder, not osteochondritis, in the disorder that carries his name.[29] The cause is thought to be injury to Sharpey's fibers at their insertion to the calcaneal apophysis.[1,17] Radiographs are not usually indicated for children with Sever's disease because of variability. The apophysis can be fragmented and lucent to solid. There is no correlation between symptoms and radiographs.[32]

Often the affected child is experiencing a rapid growth spurt and has been in a running sport. Soccer, basketball, gymnastics, and track are the sports most frequently associated with this syndrome.[24] Examination usually shows localized tenderness to compression on the medial and lateral side of the heel without erythema, edema, or skin tenderness. Ankle dorsiflexion may be limited due to pain of activity and decreased Achilles tendon mobility.

Basic treatment is the same as for Achilles tendinitis and should include gastroc-soleus stretching and anterior tibial strengthening. Heel cushions may be indicated. In some children with markedly painful heels, short-term fiberglass casting has been used, followed by an orthosis (Fig. 23-3). Cessation of the running aspect of the sport should occur. In athletes who are actively competing, non–weight-bearing workouts in a swimming pool with a water ski vest have been effective in maintaining fitness. Calcaneal apophysitis is a self-limited process if allowed to become quiescent through rest. In our series 85% of

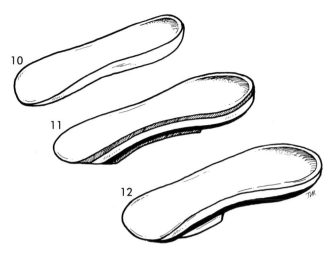

**Fig. 23-3.** Three types of semiflexible orthotic devices: *(10)* routine moldable semiflexible orthosis, *(11)* routine moldable semiflexible orthosis with antifriction sheeting and a small medial post, and *(12)* more rigid semiflexible orthosis with a medial forefoot post.

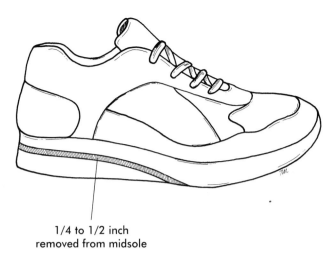

1/4 to 1/2 inch
removed from midsole

**Fig. 23-4.** Negative-heel shoe.

the children were seen only once by a physician before the problem was healed enough to allow a return to activity.

### Achilles tendinitis

Dorsiflexion aggravates the symptoms of Achilles tendinitis. Partial or complete ruptures are rare in the pediatric age group and need not enter into the differential diagnosis unless there has been severe direct trauma. The differential diagnosis does not include plantaris tear or gastric muscle tear, since these occur only rarely, being adult disorders.

Athletes are usually involved in a sport with running or jumping as a component. Physical examination often reveals a pronated foot with tightness of the tendo Achilles. Children with a high, rigid, longitudinal arch rarely have Achilles tendinitis. The problem is most often unilateral. Examining for tendon tightness requires extending the knee, inverting the subtalar joint to neutral, and dorsiflexing the ankle. There is often a 5- to 10-degree difference in ankle dorsiflexion with the heel in full valgus or in a neutral locked position.

Swelling and crepitus may be located 2 to 3 cm above the insertion. Inflammatory reduction entails rest, cold application, antiinflammatory medication, and occasionally physical therapy.

Stretches should be continued for a long period after cessation of symptoms. Rapid bone growth superimposed upon a high level of activity can lead to recurrence of the tight posterior muscle group and return of tendinitis.

A shoe with a rigid forefoot will aggravate a tendency for tendinitis. A negative-heel shoe has been helpful in chronic recurrent tendinitis; these are not commercially available but can be made easily from an old pair of athletic shoes by cutting in the midsole area (Fig. 23-4). This is then worn as an exercise sandal for several hours a day. An off-the-shelf ankle-foot orthosis worn during the night is useful in helping to maintain dorsiflexion while sleeping. If the child has a hypermobile pes planus or shortened tendo Achilles, an orthotic device with support of the longitudinal arch is recommended. This should be semiflexible, made from a thermoplastic material that can be directly molded on the foot. Initially the orthosis can have a small heel lift (1 to 1.5 cm). This should be used for training or competition while the tendo Achilles is tight or if minimal symptoms persist. It can be removed when the child becomes asymptomatic.

### Retrocalcaneal bursitis and Achilles bursitis

The examination, onset of pain, and foot anatomy are similar for retrocalcaneal bursitis and Achilles bursitis. With Achilles bursitis tendon pain is present 2 to 3 cm proximal to the tendon insertion and on the tendon sheath. Palpation of this space produces pain. Swelling or erythema is usually absent. Achilles bursitis pain will be localized approximately 1 cm from the insertion of the tendon and quite lateral superficial.

Lateral radiographs will often show a prominence of the superior angle of the calcaneus. Bursal inflammation in conjunction with this radiograph gave the term *pump bump*. Repetitive motion of the tendo Achilles over the calcaneus (retrocalcaneal bursitis) or pressure of the shoe against the tendon with the prominent bone below it (Achilles bursitis).

Dorsiflexion of the ankle causing tightness of the posterior soft tissues is the mechanical cause that triggers the pain. Limiting maximal dorsiflexion by a heel lift or orthosis can be helpful. Pressure against the tendon should be eliminated by stretching or cutting the heel counter. Surgery to remove the superior angle of the calcaneus or bony prominence is rarely indicated before epiphyseal closure.

### Calcaneal stress fractures

The mechanism of fracture is stress of the plantar fascia on the calcaneus.[6] This action produces calcaneal apophysitis in children instead of a stress fracture, accounting for its low incidence in this age group.

### Plantar fasciitis/calcaneal bursitis

Older children develop plantar fasciitis/calcaneal bursitis associated with running activity. Repetitive stretching of the plantar fascia between its origin on the calcaneus and its insertion on the metatarsal heads is thought to be the cause. Symptoms appear in the following two areas: (1) plantar fasciitis is present along the medial arch at the origin of the abductor hallucis longus muscle (commonly called a *medial arch strain*) and (2) plantar heel pain (calcaneal bursitis) is associated with pain directly under the calcaneus (often called a stone bruise). Dorsiflexion of the great toe tightens the plantar fascia by winding the insertion around the metatarsal head (Windlass effect). This often increases pain at the medial border of the fascia in plantar fasciitis pain.

Physical examination in many of these athletes shows a long arch that is rigid and elevated (cavus foot). Affected children should be in a shoe designed for shock absorption, with a full midsole at the heel. The rigid medial counter , used in antipronation shoes is not needed.

Treatment is directed toward decreasing the pull on the origin of the fascia by limiting the excursion of the fascia by decreasing the longitudinal arch motion. An orthosis can be helpful. Heel cups do not limit motion of the longitudinal arch (pronation) and are not indicated in plantar fasciitis. Heel cups may be indicated in calcaneal bursa-type pain since they act as a cushion over the painful area. An exercise program should include stretching the plantar fascia and tendo Achilles and strengthening the anterior tibial muscles. Oral antiinflammatory medications and physical therapy have been used with limited success in difficult cases.

### Fat-pad shear

Pain in fat-pad shear is diffuse throughout, medial and lateral on the heel, widespread, and not well localized. Pain is exacerbated with weight bearing and relieved with rest and cold applications. The physical examination produces pain when the fat pad is grasped and moved. Fat-pad shear is associated with a high arch and supinated foot.

## MIDFOOT PAIN

Osteochondrosis of the tarsonavicular (Köhler's disease) must be included in the differential diagnosis of children with midfoot pain. Pain along the medial border of the foot is usually a primary symptom. It also can be bilateral, with an onset similar to a juvenile rheumatoid process. Swelling and erythema in association with tenderness at the talonavicular joint and at the navicular cuneiform area are common findings. Trauma or inflammatory diagnoses should be ruled out.

The usual age of onset is between the ages of 3 and 10 years, with a high gender dominance toward boys. Plain radiographs are indicated to confirm the diagnosis. A typical radiograph demonstrates a flattening and patchy ossification of the tarsonavicular with the joint surfaces of the talus and cuneiform preserved.

Etiology of this disorder (as with all osteochondroses) is unknown. Ossification of the tarsonavicular occurs in girls between 1 and 2 years of age and in boys between 2 and 3 years of age. The tarsonavicular is the last of the tarsals to completely ossify.[19] Delayed ossification may be present in a child at age 3 to 4 and may mimic osteochondrosis. Rarely is this a problem in older children because the navicular is fully ossified at the time they begin an organized sport.

Treatment includes immobilization and rest, although long-term results appear equal for casting or arch supports.[8] Pain relief and return to activity is quicker with a short-leg walking cast. The casting period should be for 6 to 12 weeks, and then a semiflexible orthotic device should be used under the talonavicular joint. Those children followed to restoration of bony architecture require approximately 8 to 10 months before the contours of the navicular regain their normal appearance. Poor late results have occurred, necessitating arthrodesis of the talonavicular or triple arthrodesis.[20] Results in this disorder are good, with no decrease in athletic functioning or radiographic changes.

Children can be allowed to return to physical activity when symptoms have subsided and there is progression of ossification. The fact that this presents as a symptomatic pes planus supports the concept that as athletic activities occur, protection of the mediolongitudinal arch is necessary. This should be continued until radiographic restitution and size growth recur. After healing, children may have some secondary symptoms associated with running. They may experience medial tibial pain, medial ankle pain, or medial knee pain. If this continues through adolescence, an orthotic device may be needed for sport activity until total maturity. After maturity, a well-supported antipronation shoe is often recommended.

## FOREFOOT PAIN

Many considerations need to be given in the differential diagnosis of young athletes presenting with forefoot pain. Diagnoses made in the adult population of athletes also may appear in children with open epiphyses.

Differential diagnoses with forefoot pain in young adults include (1) stress fracture; (2) metatarsalagia; (3) Freiberg's disease; (4) arthropathy, infection, or tumor; and (5) sesamoid pain.

The physical examination and history should allow ruling out arthropathies, infections, and tumors; consequently the following discusses only those entities associated with athletic activities.

### Freiberg's disease

The onset of Freiberg's disease most frequently occurs between the ages of 13 and 18, with a predilection for females versus males.[30] Often there is a history of gradually increasing unilateral foot pain — usually associated with weight bearing with sports activity, and later with walking activities.

Usually there is localized tenderness at the metatarsophalangeal (MP) joint of the second toe. Less than one third of the time are symptoms present in a third MP joint and only rarely in the fourth or fifth MP joint.[17] There may be edema and erythema in the area of pain.

**Radiography.** An anteroposterior and lateral x-ray should be obtained. The first radiographic sign of Freiberg's disease is widening of the joint space, which is seen related to the effusion. This can also be present in idiopathic MP synovitis, juvenile rheumatoid arthritis, and collateral ligament injury of the MP joint. Subsequent films should show sclerosis of the rim of bone or some lucency in the subchondral bone. Smillie produced a classification based on the evolutionary process of this disorder. Stage I is a fissure fracture of the epiphysis, usually dorsally. Stages II through IV involve progressive resorption of the necrotic bone with later fracture of the epiphysis. Stage IV is associated with flattening and severe deformity of the metatarsal head (Fig. 23-5).[2,3,9]

The adult form of this disorder is more likely a different entity, being an osteochondral stress fracture.

A hypermobile foot that is repeatedly traumatized can produce intraarticular edema. Helial has a sug-

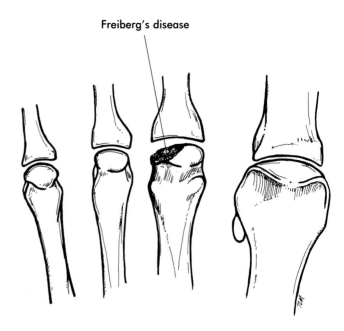

Freiberg's disease

**Fig. 23-5.** Final stage of Freiberg's disease shows degenerative changes and hypertrophic spurring.

gested that persistent edema produces incongruity of joint motion and dorsal impingement. Repetitive microtrauma to the epiphysis in conjunction with decreased blood supply in the articular cartilage of an open physis could produce this problem. These would be the mechanics occurring in an affected child performing running-type activities.

### Treatment

If the process is seen early, in Smillie stages I or II with symptoms of pain and forefoot edema, cessation of sports activity and immobilization are indicated. It is not always possible to stabilize the joint and prevent the disorder from progressing to more advanced stages. When the process is quiescent, it is advisable to use an orthotic device with a metatarsal pad to the MP joint. This should be continued for athletic activities until the epiphysis closes.

Too often athletes arrive in the physician's office after the process has evolved into the later stages. Treatment at this stage is symptomatic with protection.

Surgical treatment is not indicated in children unless symptoms persist after the cessation of activity, failure of conservative treatment, and radiographs showing a fixed stage IV or V. Stage IV is often related to loose bodies present within the joint. The original surgical treatment by Freiberg was simple debridement and removal of loose bodies.[12] The basis for surgical procedure is most frequently an incongruent joint. It is these joint surfaces on the second metatarsal head that produce the pain.

The wide variety of procedures shows a lack of superior results for any specific one. In my opinion the following procedures should not be used in the child athlete: resection of the metatarsal head, resection and joint replacement, or cancellous bone graft—all of which do not appear to have a place in the treatment of young athletes with persistent symptoms.

Resection of the joint surfaces of the proximal phalanx with MP debridement and loose body removal preserves the weight-bearing function of the second metatarsal head and permits good range of motion. A procedure that has not had widespread use but meets the criteria for surgery on a young foot is dorsiflexion osteotomy of the distal metatarsal. This procedure was described in 1979[17] and consists of a dorsally based closing wedge of the metatarsal shaft. The cut is made proximal to the metatarsal head, bringing the healthy plantar articular surface in contact with the proximal phalanx. After healing, loss of MP motion with this has not been excessive for young athletes.[21] Some metatarsal shortening occurs (3 mm maximum). Transfer lesions have not been a problem in a small series.

## STRESS FRACTURES

Fatigue fracture, insufficiency fracture, and exhaustion fracture are some of the terms describing this fracture. The etiology is usually not a single episode but an accumulation of stresses applied to the bone. Continued stresses overcome the elastic resistance of bone and a fracture occurs.[27] Often bone does not completely fracture because pain causes the athlete to stop the activity, with the result that healing occurs. In young athletes stress fractures are usually diaphyseal and rarely epiphyseal. Growth disturbances are rarely a concern, and treatment is aimed at early return to activity.[18]

Stress fractures are sports related, with running sports producing a high number of metatarsal, tibia, and fibula fractures. Fractures of the pelvis and femur are associated with jumping sports, whereas basketball is associated with fractures of the os calcis and pubis.

Radiographic and microscopic confusion between a stress fracture and a tumor in children has been discussed in the literature[7,9] and must be considered in any differential diagnosis of malignancy or infection. Stress fracture, tumor, or infections can be differentiated through magnetic resonance imaging (MRI).[31]

Stress fracture should be an early consideration in a symptomatic child athlete who is engaging in a weight-bearing sport. The most common stress fracture is the second or third metatarsal. Fibular stress fractures usually are present more proximal than in the ankle area. Injury patterns are related to age, with older children experiencing a greater frequency of metatarsal stress fractures than younger children, who experience soft tissue inflammatory problems.

Gradually increasing pain in the region of the fracture is initially present only with activity. Later it is present with any weight-bearing activity. A history of changes in activity intensity, activity frequency, or equipment type often precedes the symptom onset. Physical examination may show swelling in the area of pain. If the onset is less than 10 to 14 days, there may be no radiographic changes. The earliest changes will be minimally ossified callus at the fracture site. Bone scans are not warranted initially in the foot or ankle because the diagnosis can be made as soon as callus forms. Occasionally there is no callus or the diagnosis is in question, and then a bone scan is valuable to decide if treatment should be immobilization or activity limitation. A nondisplaced fracture can be treated with rest and decreased activity, requiring approximately 6 weeks before the child can return to weight-bearing activity. Displacement or severe pain indicates the need for cast immobilization; the recovery period may then be 10 to 12 weeks.

Stress fractures in older adolescent females have been thought to be associated with menstrual abnormalities. This has not been shown to be a directly correlated event, and when fractures occur one must look at the large number of other factors that cause stress fractures.

## Osteochondral talar lesions (osteochondritis dissecans)

The term best applied to this group of problems is *osteochondral talar lesion* rather than *osteochondritis dissecans*. Osteochondral talar lesions appear in child athletes as well as in young adults. There may be many causes, but most authors[1] agree that trauma plays a part. The term *talar transchondral fracture* has been applied to support the idea that trauma is an etiology.[13]

The male-to-female ratio in the nonmilitary population varies from approximately 3:1 to 2:1.[11] A male preponderance is noted as with many other sports injuries. With the increasing involvement of females in sports associated with foot and ankle injuries (volleyball, basketball, gymnastics), this ratio should change.

The locations of the lesions are either lateral anterior or medial posterior in the superior margin of the talus. There exists a 2:1 medial to lateral distribution of the lesions.[24] Experimental studies by Hardy support a traumatic etiology. In an anatomic specimen he reproduced a lateral anterior lesion with inversion and dorsiflexion of the foot and a medial lesion with inversion and plantar flexion. A strong history of trauma is reported in many series.[11,13-16]

Evaluation of children or adolescents with ankle pain must include this disorder in a differential diagnosis. It is not unusual for children with a diagnosis of chronic ankle sprain to later be seen and have an osteochondral lesion. Reported cases[11,13] in which ankles had normal-appearing radiographs later showed an osteochondral lesion.

The physical examination of children with acute osteochondral lesions is similar to that of a ligament injury, with edema, ecchymosis, and limited motion. Absence of localized tenderness over the anterolateral fibular ligament may raise the suspicion of osteochondral lesions instead of ligament injury. In chronic ankle pain symptoms and signs may be identical to chronic ligament instability with activity-related stiffness that improves with rest. There may also be a deep nonlocalizing aching sensation. Locking is a rare symptom. Gould has stated, "There are not pathognomonic signs or symptoms."[11] Therefore it is not possible to make the diagnosis with only a history and physical examination. Specific radiographs should be taken when an osteochondral lesion is suspected. A mortise view with the foot in full plantar flexion will bring the medial posterior lesions into view. Bringing the foot to neutral or dorsiflexion will better visualize a lateral anterior lesion on the mortise view.

## GRADING

A bone scan is a highly sensitive tool and may be indicated as a screening device before CT, MR, or arthroscopy are used. In some studies bone scans have been extremely sensitive.[10,25]

The CT scan is probably less useful than MRI in that its ability to separate stages I, II, and III is limited because there is not a free fragment.[11] MRI is a more useful tool not only because of less radiation exposure but also because of an ability to grade the lesions in a clinically relevant manner.

The Berndt-Hardy classification of these lesions is based on standard radiographs. The system defined as grade I is a depressed chondral fracture with overlying articular cartilage intact. The MR scan shows this as an intact cartilage with signal changes.

Grade II is an osteochondral fragment that is discrete, attached to bone, with a rent in the overlying articular cartilage. The MRI study shows a high signal break of the cartilage.

Grade III is a detached fragment that may have some overlying articular cartilage. This is definable on MRI with a high signal rim extending behind the fragment, indicating synovial fluid around the loose piece.

Grade IV is a displaced fragment. This shows a mixed or low signal on MRI in the center of a loose body.[25] The MR scan is least sensitive in identifying the grade IV lesion since the loose body may be entirely nonreactive. For this reason, good plain radiographs are needed.

Treatment for a lesion in a child can be nonoperative for a longer period than in an adult.[11,15] Good results have been obtained with plaster immobilization followed by physiotherapy, orthosis, or ankle support. Reports with a higher failure rate of nonoperative treatment included an increased number of adults.

The stage of an osteochondral lesion provides insight as to where the process is at that particular time. This may be an evolutionary process with a stage I lesion developing to a stage IV lesion and producing a loose body. For that reason, symptomatic grade I or II lesions with failure of conservative measures should have surgical treatment. One can usually predict what course of treatment is reasonable. A grade I lesion can usually be treated conservatively. If symptoms are present in a grade II lesion, it needs to be drilled. Grade III lesions need some type of fixation, and grade IV lesions need removal of the loose body and debridement of the crater.

Arthroscopy has changed the treatment process in this entity. One must be aware that the size of the instrument and the space available in a smaller child's ankle may make this a difficult procedure. In a child a well-performed arthrotomy heals better with better results than an "arthroscraping, traumatic arthroscope" procedure. Numerous articles are available regarding the approach to an osteochondral lesion through an arthroscope.[11,26] Generally a lateral lesion can be easily approached through an arthroscope. A medial posterior lesion may be better approached through an arthrotomy. Osteotomy of the medial malleolus in a child to approach the posterior lesion is not recommended.

## REFERENCES

1. Andrish JT: *Overuse syndrome of the lower extremity in youth sports*, Champaign, Ill, 1984, Human Kinetics.
2. Angermann P, Jensen P: Osteochondritis dissecans of the talus: long term results of surgical treatment, *Foot Ankle* 10:, 1989.
3. Boileau RA: *Advance in pediatric sports*, Champaign, Ill, 1984, Human Kinetics.
4. Brody D: Washington, DC, Runners Clinic, Personal communication, 1985.
5. DeHaven K: Athletic injuries in adolescents, *Pediatr Ann* 7:704, 1978.
6. Devas MB: Compression stress fractures in man and the greyhound, *J Bone Joint Surg* 43B:545, 1961.
7. Devas MB: Stress fractures in children, *J Bone Joint Surg* 45B:528, 1963.
8. Devine KM: Kohlers osteochondrosis of the tarsal navicular, case report with twenty-eight year follow up, *South Dakota Gen Med* 42:5, 1989.

9. Engh CA et al: Stress fractures in children, *J Trauma* 10:532, 1970.

10. Fisher C: Report from 16th annual meeting American Orthopaedic Society for Sports Medicine, Sun Valley, Idaho, 1991, *Orthop News* 13:3, 1991.

11. Flick AB, Gould N: Osteochondritis dissecans of the talus (transchondral fractures of the talus): review of the literature and new surgical approach for medial dome lesions, *Foot Ankle* 5:165, 1985.

12. Freiberg AH: Infarction of the second metatarsal bone, *Surg Gynecol Obstet* 19:191, 1914.

13. Alexander AH, Lichtman DM: Surgical treatment of transchondral talar-dome fracture (osteochondritis dissecans) long term follow-up, *J Bone Joint Surg* 62A:646, 1980.

14. Berndt AL, Harty M: Transchondral fractures (osteochondritis dissecans) of the talus, *J Bone Joint Surg* 41A:998, 1959.

15. Canale ST, Belding RH: Osteochondral lesions of the talus, *J Bone Joint Surg* 62A:97, 1982.

16. Fisher AGJ: A study of loose bodies composed of cartilage and bone occurring in joints with special reference to their pathology and etiology, *Br J Surg* 8:493, 1920-1921.

17. Gregg J, Das M: Foot and ankle problems in the preadolescent and adolescent athlete, *Clin Sports Med* 1:131, 1982.

18. Harvard JS: Overuse syndromes in young athletes, *Pediatr Clin North Am* 29:585, 1982.

19. Ippolito PT, Pollini R, Falez R: Kohler's disease of the tarsal navicular: Long term follow-up of 12 cases, *J Pediatr Orthop* 4:416, 1984.

20. Jahss M: *Disorders of the foot*, Philadelphia, 1982, WB Saunders.

21. Kinnard P, Lirette R: Dorsiflexion osteotomy in Freiberg's disease, *Foot Ankle J* 9:226, 1989.

22. McBride A: Charlotte NC, Runners Clinic, Personal communication, 1985.

23. Micheli LJ et al: Prevention and management of calcaneal apophysitis in children, *J Pediatr Orthop* 7:34, 1987.

24. Micheli LJ: Overuse injuries in childrens sports, the growth factor, *Orthop Clin North Am* 14:337, 1980.

25. Nelson DW et al: Osteochondritis dissecans of the talus and knee: prospective comparison of MR and arthroscopic classification, *J Comput Assist Tomogr* 14:804, 1990.

26. Parisien J, Serge MD: Arthroscopic treatment of osteochondral lesions of the talus, *Am J Sports Med* 14:211, 1986.

27. Pentecost RL: Fatigue, insufficiency and pathologic fractures, *JAMJ* 187:1001, 1964.

28. Rowland TW: Characteristics of child distance runners, *Physician Sports Med* 13:45, 1985.

29. Sever JW: Apophysitis of the os calcis, *N Y Med J* 95:1025, 1912.

30. Smillie IPS: Freiberg infarction, *J Bone Joint Surg* 147:553, 1957.

31. Stafford SA et al: MRI in stress fractures, *Am J Radiol* 147:553, 1986.

32. Shopfner CE, Coim CC: Effect of weight bearing on the appearance and development of the secondary calcaneal epiphysis, *Radiology* 86:201, 1966.

33. Wilkins KE: The uniqueness of the young athlete, musculoskeletal injuries, *Am J Sports Med* 8:377, 1980.

# Chapter 24

# Foot and ankle injuries in the female athlete

**Laura A. Mitchell**

Are foot and ankle injuries in the female athlete gender-specific or sports-specific? How does conditioning and training affect injury rates in female athletes? Only in the last several decades has research in sports medicine provided answers to these questions.

Before the 1970s women were not allowed to compete in long-distance running events because they were considered physiologically unsuited for such a high-demand activity. Katherine Switzer challenged the status quo in 1967 when she entered the Boston Marathon as a "K. Switzer." Officials tried to remove her bodily from the race, but she managed to run past them to a successful finish. In 1972 female athletes competed legitimately in the marathon for the first time.[19]

The enactment of Title IX of the Federal Educational Amendments of 1972 provided a major stimulus to women's participation in interscholastic sports.[19] The 1970s found female participation in athletic activities dramatically increased, and sports medicine experts began to examine gender-specific injury rates.

Early research on injuries among female athletes participating in professional and interscholastic sports found the injury rate of the female athlete was consistently higher than her male counterparts.[14,26] However, careful follow-up studies illustrate that the injury rate is sports-specific and with proper conditioning, female sports injury rates are similar to those of male athletes.[3,18]

But having stated the case for proper and adequate conditioning to prevent athletic injuries in both sexes, we are still left with the question as to whether female athletes are more likely to sustain certain injuries than are male athletes. Anthropometric studies provide raw data upon which some general statements can be made regarding anatomic differences between men and women. For example, men have relatively longer bones, with their lower extremities representing 56% of their total height, as compared with 51% in females.[11] This gives male athletes a mechanical advantage in sports that require striking, hitting, or kicking, since their longer bones act as better levers to generate greater force. Females have wider pelvises and greater genu valgus than males, which, combined with their shorter lower extremities, gives them a lower center of gravity, a distinct advantage in balance sports such as gymnastics.[11] Males must widen their stance to achieve the same degree of balance. Consequently the balance beam is an important gymnastics event for women but not even a part of men's gymnastics competition. Women also tend to have more mobile joints than men, which makes them more flexible and becomes another advantage in gymnastic activities. On the other hand, greater varus of the hips in the female and greater valgus angle of the legs at the knee may contribute to the slightly higher percentage of lower-extremity overuse syndromes in unconditioned female athletes.[11]

Women also have a weaker musculoskeletal system than men, with *less* muscle mass and *more* fat per body weight. (The muscle mass of females is approximately 23% of body weight, whereas equally trained males have approximately 40% muscle mass.[14]) The lower percentage of muscle mass handicaps the female athlete, who is unable to achieve the same power or speed as her male counterparts. However, the increased percentage of body fat in females becomes an advantage in long-distance swimming events in natural waters since it provides insulation and buoyancy.[14] It is no coincidence that a female, Penny Dean, holds the speed record for swimming the English Channel. Dean achieved the best one-way time of 7 hours and 40 minutes in 1978.[11]

Physiologic differences in female athletes place them at a slightly greater risk for stress fractures. Menstrual irregularities, sometimes caused by excessive exercise, can lead to decreased bone density, which in turn can predispose an athlete to stress fractures.[16] Although the etiology of decreased bone density is not absolutely clear, it is believed to be secondary to such factors as excessive weight loss, low body fat, and loss of hormonal estrogen stimulation.

In addition to the anatomical and physiological distinctions that pose particular risks for female athletes, other sports-specific injuries are known to occur more frequently among women for the simple reason that there are more women participating in these activities. The explosion of aerobic dance studios, which attract mainly women, is a prime example.[7]

Finally, a word must be added about footwear. Many of the forefoot problems seen in women are either caused by or exacerbated by ill-fitting shoes. Frequent wearing of high-heeled shoes leads to tight Achilles tendons and resultant heel varus, predisposing the recreational athlete to lateral ligament sprain.[10]

Lateral ligament sprain of the ankle is probably the single most common injury seen in sports activities among both men and women.[7] Kirby et al found a 27% incidence of ankle sprains in female gymnasts.[13] Because ankle sprains are so common among both male and female athletes, and because the treatment is discussed in great detail in Chapter 11, we will not concentrate on that here. However, in dealing with lateral ligament sprains in female athletes, extra attention must be paid to heelcord stretching during rehabilitation. Proprioceptive retraining and peroneal strengthening are critical in conditioning and rehabilitation regardless of the athlete's sex.

Athletic injuries tend to be more sports-specific than gender-specific; however, certain foot and ankle injuries are seen more frequently in female athletes. The reasons for this involve a variety of factors: improper footwear, anatomic or physiologic risk factors peculiar to females, and the higher ratio of female participants in the activity. In addition to ankle sprains, the other areas of frequent foot and ankle injury in female athletes are ankle impingement syndromes, posterior tibial tendinitis, bunions, and stress fractures.

## ANKLE IMPINGEMENT SYNDROMES

Ankle impingement syndromes are seen with some frequency in several sports including gymnastics and dance, which have a high proportion of female participants. These athletes work at the extremes of flexibility. As an example, impingement of the anterior ankle capsule frequently occurs in gymnasts when landing short on dismounts.[10] This hyperdorsiflexion injury presents with pain along the anterior joint line, usually without ankle effusion. The jumping demands of ice skating and diving place these athletes at risk for anterior ankle impingement as well.

In the acute phase the symptoms are treated with ice, antiinflammatory medications, and rest. Physical therapy modalities to maintain flexibility and strength are critical. A large protective pad taped anteriorly will mechanically block the ankle from extreme dorsiflexion upon return to activity.

Persistence of the anterior joint line pain upon full dorsiflexion, sometimes accompanied by swelling or popping, may require operative treatment. The hypertrophied anteroinferior tibiofibular ligament or anterior spurs may cause damage to the articular surface of the anterior talar dome. Arthroscopic debridement of the thickened ligament or spurs with chondroplasty of the articular surface injury, followed by aggressive ankle rehabilitation will relieve the symptoms of anterior impingement (see Case Studies 1 and 2).

**Case Study 1.** The patient had played soccer as a fullback for 14 years. She had suffered persistent anterior joint line pain and clicking with dorsiflexion 5 months following an inversion sprain. She had been taped and braced to finish the season. An aggressive rehabilitation program failed to relieve her symptoms. There was a palpable swelling and a click that elicited sharp pain as the ankle was moved passively from a plantar-flexed position into full dorsiflexion. Stress views failed to demonstrate significant talar tilt, and no subchondral irregularities or spurring were present.

Arthroscopic treatment of the impingement syndrome included removal of the articular surface flap on the anterolateral talar dome with abrasion arthroplasty of the defect and debridement of the hypertrophied anteroinferior tibiofibular ligament. At 4 weeks postoperatively, following an aggressive ankle rehabilitation program and resolution of the painful click, the patient was able to resume full dorsiflexion activities (Fig. 24-1).

Posterior impingement syndromes occur following plantar flexion injury to the posterior tibiotalar joint.[24] The injury may occur acutely with forceful plantar flexion that includes sudden deceleration or on a chronic basis in those sports where activity is performed on the plantar-flexed ankle. Ballerinas, for example, are at high risk for posterior

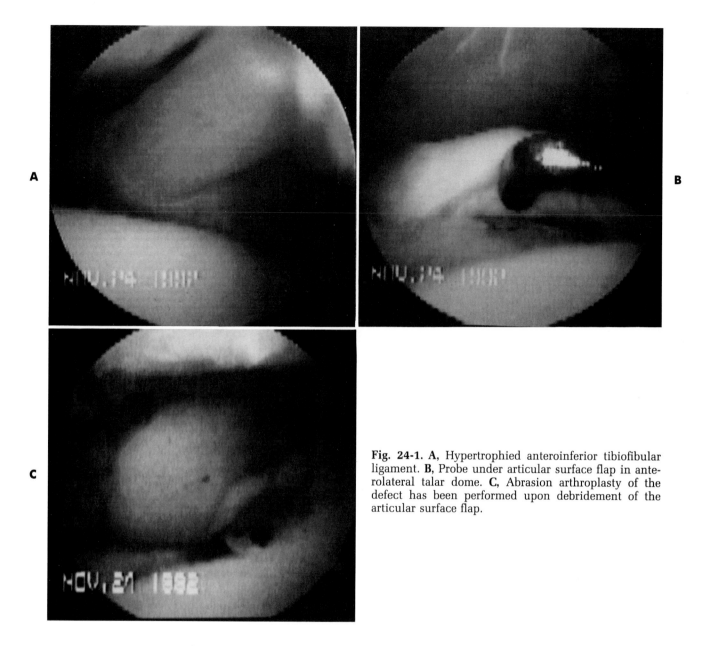

**Fig. 24-1. A,** Hypertrophied anteroinferior tibiofibular ligament. **B,** Probe under articular surface flap in anterolateral talar dome. **C,** Abrasion arthroplasty of the defect has been performed upon debridement of the articular surface flap.

impingement syndromes. The hyperextended position of the ankle demanded for pointe work may cause osteochondral loose bodies in the posterior tibiotalar joint[8] or make an incidental os trigonum highly symptomatic. Locking episodes and inability to weight bear in the plantar-flexed position may necessitate surgical removal.

**Case Study 2.** A 15-year-old Spanish dancer had a 3-month history of severe posterior ankle pain that made it impossible for her to dance on her plantar-flexed right foot. She had stopped dancing completely for 1 month. When she resumed practice, the posterior ankle pain returned. Her x-rays showed an os trigonum bilaterally, but only the symptomatic side had intense uptake posteriorly on the bone scan.

Posterior arthrotomy with excision of the separated fragment, followed by an aggressive ankle rehabilitation program specific to dance, allowed her to return to her Spanish dancing at 6 weeks postoperatively (Fig. 24-2).

## POSTERIOR TIBIAL TENDINITIS

As discussed earlier in this chapter, particular characteristics of female anatomy put women at higher risk than men for certain types of foot and ankle injuries. For example, the wider female pelvis is responsible for the relatively greater genu valgum and the resultant greater Q-angle, which places females at greater risk for malalignment syndromes. To compensate for the genu valgum, relatively greater pronation is necessary to maintain a plantigrade position. (Pronation is a combination of hindfoot eversion, forefoot dorsiflexion, and forefoot abduction.) It is no

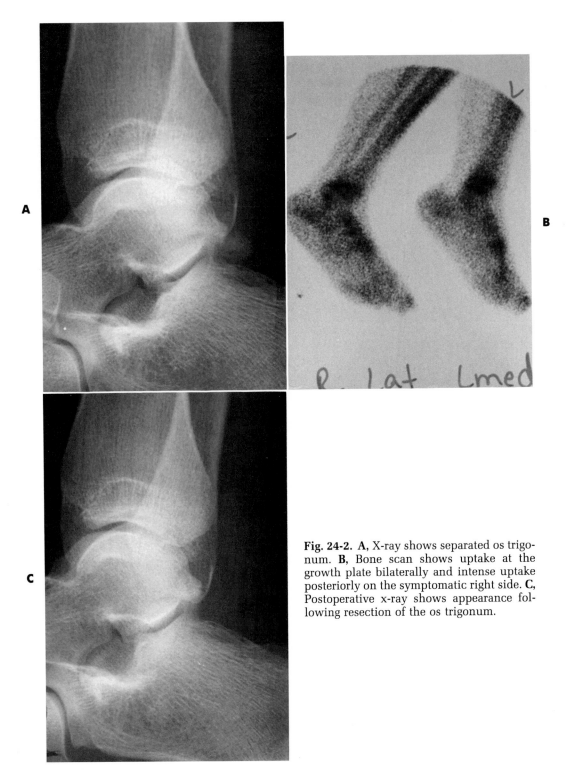

**Fig. 24-2. A,** X-ray shows separated os trigonum. **B,** Bone scan shows uptake at the growth plate bilaterally and intense uptake posteriorly on the symptomatic right side. **C,** Postoperative x-ray shows appearance following resection of the os trigonum.

coincidence that chronic posterior tibial tendinitis is more common in females who tend to be more symptomatic when hyperpronation exists.[12] Lack of strength in the female foot and ankle also may be a contributing factor.[23] A medial sole and heel wedge should be used if significant hyperpronation is present.

Female athletes with hyperpronation who are involved in running sports are at special risk for developing the insertional form of posterior tibial tendinitis. The condition usually is associated with an accessory navicular, and pain is located near the posterior tibial tendon insertion at the medial aspect of the navicular bone. Conservative treatment consists

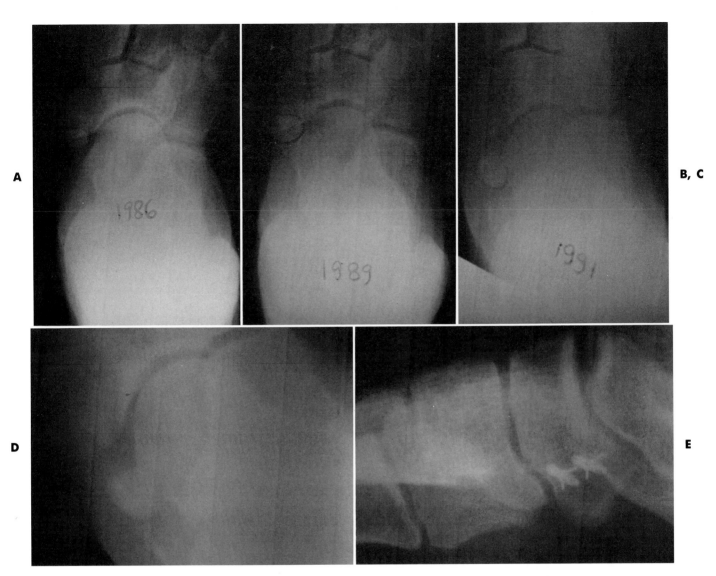

**Fig. 24-3. A,** Radiographic appearance of the accessory navicular in 1986. **B,** Radiographic appearance of the accessory navicular in 1989. **C,** Proximal migration of the accessory navicular is obvious on 1991 radiograph. **D,** Preoperative external oblique view of proximal migration of accessory navicular. **E,** Postoperative x-ray of a modified Kidner procedure with suture anchor technique. (Courtesy of Franchesca Thompson, M.D.)

of rest, intermittent ice massage, antiinflammatory medications, orthotic devices, and stretching of the Achilles and posterior tibial tendons. If conservative treatment fails after a prolonged period, surgery may be considered. With insertional tendinitis, excision of the accessory navicular may be performed. If significant tendon disruption occurs, a tendon transfer using the flexor digitorum longus may be indicated (see Case Study 3).

**Case Study 3.** An 18-year-old female college freshman had a 5-year history of left midfoot pain associated with high school and collegiate sports. Over the years the pain had been managed with cast immobilization, antiinflammatory

medications, and relative rest—all standard treatment modalities for insertional posterior tibial tendinitis. X-rays taken over the course of her treatment documented the accessory navicular bone, which migrated proximally (Fig. 24-3).

After 5 years of conservative management, the patient was treated operatively with a modification of the Kidner procedure. The accessory navicular was excised, and the posterior tibial tendon was advanced three quarters of an inch and attached to the medial osteotomized surface of the navicular with two heavy suture anchors. Postoperative management included 4 weeks of casting in inversion and equinus followed by 4 weeks of a weight-bearing short-leg cast. Aggressive rehabilitation started at 2 months postoperatively. Follow-up at 5 months after surgery found this young female athlete free from pain and able to participate in all sports without symptoms for the first time in years.

## BUNIONS

Bunions are a much greater problem among female athletes than among male athletes, just as they are a much greater problem for women in general than for men. In addition, a recent study found that the majority of women wore shoes that were too small for their feet and had not had their feet measured in over 5 years.[6] The primary cause is the design of women's shoes including athletic shoes, which are generally cut more narrowly in the forefoot than men's. This can lead to pressure over the medial side of the metatarsophalangeal (MP) joint of the great toe, eventually giving rise to the inflamed and painful swelling known as a bunion. Bony hypertrophy of the metatarsal head with an inflamed bursa accompanies the valgus deviation of the hallux. Shoes with elevated heels transfer even more pressure to the forefoot and should be avoided altogether when symptomatic hallux valgus exists.

Conservative treatment of bunions includes wearing protective pads to avoid direct pressure on the inflamed area. Taping the metatarsal joint for competition will give the hallux additional support.

If pain persists, bunionectomy can be considered for certain athletes, but great care must be taken to avoid altering foot mechanics. Some bunion procedures result in a shortening of the first ray, which increases stress on the second metatarsal head and may lead to stress fractures or metatarsalgia. It is critical to preserve proper functioning of the sesamoids, short flexor ligament, and abductor muscles since these maintain stability and flexibility in the first MP joint. The metatarsal head should not be displaced in a dorsiflexed or plantar-flexed position or balance across the metatarsal heads will be lost.

When considering a bunion procedure for an athlete, one should be aware of the increased amount of force—up to 250% of body weight—that can be generated by running activities.[17] Range of motion of the MP joint of the great toe can increase as much as 50% during running. If an osteotomy is performed in the proximal metatarsal, dorsal plantar angulation must be maintained to avoid transfer metatarsalgia.

Symptomatic bunion deformities have been treated successfully by the distal chevron type of osteotomy.[15] The procedure can be performed with minimal joint dissection and does not significantly alter foot mechanics in middle-distance and long-distance runners. Sprinters and ballet dancers are in another category, however. Their activities put increased demand on the extremes of MP joint motion

and, as a result, bunion surgery is not recommended (see Case Study 4).

**Case Study 4.** A 30-year-old female world-class middle-distance runner had a history of severe hallux valgus and metatarsus varus of the right foot. The bunion deformity on the medial aspect of the distal first metatarsal was becoming progressively more painful. She also had developed some migration of the second, third, and fourth toes laterally with subluxation of the second MP joint dorsally and nerve impingement between the second and third metatarsals. Conservative measures were not successful in relieving her symptoms, and frequent injections of cortisone were required to enable her to run. Consequently the following procedure was performed on an inpatient basis under regional anesthetic block: (1) chevron bunionectomy with osteotomy of the first metatarsal of the right foot; (2) removal of the neuroma between the second and third metatarsals; and (3) capsulotomy of the second toe to correct the second MP joint subluxation.

The patient was running at 8 weeks postoperatively. She was back at full training at 6 months and experiencing no symptoms or neuritic foot pain at 2 years postoperatively. The great toe and lesser toes were in good alignment. In the intervening time she had placed fourth in Olympic trials in European track meets and went on to break her personal record for middle-distance events (Fig. 24-4).

## STRESS FRACTURES

Stress fractures are focal structural weaknesses occurring during the bone remodeling response to repeated cyclic applications of subthreshold stresses to the bone microstructure. They occur when the rate of bone destruction from the activity is greater than the rate of bone formation. This was illustrated well in the survey of injury rates in female cadets at West Point, which showed a 10% increase in stress fractures over males during the early training weeks at the Academy. This finding was attributed to lack of conditioning and proper training techniques in the female cadets.[21] One could hypothesize that after years of training, athletes would have strong bones and be less susceptible to stress fractures. However, even in high-performance athletes, intrinsic bone weakness or mechanical alignment abnormalities can pose risks for them. In addition, other factors such as training surfaces, footwear, training variations, or temporary inactivity can predispose even well-conditioned athletes to injury.

Female athletes are more likely to have lower dietary calcium intake and lower bone density than male athletes, therefore making them more susceptible to stress fractures. Lower bone density often is linked to menstrual irregularities such as exercise-induced amenorrhea, which may result from excessive weight loss, low body fat, and loss of hormonal estrogen stimulation.[5] Females who initiate running

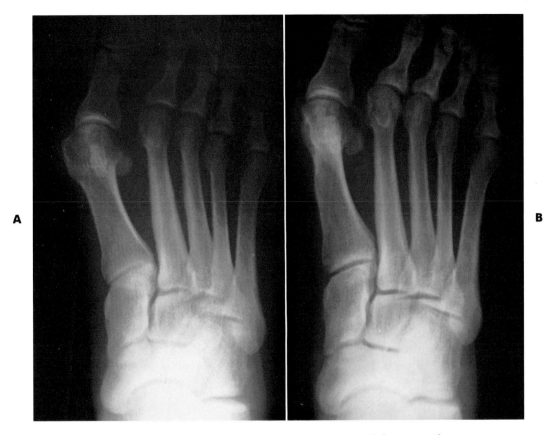

**Fig. 24-4. A,** Preoperative radiograph shows the hallux valgus deformity with a prominent medial eminence and significant sesamoid subluxation. **B,** Postoperative radiograph 2 years later shows good alignment of the hallux without significant changes in the MP joint. (Courtesy of Donald E. Baxter, M.D.)

before menarche may have delayed menarche and be at a higher risk for exercise-induced amenorrhea. The relationship between low bone density secondary to amenorrhea and stress fractures has significant implications for female runners, 50% of whom suffer from some type of menstrual irregularity.[1] Oral contraceptives, which provide a type of estrogen therapy, offer some protective effect by helping to maintain or increase bone density.[2]

Patients with stress fractures in the foot or ankle may present varied histories. Often they report a recent increase or change in a sports activity. They may have experienced pain in the injured area for weeks or months but at a level mild enough to enable them to continue their participation. There also may be mild swelling but again not prominent enough to cause alarm. Exquisite point tenderness at the location of a stress fracture is often pathognomonic. Radiographs may not be helpful at the onset of symptoms because it can take 3 to 4 weeks for changes to occur in the metaphyseal area of bone and 4 to 6 weeks for them to occur in the diaphysis.

Stress fractures in the forefoot have been reported at the base of the proximal phalanx of the great toe in athletes with hallux valgus[25] and in ballet dancers at the base of the second metatarsal at Lisfranc's joint. In the en pointe position force is concentrated on the first and second rays and, as the load is transferred proximally, Lisfranc's joint at the recessed base of the second metatarsal is relatively rigid and bears most of the stress[4,22] (see Case Study 5).

**Case Study 5.** A 23-year-old female aerobics enthusiast was employed as a personal trainer at an exercise club. She also instructed aerobics classes several times a week. She presented with a 2-week history of pain in her left foot and recalled an injury 1 week before the onset of pain, when a student stepped on the top of her foot. On further questioning, she admitted to having mild discomfort before this. It should be noted that she did an unusual amount of jumping in her profession.

Physical examination revealed tenderness along the second metatarsal with some mild swelling. There was an area of focal tenderness one third of the distance of the second metatarsal from the base and some tightness of the capsule of the second MP joint. She had a prominent hallux valgus deformity.

The x-rays revealed a prominent hallux valgus with metatarsus varus and a faint amount of callus along the tibial side of the second metatarsal near the base. She was

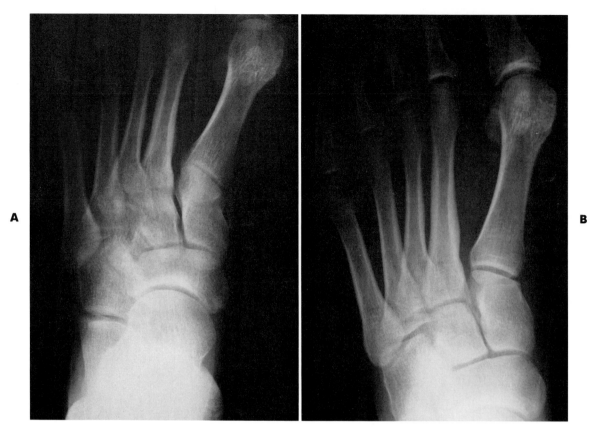

**Fig. 24-5. A,** Faint periosteal new bone along the tibial side of the second metatarsal base. **B,** Healed stress fracture at the base of the second metatarsal.

treated for a stress fracture at the base of the second metatarsal with orthotics, metatarsal pads, and taping and was advised to limit her activities. One month later her x-rays confirmed healing callus at the base of the second metatarsal. She returned to high-impact aerobics after several months (Fig. 24-5).

## SUMMARY

For any athlete, male or female, proper conditioning is a critical element in guarding against injuries to the foot and ankle. Female athletes should be particularly sensitive to the fit, support, and comfort of footwear and wear protective pads if needed. Female runners and other female athletes who are at risk for stress fractures should be evaluated and treated for amenorrhea. Although anatomic and physiologic differences between males and females may put female athletes at a disadvantage for activities that call for great strength and force, they present advantages for balance (gymnastics events) and endurance (long-distance swimming).

## ACKNOWLEDGEMENTS

I wish to thank Mary Oertel-Kirschner for her technical support.

## REFERENCES

1. Barrow GW, Saha S: Menstrual irregularity and stress fractures in collegiate female distance runners, *Am J Sports Med* 16:209, 1988.
2. Carbon R et al: Bone density of elite female athletes with stress fractures, *Med J Aust* 153:373, 1990.
3. Cox JS, Lenz HW: Women midshipmen in sports, *Am J Sports Med* 12:241, 1984.
4. Eisele SA, Sammarco GJ: *Fatigue fractures of the foot and ankle in the athlete.* In *AAOS Instructional Course Lectures,* vol 42, Park Ridge, Ill, 1993, American Academy of Orthopaedic Surgeons.
5. Fitch KD: Stress fracture of the lower limbs in runners, *Aust Fam Physician* 13:511, 1984.
6. Frey C et al: American Orthopedic Foot and Ankle Society women's shoe survey, *Foot Ankle* 14:78, 1993.
7. Garrick JG, Requa RK: The epidemiology of foot and ankle injuries in sports, *Clin Sports Med* 7:29, 1988.
8. Gelabert R: Preventing dancers injuries, *Physician Sports Med,* 8:67, 1980.
9. Haycock CE, Gillette JV: Susceptibility of women athletes to injury—myths vs. reality, *JAMA* 236:163, 1976.
10. Hunter LV: Women's athletics—the orthopedic viewpoint, *Clin Sports Med* 3:801, 1984.
11. Hunter-Griffen L, editor: *The female athlete.* In *Athletic training and sports medicine,* ed 2, Park Ridge, Ill, 1991, American Academy of Orthopaedic Surgeons.

12. Jahss MT: *Tendon disorders of the foot and ankle.* In *Disorders of the foot and ankle,* ed 2, vol 2, Philadelphia, 1991, WB Saunders.

13. Kirby RL et al: Flexibility and musculoskeletal symptomatology in female gymnasts and age matched controls, *Am J Sports Med* 9:160, 1981.

14. Klafs C, Leyon M: *The female athlete,* ed 2, St Louis, 1978, CV Mosby.

15. Lillich JS, Baxter DE: Bunionectomies and related surgery in the elite female middle distance and marathon runner, *Am J Sports Med* 14:491, 1982.

16. Lloyd T: Women athletes with menstrual irregularities have increased musculoskeletal injuries, *Med Sci Sports Exer* 18:374, 1986.

17. Mann RA: *Biomechanics of the foot and ankle.* In Mann RA, editor: *Surgery of the foot,* ed 5, St Louis, 1986, CV Mosby.

18. Meeuwiese WH, Fowler PJ: Frequency and predictability of sports injuries in intercollegiate athletes, *Can J Sports Sci* 13:35, 1988.

19. Melpomene Institute, editor: *Should ladies be active.* In *The bodywise woman,* New York, 1990, Prentice-Hall.

20. Protzman R: Physiologic performance of women compared to men, *Am J Sports Med* 7:191, 1979.

21. Protzman R, Griffis G: Stress fractures in men and women undergoing military training, *J Bone Joint Surg* 59:825, 1977.

22. Sammarco GT, Miller ET: Forefoot conditions in dancers, *Foot Ankle* 3:85, 1982.

23. Schafle MD: The child dancer—medical considerations, *Pediat Clin North Am* 37:1211, 1990.

24. Veazey BL et al: Excision of ununited fracture of the posterior process of the talus—a treatment for chronic posterior ankle pain, *Foot Ankle* 13:453, 1992.

25. Yukoe M: Stress fracture of the proximal phalanx of the great toe—a report of three cases, *Am J Sports Med* 14:240, 1986.

26. Zelisko JA et al: A comparison of men's and women's professional basketball injuries, *Am J Sports Med* 10:297, 1982.

# Chapter 25

# Treatment of the elite athlete

**Donald E. Baxter**

Elite athletes are special (Fig. 25-1). They require special treatment, keeping in mind world-class performance. Some athletes are treated differently depending on the level of activity. For example, a high school athlete would be treated more conservatively with prolonged inactivity, whereas a runner who has a chance to make the Olympic team and has a synovial impingement in the ankle or plica in the knee might have more invasive treatments.

There are policies and principles that are considered in treating high-level athletes. Most athletes need only a boost or a little help since their training and motivation is adequate. An athlete needs minimal assistance in removing minor barriers.

## KNOW THE ATHLETE

Know the athlete's event and personality. Perform a careful history and a physical examination, including a functional examination. This examination might be performed on a track while the athlete is running.

Once a 19-year-old runner described discomfort in his foot on the second lap of an 800-m run. A functional examination revealed a talonavicular spur irritating the deep peroneal nerve on the dorsum of the foot. A procedure to remove the bone spur using a regional anesthetic allowed this athlete to function at a world-class level. Eighteen months later he won an Olympic gold medal. By knowing the athlete, event, and by taking a careful history and performing a functional examination, the physician was able to provide that minor boost needed for world-class performance.

## DO APPROPRIATE TESTS

An x-ray may not identify an early stress fracture of the navicular bone or an interosseous stress fracture of the talus. The bone scan will differentiate soft tissue from bone pathology with a computed tomographic (CT) scan or magnetic resonance imaging (MRI) being more specific. MRI will delineate tendon abnormalities such as differentiating between peritendinitis and tendinosis. The CT scan is more specific for bone fractures but not as good for soft tissue lesions.

These tests are expensive, so an experienced examiner with a good history and physical examination may avoid the need for expensive tests. An example of this principle would be a professional defensive football player with pain at the insertion of the Achilles tendon. A lateral x-ray of the os calcis showed no fracture. A bone scan was positive, and a CT scan showed the outline of a stress fracture of the superior posterior os calcis, which could potentially avulse with the Achilles tendon. This football player needed immobilization and rest. Playing football with this injury would be dangerous and potentially threaten his career.

## TEAM TREATMENT FOR THE ELITE ATHLETE

The athlete needs a coach, a trainer, a physical therapist, a physician, and occasionally a psychologist and a nutritionist.

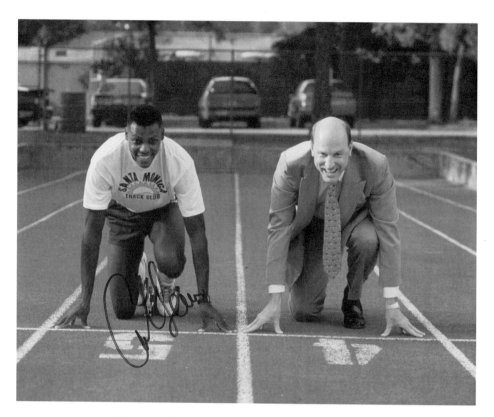

**Fig. 25-1.** Elite athlete (Carl Lewis) and physician.

Many great athletes are more concerned with appropriate diet, stretching, massage, and training than with repair of an unstable ligament. Only when conservative modalities fail does the athlete seek out more invasive treatment and evaluation.

It is important to know when the athlete needs to return to the trainer or physical therapist and when the timing is right for diagnostic testing or surgery.

### FIRST THINGS SHOULD BE CONSIDERED FIRST

After a history, physical examination and, when necessary, diagnostic studies, consider treatment options. These include changes of the surface, shoes, and orthoses. In addition, it includes correcting nutritional imbalances, training errors (overtraining often is the problem), inappropriate amounts of rest, inadequate stretching, or inadequate strength training. Also consider whether the athlete has done sufficient cross-training.

The American record holder in the 10,000-m on the road competition needed a lightweight orthosis that did not cut into his metatarsals. He had previously worn a rigid orthosis that caused neuritic pains in the plantar metatarsals. It was also a heavy orthosis that kept him from performing at his maximal capabilities. A famous baseball pitcher with recurrent hamstring tears and injuries needed to stretch his hamstring for 20 seconds seven times a day to avoid recurring injuries.

### RELATIVE REST IS IMPORTANT

There are various degrees of rest. Cross-training allows rest of gravity-affected muscles, tendons, and bones. For example, a sprinter ran in the pool using a flotation vest and a rope for resistance. This was used while recovering from a knee injury. He set the world record in 100 m 6 months later.

Training can be decreased. A cast-brace or a cast may be needed for short periods. Training can be changed using fewer sprints and a softer grass surface.

### TREAT THE ATHLETE EARLY AND VIGOROUSLY

Certain injuries need immediate attention. The navicular stress fracture needs a non–weight-bearing cast for 5 weeks when first detected. The medial malleolar stress fracture needs early immobilization. The temptation is to run through injuries or fractures. It is important to know which fractures need immediate attention.

One runner on the world-record 400-m relay team presented with a tender medial malleolus. The whole team was present when the diagnosis was given. A CT scan of the ankle revealed a medial malleolar stress fracture, which required 5 weeks in a cast and no hard training for 3 months. The team had to find a replacement for his interval of the relay.

## MINIMIZE SURGERY AND MAXIMIZE RECOVERY

Be a minimalist when it comes to surgery. Know the anatomy. Operate only in the exact area of pathology and only release part of the fascia or sheath when possible. Try to do anatomic repairs and not tendon transfers.

For example, if conservative treatment fails with an elite athlete who has plantar fasciitis, release only part of the fascia. Function can be preserved. If there is a chronic Achilles tendinosis at the insertion, split the Achilles in a small area posteriorly and remove only the calcium. Avoid damage to the normal tendon. This was necessary in a famous basketball player; by performing a minimal debridement, he was able to return to his sport without pain.

Once surgery is performed, carefully plan the recovery and the rehabilitation. Details should be worked out with the physical therapist so that no element of rehabilitation is overlooked.

## THE GOAL IS INDIVIDUAL AND TEAM PERFORMANCE

Winning is secondary. A middle-distance female Olympic runner had bunions. These bunions had been present for many years but had not caused her performance to be affected; therefore no surgery had been performed.

However, the hallux valgus became worse, and the foot developed claw toes and a neuroma as secondary features. The runner needed help. She could not run. A Lapidus procedure had been recommended to correct the 15-degree intermetatarsal angle and the 25 degrees of hallux valgus.

A chevron procedure was performed to realign the joint even though the foot postoperatively was not perfect. The first metatarsophalangeal joint was realigned to be compensated. Ten years later the runner gradually experienced recurrence of her bunion, which would not have happened with the Lapidus procedure; however, she had gone to the Olympics twice and set an American record on the roads. I feel this would not have been possible with a Lapidus procedure. The goal in this case was not a perfect bunionectomy but maximization of the athlete's performance.

## KNOW YOUR LIMITATIONS

Certain injuries cannot be corrected, and the athlete and treating team must be realistic.

A professional basketball player had a rupture of both the peroneus brevis and longus. The repair, even though good, would not allow recovery of total function. The player returned to professional basketball for 1 year, but the time of play and point average was less. The world-class sprinter with the repaired Achilles tendon can run but may lose several hundredths of a second in his time.

Severe hallux rigidus will never allow the same degree of function after a cheilectomy or a fusion.

## TIMING IS IMPORTANT FOR PEAK PERFORMANCE

Downtime must occur at appropriate intervals to allow return to full function. An arthroplasty of a joint done with precise technique is best performed 15 to 18 months before an athlete participates in a world-class event. A soft tissue procedure such as a nerve or partial fascia release is best performed no later than 6 months before a major event.

A former world record holder was training for the Olympic trials. A persistent plantar fasciitis failed to respond to nonsteroidal antiinflammatory medications, multiple cortisone injections, and therapy. Three months before the trials, a partial release of the fascia was performed. At the trials this athlete came in fourth, missing an Olympic spot by two one hundredths of a second. Had this procedure been performed 3 months earlier, I feel she would have made the team.

## PLANNING IS MOST IMPORTANT

Once an athlete sustains an injury, the treatment team needs to draw up a plan of cross-training, conservative treatment, and invasive treatment where indicated. The team includes the coach, athlete, trainer, physical therapist, physician, and often the athlete's agent. Options and outcome should be discussed and second and third opinions obtained.

Each step should be visualized and thought through. The literature should be reviewed. Timing of major events needs to be considered. This plan may necessitate meetings of the treatment team, letters, or telephone calls in addition to office visits by the athlete to the physician.

These athletes and coaches like to know the specific time required for recovery and when to initiate training after the treatment or surgery. These dates should be as precise as possible.

A major league baseball player was having tremendous problems with a fractured sesamoid. His agent called and then the team doctor. We finally decided on surgical intervention. The team physician and trainer of the team participated in the decision. The pitcher had a sesamoidectomy and has returned to full form

1.5 seasons after the surgery. The first postoperative season he had a losing season; however, the next year his earned run average was one of the five lowest in baseball.

## SUMMARY

We recommend a team approach to treating the elite athlete and meetings to plan the approach to treatment. The functional return of the athlete is most important.

Always try to repair damaged joints, tendons, and ligaments anatomically and with minimal surgery. It is important to be a minimalist.

These high-level athletes are great. They are gifted and motivated. They need only a minimal nudge, not a major reconstruction or overhaul.

# Athletic Shoes, Orthoses, and Rehabilitation

# Chapter 26

# The shoe in sports

Carol Frey

The relationship of the athlete and his shoe is extremely important to athletic performance. The desire for improved performance affects all athletes and influences not only training but also equipment research and design. Athletic shoe manufacturers rely on scientific research and prior experience in the development of their products. This chapter covers important aspects of design, technology, sports-specific needs, and medical and orthopedic considerations in the development of athletic shoe wear.

## GENERAL CONSIDERATIONS
### Construction

Although product development and marketing methods are different, most major shoe construction methods are used in the manufacturing of sport shoes (Fig. 26-1).

**The last.** The last, a three-dimensional (Fig. 26-2) form on which the shoe is made, is considered by many to be the foundation for shoe production and development. Foot shape may vary with sports activities, which is a major area of concern in the development of the last. The shape of the shoe toe box, instep, girth, and foot curvature are determined by the last. The biggest last variations occur in girth (or widest part of the forefoot) and in heel width.

**Straight and curved lasts.** Most feet have a slight inward curve. Most sport shoe companies use a last that is curved inward approximately 7 degrees. The greater the curve, the more foot mobility is allowed, which is desirable for the underpronator. The straighter the shoe, the more medial support it will provide, which can help control overpronation.

**Combination lasts.** This refers to any last that varies from a standard proportional last to lasts that

accommodate a combination of fitting or movement requirements.

## MATERIALS
### Upper materials

Leather, rubber, plastic injection molding, soft nylon, mesh nylon, PVC-coated fabrics, polyurethane-coated fabrics, and canvas have been used in the manufacture of uppers. Most uppers used in sports shoes are made of soft nylon, mesh nylon, leather, canvas, suede, and synthetic materials such as Kangoran.

### Sole materials

Rubber is the most widely used sole material because of its versatility, durability, and performance. The most commonly used forms of rubber are a highly compressed molded form or a blown microcellular form. Carbon rubber and styrene-butadiene rubber are the two most common rubber compounds used in athletic shoes. Often used in running shoe soles, black carbon rubber is the hardest wearing. Styrene-butadiene rubber is also hard and is used in tennis and basketball shoes.

### Microcellular rubber

Microcellular rubber (MCR) is a compound composed of natural rubber plus additives. MCR contains a blowing agent in powder form that decomposes during vulcanization, forming a cellular structure. MCR is mainly used for midsoles and wedges, but in some shoes it can be used as an outsole material.

### Ethyl vinyl acetate

Ethyl vinyl acetate (EVA) contains ethylene and vinyl acetate and a powdered blowing agent that

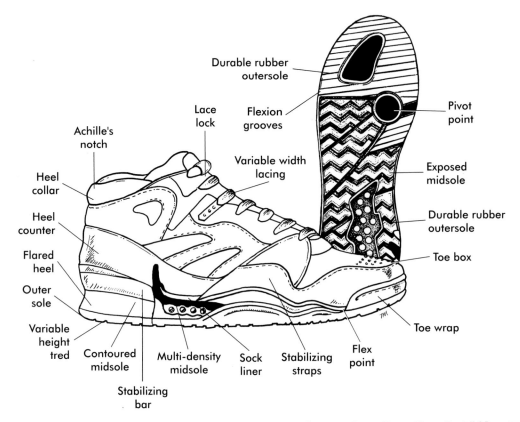

**Fig. 26-1.**  Generic athletic shoe. (From *SHAPE Magazine,* "The First Step: Know Your Feet," Nov. 1992.)

decomposes during vulcanization to form a cellular structure. Due to its lightness, flexibility, density, elongation, and impact resistance, EVA is a common material used in good-quality running shoes. EVA is available in prefabricated sheet or compression-molded forms.

### Polyurethane

Polyurethane (PU) is a liquid polyester that can be formed into a blown cellular structure. PU is versatile and can be used as a midsole and heel wedge material, and its lightness and durability make it a satisfactory outsole material. PU can be directly injected or used as a unit sole. PU can be used in the blown cellular state and as a hardened elastomer form in multi-studded soles such as golf shoes.

### Nylon

Nylon is a polyester resin with a high melting point that forms a hard outsole when injected. It is used for spike plates and as a base for screw-in studs.

The hardness grade of nylon refers to the number of carbon atoms in the nylon molecule and is graded as nylon 6, 11, and 12 (nylon 6 is the hardest).

### Leather

Split-leather and coarse full hides are used in the construction of some athletic shoes.

### LASTING TECHNIQUES

The most common methods of lasting used in shoemaking are slip lasting, board lasting, and combination lasting (Fig. 26-3).

1. *Slip Lasting*—A slip-lasted shoe is constructed by sewing together the upper like a moccasin and then gluing it to the sole. The last is usually forced into the upper, which then takes the shape of the last. A sock liner usually takes the place of an insole. This lasting method makes for a lightweight and flexible shoe with no torsional rigidity.
2. *Board Lasting*—The upper is placed over the last and fastened to the insole with cement, tacks, or staples. This construction promotes stability and torsional rigidity but decreases flexibility.
3. *Combination Lasting*—More than one lasting technique can be used on the same shoe. Usually the shoe is board lasted in the rear foot for stability but slip lasted in the forefoot for flexibility. Combination lasting can offer customized features necessary for some athletes.

### UPPER DESIGNS AND CUTS

1. *U-throat*—The U-throat offers a U-shaped full lacing system that extends down to the toes.

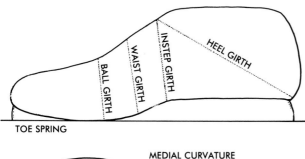

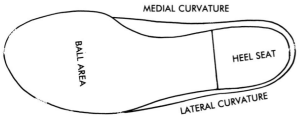

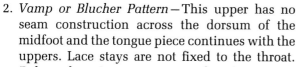

**Fig. 26-2.** Different lasts used in athletic shoes. (From *SHAPE Magazine*, "The First Step: Know Your Feet," Nov. 1992.)

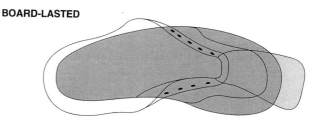

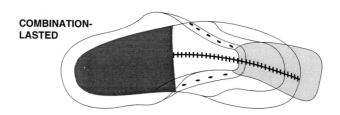

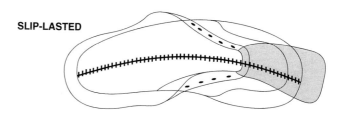

**Fig. 26-3.** Methods of lasting.

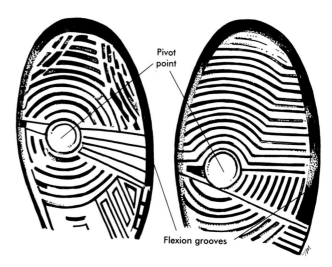

**Fig. 26-4.** Outsole patterns. (From *SHAPE Magazine*, "The First Step: Know Your Feet," Nov. 1992.)

2. *Vamp or Blucher Pattern* — This upper has no seam construction across the dorsum of the midfoot and the tongue piece continues with the uppers. Lace stays are not fixed to the throat.
3. *Balmoral or Brogue Pattern* — This design is a low-cut, laced shoe, usually with a long wing tip trimmed with pinking and perforations. The tongue, throat, and lace stays are seamed as one unit. This type of upper construction allows less space for the dorsal aspect of the midfoot and is often used in golf shoes.
4. *Lace-to-Toe Pattern* — This pattern offers lacing similar to the U-throat pattern, but in addition both quarters are pulled together across the foot for maximum support.

## BOTTOMING PROCESS

Bottoming is the process in which the sole components are attached to the upper. The upper determines the shoe fit and provides support, and the sole provides traction and cushioning.

## THE OUTER SOLE

The outsole is the most plantar surface of the shoe that makes contact with the ground and is usually attached to a midsole to form a complete sole. Most athletic shoes have outer soles of hard carbon rubber or blown rubber compounds. Blown rubber is the lightest outsole material but is not as durable as carbon rubber. Many outsoles are composed of both blown and carbon rubber, with blown rubber in the forefoot and midfoot and carbon rubber used in the high wear area of the heel. Gum rubbers are hard wearing and grip well on most surfaces. PU is less versatile but also suitable for outsole material and

seems to possess good durability. Nylon, leather, and PVC have specific outsole applications for certain sports.

### Outer sole designs

Patterns can enhance stability and traction. They can also improve shoe lightness by exposing the middle part of the midsole, thereby eliminating part of the outsole and the associated weight. The design of the outsole (Fig. 26-4) can provide cushioning, traction, pivot points, flexpaths, and wear plugs. Outsoles are specific for surface, weather condition, and sport. Outsole options include:

- Wear area reinforcement (running shoes)
- Cantilevered designs for shock absorption (running shoes)
- Pivot points (court shoes)
- Herringbone (court shoes)
- Suction cup designs (court shoes)
- Multiclaw or stud designs (field shoes)
- Radial edges (court shoes)
- Asymmetric studs (field shoes)
- Traction and wear lugs (hiking and climbing boots)

Traction provided by the outsole is an important consideration in the design of a sport shoe and is directly related to the ability of the shoe to develop frictional forces with the playing surface. Traction needs depend on the specific sports needs. Too little traction may have a negative effect on athletic performance, and too much traction may put the athlete at risk for injury.

A running shoe should create a firm enough grip with the ground so that propulsion forces created by the runner will not be lost with push-off. Push-off has the highest traction needs; therefore the forepart of the outsole should provide the most traction. The outsole rubber used in running shoes is usually blown rubber (air injected to lighten it) or hard carbon rubber.

Cleated shoes must address a compromise between performance and protection of the athlete. Rotational traction, which is expressed by the torque about a normal axis that is developed to resist rotation of a shoe on a playing surface, must be reduced to decrease the incidence of injury while providing sufficient traction. Both cleat length and outsole material affect friction. Torg and Quendenfeld concluded that the increased rotational traction characteristics of some football shoes are related to an increase in number of significant knee injuries.[6]

The necessity for lateral movement with court sports makes the traction characteristics of court shoes important. A flat outsole pattern develops the greatest frictional forces, whereas a herringbone pattern develops less.[7]

With sprinting, initial ground contact is made with the front of the shoe. At foot strike a large horizontal velocity is created, resulting in a high braking force that can cause a backward slide. Anterior spikes help to prevent slipping.

With jumping events, an athlete converts the large horizontal momentum of run-up to a vertical momentum at foot plant. The spikes prevent foot slip and allow the development of large propulsive forces necessary for long jump and triple jump.

With golf shoes motion is primarily stationary with little horizontal velocity. Golf shoes provide a base of support that allows the performance of coordinated body movements needed in hitting the ball. A nonvertical alignment of the spikes prevents slipping in this sport, which mainly requires anterior and lateral forces.

Boating shoes require a large amount of natural rubber to prevent slippage on wet surfaces.

## MIDSOLES AND WEDGES

Most of the recent advances in the athletic shoe industry have been made in midsole design and materials. The midsole and heel wedge are sandwiched between the upper and the outsole, attaching to both. These components provide cushioning, shock absorption, lift, and control.

### Unit soles

Unit soles usually contain the outsole, midsole, and heel wedge as one unit. This design is used in roller skate boots and other sports where the sole does not contact the ground. This design is usually heavy and provides little flexibility but excellent torsional rigidity.

### Combination or prefabricated soles

Midsoles are manufactured from a combination of two basic materials: EVA and polyurethane. EVA is light and has excellent cushioning properties and can be manufactured in various densities. The firmest densities in a multidensity midsole are usually designated by a darker color. These can be placed at critical points in the midsole to aid in motion control. PU is a denser, heavier and more durable material than EVA. New forms of lighter PU are being developed. Both EVA and PU are used to encapsulate other cushioning materials such as air bags (NIKE and ETONIC), gel (ASICS), silicone (BROOKS), honeycomb pads (REEBOK and PUMA), and EVA (NEW BALANCE).

Some midsoles can be contoured to the foot and are referred to as more stable "anatomical" midsoles.

## OTHER COMPONENT PARTS
### Heel counters

The heel counter is a firm cup built into the rear of the shoe that holds the heel in position and helps control excessive foot motion. Most heel counters today are made of a durable plastic, thermoplastic, stytherm, or polyvinyl. The medial side of the heel counter may be extended or reinforced for additional pronation control. Contoured or notched counters also reduce irritation of the Achilles tendon, especially in plantar flexion.

### Toe box

The toe box provides a stiff material inserted between the lining and upper in the toe area to prevent collapse and protect the toes.

### Foxing

Foxing is a stripping material that gives medial and lateral support to the outside of the shoe and is usually made of suede or rubber. In running shoes the most important foxing is at the toe, where it is called the toe cap. In court shoes the foxing runs completely around the sole for lateral support.

### Cantilevered or angled radial outsole

A cantilever outsole provides a concave outsole design in which the outer edges flare out on impact to dissipate shock. This design is used extensively by AVIA.

### Shank

The shank is the bridge between the heel and the ball area of the shoe. It is a reinforcing material that is arched and somewhat narrowed to conform roughly to the narrow underpart arch area of the midfoot. Shanks are not common in wedge-soled shoes but are important for torsional rigidity in shoes with heels to support the metatarsal arch.

### Tongues

Tongues are designed primarily to protect the dorsum of the foot from dirt, moisture, and lace pressure. Lacing loops or tongue slits help prevent the tongue from slipping.

### Sock linings, arch supports, and inserts

Sock linings cover the insole and improve comfort and appearance. A prime function of the sock lining is to serve as a buffer zone between the shoe and the foot. They are molded, soft support systems that can function in aeration, moisture absorption, hygiene, shock absorption, and motion control.

Arch supports, heel cups, and other types of padding can be added to provide support, cushioning, and motion control.

Custom-molded "foothotics" have been made popular by the ski industry. These semirigid insole devices are custom molded to the foot and may help increase comfort, shock absorption, and performance. Custom insoles can be used in any sport shoe provided there is enough room to accommodate the insert.

## NEW COMPONENTS AND DESIGNS
### Air soles

First introduced in 1979 by NIKE, this concept used encapsulated air units in the midsole to enhance cushioning. Ambient air (ETONIC) or Freon (NIKE) can also be used. Depending on the model, the air units may be in the heel, forefoot, or both. Initial reports noted that although air systems had superior shock absorption and potential energy rebound, stability was poor.[2] Stability in the context of sports refers to the ability of the shoe to resist excessive or unwanted motions of the foot and ankle. Shoes with soft well-cushioned midsoles allow significantly more motion than firmer shoes, and a poor design can encourage instability. Newer designs have addressed the stability problem with success.

Air systems are not as susceptible to compaction as EVA, PU, and other midsole materials and are therefore thought to be more durable.

### Energy return

Compression of a viscoelastic midsole material allows a small amount of strain energy to be stored in the compressed elastic components of the midsole. Theoretically, when weight is released, the elastic components spring back and stored energy is returned to the athlete. It has been suggested that by increasing the energy return of a shoe, the oxygen cost of an activity can be reduced and performance enhanced. There is little evidence to support these claims. The arch of the human foot is also a viscoelastic system and therefore can return energy.[1,4]

### The "pumps"

The "pumps" are actually inflatable linings in the tongue and other parts of the shoe that are pumped up by a device built into the top of the shoe. This provides a tight secure fit. Both NIKE and REEBOK use this fit feature.

### Replaceable plug systems

A heel plug is found in multidensity outsoles, where the most durable rubber is placed in the high-wear area of the heel. ADIDAS designed a rear-foot plug system that allows three different hardnesses of replaceable plug to be inserted into the heel wedge to improve shock absorption. BROOKS marketed a pronation control system that allows pronation to be controlled by inserting medial heel plugs of varying hardness.

### Pronation control devices

Control over pronation in runners and other athletes is a major concern of the sport shoe industry. Most of the motion control features fall into two categories: (1) a harder density material built into the medial aspect of the midsole and/or heel to counteract pronation and (2) an added medial component to the inside or outside of the shoe that limits pronation.

In the past most of the pronation control devices have focused on the rear foot. More attention is now placed on controlling the entire foot.

### Women's shoes

There has been a lot of recent interest in manufacturing women's athletic shoes, but only a few companies have tried to market shoes for women. In the past most women's models were simply men's models with cosmetic changes. It has been hard to change the common perception that men's shoes are better than women's.

## SHOE FIT

A last is a three-dimensional facsimile of a foot and the form over which the upper is fashioned. The fit of all shoes depends largely on the shape of the last.

In fitting a shoe correctly, the shape of the athlete's foot is important in that the shape of the shoe should match the shape of the foot.

Curved lasts are better suited for athletes with high arches who do not overpronate. These shoes offer less medial support but greater foot mobility. Further, a curve-lasted shoe is desirable for a faster runner who wants a more responsive shoe.

Straight lasts provide more support to the medial side of the foot and are better suited for athletes with low arches or who overpronate.

Shoes should feel comfortable and fit well the first time they are put on. Runners and athletes should shop for shoes after a run or after a training session, when their feet are at their largest. The shoe should be fit to the largest foot. There should be a finger's breadth from the end of the toe box to the end of the longest toe, and the athlete should be able to fully extend all toes.

One should keep in mind that although the most common regular shoe width is C for men and B for women, the average athletic shoe width is a D for men and C for women. This reflects additional allowances for foot expansion and movement during sport. Width fittings are not commonly available in athletic footwear. Athletic shoes are generally built on "universal" lasts and width adjustments are incorporated into lacing patterns.

When fitting new shoes, the athlete should wear the socks normally used while training. If the athlete normally wears orthotics, these should replace the sock liner of the shoe during fitting.

### Laces

Beginning at the bottom, laces should be pulled one set of eyelets at a time to tighten. This provides a more comfortable shoe fit and distributes stress evenly across the eyelets and the dorsum of the foot.

The majority of athletes can use the conventional crisscross to the top of the shoe technique, aiming for a snug but comfortable fit. But there are many lacing techniques (Fig. 26-5), and shoe manufacturers have added extra eyelets so athletes can lace them for a custom fit.

### Variable lace patterns (Fig. 26-5, *A* and *B*)

Many sport shoes incorporate a lacing system that provides a variable or wavy eyelet pattern allowing lacing to be adjusted for wider or narrower feet. The wider placed eyelets allow the lacing to pull the quarters in more tightly and are more suitable for narrow feet. The narrower placed eyelets allow for more girth and are thus more suitable for a wider foot.

### Independent lacing (Fig. 26-5, *C*)

One lace is provided near the throat of the shoe and one for the forefoot, which can be tied at different tensions for a custom fit.

### For heel spillage (Fig. 26-5, *G*)

This is a conventional pattern of lacing until the last eyelet. By looping the end of each lace and using the loop as an eyelet, one can obtain a more secure fit around the heel. This method is helpful to prevent heel slippage.

### For pain and or prominences on the dorsum of the foot (Fig. 26-5, *D*)

This lace pattern can relieve pressure over prominences and painful areas on the dorsum of the foot. The athlete starts with a conventional lacing system until just distal to the problem area. The lace is then moved vertically to the next eyelet so it does not cross over the dorsum of the foot. A conventional lacing is used to complete the shoe closure. Many soccer players prefer this lacing pattern.

### Square box lacing (Fig. 26-5, *E*)

In this method the laces never cross over the dorsum of the foot but rather pass under the eyelet. This helps distribute lace pressure more evenly over the dorsum of the foot than the crisscross lacing system. Square box lacing is useful for an athlete with a high arch, rigid feet, or a dorsal prominence.

### Single lace cross (Fig. 26-5, *F*)

The single lace cross may help the athlete having problems with black or sore toenails. One lace runs

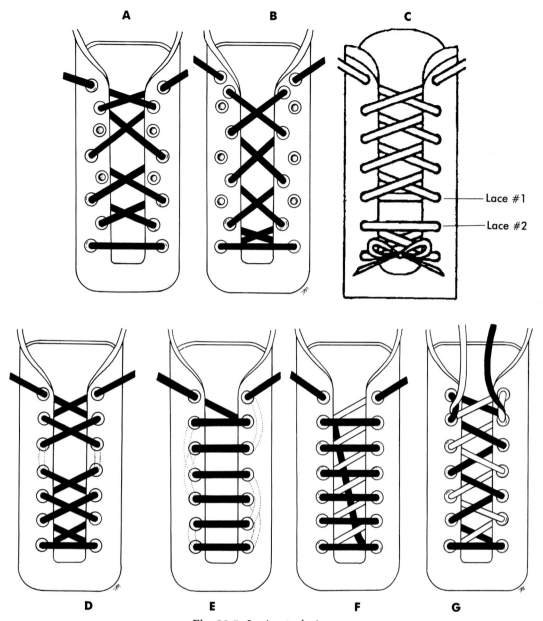

**Fig. 26-5.** Lacing techniques.

from the inside most proximal eyelet to the opposite most distal eyelet. The other end of the lace goes side to side through every remaining eyelet. This pattern pulls the toe box of the shoe up, relieving pressure on the toes.

## Show lacing

This is not practical for wearing purposes. Retailers and manufacturers use this method to show their shoes.

## Elastic lacing

Elastic laces can be beneficial to athletes with wide or expanding feet. However, with the use of elastic laces, shoes will lose some stability because as the foot rolls in, the laces will give. The elastic lace eliminates the need for lacelocks used by many triathletes as the extra stretch allows shoes to be easily pulled on.

## SPORTS-SPECIFIC SHOES

Athletic shoes are grouped by the manufacturers into the following sales categories:

1. *Running, training, and walking shoes* — includes most shoes used for running and walking
2. *Court sport shoes* — includes all shoes used for major and minor court sports
3. *Field sport shoes* — cleated, studded, and spiked shoes used in most field sports

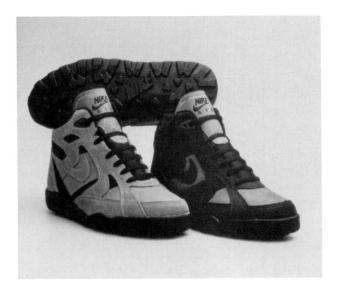

**Fig. 26-6.** Hiking boots.

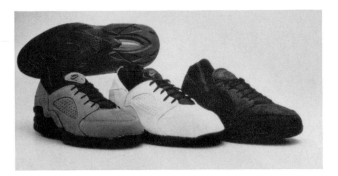

**Fig. 26-7.** Exercise walking shoes.

4. *Winter sport shoes*—shoes for all winter sports activities including skating and skiing
5. *Outdoor sport shoes*—shoes for large recreational sports like hunting, fishing, and boating
6. *Track-and-field shoes*—diverse area of sports that has its own category of shoes
7. *Specialty sport shoes*—shoes for all minor specialized sports and some major ones not covered under other groups, such as golf and aerobic dancing

### Running, training, and walking

Hiking, race walking, and exercise walking are included in this category.

**Hiking boots.** These are used on rugged terrain. The upper of a hiking boot should be water-resistant. There should be few seams for both comfort and water resistance. The soles, which are heavily lugged for traction and durability, are made of rubber PU or PVC compounds. There should be some flexibility in the forepart of the shoe at the metatarsophalangeal joints. Other features of a good hiking boot include a firm heel counter, a padded area around the ankle area, a smooth or seam-free lining, and a high wide toe box. A wedge or a heel with a shank is required. Climbing boots are different than hiking boots in that they have inflexible soles and a thicker upper (Fig. 26-6).

**Race walking shoes.** The construction of a race walking shoe is similar to that of a track shoe. A firm light midsole is important. Outsoles are made from carbon rubber or gum rubber. A firm heel counter is desirable.

**Exercise walking shoes.** The design of this shoe is similar to a training running shoe that has many of the features needed in walking such as lightness; flexible forefoot; comfortable, soft upper; and good shock absorption (Fig. 26-7).

For the urban walker weight is not as important a consideration, and leather is often used for the upper material. An ample toe box and soft sock liner are added for comfort. The sole is also different, with a wedge incorporated into the design. The tread has a smooth, low profile with a herringbone pattern. Many outsoles have a rocker profile to encourage the natural roll of the foot during the walking motion. This feature also helps reduce excessive flex at the metatarsophalangeal joints.

A walking shoe should have a firmer landing area on the heel than most running shoes. The bias-out or upswept heel of many running shoes does not offer the landing platform needed by walkers. Most walkers also benefit from the use of a more resilient compound in the rear part of the shoe. A heel height of 10 to 15 mm is recommended for exercise walking to support the correct walking motion and reduce overstretching of the Achilles tendon.

### Running

**Spikes.** Little body weight is placed on the heel in sprinting. For most track runners, even those who run the longer distances, landing and propulsion are carried out on the ball and middle part of the foot. For this reason, track shoes used in the faster and shorter races have just enough padding at the heel to prevent a contusion (Fig. 26-8).

A slight wedge in the shoes for longer races gives more torsional rigidity and support. Torsional rigidity is often omitted in track shoes for lightness. Track shoe lasts are designed to hug the foot at the heel, waist, and girth. The toe box is semipointed to prevent the toes from splaying under the pressure of landing and takeoff.

Certain specifications for track spikes may vary for different events. A maximum of six sole and two heel spikes is permitted; spikes must not project more than 25 mm or exceed 4 mm in diameter. Added spike receptacles may be present for optimal adjustment

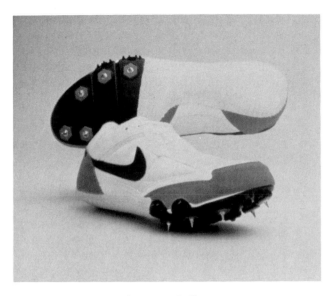

**Fig. 26-8.** Spikes.

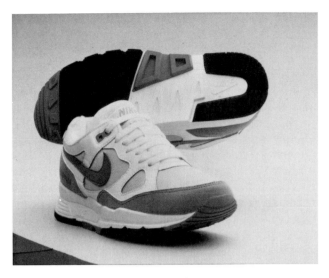

**Fig. 26-9.** Flats.

and may be filled with flat screws when not in use. Grooves, ridges, and appendages are permitted on the sole and heel.

With the use of synthetic and rubber tracks, track spikes have shortened to around 9 mm and reverted to six spikes for better traction. With the use of shorter spikes, shoe manufacturers invented removable plastic "claws." When used in conjunction with replaceable variable length spikes, track shoes have more versatility for different track surfaces.

Nylon sole plates receive the spike receptacles. These are often covered with textured rubber for added traction. For curve running (200- to 400-m races) adequate torsional stability is recommended. Lightweight MCR, PU, or EVA foams are used to give some padding, particularly in the heel area. A spikeless track shoe, usually made with a thin rubber outsole covering a midsole with a maximum heel height of 13 mm may be preferred if the track surface is hard.

Following the same pattern as sprint shoes, middle-distance shoes vary only in the midsole area. A thin wedge or shank may help control overpronation and torque during bend running.

Participants in the short and long hurdles require sprint shoes with lasts wider in the toe and shorter front spikes to avoid clipping the hurdle with the lead foot. A more heavily padded heel is desirable to cushion the landing.

**Flats.** More research and design has been done in this area than in all other areas of athletic footwear.

The features most required in a running shoe used for training on hard road surfaces are shock absorption, flexibility, control and stability in the heel counter area, torsional rigidity in the waist or shank, lightness, traction, comfort, motion control, and good fit.

Because of the specific needs of individual runners, athletic shoe wear companies now produce models for specific foot types, gait patterns, and training styles. There are designs for light runners, heavy runners, heel strikers, motion control, stability, lightweight trainers, and rugged terrain. This segmentation of the market is crossing over into other major segments of the athletic shoe market such as tennis and basketball.

Uppers are usually made of lightweight soft or mesh nylon. A rigid heel counter is a requirement because like walkers, most runners land heel first. The midsoles of training shoes should be lightweight and offer good shock-absorbing properties. PU and EVA are the most commonly used materials, but ambient air, Freon, and silicone can also be used. All these materials have good to excellent shock absorbency and are built into heel wedge and midsole combinations. The shape of the sole is wedged from heel to toe, with approximately a double thickness at the heel to the metatarsophalangeal joint flexion points. A flared heel increases stability in the heel area (Fig. 26-9).

Traction is obtained by rubber outsole materials and a good tread design. To obtain the best traction on loose or open terrain surfaces, a deeper sole tread is desired. On smoother, harder surfaces such as pavement, a lower profile sole offers better stability and adequate traction. Flexpath designs on the outsole increase flexibility.

### Throwing events

Shoes for throwing events, where athletes tend to be larger, are primarily made of leather or suede for maximal durability and support. Because of tremendous stresses applied to the medial and lateral portion of the shoe, the uppers are made with extra support around the girth. A shot-put shoe should have reinforced leather uppers, a sturdy heel counter, firm toe box and reinforcement in the quarter for lateral support. A good grip from a rubber sole and adequate shank provides some control for anterior and lateral movements across the circle. Discus shoes are similar to shot-put shoes but have more flexibility in the forefoot and a wrap-up sole for improved turning motion in the circle. Javelin boots are the only throwing shoes made with spikes for run-up and planting. Soles have a heavy-duty forefoot and heel spike plates containing six front and two back spikes, which may be as long as 25 mm for competition on grass runways. A buckle or strap may be used across the girth to provide additional support.

### Jumping events

For jumping events the spike placement changes from the asymmetric pattern, with two spikes in front for stability (the IAAF rules that there may be a maximum of six forepart spikes and two heel spikes). Most long jumpers do not use heel spikes. The forepart spike plate is sturdy for extra support. Heel cushioning is used for shock absorption.

Similar to long-jump shoes, triple-jump shoes vary only in the midsole, where a sturdy wedge gives better support for landing during the midstance and toe-off stress during this event. Most triple jumpers use heel spikes.

Regardless of their style, high jumpers use a one-foot takeoff. Because foot plant and takeoff are critical for a successful jump, the "jump foot" shoe is emphasized by designers. The takeoff shoe is made in right and left foot versions. Forward and backward ascent styles ("Fosbury Flop") have different spike placements and gradient on the sole for takeoff. The jump shoe can be built with a maximum elevation of 10 mm in the forepart to aid lift-off. Six forepart spikes and two heel spikes may be used. Most shoe companies now produce counterpart trailing shoes that are lighter, with fewer spikes and more flexibility to assist the run-up.

### COURT SPORT SHOES
### Racquet sports

These sports require forward, backward, and side-to-side movements. The body must be moved with control in all directions. Wear patterns produced in even a short time show that court shoes used in racquet sports are subjected to heavy abuse.

### Tennis

Tennis requires body control with quick side-to-side movement, sprinting, jumping, and stretching.

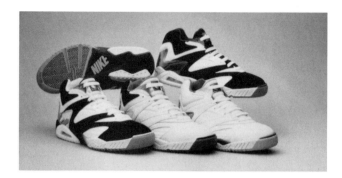

**Fig. 26-10.** Tennis shoes.

The sport is played on lawn, clay, asphalt, and synthetic and rubberized courts. The selection of an appropriate sole must be made for each surface. On clay courts soles with too deep a tread pattern may be prohibited because of excessive court maintenance, even though most players would prefer the traction. On artificial or synthetic surfaces, harder soles with high rubber content or dual-density PU are preferred for durability.

A tennis shoe should provide good lateral support, light-to-medium weight, a flat sole with a good heel wedge, a firm heel counter, a well-cushioned insole and midsole, ample toe box, good ventilation, nonslip traction, a pivot point, and reinforcement for toe drag.

The upper should provide a sufficiently high quarter pattern to provide good ankle and lateral foot support. Over the ankle line midcut models are available for those players who prefer more ankle support.

Manufacturers of tennis shoes recommend more cushioning in the ball of the foot for the serve-and-volley player. For the baseline player, a solid heel counter, strong reinforcement in the heel and midfoot area, and good rear-foot stability are recommended (Fig. 26-10).

### Basketball

Basketball requires backward, forward, and vertical accelerations; quick stops; and side-to-side movements. The playing surface is usually wood but may be synthetic or rubberized material. The shoe should provide good lateral and medial support, light-to-medium weight, a flat sole, a slight heel wedge, good cushioning, a large firm heel counter, toe drag reinforcement, ventilation, a pivot point, and good traction. High rubber content in the sole is recommended. Soles with multiple-edge patterns, such as circles, squares, or diamonds, offer better traction than herringbone patterns (which are excellent for forward stops but not for good lateral stops). High-cut designs are available for full ankle support. In addition to offering added ankle support, high-cut uppers must

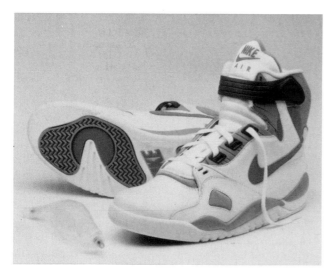

**Fig. 26-11.** Basketball shoes.

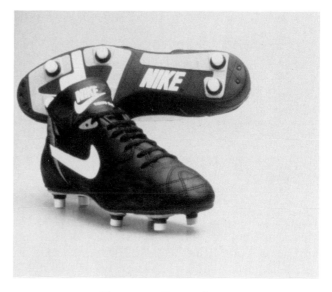

**Fig. 26-12.** Soccer shoes.

not restrict ankle flexion. Proprioceptor straps are popular. Low-cut uppers are preferred by some players for better ankle flexibility, but the incidence of ankle injuries may increase with use of these shoes[3] (Fig. 26-11).

The emphasis of recent design research in basketball shoes has been the reduction of inversion injuries to the ankle. Shoes with increasing amounts of ankle restriction in the upper significantly reduce ankle joint inversion.[5] However, with increasing amounts of ankle restriction, movements are not only restricted in the sagittal plane but also the frontal plane, which leads to reduced agility. Therefore a design compromise must be met between performance and protection of the athlete from injury.

### Volleyball

Volleyball requires quick movements, sudden stops, jumping, and side-to-side motion. The indoor sport is usually played on wood surfaces. The shoe should provide lateral support, be lightweight, provide a flat herringbone or deep ripple rubber sole, good cushioning, ventilation, firm heel counter, and toe-drag protection.

### FIELD SPORT SHOES

Field sports combine many types of movement and a variable degree of body contact. Running is basic to all these sports.

Spike and stud formations vary from sport to sport but are almost all replaceable or detachable cleats, studs, or spikes affixed into nylon soles. Generally, smaller studs in a denser formation help prevent ankle and knee injuries secondary to less penetration of the cleat into the playing field. In addition, weight distribution is better in multistudded designs.

### Soccer

Soccer involves mainly running, kicking, jumping, sliding, stretching, and multidirectional movements. The playing surfaces are natural grass and artificial turf. Soccer is played almost entirely by the feet with the ball being kicked off the medial, lateral, and dorsal aspects of the foot. Soccer shoe lasts tend to be snug fitting, often using European lasts, which are somewhat more narrow than American lasts. Thinner soft leathers are preferred for the upper as players like to feel the ball, but the tongue should be well padded to reduce lace pressure and cushion the dorsal kicking area of the foot. Some players use the tongue and lace area to produce spin and control the ball (Fig. 26-12).

Soles should be flexible at the metatarsophalangeal joints for running and have torsional stability.

### Football

Running is the primary motion in football along with quick lateral movements and the production of great forces secondary to blocking and hitting. Studies have shown that injuries may be caused from wearing fewer, longer cleats which produce excessive pressure beneath the cleats from increased foot fixation.[6] More specifically, the excessive resistance to rotation causes knee injuries during the twisting motions of football. The maximum diameter of a cleat tip should be seven sixteenths of an inch and a maximum overall length one half inch. A seven stud pattern is preferred on natural grass. Nylon soles are preferred as they shed dirt easily and prevent caking of mud between the studs. Multistudded rubber soles are common on natural grass.

Shoe wear exists for linemen, backs, and kickers.

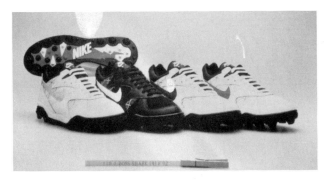

**Fig. 26-13.** Football shoes.

Uppers for linemen must provide support and protection. High-cut or semi–high-cut boot designs are preferred. A sturdy toe box and firm heel counter are recommended. Astroturf linesmen's shoes are multi-studded for grass with shorter, more numerous studs for traction and stability.

The uppers used for backs are similar as for linemen. For added mobility, a low-cut design is usually preferred. Lightweight astroturf shoes with nylon or cotton mesh uppers reinforced with suede are popular. These shoes usually have a rubber outsole with a waffle design that wraps up at the toe and front quarter for better lateral support.

For place-kickers a shoe with a square toe box is usually hand-made for the kicking foot and conventional for the nonkicking foot. The shoe is usually custom made for the individual kicker at the professional level. A soccer shoe is usually preferred for kickers who kick from the side of the foot. For punting, either a soccer or a back's shoe is used. Some players kick in a traditional football back's shoe (Fig. 26-13).

## Baseball

The sport of baseball requires sprinting, throwing, and complex batting movements. The playing surface is usually natural but may be artificial turf with dirt or clay on infield basepaths. A traditional baseball shoe has a U-throat, and a conventional lacing system is the ultimate design. Lasts are similar to a football shoe. On natural turf steel cleats with a design of three in the front and two in the heel is used extensively. Removable cleats are available in steel, PU, and nylon. For pitchers, a pitching toe is often added for toe-drag reinforcement.

## Rugby

The movements in rugby are similar to a football lineman and back. A drop kick is used, but the ball must touch the ground before it is kicked. The surface is natural grass. The rugby boot is similar in design to a soccer shoe with four front cleats and two heel cleats. A semicut or three-quarter–cut style is com-

monly used for ankle protection. For linemen and some wing quarterbacks, a hard square toe box is used. Multistudded versions of rugby boot models are also made for firm playing surfaces.

## WINTER SPORTS
### Skating

Skating mechanics are similar for all skating events, although footwear and blades are specialized. Ankle movement and support are essential to skating performance. However the subtalar joint must be free to allow positioning of the blade on the ice.

The traditional leather boot and the injection-molded model are the two main types of boots available. A leather boot should have good ankle support and a firm heel counter with elongation of the medial side. Uppers are made from thick-grade leather or split leather, with a leather or textile lining that gives the foot and ankle stability but allows some flexibility. Metal eyelets are used in the lower portion of the throat and metal hooks above the ankle.

Ice hockey skates were the first to use injection-molded models. A viscous plastic is injected under pressure into molds to form the lower and upper parts of the boot. The two parts are placed together, completing a hinged outer shell. A soft foam liner is then added.

The hinged two-piece design gives the boot some lateral flexibility needed in ice skating. Leather boots tend to become more flexible with age.

### Figure skating

Figure skating requires the athlete to jump, skate, balance, spin, dance, and lift. The performing surface is the ice on artificial or natural rinks.

The upper is either full- or top-grain cowhides. Good-quality boots are lined with lightweight top-grain leather or suede. A firm heel counter, usually elongated on the medial side for added arch support, is important. Soles are PVC or PU molded units with a shank for added support. Screw-in blades are often used so that the position of the blades may be changed. The lasts used in figure skating are semi-pointed, with a narrow shank and heel to contain the foot and maintain position.

The quality of the blades helps determine the quality of the skate. Blades are commonly made of tubular steel or plastic frame with high-tempered steel that is hollow ground to give two skating edges to the blade. The blades can be nickel- or chrome-plated. Figure skating and free-style blades have a front to back curvature called a radius or rocker. The placement of the blades is usually slightly medial to the midline of the sole. For jumps or spins, a toe rake or pick is used. With forward motion the picks can also help prevent the blade from sliding sideways. For figures, a pair of skates without a pick and less sharply ground blades is often preferred.

### Ice hockey

Ice hockey requires skating, quick stops, quick turns, and balance on the ice of artificial and natural rinks. A high-cut model of leather or ballistic nylon with leather reinforcement is available. A good skating boot requires a firm protective leather toe box of polyethylene or firm fiber and comfortable ankle padding, with a high cut over the Achilles tendon for protection. A molded boot with a hinged upper can provide additional protection and durability. High-grade boots have a leather lining.

The goalie wears a specially designed molded or leather boot with a protective casing. The boots have a low-cut design at the ankle, which allows increased flexibility and also accommodates goalie pads. The blades are thick and reinforced, with increased surface area in contact with the ice to block shots at the goal.

### Speed skating

Speed skating requires balanced skating with a low center of gravity in the lunge position. Skaters often compete with bare feet in skates. The skating surface is ice on artificial or natural ice tracks. The uppers have a deep-cut U-throat with a full lacing pattern to the toes. A three-quarter ankle boot is the preferred design, with a firm heel counter elongated on the medial side.

Thin (one-sixteenth-inch) straight blades are used of either tubular steel or plastic frames. The blade is long (30 to 45 cm) and is placed distal to the skating boot via a high-profile frame to allow a lean of low angle between the skate and the track. Higher-quality blades are chrome plated.

### Alpine skiing

Alpine skiing requires ankle and knee flexion, forward lean, and balance on snow-covered surfaces. Ski boots provide a high-cut upper of a hinged or one-piece injection-molded plastic outer shell to support the lower leg. The boot should provide rigid support for the foot and ankle and allow forward ankle flexion. Adjustable buckles, dial closure devices, or straps are used for instep support and a comfortable snug fit. More recently rear-entry and midentry boots have eliminated buckles and overlaps on the vamp, instep, and ankle regions to reduce pressure. Inner liners can contain a foot bed, a variety of wedges, or adjustable canting devices. To relieve pressure, conforming foam or pressure-flow bags can be used (Fig. 26-14).

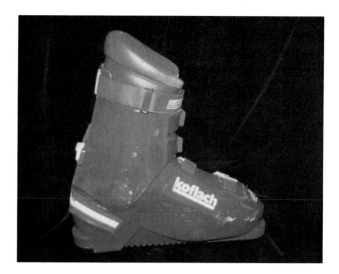

Fig. 26-14. Ski boots.

Ski boots are one of the last categories of athletic footwear to accommodate the female athlete. Important design differences include an elevated heel for a shorter female Achilles tendon, easier forward flexion, and a more flared ankle cuff.

### Cross-country skiing

Cross-country skiing requires fast walking movements, running, jogging, downhill skiing, and balance on snow-covered terrain. Boot and bindings act together as a hinge between the foot and the ski and must be compatible. Boots are made of leather, Gore-tex, nylon, or poromeric materials that allow air to circulate and transpire. Boots should be waterproof, as seam-free as possible, with rigid heel counters. Good forefoot flexion is essential. Rubber soles are preferred for use on snow and ice.

## OTHER SPORTS
### Aerobic dancing

Aerobic dancing requires stationary running, skipping, jumping, stretching, dancing, and stair climbing. The dance surface is on carpet or covered surfaces. The shoe requirements are a combination of a lightweight shock-absorbing running shoe and a modified indoor court shoe. Medial and lateral support is needed as well as a wrap-up toe and heel protection. The forefoot requires stabilization and good shock absorption. EVA and PU combinations, air systems, and gel are used in shock-absorbing forefoot pads. Flexibility in the forepart is important.

### Bicycling

Bicycling involves use of the gluteus, quadriceps, hamstrings, and calf muscles to generate the power necessary to perform upward and downward thrusts

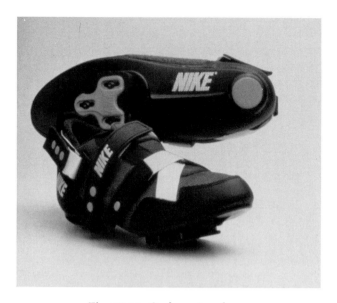

**Fig. 26-15.** Cycle racing shoes.

through the forefoot. The foot is often placed into a valgus or varus position on the pedal, causing pressure to develop on the lateral or medial sides of the foot. Cleat and pedal placement can be changed to prevent this canting.

A cycle racing shoe has a last similar to a sprinting shoe with a wide girth, semipointed toe, narrow waist, and narrow heel. A high toe box is required for toe movement. Uppers are usually made of smooth calf or kid leather with perforations for ventilation. Racing shoes are usually unlined and tend to stretch. Rigid soles are made of reinforced steel, nylon, or PU and can protect the foot from pedal pressure. Depending on the system, shoes are affixed to pedals by cleats, which improve cycling efficiency by locking the foot to the pedal for upward and downward thrust. Most shoes have adjustable cleats permitting angular and fore and aft adjustments (Fig. 26-15).

Clips hold the foot to the pedal, but clipless systems are available.

## INJURIES RELATED TO ATHLETIC FOOTWEAR

A properly designed and constructed athletic shoe can help protect athletes from both external and internal forces that may lead to injury.

### Toes

Ingrown and black toenails (subungual hematoma) are common problems seen in athletes and are usually the result of tight-fitting shoes or shear forces causing the toes to abut the end of the toe box. An adequate high and wide toe box and proper shoe fit should reduce the incidence of this injury.

Corns result from pressure on the toes from the toe box. If the athlete has hammertoes, then the proximal

interphalangeal joint is more prominent, and a corn can result in this location. A high toe box and proper shoe fit usually eliminate this problem. The use of various pads, splints, and lamb's wool can be helpful.

### Forefoot

**Blisters.** Blisters are caused by friction of the skin rubbing against a shoe, sock, or other material. Applying a piece of moleskin or paper tape can be helpful. A cushioned liner such as Spenco may help cut down on shearing and sliding inside the shoe.

**Calluses.** Similar to corns, calluses are hyperkeratoses caused by friction and pressure which may or may not be painful. Calluses may occur over the ball of the foot at sites of pressure on the skin from underlying bone. A cushioned shock liner can help equalize the weight load. Calluses may be pared and pads made from adhesive felt or foam rubber placed proximal to the callus. A Spenco insole, contoured anatomic foot bed, or other shock-absorbing and friction-reducing materials are used in many athletic shoes to prevent calluses. Following proper lacing techniques will help improve foot stability and reduce shear forces between the foot and the shoe.

**Metatarsalgia.** Metatarsalgia is a nonspecific diagnosis that describes pain in and about the head of the metatarsal, metatarsophalangeal joint, and adjacent soft tissue structures. Metatarsalgia can result from atrophic fat pad, basic anatomy of the metatarsals, increased pressure on the metatarsal heads, neurological dysfunction, postsurgical changes, metabolic disorders, and inflammation. A well-cushioned liner and midsole material in addition to a rocker sole, which allows the athlete to roll off the painful forefoot, can be useful.

**Sesamoiditis.** Because of their location under each big toe joint, the sesamoid bones are prone to injury. Cavus feet, equinus of the first metatarsal, or rigid foot can cause excessive pressure to be placed on the sesamoids. A shoe with a good shock-absorbing midsole material extending out into the forefoot must be worn to protect the area. A rocker sole can be helpful. Orthotics that incorporate a sesamoid pad placed just proximal to the injured sesamoid to float the painful area is a useful way to treat this problem.

**Interdigital neuroma.** The most common location for an interdigital neuroma is in the third web space. Excessive pressure on the ball of the foot or a shoe that does not fit well in the girth may contribute to this problem. A shoe with excellent shock-absorbing properties that extend out into the forefoot must be worn to protect the area. A rocker sole can be helpful. Orthotics incorporating a metatarsal pad placed just proximal to the involved web space to help spread the metatarsal heads can take pressure off of the inflamed nerve.

**Nerve entrapment.** Cutaneous nerves including the sural, saphenous, and superficial peroneal nerve can lie under pressure areas of an athletic shoe and result in a painful nerve irritation. Their location makes them vulnerable to compression. Nerve compression is a direct result of wearing irritating or tight-fitting shoes. Ski boots and ice skates are the two major types of athletic footwear that produce this problem. To avoid this problem, shoes should be padded, lacing techniques modified, and careful shoe fit followed.

## Heel

**Plantar fascia.** To prevent this common injury, a shoe must have excellent shock-absorbing abilities in the heel. A varus heel pad or wedge can also be indicated to decrease forces on the medial aspect of the heel. Once the problem develops, heel cups, foam pads with a cut-out, or orthotics with a well-cushioned heel and a well to float the painful area can be indicated. A shoe with a firm medial heel counter can decrease pronation and stress on the plantar fascia.

**Bursitis.** The retrocalcaneal and pre-Achilles bursa can be irritated during sports. This disorder can result from poor shoe fit, a ill-padded heel counter, or excessive heel motion. The athlete should be advised to buy a shoe with well-padded heel counter, an Achilles notch that accommodates the Achilles tendon in plantar flexion, and an adequate heel height of at least 15 mm.

**Achilles tendon.** Low heel elevation in an athletic shoe is often a factor in the development of Achilles tendinitis. To prevent irritation of the tendon, a shoe with a well-padded Achilles tendon pad or notch should be worn. Heel lifts can be worn to elevate the foot in the shoe and reduce tension on the tendon. A firm heel counter can reduce the side-to-side motion of the heel and the Achilles tendon, thus reducing irritation of the tendon.

## Ankle

Sports involving walking, running, or jumping frequently can result in inversion injuries to the ankle. If an athlete has a tendency to inversion injuries of the ankle, a shoe should be worn that has a firm heel counter, a moderately flared heel for a runner, and the stability of a high-cut model rather than a low-cut model for field or court sports. Hockey skates and alpine ski boots should provide good ankle support. Taping, various shoe wedges, braces, and orthoses are all used in the treatment and prevention of ankle sprains.

## REFERENCES

1. Alexander RM: How elastic is a running shoe? *New Sci* 123:45, 1989.
2. Clarke TE et al: The effects of shoe design parameters on rear foot control in running, *Med Sci Sports Exer* 15:376, 1983.
3. Garrick JG, Requ RK: Role of external support in the prevention of ankle sprain, *Med Sci Sports Exer* 5:200, 1973.
4. Kerr RF et al: The spring in the arch of the human foot, *Nature* 325:147, 1987.
5. Robinson JR, Frederick EC, Cooper LB: Systematic ankle stabilization and the effect on performance, *Med Sci Sports Exer* 18:625, 1986.
6. Torg JS, Quendenfeld T: Effect of shoe type and cleat length on incidence of severity of knee injuries among high school football players, *Res Q* 42:203, 1971.
7. Valiant GA: *The effect of outsole pattern on basketball shoe traction.* In Terauds J, Gowitzke BA, Hole LE, editors: *Biomechanics in sports III & IV,* Del Mar, Calif, 1986, Academic Publishers.

# Chapter 27

# Foot orthoses

**Donald C. Jones**
**Stan L. James**

A wide variety of over-the-counter arch supports, prefabricated orthotic systems, and custom-made orthoses are available to the runner. Foot orthoses are frequently viewed by the injured runner as a "simple salve" for problem feet. Little thought is given to the actual need for the device. The general population is aware of orthoses. In many cases people demand an appliance because they believe an orthosis will improve their function. This chapter seeks to provide sufficient information to allow a physician to make a sound decision as to whether an orthosis will benefit a patient. When one looks randomly at the accumulated literature addressing orthoses, the information available can be confusing. However, if the literature is reviewed in a systematic fashion, the information and justification for the use of orthotic devices becomes far less nebulous.

The subject is best addressed by using the following four steps: (1) examining definitions, (2) understanding the biomechanics of the lower extremity, (3) reviewing the assertions concerning orthoses to determine their scientific validity, and (4) reviewing the types of orthoses and purposes of each.

## DEFINITIONS

Considerable confusion exists concerning terms to denote hindfoot and forefoot positions and motions. For example, the terms supination and pronation are often used interchangeably with the terms inversion and eversion. This crossover usage is often confusing and can impair meaningful communication between the orthopedist and the pedorthist. A clear definition of these and other terms provides a common ground for discussion of foot problems.

## Terms

**Pronation and hyperpronation.** These are perhaps the most frequently used biomechanical terms in the runner's jargon. Pronation has, in some instances, been associated with abnormal motion in the subtalar metatarsal joint complex. This is not the case. Pronation is a normal biomechanical phenomenon. Only when there is an excessive or prolonged amount of pronation do problems relative to pronation occur. This is a single motion of the foot with components consisting of hindfoot eversion, forefoot dorsiflexion, and forefoot abduction. This term describes a dynamic event, not a position of the foot.

**Supination.** Supination is the opposite of pronation and is a single motion consisting of hindfoot inversion, forefoot plantar flexion, and forefoot adduction. Like pronation, supination is a dynamic occurrence and the word should not be used to describe a position of the foot.

**Subtalar joint neutral.** An understanding of the definition of subtalar joint neutral is essential for the satisfactory fabrication of most orthoses. One definition states that subtalar joint neutral is the position in which the heel is aligned with the midline of the tibia (Fig. 27-1).[1] This convenient definition is accurate in most instances. There are, however, a few anatomic variations that can make this definition less than valid.

Subtalar joint neutral is the most effective and efficient position of the hindfoot. In subtalar joint neutral the foot is neither supinated nor pronated. As a result, this is the position from which the foot can be maximally supinated or maximally pronated.

Subtalar joint neutral is established by placing the

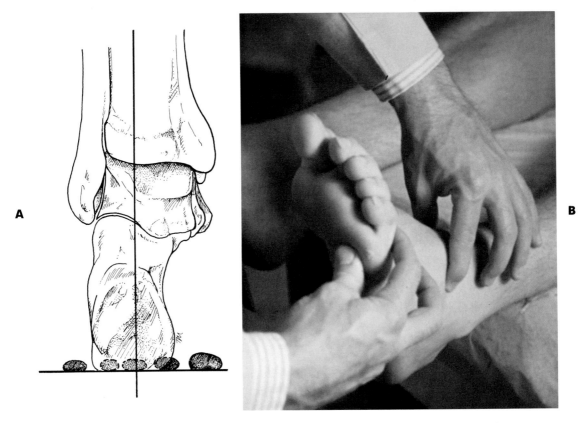

**Fig. 27-1. A,** In subtalar joint neutral, the heel is aligned with the midline of the tibia. **B,** Establishing subtalar joint neutral.

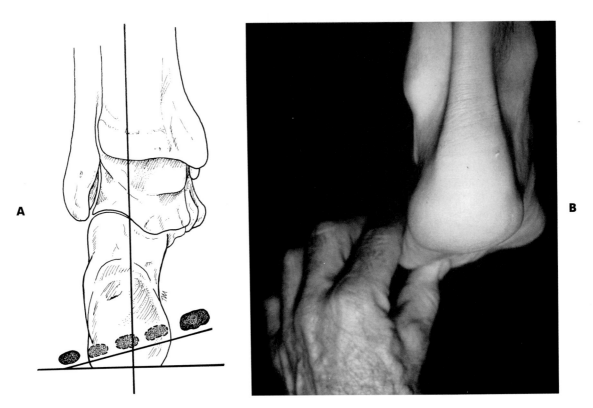

**Fig. 27-2. A,** In forefoot varus the forefoot is in structural inversion. **B,** Appearance of forefoot varus.

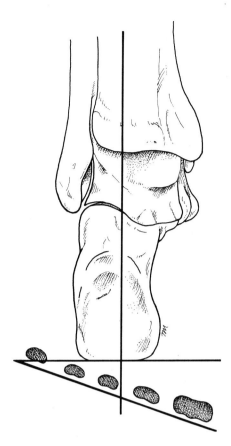

**Fig. 27-3.** In forefoot valgus, the forefoot is in structural eversion.

patient in the prone position and dorsiflexing the ankle to a soft end point. The foot is then supinated and pronated alternately until the talar head is centrally located within the navicular cup (Fig. 27-1). In unskilled hands this position is difficult to duplicate, and Elveru et al[14] have stated that even the skilled individual may find it difficult to reproduce this position consistently.

**Forefoot varus.** One of the more common deformities of the foot, forefoot varus is defined as a constant structural inversion of the forefoot with the hindfoot in subtalar joint neutral (Fig. 27-2).

**Forefoot valgus.** In forefoot valgus there is a constant structural eversion of the forefoot with the hindfoot in subtalar joint neutral (Fig. 27-3).

**Subtalar varus.** Subtalar varus is one of the exceptions to the previously noted definition of subtalar joint neutral. With the subtalar joint in the neutral position, subtalar varus is present when there is an inversion deformity of the calcaneus (Fig. 27-4).

## BIOMECHANICS

Without a firm understanding of the biomechanics of the lower extremity, knowing how an orthosis

functions and providing an accurate description of the appropriate orthosis is impossible. Patients are always amazed when they learn how much weight is transferred across the foot during walking and running activities. While walking, 110% of the body weight is transferred across the foot with each step; while running, 250% of the body weight is transferred. If a 150-lb individual walks 1 mile, each foot absorbs approximately 63.5 tons of weight over this distance. If the same individual runs the mile, the weight absorbed at ground contact increases to 110 tons for each foot. If the same individual were to run a marathon, more than 2800 tons of force per foot would be absorbed during the race. Therefore it is extremely important that the body have mechanisms to absorb this degree of impact to prevent functional and structural breakdown of the lower extremities. The fat cells contained in the chambers formed by the fibrosepta in the heel pad act as shock absorbers, providing one such mechanism. The normal biomechanics of the foot during the gait cycle are even more important, however.

In the initial phase of gait, the foot contacts the ground in supination (Fig. 27-5). During supination, the subtalar and midfoot joint are locked and form a highly rigid structure. This rigidity of the foot provides the sturdy platform needed to absorb the tremendous amount of force transferred across the heel. Immediately after heel strike, the runner's body weight progresses over the foot and passive pronation is initiated (Fig. 27-6). The calcaneus moves laterally, the talus drops off medially, and the forefoot begins to abduct. As this occurs, the foot becomes more flexible. This flexibility results in the foot becoming a "bag of bones" and allows the foot to adapt to uneven running surfaces. Then as the foot approaches the toe-off position, it again supinates, becoming a rigid lever poised for the function of push-off. According to Bates et al,[3] the total range of motion of the subtalar joint is 31 degrees: 31 degrees of inversion and 8 degrees of eversion. In a person walking at a normal pace, full pronation occurs within 150 ms. In a runner at a 6-minute-per-mile pace, this event occurs in about 30 ms. Three important parameters must be determined during the gait cycle: (1) maximum pronation (Fig. 27-7) or the number of degrees the hindfoot moves when progressing from supination to pronation, (2) the time required for this event to occur, and (3) the total period of pronation during the support phase. A prolonged period of pronation during support will extend into the propulsive phase of the running stride when the foot should be supinating to become a more rigid lever for push-off. The importance of these parameters is discussed later.

What happens to the tibia during pronation and

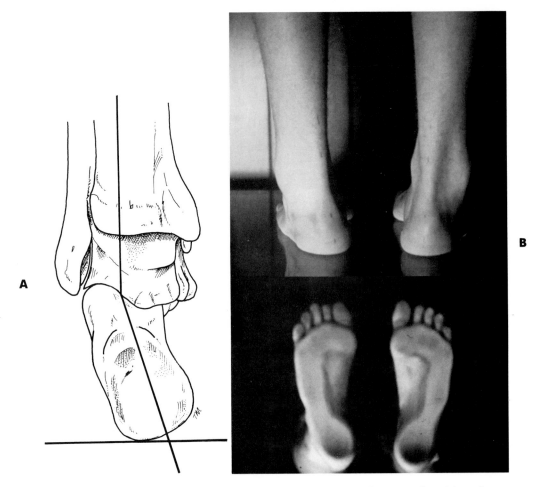

**Fig. 27-4. A,** Subtalar varus. Although the subtalar joint is in the neutral position, there is an inversion deformity of the calcaneus. **B,** Patient with subtalar varus.

supination? The mitered-hinge theory states that with pronation of the foot, there is an obligatory internal rotation of the tibia. The greater the maximum degree of pronation, the greater the excursion of the tibia. Conversely, with supination of the foot, there is an obligatory external rotation of the tibia.

Volumes of literature have been written stating that pronation of the foot has a deleterious effect on the knee. Symptoms associated with anterior knee pain, such as chondromalacia of the patella, are believed to increase in the patient who experiences hyperpronation during running. Therefore researchers sought to find how the patella is affected by hindfoot motion.

In a study performed by Lafortune,[20] cortical pins were inserted into the tibia, patella, and femurs of volunteers. The patients were then fitted with valgus-wedged shoes. Ten degrees of lateral wedging in the

shoe provided a significant pronation stress, and patellar deviation was 10 mm. The patients were then fitted with 10-degree varus shoes. With these shoes patellar deviation was 8.4 mm. Therefore the difference in patellar deviation with a 20-degree change in hindfoot wedging was only 1.6 mm of motion. It seems somewhat curious that such a small change in patellar deviation can be held accountable for the significant symptoms ascribed to hyperpronation of the foot.

## ASSERTIONS CONCERNING ORTHOSES

A number of assertions have been made concerning orthoses and the benefit to be derived from their use. It has been stated that

1. Patients are extremely satisfied with orthoses.
2. Permanent bone and ligamentous alterations can be expected with their long-term use.

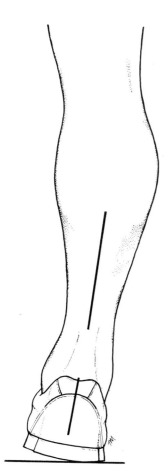

**Fig. 27-5.** Supination in the initial phase of gait. The foot contacts the ground in supination and is rigid.

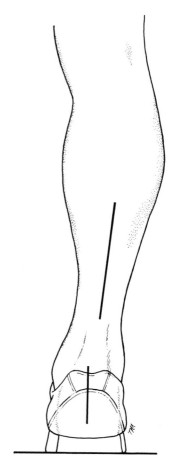

**Fig. 27-6.** Passive pronation. As the runner's weight progresses over the foot, the foot becomes more flexible.

3. Oxygen consumption is altered with the use of orthoses.
4. The pressure on the plantar aspect of the foot can be altered by appropriate use of orthoses.
5. Orthoses can alter foot biomechanics.

Are patients satisfied with orthoses? Surveys have shown that 70% of runners exiting from running clinics leave with some type of foot orthosis. There appears to be a high level of satisfaction with these devices. Estimates of patients' relief of symptoms quoted in literature vary from 64% to an astonishing 96%.[23] Lutter reviewed 899 patients provided with orthoses. He found that 60% of the patients were still using the orthoses when reviewed. The average length of use was approximately 37 months. Of patients who ceased use of the orthoses, 20% stopped because of perceived lack of value. However, one must remember that these series were not controlled studies, and it is highly likely that many of the patients received other forms of treatment in addition to the orthotic device. Some received antiinflammatory medications, others received physical therapy treatment, and still others

had changed their exercise programs. As a result, it is difficult to determine which patients actually benefited from the use of the orthotic device and which patients benefited from the other forms of treatment.

Can long-term use of an orthosis permanently alter the bone and ligament configuration of the foot? There has been a long-time search for a device that, when inserted into the shoe, would hold the pes planus foot deformity in a more anatomic position, with the major benefit being long-term alteration of the arch. Bleck and Berzins[6] evaluated the use of UCBL inserts and the Healthfit heel seat in treatment of children with pes planus. When using these orthoses in children up to 3 years of age, they found that 79% of the patients had improved clinical and radiographic appearance of the foot. Following their use, 32% of the children had normal feet. Bordelon[7] found that the use of an insert produced a correction of 5 degrees per year in the lateral metatarsal angle.

However, Penneau et al[22] evaluated 10 children with bilateral pes planus. They radiographed the feet both with and without the orthosis. Their conclusion was that the immediate radiographic appearance of

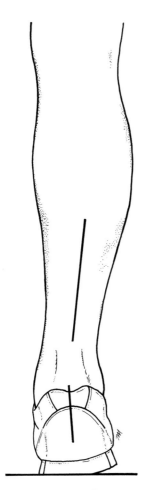

**Fig. 27-7.** Maximum pronation. The runner's weight is over the midline of the foot and the foot is highly flexible.

the flexible planus foot is not significantly changed by the addition of these devices. The question raised by this study is: How can a long-term benefit and permanent change be expected if there is no immediate change of the appearance of the flexible foot while wearing the device?

An important question for distance runners is whether the use of an orthosis can change oxygen consumption. Otman et al[21] evaluated 20 patients with flat feet without orthoses and with orthoses. Although the mechanism of arch support in the foot remains controversial despite years of investigation, one theory implies that the arch is maintained by contraction of muscles and by strength of passive tissue. The assumption is that energy costs of locomotion can be decreased if muscular effort to accommodate the strain of the abnormal foot is decreased. Following this study the conclusion was that $O_2$ consumption can be decreased in the walking patient with pes planus simply by applying a suitable orthosis.

Clement et al[13] had previously determined that the

effect of an orthotic device on steady-state oxygen consumption in athletes is not significant. On the other hand, Stipe[26] found an increase in oxygen consumption in individuals who ran while wearing a pair of orthoses. He attributed this increase in oxygen consumption to the weight of the orthosis. Frederick et al[15] demonstrated that a weight as small as 75 g, when added to each running shoe, can produce a significant change in the aerobic demands of treadmill running. Likewise, Burkett et al[8] demonstrated that the use of orthoses requires increased oxygen consumption. However, they stated that if there is a question regarding whether a runner should wear an orthosis for training, recreation, or competition, it is probably better answered by the runner's ability to run free of pain, rather than because of some expected alteration in oxygen consumption.

There has also been a question regarding whether or not orthosis use is beneficial for cyclists. Hice et al[17] found it beneficial to use orthoses in biking shoes. However, Anderson and Sockler[2] were critical of Hice's study, and Anderson found the benefit of orthoses use while biking to be minimal.

Can a pair of orthoses alter the pressure patterns on the plantar aspect of the foot? Before discussing whether this is the case, normal pressure patterns of the foot should be reviewed. Over the years the presence or absence of a transverse metatarsal arch has been widely debated. The tripod theory of weight distribution contends that there are three major weight-bearing points on which the foot rests: the tuberosity of the os calcis proximally, and the first and fifth metatarsal heads distally. On the other hand, Giannestras[16] believes that there is no transverse metatarsal arch. The studies of Cavanagh et al[9] have resolved this issue by clearly demonstrating that the tripod theory is erroneous. They found that 60% of the load is carried by the rear foot, 8% by the midfoot, and 28% by the metatarsal heads. The load borne by the toes is minimal, averaging less than 4%. The largest pressure area in the forefoot is located under the second and third metatarsal heads, not under the first and fifth metatarsal.

The pattern of ground reaction forces during distance running varies. There are two types of runners. In one group the first point of contact with the ground is made by the heel. These are referred to as rear-foot strikers. The second group makes ground contact more distally in the foot. These are referred to as midfoot or forefoot strikers. Approximately 80% of runners are rear-foot strikers; the other 20% of runners make initial ground contact with the midfoot or forefoot. In rear-foot strikers the initial pressure is focused exclusively on the lateral border of the heel. Shortly after initial contact, the center of pressure migrates medially and anteriorly. Once it is 50% of the shoe length from the heel, there is virtually no mediolateral movement of the center of pressure.[11] In the midfoot striker the initial ground contact is made by the midportion of the foot laterally, with rapid progression medially and distally.

Unfortunately little information is available that shows how the use of orthotic devices alters pressure patterns on the plantar aspect of the foot. However, some useful information can be gleaned from the literature. Holmes and Timmerman[18] studied the effect of a simple metatarsal pad on the pressures transmitted to the metatarsal heads. They found that a metatarsal pad placed appropriately in the shoe is highly effective in reducing metatarsal pressure. The reduction in peak metatarsal pressure ranged from 12% to 60%. Bieber et al[5] studied the effect of orthoses on ground reaction forces under the foot while walking. They found that with orthoses the center of pressure is more medial at heel contact and more lateral at 25% of contact and beyond than it is without orthoses. Scranton et al[24] have stated that a medial arch support shifts the concentration of forces but does not diminish the duration of forces under the foot.

Can a foot orthosis alter the biomechanics of the foot? It has been hypothesized that excessive pronation of the subtalar joint during the support phase of running is linked to various injuries of the hip, knee, Achilles tendon, and foot.[19] Normally the relationship between the hindfoot and forefoot is such that when the rear foot is in subtalar joint neutral, the forefoot is situated transversely to the long axis of the calcaneus. In pathologic conditions, such as cavovarus and pes planus, this relationship is altered. Realizing that excessive hindfoot motion is not desirable, it is important to determine whether an orthosis can be used to control rear-foot kinematics in walking and running. To evaluate this, two parameters must be investigated. One must first look at the degree of maximum pronation during the stance phase. Maximal pronation is the degree of hindfoot motion as measured from the position of the heel at heel strike to the position of the heel at maximal eversion. A number of studies have shown that orthoses of various designs and placements can reduce maximum pronation.[4,10-12,25,27] In these studies the reduction in maximal eversion ranged from 6% to 12%. Theoretically speaking, these seem to be small changes to offer such large benefits. However, perhaps the statement of Cavanagh et al that "many of the mechanical changes that represent the difference between running in pain and running pain free may be at a level of subtlety that we have not yet explored" could help explain this phenomenon. The change in the maximum velocity of pronation

achieved through the use of orthoses seems to be greater, both in percentage and importance. In fact, Smith et al[25] indicated that controlling the velocity of pronation may be more important in preventing running injuries than controlling the extent of pronation. Several studies clearly indicate that the change in the maximum velocity of pronation while wearing an orthosis can range from 20% to 70%.[4,25]

In addition to the maximum velocity of pronation and the amount of pronation, the total *time of pronation* during the support phase is probably of significance also. When the subtalar joint is maintained in a maximum position of pronation, which may be excessive and prolonged, disruption of the normal tibiofemoral rotation at the knee likely occurs, resulting in many runner-related problems. Increased leg varus beyond 10 degrees standing, a tight gastroc-soleus group, increased heel varus, and forefoot supination can all cause compensatory pronation with a prolonged period of pronation during support. The time of total pronation becomes significant when considering that the tibia is held in the internally rotated position during the period of pronation, and if this is a prolonged event, one can postulate that abnormal rotational events of the knee may be disrupted because of this relative internal rotated position of the tibia during the propulsive phase, when it should be moving into external rotation. This may be one of the factors in numerous knee injuries associated with distance runners and particularly in those individuals demonstrating compensatory pronation.

## TYPE OF FOOT ORTHOSIS

Before prescribing an orthosis, it is necessary to define the type of foot deformity, biomechanical abnormality, and scientifically based proposed benefit of the orthosis. The ideal orthosis should be a flexible, easily moldable, shock-absorbing device that decreases torque on the plantar aspect of the foot while controlling the forefoot, hindfoot, and midfoot. Understandably it is impossible to obtain all of these qualities in a single material, resulting in the need for three basic types of orthoses. Each has its appropriate application and benefits. The three categories are soft orthoses, semirigid orthoses, and rigid orthoses.

Soft orthoses are constructed of a soft, low durometer material. These inserts have the distinct advantage of providing cushioning and reducing plantar surface shear. They also relieve stress to intolerant pressure areas on the plantar aspect of the foot. These inserts are generally not custom-made and their fabrication is quite simple. The material most widely used for this type of orthosis is Plastizote. However, the disadvantages of a soft insert are numerous. The soft orthosis provides minimal biomechanical alteration of the hindfoot and forefoot. To be effective, the material must be at least 3 mm in thickness, and this thickness precludes its use in dress-type shoes. Also these orthoses do not hold up well. Depending on the material used, a soft orthosis can be expected to wear out in 2 to 6 months.

Semirigid orthoses are the most common type and are constructed of a combination of materials that range from relatively soft to relatively firm. These orthoses have significant advantages in that they facilitate weight transfer and provide biomechanical alteration to the hindfoot and midfoot. Semirigid orthoses provide enough cushioning for the rigid cavovarus foot and are rigid enough to provide biomechanical change in the pes planus foot. The main disadvantage of these orthoses is that they require skilled molding. Materials used to construct semirigid orthoses include cross-linked polyethylene foam, cellular rubber, and viscoelastic polymers.

Rigid orthoses are made from materials that provide maximal tensile strength and firmness and minimal flexibility. The benefit of rigid orthoses is that they provide maximal support and are of thinner construction, usually less than three-sixteenths-inch in thickness. However, rigid orthoses have a large list of disadvantages, including minimal reduction of impact shock. For this reason, in my opinion, they should not be used in high-impact activities such as basketball and volleyball. Also, if they are not carefully made, rigid orthoses can add pressure to bony prominences, resulting in additional problems. These orthoses require highly skilled technicians trained to measure, cast, and fabricate them. Because of their rigidity, they leave little room for error. It is my belief that rigid orthoses should be used much less frequently than semirigid orthoses.

Although the literature provides a basis for the use of scientifically prescribed foot orthoses, it still seems likely that the proposed benefit from the use of orthoses is greater than scientific evidence would indicate. Some of these discrepancies between perceived benefits and the results of studies may be attributed to (1) a placebo effect, (2) the possibility that some of the changes that should be measured cannot be detected by the instruments currently in use, and (3) the possibility that at the present time some of the parameters being measured are not valid.

**Case Study 1.** A 30-year-old NBA professional basketball player was seen for bilateral painful heels with a 2-year history of gradually increasing plantar heel pain. Previous treatment consisted of various types of taping and orthoses as well as several injections into the tender areas, more on the right foot than the left. During midseason, a marked increase in his discomfort resulted in discontinuation of competitive basketball.

Physical examination revealed a mild genu varum with 12 degrees of leg varus. He had mild pes planus bilaterally with ankle dorsiflexion of 10 degrees bilaterally. His heel position was neutral. The subtalar joint examination revealed 10 degrees of inversion/eversion on the right and 15 degrees inversion/eversion on the left. Heel/forefoot alignment revealed a supinated forefoot on the right with normal alignment on the left. He was markedly tender over the plantar fascia insertion into the right calcaneus, with much less tenderness over the similar area on the left.

Lateral standing x-rays of the feet revealed a break in the Cyma line. The impression was of chronic, bilateral plantar fasciitis secondary to compensatory pronation of the feet.

He had been wearing rigid orthotics to no avail; therefore semi-rigid orthotics were subsequently prescribed. The orthotics had a medial heel post of 4 degrees on the right and a ³⁄₁₆ inch metatarsal bar between the second and fifth metatarsals.

The patient required a 10-day break at midseason to accommodate to the orthotics; his plantar fasciitis subsequently resolved, allowing him to successfully complete the season.

**Case Study 2.** A 23-year-old Olympic-caliber distance runner began complaining of left leg pain 2 months before the Olympic trials. Pain was seriously hampering his training.

Examination revealed a mild bilateral genu varum, leg varus on the right of 10 degrees and on the left of 6 degrees with a slight externally rotated foot progression angle. He had no tibial torsion. Ankle dorsiflexion on the left was 10 degrees with the knee extended and was 12 degrees on the right. Leg/heel alignment revealed a varus of about 2 to 3 degrees and a heel/forefoot alignment with 4 degrees of supination. There was tightness of the gastoc-soleus group or hamstrings.

Semirigid orthoses were prescribed with a 2-degree medial forefoot post and a 2-degree medial heel post.

The patient's leg pain resolved and he qualified for the Olympic team at 5000 m.

**Case Study 3.** A 25-year-old distance runner had a 1 year history of bilateral Achilles tendinitis, with the pain localized 4 to 5 cm proximal to his calcanei. Conservative treatment consisted of changes in the training program, periods of relative rest, various physical therapy modalities, but without relief of discomfort. At times, he had noted swelling in both Achilles, but no crepitus or nodularity had ever been detected.

Examination revealed a slight genu varum bilaterally. He had a mild cavovarus-type foot and stood with the calcaneus oriented vertically to the support surface. Leg angle to the support surface was approximately 10 degrees. Subtalar joint position standing was fully pronated, although the arch still appeared to be higher than normal. (The point here is that an individual may stand fully pronated in the subtalar-midtarsal joint complex, but still have the appearance of a high arch.) Examination revealed reduced range of motion in the subtalar joint with total excursion of 20 degrees, and neutral position revealed a 3-degree heel varus.

The heel/forefoot alignment with the heel in neutral position displayed a pronated forefoot. There were heavy calluses under the first metatarsal head with relatively even callus distribution across the remainder of the forefoot. The first ray demonstrated diminished range of motion. Both Achilles tendons were tender 5 cm proximal to the insertion site, but no swelling or crepitus was detected. Dorsiflexion with the foot in neutral position and the knee extended was limited to zero.

In addition to training changes that reduced mileage and intensity of running, a cushioned shoe was recommended for additional shock absorption and accommodative orthotic devices were prescribed. The orthotics had a 3-degree medial heel post and 1- to 2-degree lateral forefoot post. With these changes the runner became asymptomatic within 6 to 8 weeks of resumption of training.

**Case Study 4.** A 34-year-old world-class distance runner complained of chronic, recurrent left Achilles tendinitis and also the sense that his right lower extremity was not functioning normally. His problems began some 2 years earlier when his primary competitive distance changed from 1500/5000-m runs to marathons. This was accompanied by a marked increase in training mileage, which was a dramatic change compared with his previous training mileage.

The examination revealed a significant pelvic tilt to the right, and leg length x-rays showed a 2.4-cm shortening of the right lower extremity. His left Achilles tendon was enlarged and tender some 5 cm proximal to the insertion site. Cybex testing showed the left gastroc-soleus muscles to be stronger than the right. On standing, he had a mild cavus type of feet and stood in a fully pronated position with the vertical axis of the calcaneus perpendicular to the floor. Subtalar joint motion was diminished, and neutral position revealed a 3-degree varus. His standing position was full pronation through the subtalar midtarsal joint complex. Heel/midfoot alignment was neutral. Dorsiflexion of the foot was limited to zero.

In this situation biomechanical studies were available. Treadmill running with lightweight accelerometers on the lower tibia were used to measure peak deceleration at foot strike as an index of the "shock" transmitted to the foot and lower leg, rear-foot movements also were analyzed. The left leg (involved extremity) experienced on average 19% more shock at foot strike than the shorter right lower extremity. Left foot contact was on the heel, whereas on the right, shorter extremity, it was midfoot. Rear-foot motion analysis revealed more supination on the right at touchdown, whereas maximal pronation was greater on the left (an accommodation to greater length).

The insertion of orthosis generally increased supination and decreased maximal pronation on both feet. There was a consistently longer contact time on the left and longer flight time when pushing off with the right foot. Both phenomena were believed to be an accommodation to the leg length discrepancy. The runner also exhibited an exceptionally large distance between the right and left foot placement along the midline. These studies showed a significant asymmetry in lower extremity function due to considerable compensation on the left, which resulted in increasing stress on the Achilles tendon.

The treatment program was to modify his training program by diminishing mileage and adjusting the right shoe midsole height to half the leg length discrepancy. It was thought that a full correction would not be tolerated since he had accommodated to this discrepancy for a number of years. Accommodative orthotics were also used for additional shock absorption and to decrease the maximum pronation in both feet as demonstrated during biomechanical testing. The orthotics had a 3-degree medial heel wedge with a neutral forefoot.

## REFERENCES

1. American Academy of Orthopaedic Surgeons: *Joint motion: method of measuring and recording,* Chicago, 1965, American Academy of Orthopaedic Surgeons.
2. Anderson JC, Sockler JM: Effects of orthoses on selected physiologic parameters in cycling, *J Am Podiatr Med Assoc* 80:161, 1990.
3. Bates BT et al: *Lower extremity function during the support phase of running.* In Asmussen E, Jorgensen K, editors: *Biomechanics,* University Park, Pa, Baltimore, 1978.
4. Bates BT, James SL, Osternig LR: Foot function during the support phase of running, *Am J Sports Med* 7:328, 1979.
5. Bieber JM et al: The effects of pronation-controlling orthotic devices on pressure and force under the foot during dynamic stance, *Phys Ther* 68:805, 1988.
6. Bleck E, Berzins T: Conservative management of pes valgus with plantar flexed talus flexible, *Clin Orthop* 122:85, 1977.
7. Bordelon LR: Correction of hypermobile flatfoot in children by molded insert, *Foot Ankle* 1:143, 1980.
8. Burkett LN, Kohrt W, Buchbinder R: Effects of shoes and foot orthotics on $CO_2$ and selected frontal plane knee kinematics, *Med Sci Sports Exer* 17:158, 1985.
9. Cavanagh PR, Rodgers MM, Iiboshi A: Pressure distribution under symptom free feet during barefoot standing, *Foot Ankle* 7:262, 1987.
10. Cavanagh PR: *The running shoe book,* Mountain View, Calif, 1980, Anderson World.
11. Cavanagh PR et al: An evaluation of the effect of orthotics on pressure distribution and rearfoot movement during running. Presented at the meeting of the American Orthopaedic Society for Sports Medicine, Lake Placid, NY, June 1978.
12. Clarke TE, Frederick EC, Cooper LB: *Biomechanical measurement of running shoe cushioning properties.* In Nigg BM, Kerr BA, editors: *Biomechanical aspects of sports shoes and playing surfaces,* Calgary, AB, 1983, University of Calgary.
13. Clement DB et al: *The corrective orthotic device on $O_2$ uptake during running.* In Bachl, Prokop, Suckert, editors: *Current topics in sports medicine,* Baltimore, 1984, Urban & Schwarzenberg.
14. Elveru RA et al: Methods for taking subtalar joint measurements: a clinical report, *Phys Ther* 68:678, 1988.
15. Frederick EC, Robinson JR, Hamill CL: *Rearfoot kinematics and ground reaction forces in elite caliber twin runners.* In Jonsson B, editor: *Biomechanics,* Champaign, Ill, 1987, Human Kinetics.
16. Giannestras N: *Foot Disorders,* Philadelphia, 1973, Lea & Febiger.
17. Hice GA, Kendrick Z, Webber K: The effect of foot orthosis on oxygen consumption while cycling, *J Am Podiatr Med Assoc* 80:161, 1990.
18. Holmes GB Jr, Timmerman L: A quantitative assessment of the effect of metatarsal pads on plantar pressures, *Foot Ankle* 11:141, 1990.

19. James SL, Bates BT, Osternig LR: Injuries to runners, *Am J Sports Med* 6:40, 1978.
20. LaFortune MA: The use of intracortical pins to measure the motion of the knee joint during walking, Doctoral dissertation, University Park, Pennsylvania State University, 1984.
21. Otman S, Basgoze O, Gokcek-Kutsal Y: Energy cost of walking with flat feet, *Prosthet Orthot Int* 12:73, 1988.
22. Penneau K, Lutter LD, Winter RD: Pes planus: radiographic changes with foot orthoses and shoes, *Foot Ankle* 2:299, 1982.
23. President's Symposium: The use and abuse of orthotics, Presented at the American Orthopaedic Foot and Ankle Society, Las Vegas, Nev, February 1989.
24. Scranton PE Jr, Pedegana LR, Whitesel JP: Gait analysis: alterations in support phase using supportive devices, *Am J Sports Med* 10:6, 1982.
25. Smith L et al: The effect of soft and semi-rigid orthoses upon rearfoot movement in running, *Podiatr Sports Med* 76:227, 1986.
26. Stipe P: The effects of orthotics on rearfoot movement in running, *Nike Res Newsletter* 2:1983.
27. Taunton JE et al: A triplanar electrogoniometer investigation of running mechanics in runners with compensatory overpronation, *Int J Sports Med* 2:31, 1982.

# Chapter 28

# Rehabilitation of the elite athlete

Donald E. Baxter
Pamela F. Davis

Rehabilitation is often neglected after an injury. If rehabilitation is done, often it is not well planned and short on scientific basis. In dealing with elite athletes, the treating physician and trainer place a high priority on prevention, making sure the athlete has adequate shoes, appropriate surface for training, comprehensive program of flexibility and strengthening exercises, and appropriate bracing or taping for weak ankles or feet.

An accurate diagnosis is the key to rehabilitating an injured athlete. Specific history of the injury, the type and intensity of training including changes in the training regimen before the injury, and all previous injuries should be documented. A thorough physical examination includes both a static examination and a functional examination. The functional examination requires the athlete to jog or run while the examiner evaluates the lower extremity for biomechanical problems. Functional examination of the athlete with injuries caused by jumping or dancing may also be carried out with the athlete performing the problematic task. Radiographs, bone scans, computed tomographic (CT) scans, magnetic resonance imaging (MRI), nerve studies, and laboratory tests are performed, when indicated, to make the appropriate diagnosis.

## PREVENTION

In considering prevention of injuries to elite athletes, athletic trainers are aware that flexibility is important. Flexibility is particularly important in athletes with tight muscles. Some athletes have isolated tightness in the hamstrings, calf, or toes; others have a combination of all three. Each of these areas should be evaluated and an appropriate stretching program instituted. Stretching three to four times a week or once a day is not sufficient. Increased flexibility is best achieved by doing stretching exercises five to six times a day for 20 to 30 seconds each session. Stretching should be performed in a smooth, controlled manner to avoid injury to the muscle or tendon. This is especially important in stretching hamstrings or the gastroc-soleus muscles.

The second area that needs attention is strengthening exercises. The anterior leg muscles (ankle dorsiflexors) are approximately one sixth as strong as the posterior leg muscles (plantar flexors). The ankle evertors must be strengthened in athletes with a history of ankle sprains.

Proprioception is extremely important, not only in treating injuries but also in preventing injuries. Exercises such as jumping rope or balancing on one foot gain proprioception for the elite athlete. Walking on the heels, toes, medial and lateral borders of the foot, as well as walking backward and side to side also promote rehabilitation of proprioceptive mechanisms. In the injured athlete, careful progression of exercises to increase demands without risking injury is necessary. Equipment that promotes side-to-side and rotational balancing includes the rocker board, ankle disc, and biomechanical ankle platform system (BAPS) board. Functional exercises such as running in place or hopping with controlled resistance, and weight shifting with external forces and cues are advanced exercises for improving proprioception.

In elite athletes nutrition can make the difference between winning an Olympic gold medal and not even making it to the finals. A recent study showed that heavy training depresses the immune function, leaving the body more vulnerable to infection. Anemia, a negative nitrogen balance,[17] glycogen depletion, and electrolyte depletion contribute to poor performance. There is a great frontier for researchers looking into these elements of training and prevention of injuries.

Another important consideration in preventing injuries of the lower extremity includes using proper shoes and correcting the biomechanics of the foot. The foot and ankle should be analyzed from a biomechanic viewpoint. Too much pronation or supination, abnormal heel strike, or abnormal weight-bearing pattern of the forefoot cause chronic overload more proximal in the kinetic chain at the knee or hip. Appropriate orthoses may be prescribed to ameliorate each of these problems. By guiding the athlete in appropriate selection of shoes and the use of orthotic devices and supportive taping, both acute and overuse injuries are prevented.

Avoiding training errors is one of the easiest ways to prevent injuries. Warm-up exercises should be a ritual before all athletic endeavors. The training regimen should be progressed carefully, increasing demands slowly to gradually condition the athlete. Abrupt increases in intensity, duration, or number of training sessions markedly increase the athlete's susceptibility to injuries. Simple considerations can often make a difference. The direction of running on a track or road should be alternated so that the tilt of the track or road alternates stresses on the lower extremities. Rotating two or three pairs of shoes and varying terrain also changes the pattern of biomechanical stresses and avoids overuse syndromes.

## REHABILITATIVE STRATEGIES

When there is a persistent problem, the elite athlete should seek consultation with a first-rate sports medicine physician such as an orthopedic surgeon or physical medicine physician who specializes in evaluating sports-related injuries. A physician knowledgeable in sports injuries, appropriate treatment, and possible complications of both treatment and premature return to competition should direct the rehabilitation program. Professionals helpful in rehabilitating the elite athlete include athletic trainers, sports physical therapists, and massage therapists. The key to providing first-rate rehabilitation is an accurate diagnosis.

When an injury occurs, training and playing should cease until the exact diagnosis is made. Once the nature and extent of the injury has been determined, a decision can be made by the examining physician about whether play and training may be resumed. The physician's decision depends on the possibility for exacerbation of the injury. For example, if the elite athlete has a stress fracture of the navicular bone of the foot, he should not be allowed to practice or compete until full recovery. The risk of completing the navicular fracture can be a career-ending injury. Therefore appropriate treatment is a short-leg non–weight-bearing cast until bony union occurs. However, athletes with a chronically unstable ankle or chronic plantar fasciitis might be allowed to play with appropriate taping and strapping of the foot and ankle.

Elite athletes with an injury such as a sprained ankle or Achilles tendinitis that they have never before experienced should be treated aggressively. If treatment is carried out expeditiously with the appropriate regimen, chronic recurring problems are avoided. After the initial period of rest or immobilization, cross-training should be initiated using swimming and bicycling to maintain aerobic capacity while providing relative rest to the injured part. Carrying out a well-directed rehabilitation program specific to the injury expedites return to competition and prevents repeated injury.

### Therapeutic exercise

Achieving and maintaining flexibility is an important part of injury prevention as well as rehabilitation. The incidence of severe ankle sprain has been decreased after a program of Achilles tendon stretching and peroneal muscle strengthening was initiated. Following a period of immobilization, muscular tenderness units and joint capsules and ligaments are contracted. Therapeutic stretching to regain normal range of motion and flexibility is required to allow normal functioning of the limb. Stretching should be performed in a smooth, slow, controlled manner to avoid injury to the muscle or tendon. The heel cord wedge is an excellent tool for stretching the Achilles tendon. The wedge may be used in at least two ways. First, the wedge is placed with the vertical side against the wall and the athlete stands facing the wall with the feet directed up the incline. Second, the wedge is turned around so that the apex is against the wall. The athlete stands with the back against the wall and the feet directed up the incline for a longer sustained stretch. A useful tool for stretching the heel cord and plantar fascia together is the ProStretch. Of course, stretching the heel cord can also be accomplished without any special equipment by standing on ground level and leaning the body toward the wall or standing with the ball of the foot on a step and allowing the heel to lower. While doing any of these exercises, the athlete should intermittently bend the knee slightly to achieve additional stretch of the soleus muscle.

Joint mobilization addresses the accessory motions of the synovial joints. These accessory motions, termed "joint play," are not volitional but accompany voluntary movements and occur passively in response to the ground or other forces. After prolonged immobilization, accessory motions of the synovial joints are limited. Muscle tightness, inflammation, and edema also limit accessory motions. Mobilization techniques are used by physical therapists to increase limited joint play. Mobilization techniques involve oscillating, gliding movements of the joints within the planes of accessory motions. The range of oscillation and gliding is graded but always occurs within the physiologic limits within the joint.

Cross-training is valuable in rehabilitating many types of injuries. One of the best forms of exercise used by many elite athletes is aquatraining. The athlete wears a buoyant vest and hooks a rope from the vest to the side of the pool and runs against the resistance of the rope. Paddles and flippers increase the resistance of arm and leg movements. The heart rate can be elevated for sustained periods with this type of exercise. Aquatraining is extremely useful for athletes who need to maintain their endurance but are unable to weight bear because of an injury of the lower extremity.

Strengthening exercises may be performed throughout the rehabilitation process, beginning with isometric contractions to maintain muscle tone during the period of immobilization. Once immobilization is discontinued, strengthening is accomplished by a program of progressive resistance exercises. When rehabilitating the foot and ankle, weights tend to be cumbersome; therefore TheraBand or Theraband tubing is used for providing progressive resistance to the peroneal and anterior tibialis muscles.

Proprioception, the sense of joint position, is altered by injury, immobilization, and non–weight bearing. Nerve receptors for proprioception are located in tendons, muscles, ligaments, and joint capsules and prevent excessive excursion of the joints and musculotendinous units by causing reflex muscle contractions. Although normal proprioception may be permanently altered by an injury to one component of the proprioceptive mechanism, rehabilitation of the other components allows compensation. Exercises that emphasize proprioceptive retraining include walking on the heels, toes, medial and lateral borders of the foot, as well as walking backward and side to side. The BAPS board, ankle disc, and rocker board are excellent tools that require proprioceptive sense for the athlete to maintain balance. Proprioceptive

training progresses to weight shifting and counterbalancing with the use of external forces.

Plyometrics, a concept gaining popularity in sports rehabilitation, refers to exercises and drills based on a science of the stretch reflex. Jumping and springing activities prestretch the muscle, enabling greater force generation via neuromuscular integration of the myotatic stretch reflex. Plyometric exercises load the muscle tendon unit with a lengthening force, requiring an eccentric contraction that immediately precedes a concentric contraction. This combination of contractions increases the force produced by the concentric contraction. Sled-on track-type equipment such as the Plyotrack and Pilates board have been specially designed to make use of the plyometric concept. Simple trampoline activities provide plyometric training to the foot and ankle muscles. From the trampoline, exercises progress to skipping rope, stair hopping, one-legged hops, vertical and broad jumping. The intensity of each drill is increased. As fitness increases, athletes develop increased speed and decreased reaction time.

### Therapeutic modalities

During rehabilitation physical therapy modalities are used to decrease edema, relieve pain, decrease muscle spasm, and occasionally to deliver topical medications. The literature lacks well-designed scientific studies documenting the effectiveness of each modality for specific indications. Therefore the choice of which modality to use for each indication is often empiric and depends on therapist preference and patient response (Table 28-1).

Cryotherapy is typically used to relieve pain, reduce swelling and hemorrhage, and decrease inflammatory infiltrates. Cold is the most appropriate modality to use following an acute injury and may be applied by immersion in an ice water bath or directly with ice packs and ice massage. For the acute injury, recommended treatment frequency is three times a day for 20 to 30 minutes each sitting. Cold may also be used after a vigorous workout when the athlete has returned to activity following an injury. Contrast treatment of heat alternating with cold has been promoted to decrease swelling in the subacute and chronic stage of injury. Theoretically the mechanism responsible for decreasing swelling is a pumping action occurring from the alternating vasodilatation and vasoconstriction to alternating heat and cold. However, the effectiveness of contrast bath treatments in decreasing edema has not been well documented scientifically.

Complications of ice application include frostbite and nerve palsy. Nerve palsy is rare and can be prevented by limiting the treatment duration to less

**Table 28-1.** Physical therapy modalities

| Modality | Acute edema | Chronic edema | Muscle spasm | Acute pain | Chronic pain | Soft tissue tightness |
|---|---|---|---|---|---|---|
| Cold immersion | X | X | | X | | |
| Ice pack | X | X | X | X | | |
| Ice massage | X | | X | X | X | |
| Hot packs | | | X | | X | X |
| Whirlpool | | | X | | X | X |
| Shortwave | | X | X | | X | X |
| diathermy | | X | X | | | X |
| Ultrasound | | X | X | | | |
| Electrical muscle stimulation | X | X | X | | | |
| TENS | | | | X | X | |
| Interferential stimulation | X | X | | X | X | |

*TENS,* Transcutaneous electrical nerve stimulation.

than 20 to 30 minutes and protecting the superficial nerves from excessive compression.[1] Contraindications to cryotherapy include Raynaud's phenomenon, cold urticaria, cold agglutinin disease, and hemoglobinuria. A relative contraindication is patient intolerance of the discomfort associated with the burning or aching sensation during the application of cold.

Therapeutic heat is indicated in the treatment of injuries after the acute period ends and when residual joint stiffness and chronic pain are present. The physiological effects of heat include vasodilatation, clearance of inflammatory infiltrates, and increased metabolic rate of the warm tissues. Heating increases blood flow and capsular permeability, which potentially increases edema. Because of this, heat should not be used during the acute stage of an injury. Athletes typically use superficial heat to warm up before a workout when they are "nursing" a mild or chronic injury. They perceive that heating the bothersome tissues before activity assists in gaining flexibility. A complication of superficial heat is burning of the skin. Therefore contraindications to heat therapy include insensate skin and sleeping patients. Heat-induced urticaria is another contraindication.

Superficial heat is applied by a hydrocolator or "hot" packs or hydrotherapy (whirlpool). Hot packs are wrapped in several dry cotton terrycloth towels and applied for 20 to 30 minutes. Maximum skin temperature is reached at approximately 8 minutes after application. Whirlpools make use of agitated water to achieve heating. Duration of treatment is 20 to 30 minutes. A disadvantage of using whirlpool treatment is that the extremity is usually placed in the dependent position, which encourages swelling. Indications for whirlpool therapy include joint stiffness and muscle soreness. Whirlpool therapy may also be used to facilitate callus removal by softening the skin before trimming.

Deep heat may be applied by shortwave diathermy and ultrasound. Deep-heating modalities cause a rise in temperature of fat, muscle, and connective tissue well below the skin. With deep-heating modalities, the temperature rise in deep tissues results from conversion of energy into heat by resistance of the tissues to passage of the energy delivered by the modality. Tissue temperatures of 40 to 45° C are required to achieve therapeutic effect.

Shortwave diathermy uses high-frequency electromagnetic fields to produce heat at a depth of as much as 3 to 5 cm. Although shortwave diathermy is excellent at heating deep tissues, especially those with high electrolyte content such as muscle, the skin is not heated, so the athlete will not have a sensation of warmth. Complications of shortwave diathermy include burns of the skin and subcutaneous fat necrosis from overheating. Contraindications of shortwave diathermy are the presence of metal implants, open growth plates of the bone, and presence of electronic devices (watches or hearing aids) or transistorized units (radios or stereos) within the treatment area.

Ultrasound is another modality used to deliver deep heat. Ultrasound makes use of acoustic vibrations to cause heating. Although ultrasound has both thermal and nonthermal effects, most research suggests that the clinically useful effects of ultrasound are due to the temperature rise by the absorption and conversion of ultrasonic energy to heat. Exposure to ultrasound increases tendon and capsular extensibility and therefore is highly useful before stretching or joint mobilization.

Indications for ultrasound are similar to those for other heat modalities, especially when heating of deep tissues is necessary. In the treatment of foot and ankle

**Table 28-2.** Application of TENS

|  | High-frequency TENS | Low-frequency TENS |
| --- | --- | --- |
| Mechanism of action | Spinal gait | Endorphins, enkephalins |
| Pulse frequency | 50-100 Hz | 1-4 Hz |
| Pulse duration | 20-60 ms | 20-30 ms |
| Amplitude | Pins and needles, paresthesia | Muscle contraction |
| Treatment duration | 30 min to 24 hr/day | 30-45 min |
| Duration of analgesia | During treatment only | 3 hr to 3 days |

problems, ultrasound may be useful for plantar fasciitis, tendinitis, and joint capsule tightness because fascia, tendons, ligaments, and joint capsules are selectively heated. For the foot and ankle application of ultrasound is usually performed in a water bath because of the uneven surfaces of the foot. If ultrasound is applied to the calf or other regions in which there is a broad flat surface, an aqueous gel or lotion is used as a coupling agent. A sensation of mild warmth is aimed for when applying ultrasound. Overheating the periosteum causes a deep aching or piercing sensation and should be avoided. Treatment duration is 5 to 10 minutes, depending on the size of the area being treated. Contraindications for ultrasound are the same as those for heat in general. Metal implants are not a contraindication to ultrasound; however, implants containing plastics contraindicate the use of ultrasound because the plastic may be selectively heated to the point of damage. Ultrasound should not be applied to areas of fluid collection or open growth plates.

Phonophoresis is the use of ultrasound to deliver antiinflammatory medication and/or local anesthetic directly into the tissues below the skin without discomfort of an injection. The nonthermal effects of ultrasound include streaming of extracellular fluids, increased diffusion rates, and increased permeability of membranes to ions responsible for the movement of large molecules through tissues. Medications such as 1% to 10% hydrocortisone cream, dexamethasone, 2% lidocaine gel, and 10% salicylate may be used for phonophoresis.

Electrotherapy modalities such as electrical muscle stimulation, interferential current therapy, and transcutaneous electrical nerve stimulation (TENS) are used in rehabilitating athletes. Electrical muscle stimulation and interferential current therapy are primarily used for edema reduction and prevention of muscle atrophy. TENS is primarily used for pain reduction. Contraindications to the use of electricity include pacemakers and cardiac arrhythmias, rarely a problem in the athletic population. Electrodes should not be placed on abnormal skin because the skin impedance to the electrical current may be increased

or decreased which changes the necessary current intensity and predisposes the skin to being burned, especially when direct current is being used.

Electrical muscle stimulation is used to retard disuse atrophy, decrease reflex inhibition of muscles, and decrease muscle spasms. Specific recommendations for type of current, intensity, and waveform characteristics to achieve maximal benefit of electrical muscle stimulation for each indication can be obtained from the manufacturers of the various machines available. Generally, electrical muscle stimulation treatment durations are 15 to 30 minutes, two to five times daily depending on the goals of treatment.

TENS is used for pain relief. There are two theories as to how TENS achieves pain control. The first is the gait control theory of pain developed by Melzak and Wall.[9] A second mechanism of pain modulation is based on the endogenous opiates called endorphins and enkephalins.[14] TENS units are small battery-powered units with adjustable current intensity, pulse frequency, and pulse duration for different modes of application. Most machines produce a balanced biphasic waveform to avoid skin irritation. TENS may be applied in either a high-frequency mode or low-frequency mode to achieve pain relief by the gait theory or endogenous opiates, respectively (Table 28-2).

Interferential current therapy is similar to electrical muscle stimulation in terms of its indications and treatment duration. Interferential current therapy is different from electrical muscle stimulation in that it uses two biphasic currents that are delivered to the tissues and result in a third current, the interferential current. The medium frequency of the two primary currents causes less skin nociceptor stimulation, which allows the use of more voltage. The greater the voltage delivered, the greater the penetrance of the current.

In rehabilitating the athlete a combination of a well-directed exercise program, as well as the application of therapeutic modalities, enables the treating physician, athletic trainer, and physical therapist to return the athlete to play in the most expeditious manner. Care should be taken throughout rehabilitation to gradually increase the demands of the athlete's activity without risking reinjury. Modalities should be used judicially to promote tissue healing and avoid masking symptoms of overuse.

## REHABILITATION PROTOCOLS (NONSURGICAL)
### Lateral ankle sprain

When elite athletes sprain their ankle for the first time, an assessment of whether the ankle sprain is a first-, second-, or third-degree sprain is necessary. Physical examination includes palpation of the regional bony anatomy, ligaments (anterior talofibular ligament, calcaneofibular ligament, anterior syndesmosis, deltoid ligament) as well as the sinus tarsi, and calcaneocuboid joint to localize the injury and define the extent of the injury. The most common ankle sprain includes injury to the anterior talofibular ligament and calcaneofibular ligaments only. Radiographic examination is performed to exclude fractures. In a first-degree sprain, immediate pain is followed by delayed swelling; there is no instability and the athlete is usually able to bear weight. Usually with a third-degree sprain, there is immediate pain, swelling, instability, and inability to bear weight; marked ecchymosis appears several hours after the injury. Second-degree sprains can be more difficult to assess and often need a stress test to determine if there is any difference in the anterior drawer or talar tilt comparing the normal ankle with the abnormal ankle.

The initial treatment of all ankle sprains includes rest, ice, compression, and elevation. Rehabilitation following an ankle sprain emphasizes Achilles tendon stretching, peroneal muscle strengthening, and proprioceptive retraining. First-degree sprains are treated with an Aircast brace, early motion, and weight bearing as tolerated. Plantar flexion should be avoided. Exercises including strengthening the peroneals and stretching the Achilles tendon are begun as soon as the athlete is able. Occasionally injection of tender areas with Marcaine to decrease the pain cycle is indicated. Interrupting the pain cycle improves rehabilitation and allows for more rapid recovery but should not be used to allow the athlete to return to competition prematurely. More severe second-degree and third-degree sprains are treated with a short-leg walking cast with ankle dorsiflexion[13] for 3 weeks followed by a dynamic splint to allow for protected rehabilitation.

For chronic recurring ankle sprains, an Aircast brace, ankle strapping with tape, or other ankle support is applied and physical therapy is initiated immediately. Recovery is much quicker for chronic recurring ankle sprains than for acute ankle sprains. Subtalar sprains are treated with the same rehabilitation protocol, but the physical examination is different in that the tenderness is in the sinus tarsi rather than at the ankle joint.

### Heel pain syndrome

The athlete with plantar fasciitis usually presents with heel pain localized to the plantar medial aspect of the heel at the insertion of the plantar fascia on the medial tubercle of the calcaneus. Symptoms may follow training errors such as an abrupt change in terrain, shoes, mileage, and intensity or frequency of workouts. Affected athletes usually have pain with the first several steps upon arising in the morning or after a period of rest. During workouts, pain may be intense upon the start of exercise, then diminish during the exercise period, only to return after the activity. Pain may become constant, occurring with every step, a symptom requiring the physician to rule out a stress fracture of the calcaneus.

Physical examination includes palpation of the entire plantar fascia and its insertion on the medial tubercle of the calcaneus. Tenderness along the first branch of the lateral plantar nerve as it courses under the abductor hallucis muscle signifies possible entrapment of this nerve. Examination of the range of motion of the ankle usually reveals a tight Achilles tendon. Biomechanical examination of the foot may reveal a rigid or flexible high arch or sometimes a flat foot.

Treatment is initiated with gentle stretching of the Achilles tendon and plantar fascia, ice treatments, and taping of the heel and arch to support the plantar fascia. Heel pads or cushions can be used in the shoe. Occasionally an orthotic is helpful to normalize foot biomechanics. If symptoms are severe, an injection of Marcaine and a cortisone preparation to decrease the inflammation, followed by intensive physical therapy, may shorten the symptomatic period. Ultrasound is used by therapists with some success. This problem can be short-lived and become asymptomatic within 6 weeks or it can last 10 to 12 months. Rarely does plantar fasciitis remain symptomatic beyond 10 to 12 months; therefore surgery should be avoided until the athlete has had pain for a year. Surgical management is discussed in the section on Heel Pain Surgery. Most patients with plantar fasciitis recover without surgery.

### Shinsplints

Shinsplints is a term that includes multiple etiologies. These problems include stress fractures, compartment syndromes, and periostitis. The exact type of problem should be determined by the examining physician.

The athlete with a stress fracture of the tibia relates a history that begins with diffuse pain occurring late in the workout. As the problem worsens, the pain becomes more localized and occurs earlier in the workout and finally throughout the day. However, the athlete is pain-free when he/she is not bearing weight on the injured extremity. On examination, the athlete with a stress fracture will have exquisite point tenderness. The radiograph may or may not show a fracture, but bone scans always show a localized area of increased activity.

The athlete with exercise-induced compartment syndrome complains of pain occurring toward the end of a training session that persists after activity ceases. On physical examination, tenderness is elicited by palpating the involved muscle compartment, not the tibia.

The athlete with periostitis complains of diffuse pain along the tibia when he/she begins to exercise; however, the pain diminishes during the workout. Activities that require active ankle dorsiflexion such as stair or hill climbing exacerbate the discomfort of periostitis. On physical examination, the athlete with periostitis has diffuse tenderness of the medial border of the tibia, and ankle range of motion may exacerbate the tenderness. Radiographs are negative and bone scan shows diffuse linear increased uptake along the middle to distal posteromedial tibia.

If there is a stress fracture, the athlete should rest until symptoms subside and there is no tenderness of the bone. Nonunion of stress fractures of the tibia occur, and the tibia may shatter or break through the area of stress fracture.[6] For these reasons, the athlete should be protected until the stress fracture heals. For exercised-induced compartment syndrome symptoms or periostitis, calf stretching exercises, antiinflammatory medications, and orthoses with medial wedges are prescribed. Occasionally athletes with persistent exercise-induced compartment syndrome require surgical release of the compartment involved.

### Tendinitis and tendinosis

The peroneal tendon, posterior tibial tendon, and the flexor hallucis longus tendon can develop peritendinitis, which occasionally evolves to tendinosis with or without a longitudinal tear within the tendon. If the problem is peritendinitis, it should be treated conservatively with appropriate immobilization using a removal cast-brace or a walking cast. Antiinflammatory medication is prescribed. On occasion, Marcaine can be injected into the sheath of the tendon to decrease pain about the tendon. Steroids should not be injected because of their long-term deleterious effects. If the athlete fails to respond to the usual conservative treatment of antiinflammatory medications, physical therapy, and immobilization, an MRI can be performed to determine if there is tendinosis. If tendino-

sis develops, the prognosis is worse for a rapid recovery; often these athletes need surgical intervention to debride the tendon and thus initiate healing.

The same holds true with the Achilles tendon. If there is peritendinitis and crepitus about the Achilles tendon, conservative antiinflammatory medications and physical therapy modalities are used. The athlete is immobilized until the crepitus and the inflammation subside. If it persists or progresses to tendinosis, more aggressive treatment is considered. When symptoms do not resolve with nonoperative treatment, an MRI is performed to determine the extent of damage. If there is extensive Achilles tendinosis that has failed to respond to conservative care, surgical debridement of the necrotic tendon is carried out with appropriate postoperative rehabilitation.

### Stress fractures

Fractures of the base of the fifth metatarsal distal to the tuberosity may occur as an acute fracture or as a result of completing a preexisting stress fracture.[4] These fractures are prone to delayed union and nonunion because of the tenuous blood supply in the area of the fracture. Torg[15] delineated radiographic criteria to classify fractures of the base of the fifth metatarsal distal to the tuberosity into three types: (1) acute fracture, (2) fracture with delayed union, and (3) nonunion.

The acute fracture occurs as a result of a traumatic event and may be treated nonoperatively with a short-leg non–weight-bearing cast until union. However, there is support in the literature for treating this fracture surgically[4] because of the high incidence of delayed union and nonunion. Treatment of bonafide delayed union and nonunion of the fifth metatarsal is discussed in the section on Surgical Problems.

For stress fractures of the navicular without displacement, at least 6 to 8 weeks of immobilization in a non–weight-bearing cast is the treatment of choice.[16] If there is any sign of displacement, open reduction with internal fixation is indicated. We prefer two screws placed from lateral to medial, entering at the sinus tarsi.

Recently a ballet dancer with a vertical stress fracture of the talus was seen. She was disabled by diffuse pain in the midfoot area; therefore an MRI was obtained that showed a vertical stress fracture of the body of the talus. The dancer was maintained in a short-leg cast-brace with non–weight bearing; as recovery occurred, progressive weight bearing was allowed.

Another common stress fracture in dancers is a stress fracture of the base of the second metatarsal. These are slow to recover because there is so much force placed on the second metatarsal. It is not unusual for a stress fracture of the base of the second metatarsal to take twice as long to heal as stress fractures in the distal metatarsals.

Sesamoid stress fractures are also slow to heal, creating a chronic problem. The fractured sesamoid should first be treated conservatively with restricted activities that might aggravate the problem. A rigid insole is placed in the training shoe with appropriate padding to relieve the first metatarsal head and sesamoids from bearing weight. A rocker bottom can be placed on the outer aspect of the shoe to lessen stress on the sesamoid fractures.

## Turf toe

Sprain of the first metatarsophalangeal joint, commonly known as "turf toe," has increased in incidence over the past 20 years with the advent of more flexible sporting shoes and artificial turf. American football players have the highest incidence of this injury. The mechanism of injury is forced hyperdorsiflexion, which causes tearing of the joint capsule at its insertion on the plantar aspect of the metatarsal head and neck. The most severe injuries also have a dorsal compression fracture that occurs as the base of the proximal phalanx jams into the metatarsal head. Other pathology associated with turf toe injury include sesamoid fractures, ligament avulsion fractures, fractures of the metatarsal or proximal phalanx, or dislocation of the joint.

Sprains of the first metatarsophalangeal joint have been categorized into three grades. Treatment protocol based on this grading system has been proposed.[3] Grade I sprains have localized tenderness, minimal swelling, no ecchymosis, and weight bearing is tolerated. Grade II sprains have diffuse tenderness, mild to moderate swelling and ecchymosis, and weight bearing may or may not be tolerated. Grade III sprains have severe tenderness, especially dorsally, marked swelling and ecchymosis, and weight bearing is not tolerated. Initial treatment for all degrees of injury is rest, ice, compression, and elevation to minimize swelling and protect the tissues from additional trauma. Grade II and III injuries should be evaluated radiographically to rule out fractures and soft tissue interposition within the joint, which may occur in the case of a spontaneously reduced dislocation. The toe should be taped to limit dorsiflexion and a rigid full-length longitudinal support added to the shoe. Weight bearing is allowed as tolerated. Athletes with grade II and III injuries may require crutches for several days to 2 weeks. Athletes with a grade I injury may not miss any playing time, whereas those with a grade II injury may miss 1 day to 2 weeks, and those with a grade III injury may miss 3 to 6 weeks.[3] Return to sports participation

should be delayed until the athlete has minimal pain and swelling and running does not cause pain. Those athletes who resume play too soon may suffer a more severe reinjury and resultant prolonged disability.

## Impingement syndromes

Posterior or anterior impingement or sinus tarsi impingement in the elite athlete should be treated with appropriate elevation of the heel of the shoe or the medial aspect of the sole to take pressure off the area of impingement. Ankle braces and rehabilitation exercises help to stabilize the ankle. Upon failure of conservative treatment, anterior tibiotalar bony impingement is treated by either open or arthroscopic techniques.[12] Posterior impingement secondary to a large or fractured os trigonum is treated by open excision of the os trigonum.

## Nerve entrapment

The most common nerve entrapment encountered in athletes is the interdigital neuroma (Morton's neuroma). Other nerve entrapments include tarsal tunnel syndrome, entrapment of the first branch of the lateral plantar nerve, medial plantar nerve entrapment (jogger's foot), superficial peroneal nerve entrapment, and deep peroneal nerve entrapment (anterior tarsal tunnel syndrome). Each of these nerve entrapments can be treated nonoperatively, usually with successful results.

An interdigital neuroma causes pain and numbness of adjacent toes—most commonly the third and fourth, or second and third. Entrapment of the interdigital nerve occurs as the nerve courses plantar to the deep transverse metatarsal ligament. Symptoms may be controlled by using an insole with a metatarsal pad or by modifying the sports shoe with a metatarsal bar on the outer sole. When nonoperative treatment fails, surgical excision of the neuroma is performed. Although popular technique includes releasing the intermetatarsal ligament, an attempt is made to preserve at least one half to one third of this ligament in athletes.

Tarsal tunnel syndrome is entrapment of the tibial nerve by the lancinate ligament. It is rare in athletes and usually occurs following an injury such as an ankle sprain. Occasionally bony anomalies or ganglion cysts impinge on the tibial nerve. Shoe modifications such as an enlarged medial flare of the sole of the shoe or a longitudinal medial arch support may help to decrease eversion of the foot, which decreases stretch on the nerve. When tarsal tunnel syndrome becomes chronic and unresponsive to nonoperative treatment, surgical release is indicated.

Entrapment of the first branch of the lateral plantar

nerve is discussed in the section on Heel Pain Syndrome.

Entrapment of the medial plantar nerve occurs at the area of the master knot of Henry. It is most commonly seen in joggers, especially those who run with increased heel valgus or hyperpronation of the foot. A medial longitudinal arch support usually exacerbates the symptoms by compressing the nerve. Most patients respond to a rehabilitation program that focuses on increasing strength of the invertors (posterior and anterior tibialis muscles).[11] The athlete is also encouraged to strike the lateral aspect of the heel and forefoot during the running gait cycle. If symptoms do not resolve, surgical release is considered.

Superficial peroneal nerve entrapment occurs as the nerve exits the lateral compartment, piercing the deep fascia. The fascial edge impinges on the exiting nerve, especially if muscle herniation is present at the fascial hiatus. Some athletes relate a history of previous ankle sprain and describe vague pain over the anterolateral leg. Sometimes there is numbness and paresthesia over the dorsum of the foot. Symptoms are exacerbated with activity. Relief of symptoms by nonoperative means is uncommon. Surgical release of the nerve involves incising the fascia proximal and distal to the nerve as it exits the lateral compartment.

Entrapment of the deep peroneal nerve occurs as it courses under the inferior extensor retinaculum, as it passes under the tendon of the extensor hallucis brevis, or as it passes under the extensor hallucis longus tendon at the superior edge of the extensor retinaculum. Compression may also occur secondary to osteophytes of the talonavicular joint or an os intermetatarseum (between the bases of the first and second metatarsals). Symptoms may be initiated by the added compression of tight-fitting ski boots, tying shoelaces too tight, or hooking the feet under a bar to do sit-ups. The remedy in these cases is to remove the source of external compression. Changing the lacing of the shoes by skipping the eyelets in the region of the compression is a simple remedy that may be indicated whether the source of compression is internal or external. If symptoms become chronic, surgical release of the offending portion of the retinaculum and excision of any osteophytes or os intermetatarseum is performed.

## Skin and nail problems

Blisters form because of friction and shearing of the layers of the skin. Usually blisters form at the beginning of the training season, after shoe change, or from wearing ill-fitting shoes. A horizontal tear forms within the epidermis and serous fluid sometimes mixed with blood accumulates between the skin layers. Blisters usually occur in skin that is fixed to the underlying tissues, such as the plantar skin in the metatarsal head area or the medial border of the great toe at the base of the distal phalanx. Another area prone to blisters is the posterior heel where the shoe counter rubs.

The first step in treatment of blisters is prevention. Athletic shoes should always fit properly with plenty of room and adequate support. New shoes should be "broken in" by wearing them for nonsporting activities first, then wearing them for limited periods during sporting activities. Shearing forces of the skin can be decreased by wearing two pairs of socks, applying petroleum jelly over areas prone to blistering, or using toe glides. Toe glides are coated paper with a low coefficient of friction that allow the foot to slide instead of building sheer stresses in the skin.

A rational, practical treatment regimen for blisters has been outlined recently in the literature.[7] The fluid is drained under sterile conditions, and the overlying skin of the blister is left in place to protect the tender layer of skin below. An antibiotic cream with or without local anesthetic can be injected into the potential space once filled with fluid. The blistered area is then sprayed with a pre-tape adhesive and protected with a supportive layer of adhesive padding that is left in place for 3 days. The adhesive padding is only removed if there is increased pain, drainage, or erythema, all of which may signal complication by infection. At the end of 3 days, the dressing is removed, the blistered area is cleansed, then sprayed with pre-tape adhesive. The adhesive padding is reapplied for another 3 days. The procedure is repeated until the blistered area is nontender. The most common complication of blisters is infection, which should be treated by local cleansing and appropriate antibiotics.

Calluses are areas of increased thickness of the keratinized layer of the skin that occur as a response to increased pressure or friction. They are usually located on weight-bearing skin of the foot such as the plantar skin under metatarsal heads or interphalangeal joint of the great toe. Increased pressure may be secondary to external causes such as ill-fitting shoes, orthotics, or incorrectly placed shoe pads. Internal causes of increased pressure include abnormal foot alignment or mechanics. An example is hallux valgus with a hypermobile first metatarsal causing decreased weight bearing of the first metatarsal head with transfer of weight bearing to the second metatarsal head. Other internal causes include a plantar-flexed ray, claw toe deformity, or malunited fracture.

The first step in treating a symptomatic callus is modifying external causes of increased pressure. The thickness of the skin is at first decreased by daily trimming, then trimmed on a weekly basis to control buildup of skin. To facilitate trimming, the foot is soaked in warm water to soften the skin, then the callus is trimmed by rubbing the area with a pumice stone or carefully removing the excess skin with a callus razor or a safety razor (the same type of razor used to shave a beard). Great care is taken to avoid injury to the underlying normal skin. Trimming should cease before seeing pink skin, and one should never cause bleeding. The athletic trainer should teach proper callus trimming technique so that callus care is incorporated into the athlete's personal hygiene routine.

If modification of external causes and simple callus care does not alleviate the symptoms, internal causes of callus formation should be addressed. Unweighting the area of increased pressure by padding may be helpful. For example, a metatarsal pad is placed just behind the metatarsal head to decrease the weight borne by the metatarsal head. Athletes involved in sports requiring abrupt starts and stops may prefer a full-length insole that incorporates a metatarsal pad so that the pad is maintained in the proper position. Flexible claw toes may be treated with exercises to increase metatarsophalangeal plantar flexion and strengthen intrinsic muscles. A special metatarsal pad with a distal extension and strap to hold the proximal phalanx in normal alignment with the metatarsal head may also be indicated. If exercises and shoe modifications are not helpful in relieving symptoms, occasionally surgical correction of the underlying cause may be necessary.

A corn, like a callus, is secondary to increased pressure and consists of a discrete area of thickening of the keratinized layer of skin. The thickened keratin layer is conical with the apex of the cone deep and broad base at the surface of the skin. There are two types of corns, hard and soft. Hard corns occur over bony prominences that rub on the shoe. The most common location is over the lateral aspect of the head of the proximal phalanx of the fifth toe. Other common areas are over the dorsal aspect of the proximal or distal interphalangeal joints of the toes. Soft corns occur in the web spaces of the toes, most commonly the space between the fourth and fifth toes. They may be exquisitely painful if the thickened keratin causes pressure on an underlying digital nerve. Soft corns are soft because moisture collects in the web space. Corns typically occur because of ill-fitting shoes. The toe box of the shoe may be too narrow or not deep enough.

Treatment begins with assessing the shoe and remedying any problems with the fit. The hard and soft corn may be trimmed carefully with a scalpel to enucleate the deep apex of keratin. Sometimes a local anesthetic is necessary. Occasionally corns harbor an underlying subclinical infection that is discovered when purulent material is encountered during trimming. Most often underlying infection is heralded by a marked increase in pain and the development of persistent surrounding erythema. After unroofing an infected corn, additional dissection should not be done and the patient should be given wound care instructions and a course of oral broad-spectrum antibiotics. After trimming the corn, a pad or spacer should be used to prevent recurrence. Sometimes trimming, pads, and improvement of shoe fit does not alleviate the symptoms, and surgical management of the underlying bony prominence or deformity is necessary.

Fungal infection of the toenails (onychomycosis) is categorized into four types: (1) distal subungual onychomycosis, (2) white superficial onychomycosis, (3) proximal subungual onychomycosis, and (4) *Candida* onychomycosis.[18] *Candida* onychomycosis occurs rarely in the athletic population because it is an opportunistic infection seen in immunocompromised patients; therefore it will not be discussed. Distal subungual onychomycosis is the most common form of fungal nail infection seen in the athlete and is commonly associated with athlete's foot. The fungi gain access to the nail bed at the lateral nail fold or the end of the nail plate (hyponychium). The infection then causes a buildup of white grainy debris, yellowing and thickening of the nail plate, and separation of the nail plate from the nail bed (onycholysis). Proximal subungual onychomycosis causes similar changes at the proximal aspect of the nail and may cause the nail plate to separate from the nail matrix (onychomadesis), resulting in shedding of the whole nail plate. Proximal subungual onychomycosis is a rare problem. White superficial onychomycosis is a fungal infection of the superficial nail plate itself, causing the nail to become white and crumbly.

Distal subungual onychomycosis in its early mild form and white superficial onychomycosis may be treated by first trimming away as much of the nail plate and debris as possible, then applying either Betadine, a drying agent, or naftifine hydrochloride 1% gel (topical fungicide) two to three times daily.[10] Usually 6 to 12 months of treatment is necessary.

Proximal subungual onychomycosis and severe forms of distal subungual onychomycosis may be treated with oral antifungal agents such as griseofulvin ultramicrosize or ketoconazole. These medications have potential adverse effects, significant drug interactions, and require routine monitoring of blood chemistry and complete blood cell counts; therefore oral antifungal treatment should be initiated and supervised by a dermatologist or internist who is familiar with these drugs.

Although most athletes are able to manage fungal infections of the toenails with topical agents and trimming, some may prefer to have the nail permanently surgically excised. Surgical excision of the nail and matrix is the most expedient route to curing the fungal infection and preventing its recurrence.

## PRINCIPLES OF SURGERY OF THE FOOT AND ANKLE

During the preoperative period the elite athlete should have appropriate nutritional supplements including vitamin C and iron. The athlete should discontinue vitamin E, aspirin, and other nonsteroidal antiinflammatory medications for at least 2 weeks if possible. This will prevent swelling and bleeding postoperatively. Surgery preferably is performed without a tourniquet, using gentle techniques with minimal dissection of the tissues. A regional anesthetic is used. When releasing nerves, the perineural fat is left in place to avoid postoperative scarring. Repairs of bones, tendons, or ligaments should be performed anatomically to reduce and repair the tissues. By performing anatomic repairs, less joint stiffness occurs, and the elite athlete has a better chance of returning to his preinjury status.

The first 72 hours after surgery is a critical time to prevent and decrease postoperative swelling by elevation, compression, and icing. Postoperative immobilization with a cast should be done when indicated, but the immobilization time should be minimized to avoid muscle atrophy. Isometric exercises during immobilization retard muscle atrophy. Functional rehabilitation programs using a splint or a cast-brace expedite return of muscle strength while protecting the injured tissues and should be initiated as soon as possible. Cross-training is begun early even if the athlete is restricted to upper-extremity exercises and leg lifts. A comprehensive postoperative rehabilitation plan including dates for dressing changes, suture removal, and the initiation and progression of an exercise program should be outlined by the surgeon so that the athlete, coaches, trainers, and therapists know what to expect. The exercise program must be progressed gradually with close supervision to increase activity demands without compromising healing or predisposing the healing tissues to injury.

With elite athletes the physician is often pushed into trying to rush the surgery and rehabilitation, which can lead to a longer convalescence and more complications. The athlete should be analyzed not just in terms of one season or one game but his/her entire career. For instance, by missing an entire season, the athlete may ultimately have better return of function and a more successful, longer career than if he/she rushes back to competition before complete healing and rehabilitation have occurred.

## POSTOPERATIVE REHABILITATION PROTOCOLS
### Ankle ligament reconstruction

Ankle ligament reconstruction is performed after all conservative treatment fails, and the athlete has continued complaints of repeated ankle sprains despite taping or bracewear. Instability is documented objectively by physical examination and radiographic stress tests. Appropriate ankle ligament surgery is performed, followed by immobilization in a short-leg weight-bearing cast for 3 weeks, then a removal cast-brace for an additional 3 weeks. During the first 3 weeks, isometric exercises of the ankle dorsiflexors and evertors are performed. During the second 3 weeks, Achilles tendon stretching and peroneal strengthening are initiated. Plantar flexion range-of-motion exercises are avoided. Proprioceptive retraining consisting of balancing on one foot and using an ankle disc while grasping parallel bars is also begun. At 6 weeks postoperatively a functional rehabilitation program is initiated. Agility exercises are progressed gradually from straight jogging to running to figure-eight jogging to cutting. Other agility exercises such as hopping from side to side without resistance, then with resistance, are incorporated into the program as the athlete gains confidence in the ankle.

### Heel pain surgery

Plantar fasciitis may become chronic and may be associated with entrapment of the first branch of the lateral plantar nerve. After the heel has been symptomatic for 10 to 12 months despite aggressive nonoperative treatment, surgery is considered. Chronic plantar fasciitis, heel spur, and entrapment of the first branch of the lateral plantar nerve is addressed surgically through an oblique vertical incision on the medial aspect of the heel. A partial plantar fascia excision, resection of the heel spur, and release of the first branch of the lateral plantar nerve is performed as indicated. After surgery the patient is non–weight bearing for 4 days, then begins touch-down weight bearing on the ball of the foot. Over the next week the patient begins to bear weight on the whole foot as tolerated. By 1 week the athletes are usually able to walk with a heel-toe gait, and by 4 weeks they start a jogging program. It is important to start ankle range-of-motion exercises emphasizing ankle dorsiflexion immediately after surgery to prevent Achilles tendon tightness. Recovery takes an average of 3 months and as much as 6 months in some patients.

## Selected injuries

The Lisfranc injury (tarsometatarsal fracture dislocation) usually occurs when the foot is axially loaded while the ankle is plantar flexed. However, some athletes report a twisting mechanism of injury. The other common mechanism of injury is a severe crush injury to the foot that occurs as a result of a motor vehicle accident or industrial accident. Severe crush injuries are easy to diagnose because of associated fractures and soft tissue trauma. In the athletic population the physical and radiographic findings may be subtle, and a high index of suspicion is necessary to make the diagnosis. Severe swelling of the midfoot and inability to bear weight are clues that there may be a Lisfranc injury. Radiographic findings are subtle, but on careful inspection radiographs reveal subluxation of the tarsometatarsal joints with widening of the space between the bases of the first and second metatarsals. A fleck fracture of the base of the second metatarsal is frequently present. History and physical examination are suggestive of an injury, and if radiographs are inconclusive, the athlete should be immobilized and standing radiographs repeated in 1 week with contralateral comparison views.

Once a Lisfranc injury is diagnosed, surgical management is indicated. The Lisfranc joint is stabilized with two or three screws that are left in place for 16 weeks. After 5 weeks non–weight bearing, weight bearing in a supportive shoe is begun. Aerobic fitness is maintained with cross-training (swimming, aqua-training) during the recovery phase. After the screws are removed, the athlete is gradually progressed to their usual training regimen.

An isolated injury to the syndesmosis of the ankle is caused by forced external rotation of the foot or leg. Forced ankle dorsiflexion may also cause the injury. Syndesmosis injuries of the ankle are usually associated with fractures of the ankle and in that setting are relatively easy to diagnose. Often the isolated syndesmosis sprain or diastasis of the ankle is not diagnosed until the athlete who is thought to have a simple lateral ligament sprain of the ankle is unable to resume sport activity in a reasonable period. Clinical suspicion is necessary to make the diagnosis. On physical examination, the athlete has point tenderness at the syndesmosis. There are two provocative tests to confirm suspicion of a syndesmosis injury. The first is the "squeeze test" performed by squeezing the fibula toward the tibia at the midcalf, which elicits pain at the syndesmosis if an injury is present.[8] The second is a stress test performed by externally rotating the foot on the stabilized leg, which causes pain in the presence of an injury.[5] Radiographs may be normal or may have widening of the ankle mortise. The stress test can be performed and recorded radiographically to demonstrate widening of the mortise.

When ankle syndesmosis injury with diastasis is diagnosed, surgical stabilization of the syndesmosis is indicated. Usually a cortical screw is used to purchase three cortices while the syndesmosis is reduced with the ankle in neutral dorsiflexion, with care being taken not to overtighten the syndesmosis. The syndesmosis screw is removed after 12 weeks; however, the athlete is permitted to weight bear and begin a rehabilitation program (similar to the ankle sprain protocol) after 6 weeks.

Fractures of the fifth metatarsal distal to the tuberosity with delayed union and nonunion are treated surgically. We prefer intramedullary fixation using an AOSIF malleolar screw,[4] which is left in place until the athlete's competitive career is over. If the screw is removed after the bone heals, a new fracture can occur. Many patients have a mild fixed cavovarus deformity that predisposes them to increased stresses on the fifth metatarsal and subsequent stress fracture.

## Forefoot problems

Usually bunion deformities are not addressed surgically until the athlete's career is over. For athletes who have pain so severe that they cannot perform, or if the bunion has progressed significantly over a short time, a bunionectomy with a distal chevron osteotomy is performed.

Surgery may be considered for the athlete with pain and disability secondary to hallux rigidus. An arthroplasty of the first metatarsophalangeal joint through an incision on the dorsolateral aspect of the joint is performed. Osteophytes on the lateral, dorsal, and medial aspects of the first metatarsal head and dorsal base of the proximal phalanx are removed. Postoperatively active and gentle passive range-of-motion exercises of the first metatarsophalangeal joint are initiated as soon as possible.

Chronic sesamoiditis of the tibial sesamoid is treated by partial or complete sesamoidectomy. Sesamoidectomy is performed through a medial capsulotomy, with care being taken to preserve the abductor hallucis insertion. If the entire sesamoid is avascular and has fragmented, the entire bone is removed. If the athlete has a tendency to develop a hallux valgus, the adductor tendon is released and the great toe is held in neutral position for 8 weeks.

Chronic symptomatic claw toes with hyperkeratotic lesions that have failed nonoperative treatment are operated during the off season. Bony prominences are excised and the toes are realigned. The toes are supported with dressings until the swelling subsides and the soft tissues are healed.